Principles of Nutritional Assessment

Principles
of Nutritional
Assessment

ROSALIND S. GIBSON

New York   Oxford
OXFORD UNIVERSITY PRESS
1990

Oxford University Press

Oxford   New York   Toronto
Delhi   Bombay   Calcutta   Madras   Karachi
Petaling Jaya   Singapore   Hong Kong   Toyko
Nairobi   Dar es Salaam   Cape Town
Melbourne   Auckland
and associated companies in
Berlin   Ibadan

Copyright © 1990 by Rosalind S. Gibson

Published by Oxford University Press, Inc.,
200 Madison Avenue, New York, New York 10016

Oxford is a registered trademark of Oxford University Press

Library of Congress Cataloging-in-Publication Data
Gibson, Rosalind S.
Principles of nutritional assessment
by Rosalind S. Gibson.
p.   cm.
Includes bibliographies.   ISBN 0-19-505838-0
1. Nutrition—Evaluation.   I. Title.
RC621.G52   1990   613.2—dc20   89-3411   CIP

Typeset in Adobe Times Roman, 10.5/12 and 8.5/10.5; figures are annotated in Adobe
Helvetica. The text and diagrams were prepared on an IBM-XT with a Quad386XT card,
using Professor Donald E. Knuth's program TₑX, Dr. Leslie Lamport's package LATₑX,
Harvard Graphics, and Adobe Illustrator. The material was typeset on a Linotronic-300
at the University of Waterloo, Ontario, Canada. Book design by Ian L. Gibson and
Philip Taylor, with the assistance of Oxford University Press.

9   8   7   6   5   4   3   2   1

Printed in the United States of America
on acid-free paper

Preface

Nutritional assessment is of increasing importance in today's world, both in examining the nutritional health of populations in less industrialized and industrialized countries and in determining the nutritional status of individuals in hospitals and in the community. This book, designed and written as a reference text on all aspects of nutritional assessment, provides an up-to-date, comprehensive, and detailed account of the major assessment methods — dietary, anthropometric, laboratory, and clinical — currently being used. Its detailed treatment of nutritional assessment procedures currently used in hospitals and the community, combined with its international perspective, will make it a valuable reference text for all senior undergraduate and graduate students studying dietetics, nutritional sciences, medicine, public health, nursing, and home economics; health professionals involved in nutritional assessment in hospital and community settings in both industrialized and less industrialized countries will also find the book useful.

The decision to write the complete text myself was made in an effort to enhance the cohesiveness of the book, and to enable detailed cross-referencing to be incorporated throughout the text. In all areas, I have emphasized the scientific principles, the advantages, limitations, and applicability of the various methods, and the use of appropriate reference data. Too often nutritional assessment is marred by an inadequate appreciation of confounding factors that may affect a proper interpretation of the results, as well as the use of inappropriate procedures and reference data. I have attempted to discuss these problems at appropriate points in the book, to highlight confounding factors where these are known to exist, and to provide guidance on the selection of the most suitable procedures and reference data.

Dietary, anthropometric, and laboratory methods are major forms of nutritional assessment. Each topic constitutes about one third of the book; clinical assessment and assessment of the nutritional status of the hospitalized patient are discussed in the final two chapters. Each chapter is followed by a comprehensive and current list of references that will provide a useful basis for a more extensive review of the literature pertinent to each topic.

In the dietary section, particular attention has been paid to the more quantitative assessment procedures, and to methods for assessing and improving both the precision and validity of assessment. A brief description of the statistical methods appropriate for measuring precision and validity is also included; more detailed accounts are available in the references cited. The current emphasis on diet in relation to health and disease highlight some of the difficulties associated with assessing relationships between these two variables. This book includes discussions of some of the numerical problems and procedures involved in evaluating these relationships.

In the anthropometric section an attempt has been made not only to describe the major anthropometric indices used in nutritional assessment but also to discuss the many different sets of reference data available for comparative purposes. The limitations of some of these reference sets are highlighted, and their use in different assessment protocols is discussed. A separate chapter is devoted to the more recent laboratory methods utilized for assessing body composition.

The laboratory assessment section is divided into ten chapters each dealing with a specific nutrient or group of nutrients. Given the growing interest in functional indices of nutritional assessment, details of both biochemical and physiological/behavioral functional indices have been included where applicable. For all nutrients, emphasis has been placed on those methods appropriate for community surveys and hospital clinical chemistry laboratories; methods better suited to specialized research settings have been discussed only briefly. Each of these laboratory methods is presented in detail, together with comments on their relative merits, sensitivity and specificity. The biochemical basis for each method is also discussed, thus enabling the reader to gain an understanding of the scientific principles of the assessment procedures. Special emphasis has been placed on the assessment of trace-element status, since deficiencies of these micro-nutrients are increasingly being recognized in hospital and community environments of both industrialized and less-industrialized countries.

The final two chapters provide an overview of assessment in the clinical environment; details of the specific tests included in hospital nutritional assessment protocols are provided in the earlier chapters.

Appendix A includes tables and figures of current Canadian, United Kingdom, and United States anthropometric reference data, tables of the recommended nutrient intakes for these countries, and interpretive criteria for selected laboratory indices. These form a convenient companion to the text and spare the reader having to search for original information. A computer database containing all references cited in the text as well as references to material that has appeared since the preparation of the individual chapters, will be available from the author following publication of this book (see Appendix B).

It will be obvious to the reader that this volume is based on the research and reports of many investigators, but I am particularly grateful to the private individuals, editors, and publishers who granted permission to reproduce figures and tables containing numerical data. In most cases these tables have been reset and the figures redrawn; the sources have been acknowledged in the text, usually in the caption. I am also indebted to my colleagues at the University of Guelph and elsewhere — Dr. C. Casey, Dr. H. H. Draper, Dr. M. Hadley, Dr. O. B. Martinez, Dr. D. O'Connor, Dr. J. E. Miles, Dr. J. H. Sabry, Dr. A. Stephens, and Dr. W. W. Woodward, who kindly read drafts of one or more of the individual chapters and suggested improvements; I would also like to thank Faith Alexander, Susan Atlin, Judy Kitchen, and Annamaria Rosas for their invaluable assistance in checking references and proofs, although I alone remain responsible for defects of fact, treatment, judgment or style. Inconsistencies in usage and spelling are probably the result of my British education and Canadian residence, combined with the expressed wishes of my American publisher.

To speed publication, the book has been printed from computer-typeset material prepared by myself and my husband, Ian L. Gibson. I am particularly grateful to Mr. Philip Taylor, Royal Holloway and Bedford New College, University of London, for proofreading the entire text and providing advice and assistance with typesetting. Mr. Jeffrey House and the staff at Oxford University Press, New York, not only agreed to our typesetting the book, but kindly provided appropriate guidance; I am grateful for this help from the publisher.

R. S. G.
Guelph, Ontario, Canada.
September, 1989.

Contents

Contents   xv

Principles of Nutritional Assessment

Chapter 1

Introduction

Nutritional assessment procedures were first used in surveys designed to describe the nutritional status of populations on a national basis. The methods used were initially described at a conference held in 1932 by the Health Organization of the League of Nations. In 1955, the Interdepartmental Committee on Nutrition for National Defense (ICNND) was organized to assist developing countries in assessing their nutritional status and in identifying problems of malnutrition and the ways in which they could be solved. The ICNND teams conducted medical nutrition surveys in twenty-four countries, and consisted largely of clinical nutritionists, dentists, biochemists, food technologists, and agricultural, public health, and sanitation specialists; sometimes pediatricians, dermatologists, and ophthalmologists were also involved. The ICNND produced a comprehensive manual in 1963 describing their methods and interpretive guidelines (ICNND, 1963), with the intention of standardizing both the methods used for the collection of nutrition survey data and the interpretation of the results. On the recommendation of the WHO Expert Committee on Medical Assessment of Nutritional Status in 1963, a second publication was prepared by Jelliffe (1966) in consultation with twenty-five specialists in various countries. This monograph was directed specifically at the assessment of the nutritional status of vulnerable groups in developing regions of the world. The methods described in this monograph are still applicable today.

Nutritional assessment has also become an essential component of the nutritional care of the hospitalized patient. The important relationship between nutritional status and health, and particularly the critical role of nutrition in recovery from acute illness or injury, is well documented, but although it is now almost fifteen years since the prevalence of malnutrition among hospitalized surgical and medical patients was first reported (Bistrian et al., 1974; 1976), such malnutrition still occurs. The failure to identify and treat malnourished patients in hospitals appears to be associated with a lack of physician-awareness (Roubenoff et al., 1987; Anon., 1988). Consequently it is essential that physicians appreciate

3

the most effective means of diagnosing, evaluating, and monitoring the nutritional status of high-risk hospital patients.

As health-care administrators and the community in general make increasing demands for demonstrable benefits from the investment of public funds in nutrition intervention programs, efforts to improve nutritional assessment techniques will continue. The aim of this book, therefore, is to provide a comprehensive and critical appraisal of both well-established and new methods in nutritional assessment.

1.1   Nutritional assessment systems

Nutritional assessment can be defined as:

> The interpretation of information obtained from dietary, biochemical, anthropometric and clinical studies.

The information is used to determine the health status of individuals or population groups as influenced by their intake and utilization of nutrients. Nutritional assessment systems can take one of three forms: surveys, surveillance, or screening (WHO, 1976a).

Nutrition surveys

The nutritional status of a selected population group may be assessed by means of a cross-sectional survey. This nutrition survey may establish baseline nutritional data and/or ascertain the overall nutritional status of the population. Cross-sectional nutrition surveys can also identify and describe those population subgroups 'at risk' to chronic malnutrition. They are less likely to identify acute malnutrition or to provide information on the possible causes of malnutrition. Information on the extent of existing nutritional problems is obtained, which can be used to allocate resources to those population subgroups in need, and to formulate policies to improve the overall nutrition of the population.

Nutrition surveillance

The characteristic feature of surveillance is the continuous monitoring of the nutritional status of selected population groups. Surveillance studies therefore differ from nutrition surveys because the data are collected, analyzed, and utilized, for an extended period of time. Sometimes, only data for specific at-risk subpopulation groups, identified in earlier nutrition surveys, are collected. Unlike cross-sectional nutrition surveys, surveillance studies identify the possible causes of malnutrition, and hence can be used to formulate and initiate intervention measures at the population or subpopulation level. Additional objectives of nutrition surveillance, summarized in the report of the United Nations Expert Committee on

Methodology of Nutrition Surveillance (WHO, 1976b), include the promotion of decisions by governments concerning priorities and the disposal of resources, the formulation of predictions on the basis of current trends, and the evaluation of the effectiveness of nutrition programs. Nutrition surveillance can be carried out on selected individuals, in which cases the term 'monitoring', rather than surveillance, is used.

Nutrition screening

The identification of malnourished individuals requiring intervention can be accomplished by nutrition screening. This involves a comparison of an individual's measurements with predetermined risk levels or 'cutoff' points. Screening can be carried out at the individual level as well as on specific subpopulations considered to be at risk. In the United States, for example, screening was used to identify individuals for the Food Stamp Program and the Women, Infants and Children Special Supplemental Food Program (WIC) (Habicht et al., 1982). Screening programs are usually less comprehensive than surveys or surveillance studies.

Each of these three types of nutritional assessment systems has been adopted in clinical medicine to assess the nutritional status of hospitalized patients. This practice arose because of reports of a substantial prevalence of protein-energy malnutrition among surgical patients in North America (Blackburn et al., 1977). Today, nutritional assessment is often performed on patients with acute traumatic injury, on those undergoing surgery, on chronically ill medical patients, and on elderly patients. Screening can initially be carried out to identify those patients requiring nutritional management, after which a more detailed and comprehensive baseline nutritional assessment of the individual may take place. This assessment will clarify and expand the nutritional diagnosis, and will establish the severity of the malnutrition. Finally, a nutritional monitoring system is often initiated to follow the response of the patient to nutritional therapy.

1.2 Methods used in nutritional assessment

Nutritional assessment systems utilize a variety of methods to characterize each stage in the development of a nutritional deficiency state (Table 1.1). The methods are based on a series of dietary, laboratory, anthropometric, and clinical measurements, used either alone or, more effectively, in combination.

Dietary methods

The first stage of a nutritional deficiency is identified by dietary assessment methods. During this stage, the dietary intake of one or more nutrients is inadequate, either because of a primary deficiency (low levels in the diet), or because of a secondary deficiency. In the latter case,

Stage	Depletion Stage	Method(s) Used
1	Dietary inadequacy	Dietary
2	Decreased level in reserve tissue store	Biochemical
3	Decreased level in body fluids	Biochemical
4	Decreased functional level in tissues	Anthropometric/Biochemical
5	Decreased activity in nutrient-dependent enzyme	Biochemical
6	Functional change	Behavioral/Physiological
7	Clinical symptoms	Clinical
8	Anatomical sign	Clinical

Table 1.1: Generalized scheme for the development of a nutritional deficiency. Modified from Table 4.1 in: Methods for the Evaluation of the Impact of Food and Nutrition Programmes. Sahn DE, Lockwood R, Scrimshaw NS (eds) © 1984 by the United Nations University.

dietary intakes may appear to meet nutritional needs, but conditioning factors (such as certain drugs, dietary components, or disease states) interfere with the ingestion, absorption, transport, utilization, or excretion of the nutrient(s).

Laboratory methods

Several stages in the development of a nutritional deficiency state can be identified by laboratory methods. In primary and/or secondary deficiencies, the tissue stores become gradually depleted of the nutrient(s). As a result of this depletion, reductions may occur in the levels of nutrients or in the levels of their metabolic products in certain body fluids and tissues, and/or in the activity of some nutrient-dependent enzymes. This depletion may be detected by biochemical tests, and/or by tests that measure physiological or behavioral functions dependent on specific nutrients (Solomons, 1985). Examples of such functions include: dark adaptation (vitamin A); taste acuity (zinc); capillary fragility (vitamin C); and cognitive function (iron). Functional tests provide a measure of the biological importance of a given nutrient because they assess the functional consequences of the nutritional deficiency (Solomons and Allen, 1983). In general, physiological functional tests are not suitable for field surveys; they are too invasive, and often require elaborate equipment.

Anthropometric methods

Measurements of the physical dimensions and gross composition of the body are used in anthropometric methods (Jelliffe, 1966). The measurements vary with age and degree of nutrition and, as a result, are particularly useful in circumstances where chronic imbalances of protein and energy are likely. They can be used, in some cases, to detect moderate as well as severe degrees of malnutrition. Anthropometric measurements have the additional advantage of providing information on past nutritional history, which cannot be obtained with equal confidence using the other assessment techniques.

Clinical methods

A medical history and a physical examination are clinical methods used to detect signs (i.e. observations made by a qualified examiner) and symptoms (i.e. manifestations reported by the patient) associated with malnutrition. These signs and symptoms are often nonspecific, and only develop during the advanced stages of nutritional depletion; for this reason, diagnosis of a nutritional deficiency should not rely exclusively on clinical methods (McGanity, 1974). It is obviously desirable to detect marginal nutrient deficiencies before a clinical syndrome develops, and as a result, laboratory methods should also be included as an adjunct to clinical assessment.

Nutritional assessment methods may also involve the collection of information on variables known to affect the nutritional status of a population, including relevant economic and sociodemographic data, cultural practices, food habits, food beliefs, and food prices. Information on marketing, distribution, and storage of food may also be collected, as may health and vital statistics; the latter may involve information on the percentage of the population with ready access to a good source of drinking water, the proportion of children immunized against measles, the proportion of infants born with a low birth-weight, the percentage of mothers breast-feeding, and age- and cause-specific mortality rates.

Some non-nutritional variables are so strongly related to malnutrition that they can also be used as variables to identify at-risk individuals in surveillance studies (Habicht et al., 1978). For example, Morley (1973) identified birth order over seven, breakdown of marriage, death of either parent, and episodes of infectious diseases in early life, as being important factors in the prediction of children nutritionally at risk in West Africa.

Raw measurements derived from each of the four methods used in nutritional assessment systems are often combined to form 'indices' (singular: 'index'). Examples of such combinations include weight for age, weight for height, mid-upper-arm muscle circumference (i.e. mid-upper-arm circumference and triceps skinfold), hemoglobin in relation to age and sex, and mean corpuscular hemoglobin concentration (i.e. hemoglobin and hematocrit). Indices are used to interpret and group measurements (WHO Working Group, 1986).

1.3   The design of nutritional assessment systems

The design of the nutritional assessment system is critical if time and resources are to be used effectively. The assessment system used, and the type and number of measurements selected, will depend on a variety of factors.

Study objectives

The general design of the assessment system and the measurements or indices selected should be dictated by the study objectives. For example, if information on the current overall nutritional status at the national level is needed to estimate the prevalence of malnutrition, a comprehensive baseline cross-sectional nutrition survey, involving all four methods of nutritional assessment, may be necessary. Alternatively, to evaluate the impact of nutrition intervention on a specific high-risk group, a nutritional surveillance system, designed to monitor acute (i.e. short-term) changes in nutritional status, may be employed. To identify malnourished individuals, a screening system using indices which reflect both past and present nutriture, may be selected.

Sampling protocols

It is important that sampling protocols be designed and rigorously adhered to throughout the study to avoid systematic bias in the sample selection, and to ensure that the sample is random and representative of the target population. Extrapolation of the results to the population at large will then be valid. Self-selection (i.e. survey participation by consent) produces unrepresentative samples and, sometimes, systematic bias; for example, only those with a higher level of education may volunteer to participate. In these circumstances, it is essential to identify the probable direction and magnitude of the bias arising from the sample design and nonresponse rate (Elwood, 1983).

The sample design may necessitate the use of random number tables or generators to produce a randomly selected representative sample. Alternatively, stratified and/or multi-stage random sampling may be required. In stratified sampling, the target population is divided into a number of categories or strata (e.g. urban and rural populations, different ethnic groups, various geographical areas or administrative regions) from each of which is drawn a separate random sample. In multi-stage random sampling, a number of levels of sampling are defined, from each of which is drawn a random sample.

In the Nutrition Canada National Survey, the sample was selected in three stages. The first stage involved the selection of 80 enumeration areas reflecting the different regions, population types (40 metropolitan, 24 urban, and 16 rural), income levels (low and other), and seasons (January to May and June to December). The second stage of sampling involved the selection of a random sample of households from within each enumeration area, and the third stage involved the selection of persons from within households. The latter were randomly selected from each of 10 age-sex categories (Health and Welfare Canada, 1973). The United States First and Second National Health and Nutrition Examination Surveys (NHANES I and II) (NCHS, 1981) also used a combination of stratified and multi-stage random sampling techniques to obtain a sample representative of the U.S. population.

Validity

Validity is important in the design of nutritional assessment systems because it describes the *adequacy* with which any measurement or index reflects the nutritional parameter of interest. For example, if information on the long-term nutritional status of an individual is required, the dietary measurement should provide a valid reflection of the true 'usual' nutrient intake, rather than the intake over a single day (Block, 1982). Similarly, the biochemical index should be a valid measure of the total body content of a nutrient or the size of the tissue store most sensitive to deficiency, and not reflect the recent dietary intake (Solomons, 1985). The design of the nutritional assessment system must include consideration of the validity of all the indices selected.

Precision

The degree to which repeated measurements of the same variable give the same value is a measure of precision — also referred to as reproducibility or reliability. The study design should always include some replicate observations (repeated but independent measurements on the same subject/sample). In this way, the precision of each measurement procedure can be calculated and expressed as the coefficient of variation (CV%).

$$CV\% = \text{standard deviation} \times 100\% \,/\, \text{mean}$$

The precision of a measurement is a function of the random measurement errors, and, in certain cases, true variability in the measurement that occurs over time. For example, the nutrient intakes of an individual vary over time (intra-subject variation) and this results in uncertainty in the estimation of usual nutrient intake. This variation characterizes the true 'usual intake' of an individual. Unfortunately, intra-subject variation cannot be distinguished statistically from the random measurement errors, irrespective of the design of the nutritional assessment system.

Random measurement errors

An insensitive instrument or variations in the measuring and recording technique produced by random measurement errors reduce the *precision* of a measurement by increasing the variability about the mean. They do not influence the mean or median value. Random measurement errors may occur when the same examiner repeats the measurements (within- or intra-examiner error) or when several different examiners repeat the same measurement (between- or inter-examiner error). Unfortunately, such errors produce measurements which are imprecise in an unpredictable way, resulting in less certain conclusions. Random measurement errors can be minimized by incorporating standardized measurement techniques and the use of trained personnel in the nutritional assessment system, but can never be entirely eliminated.

Accuracy

Accuracy is a term best used in a restricted statistical sense to describe the extent to which the measurement is close to the true value. It therefore follows that a measurement can be precise, but, at the same time, inaccurate — a situation which occurs when there is a systematic bias in the measurements (see below). Accurate measurements, however, necessitate high precision. The design of any biochemical assessment protocol should include the use of reference materials, with certified values for the nutrient of interest, to control the accuracy of the analytical methods. The control of accuracy in other assessment methods is difficult and is discussed in more detail in later chapters. It is preferable to avoid statements such as: 'Weight for age is an "accurate" reflection of acute protein-energy malnutrition'. The term 'valid' is more appropriate here, and confusion with the well-accepted statistical usage of 'accurate' is avoided.

Systematic measurement errors or bias

Unfortunately, systematic measurement errors may arise in any nutritional assessment method. Such errors reduce the *accuracy* of a measurement by altering the mean or median value. They have no effect on the variance, and hence do not alter the precision of the measurement (Himes, 1987). Examples of measurement bias include dietary scales which always over- or underestimate weight, skinfold calipers which systematically over- or underestimate skinfold thickness, and a biochemical method for assaying vitamin C in foods which systematically underestimates the vitamin C content because only the reduced form of vitamin C (L-ascorbic acid) is measured. Interviewer and respondent bias may also reduce the accuracy of dietary assessment results (Anderson, 1986). For example, social desirability bias by respondents may occur if they consistently underestimate their alcohol consumption in a food-frequency questionnaire or dietary record method. Bias is important as it cannot be removed by subsequent statistical analysis (NRC, 1986). Consequently, care must be taken to reduce and if possible eliminate all sources of systematic errors in the design of the nutritional assessment system, by careful attention to the equipment and methods selected. This is particularly important in cross-sectional surveys, where the absolute values of the parameters are often compared with reference data.

Sensitivity

The sensitivity of an index refers to the extent to which it reflects nutritional status, or predicts changes in nutriture. Sensitive indices show large changes as a result of only small changes in nutritional status, and, as a result, have the ability to identify and classify those persons within a population who are *genuinely* malnourished. An indicator with 100% sensitivity correctly identifies all those individuals who are genuinely malnourished: no malnourished persons are classified as 'well' (i.e. there are no false negatives). Numerically, sensitivity (Se) is the proportion of individuals with malnutrition who have positive tests (true positives divided by the sum of true positives and false negatives) (Table 1.2). Unfortunately, the term 'sensitivity' is also used to describe the ability of an analytical method to detect the substance of interest. The term 'analytical sensitivity' should be used in this latter context (Chapter 15).

Specificity

The specificity of an index refers to the ability of the index to identify and classify those persons who are *genuinely* well-nourished. If an indicator has 100% specificity, all genuinely well-nourished individuals will be correctly identified: no well-nourished individuals will be classified as 'ill' (i.e. there are no false positives). Numerically, specificity (Sp) is the proportion of individuals without malnutrition who have negative tests (true negatives divided by the sum of true negatives and false positives) (Table 1.2).

The specificity (and sensitivity) of an index depend both on the extent of the random errors associated with the raw measurement and on the influence of non-nutritional factors such as diurnal variation and the effects of disease (Habicht et al., 1979). If the former is large, the index will be imprecise and the specificity (and sensitivity) will be reduced. Similarly, if the latter is important, the specificity (and sensitivity) will also be reduced. In these circumstances, the index will show a change which is not associated with a nutritional effect, and misclassification may occur; individuals may be designated 'at risk' when they are actually

	The True Situation	
	Malnutrition present	No malnutrition
Positive Test Result	True positive (TP)	False positive (FP)
Negative Test Result	False negative (FN)	True negative (TN)

Sensitivity (Se) = TP / (TP + FN)

Specificity (Sp) = TN / (FP + TN)

Predictive value (V) = (TP + TN) / (TP + FP + TN + FN)

Positive Predictive value (V+) = TP / (TP + FP)

Negative Predictive value (V–) = TN / (TN + FN)

Prevalence (P) = (TP + FN) / (TP + FP + TN + FN)

Table 1.2: Numerical definitions of sensitivity, specificity, predictive value, and prevalence for a single index used to assess malnutrition in a sample group. Modified from Habicht (1980). © Am. J. Clin. Nutr. American Society for Clinical Nutrition.

unaffected (false positives), or individuals may be designated 'not at risk' when they are truly affected by the condition (false negatives). The ideal index has a low number of both false positives (high specificity) and false negatives (high sensitivity).

The choice of a cutoff point to differentiate between malnourished and well-nourished states for a particular index critically affects both the sensitivity and specificity. In cases where lower values of the index are associated with malnutrition, reducing the cutoff point increases specificity and decreases sensitivity for a given index. Table 1.3 shows the influence of a change in cutoff point on sensitivity and specificity. For example, when the cutoff point for mid-upper-arm circumference is reduced from < 14.0 cm to < 12.5 cm, the specificity in predicting malnutrition (based on weight for height $< 60\%$ of median) increases from 82.7% to 98.0%, whereas the sensitivity falls from 90.4% to 55.8% (Trowbridge and Staehling, 1980). Similarly, when the cutoff point for total iron binding capacity (TIBC) is lowered from $< 310\,\mu$g/dL to $< 270\,\mu$g/dL, the specificity in predicting postoperative sepsis increases from 68% to 87%, but the sensitivity falls from 55% to 30% (Bozzetti et al., 1985).

The term 'specificity' is also used in analytical work to describe the degree to which a particular laboratory procedure measures only the component of interest. 'Analytical specificity' should be used to clearly distinguish this more specialized use of the term (Chapter 15).

Parameter	Cutoff	Sensitivity	Specificity	Author
Arm Circ. (cm)	< 14.0 < 12.5	90.4% 55.8%	82.7% 98.0%	Trowbridge & Staehling (1980)
TIBC (μg/dL)	< 310 < 270	55% 30%	68% 87%	Bozzetti et al. (1985)

Table 1.3: Influence of change in the cutoff point on the sensitivity and specificity of mid-upper-arm circumference and total iron binding capacity (TIBC) as predictors of outcome.

Prevalence

The number of persons with malnutrition or disease during a given time period is measured by the prevalence. Numerically, the actual prevalence (P) is the proportion of individuals who really are malnourished or infected with the disease in question (the sum of true positives and false negatives) divided by the sample population (the sum of true positives, false positives, true negatives and false negatives) (Table 1.2). Prevalence influences the predictive value of a nutritional index more than any other factor.

Predictive value

The predictive value can be defined as the likelihood that an index correctly predicts the presence or absence of malnutrition or disease (Galen and Gambino, 1975). Numerically, the predictive value of a test is the proportion of all tests that are true (the sum of the true positives and true negatives divided by the total number of tests) (Table 1.2). The predictive value can be further subdivided into the positive predictive value and the negative predictive value. The positive predictive value of a test is the proportion of positive tests that are true (the true positives divided by the sum of the true positives and false positives). The negative predictive value of a test is the proportion of negative tests that are true (the true negatives divided by the sum of the true negatives and false negatives).

The predictive value of any index is not constant but depends on the sensitivity, specificity, and the prevalence of malnutrition or disease. Table 1.4 shows the influence of prevalence on the positive predictive value of an index when the sensitivity and specificity are constant. When the prevalence of malnutrition is low, even very sensitive and specific tests have a relatively low positive predictive value. Conversely, when the prevalence of malnutrition is high, indices with rather low sensitivity and specificity may have a relatively high positive predictive value. Determination of predictive value is the best test of the usefulness of any index of nutritional status. An acceptable predictive value for any index depends on the number of false-negative and false-positive results

Predictive Value	Prevalence					
	0.1%	1%	10%	20%	30%	40%
Positive	0.02	0.16	0.68	0.83	0.89	0.93
Negative	1.00	1.00	0.99	0.99	0.98	0.97

Table 1.4: Influence of disease prevalence on the predictive value of a test with sensitivity and specificity of 95%. From DT Dempsey and JL Mullen, Prognostic value of nutritional indices. Journal of Parenteral and Enteral Nutrition, 11: 109S–114S © by Am. Soc. for Parenteral and Enteral Nutrition, 1987.

that are considered tolerable, taking into account the prevalence of the disease or malnutrition, its severity, the cost of the test, and, where appropriate, the availability and advantages of treatment. In general, the highest predictive value is achieved when specificity is high, irrespective of sensitivity (Habicht, 1980).

Additional factors

There are many other factors affecting the design of nutritional assessment systems. These include respondent burden, equipment and personnel requirements, and field survey and data processing costs. The methods selected should aim at keeping the respondent burden to a minimum, thus reducing the nonresponse rate, and avoiding bias in the sample selection. In the early United Kingdom National Food Survey, for example, the inventory method was used to assess household food consumption; the method was found to have too high a respondent burden, and was abandoned in 1951 in favor of the food accounts method (Derry, 1984). Alternative methods for minimizing the nonresponse rate include the offering of material rewards and the provision of incentives such as regular medical checkups, feedback information, social visits, and telephone follow-up.

The requirements for equipment and personnel should also be taken into account when designing a nutritional assessment system. Measurements requiring elaborate equipment and highly trained technicians may be impractical in a field survey setting; instead, the measurements selected should be relatively noninvasive, and easy to perform accurately and precisely, using unskilled but trained assistants. The ease with which equipment can be maintained and calibrated must also be considered.

The field survey and data processing costs are also important factors. In surveillance systems, the resources available may dictate the number of malnourished individuals who can subsequently be treated in an intervention program. In such circumstances, the cutoff point for the index (Section 1.4.3) can be manipulated to select only the number of individuals who can be treated.

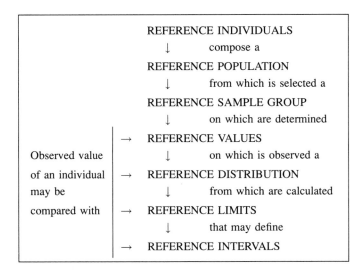

REFERENCE INDIVIDUALS
↓   compose a
REFERENCE POPULATION
↓   from which is selected a
REFERENCE SAMPLE GROUP
↓   on which are determined
→   REFERENCE VALUES
↓   on which is observed a
→   REFERENCE DISTRIBUTION
↓   from which are calculated
→   REFERENCE LIMITS
↓   that may define
→   REFERENCE INTERVALS

Observed value of an individual may be compared with

Table 1.5: The concept of reference values and the relationship of recommended terms. Reproduced with permission from Clinical Chemistry (1979) Volume 25, No. 8, page 1507, Scheme 1. © American Association for Clinical Chemistry, Inc.

1.4 Evaluation of nutritional assessment indices

Nutritional assessment indices can be evaluated by comparison with a distribution of reference values, or with reference limits drawn from the reference distribution. Alternatively, predetermined cutoff points (based on data that relate the levels of the indices to low body stores of the nutrient, impaired function, and/or clinical signs of deficiency) can be used. In some large-scale surveys, some indices have been linked to mortality risk.

1.4.1 Reference distribution

Reference values are obtained from a healthy reference sample group. The distribution of these reference values forms the reference distribution. The relationship between these terms is shown in Table 1.5. For comparison of the observed values of an individual with data derived from the reference sample group, the person under observation should be matched as closely as possible to the reference individuals by the factors known to influence the measurement. Frequently, these factors include age, sex, race, physiological state, and may also, depending on the index, include exercise, body posture, fasting, and the procedures used for specimen collection and analysis. Only if this criterion is met can the observed value be correctly interpreted.

Age	Arm Muscle Circumference Percentiles (mm)						
(yr)	5	10	25	50	75	90	95
Males							
35–44.9	247	255	269	286	302	318	327
45–54.9	239	249	265	281	300	315	326
Females							
35–44.9	186	192	205	218	236	257	272
45–54.9	187	193	206	220	238	260	274

Table 1.6: Part of the reference percentiles for mid-upper-arm muscle circumference (mm) for US males and females derived from the combined NHANES I and II data sets. From Frisancho (1981). © Am. J. Clin. Nutr. American Society for Clinical Nutrition.

Various methods are used to compare the observed values with the distribution of the reference values. In population studies, the distribution of the observed values can be compared using percentiles and/or standard deviation scores derived from the reference data. The latter are frequently based on measurements from large national nutrition surveys (e.g. NHANES II or Nutrition Canada). Table 1.6 presents a small sample of selected percentile values for mid-upper-arm muscle circumference derived from the NHANES I and II surveys (Frisancho, 1981), which can be used to evaluate observed values for mid-upper-arm muscle circumference. Such an approach is discussed more fully in Section 13.1.

1.4.2 Reference limits

The reference distribution can also be used to derive reference limits and a reference interval. Reference limits are generally defined so that a stated fraction of the reference values would be less than or equal to the limit, with a stated probability. Two reference limits are usually defined, the interval between and including them being termed the reference interval. Observed values for individuals can then be classified as 'unusually low', 'usual', or 'unusually high' according to whether they are situated (a) below the lower reference limit; (b) between or equal to either of the reference limits; or (c) above the upper reference limit (International Federation of Clinical Chemistry, 1979; 1984). For anthropometric growth indices, the 5th and 95th percentiles are frequently the two reference limits used to designate individuals with unusually low or unusually high anthropometric indices (Section 13.2.1). It is preferable not to use the terms 'abnormal', 'pathological', or 'normal' when this approach is used because an unusually high or low value for an index

Number of subjects

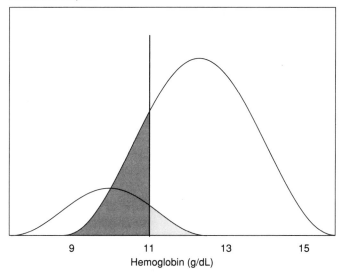

Hemoglobin (g/dL)

Figure 1.1: The distribution of hemoglobin values among persons with adequate intakes of iron (right curve) and those known to be responsive to an iron supplement (left curve). The two distributions are superimposed and overlap, showing that no single cutoff value can separate individuals with adequate from those with inadequate iron status. From Cook et al. (1971). Reproduced by permission of Grune and Stratton.

is a purely statistical occurrence, not necessarily associated with any impairment in health status (Smith et al., 1985).

1.4.3 Cutoff points

Cutoff points, unlike reference limits, are based on the relationship between nutritional assessment indices and functional impairment and/or clinical signs of deficiency. Their use is less frequent than that of reference limits because information relating indices and signs of deficiency is often not available.

Sometimes two cutoff points are used to define three intervals, in which case the three intervals can be designated deficient, marginal, and adequate (or deficient, low, and acceptable), representing a concept of degree of depletion (ICNND, 1963). Alternatively, a concept of likelihood or risk of deficiency can be used in which the three intervals are designated high-risk, low-risk, and adequate. The Nutrition Canada National Survey (Health and Welfare Canada, 1973) adopted this latter method as the basis for their interpretive standard for biochemical and clinical indices. This approach is also used in dietary assessment, when the cutoff points are often based on the recommended nutrient intakes. Nevertheless, as discussed in Section 1.3, cutoff values can never separate the 'deficient' and the 'adequately nourished' without some misclassification occurring. In Figure 1.1, for example, the light-shaded area to the right of 11 g/dL (110 g/L) and below the left curve represents persons who are anemic but who are classified as normal according to the cutoff point (11 g/dL; 110 g/L) defined by the World Health Organization (WHO, 1972). The dark-shaded area to the left of 11 g/dL (110 g/L) and below the right curve comprises persons classified as anemic by the WHO cutoff point but who are not found to be responsive to iron administration. Hence, the dark-shaded area represents those well-nourished persons who were incorrectly classified as 'anemic'. Misclassification arises because there is always biological variation among individuals (and hence in the physiological normal levels of any indices) depending on the nutrient requirements of an individual (Beaton, 1986). Specific procedures used for the evaluation of dietary, anthropometric, laboratory, and clinical methods of nutritional assessment are discussed more fully in Chapters 8, 13, 15, and 25, respectively.

References

Anderson SA. (1986). Guidelines for Use of Dietary Intake Data. Life Sciences Research Office, Federation of American Societies for Experimental Biology, Bethesda, Maryland.

Anonymous (1988). Hospital malnutrition still abounds. Nutrition Reviews 46: 315–317.

Beaton GH. (1986). Toward harmonization of dietary, biochemical, and clinical assessments: the meanings of nutritional status and requirements. Nutrition Reviews 44: 349–358.

Bistrian BR, Blackburn GL, Hallowell E, Heddle R. (1974). Protein status of general surgical patients. Journal of the American Medical Association 230: 858–860.

Bistrian BR, Blackburn GL, Vitale J, Cochran M. (1976). Prevalence of malnutrition in general medical patients. Journal of the American Medical Association 235: 1567–1570.

Blackburn GL, Bistrian BR, Maini BS, Schlamm HT, Smith MF. (1977). Nutritional and metabolic assessment of the hospitalized patient. Journal of Parenteral and Enteral Nutrition 1: 11–22.

Block G. (1982). A review of validations of dietary assessment methods. American Journal of Epidemiology 115: 492–505.

Bozzetti F, Migliavacca S, Gallus G, Radaelli G, Scotti A, Bonalumi MG, Ammatuna M, Sequeira C, Ternø G. (1985). Nutritional markers, as prognostic indicators of postoperative sepsis in cancer patients. Journal of Parenteral and Enteral Nutrition 9: 464–470.

Cook JD, Alvarado J, Gutnisky A, Jamra M, Labardini J, Layrisse M, Linares J, Loria A, Maspes V, Restrepo A, Reynafarje C, Sanchez-Medal L, Velez H, Viteri F. (1971). Nutritional deficiency and anemia in Latin America. Blood 38: 591–603.

Dempsey DT, Mullen JL. (1987). Prognostic value of nutritional indices. Journal of Parenteral and Enteral Nutrition 11: 109S–114S.

Derry B. (1984). Food purchases — strengths and weaknesses of the National Food Survey. In: The Dietary Assessment of Populations. Medical Research Council Scientific Report No. 4: 22–25.

Elwood PC. (1983). Epidemiology for nutritionists. 2. Sampling. Human Nutrition: Applied Nutrition 37A: 265–269.

Frisancho AR. (1981). New norms of upper limb fat and muscle areas for assessment of nutritional status. American Journal of Clinical Nutrition 34: 2540–2545.

Galen RS, Gambino SR. (1975). Beyond Normality: The Predictive Value and Efficiency of Medical Diagnosis. John Wiley and Sons, New York.

Habicht J-P. (1980). Some characteristics of indicators of nutritional status for use in screening and surveillance. American Journal of Clinical Nutrition 33: 531–535.

Habicht J-P, Lane JM, McDowell AJ. (1978). National Nutrition Surveillance. Federation Proceedings 37: 1181–1187.

Habicht J-P, Meyers LD, Brownie C. (1982). Indicators for identifying and counting the improperly nourished. American Journal of Clinical Nutrition 35: 1241–1254.

Habicht J-P, Yarbrough C, Martorell R. (1979). Anthropometric field methods: criteria for selection. In: Jelliffe DB, Jelliffe EFP (eds) Nutrition and Growth. Plenum Press, New York, pp. 365–387.

Health and Welfare Canada (1973). Nutrition Canada National Survey. Health and Welfare, Ottawa.

Himes JH. (1987). Purposeful assessment of nutritional status. In: Johnston FE (ed) Nutritional Anthropology. Alan R. Liss Inc., New York, pp. 85–99.

ICNND (Interdepartmental Committee on Nutrition for National Defense) (1963). Manual for Nutrition Surveys. Second edition. Superintendent of Documents, U.S. Government Printing Office, Washington, D.C.

International Federation of Clinical Chemistry (1979). Provisional recommendation on the theory of reference values (1978) Part 1. The concept of reference values. Clinical Chemistry 25: 1506–1508.

International Federation of Clinical Chemistry (1984). The theory of reference values, Part 5. Statistical treatment of collected reference values. Determination of reference limits. Clinica Chimica Acta 137: 97F–114F.

Jelliffe DB. (1966). The Assessment of the Nutritional Status of the Community. WHO Monograph No. 53. World Health Organization, Geneva.

McGanity WJ. (1974). The clinical assessment of nutritional status. In: Hawkins WW (ed) Assesment of Nutritional Status. Miles Symposium II. Miles Laboratories Ltd., Rexdale, Ontario, pp. 47–64.

Morley D. (1973). Pediatric Priorities in the Developing World. Butterworth, London.

NCHS (National Center for Health Statistics), Office of Health Research, Statistics and Technology (1981). Plan and operation of the Second National Health and Nutrition Examination Survey, 1976–80. (Vital and health statistics: Series 1, no. 15) (DHEW publication; no. (PHS) 81-1317), Washington, D.C.

NRC (National Research Council) (1986). Nutrient Adequacy. Assessment using Food Consumption Surveys. Subcommittee on Criteria for Dietary Evaluation, Coordinating Committee on Evaluation of Food Consumption Surveys. Food and Nutrition Board, Commission on Life Sciences. National Academy Press, Washington, D.C.

Roubenoff R, Roubenoff RA, Preto J, Balke CW. (1987). Malnutrition among hospitalized patients. A problem of physician awareness. Archives of Internal Medicine 147: 1462–1465.

Sahn DE, Lockwood R, Scrimshaw NS (eds). (1984). Measuring the Impact of Nutrition Intervention on Physical Growth. The United Nations University, Tokyo, Japan, pp. 65–93.

Smith JC, Jr, Holbrook JT, Erhard Danford D. (1985). Analysis and evaluation of zinc and copper in human plasma and serum. Journal of the American College of Nutrition 4: 627–638.

Solomons N. (1985). Assessment of nutritional status: functional indicators of pediatric nutriture. Pediatric Clinics of North America 32: 319–334.

Solomons N, Allen LH. (1983). The functional assessment of nutritional status: principles, practice and potential. Nutrition Reviews 41: 33–50.

Trowbridge FL, Staehling N. (1980). Sensitivity and specificity of arm circumference
    indicators in identifying malnourished children. American Journal of Clinical
    Nutrition 33: 687–696.
WHO (World Health Organization) (1972). Nutritional Anemia. WHO Technical Report
    Series No. 3. World Health Organization, Geneva.
WHO (World Health Organization) (1976a). Anthropometry in Nutritional Surveillance:
    An overview. United Nations Protein Advisory Group Bulletin 6: 2.
WHO (World Health Organization) (1976b). Methodology of Nutrition Surveillance.
    WHO Technical Report Series No. 593. World Health Organization, Geneva.
WHO (World Health Organization) Working Group (1986). Use and interpretation
    of anthropometric indicators of nutritional status. Bulletin of the World Health
    Organization 64: 929–941.

Chapter 2

Food consumption at the national and household level

Food consumption assessment methods produce qualitative or quantitative information from food consumption surveys. The survey data, collected at the national, household, or individual levels, can be expressed in terms of nutrients and/or foods. This chapter will consider methods suitable for measuring food available for consumption at the national level and at the household level. Chapter 3 includes a detailed discussion of methods suitable for measuring food consumption at the individual level.

2.1 Measuring food consumption at the national level

The most widely used method of assessing the nationally available food supply (food which is available for consumption, but not necessarily consumed) is based on food balance sheets. The data are presented on a *per capita* basis using population estimates, but provide no information on the distribution of the available food supplies within the country, or the extent to which individuals within populations vary in food intake. The data can be used to compare the available food supply between countries, and to monitor trends over time. The accuracy of the estimates of available food supplies varies among countries, and systematic errors may occur, which increase as the food system becomes more sophisticated; the limitations of the data should be clearly understood. Attempts to link trends in national food consumption data to trends in disease or mortality must be viewed with caution.

2.1.1 Food balance sheets

Food balance sheets are most commonly used to assess food consumption at the national level, and provide data on the food available for consumption, (i.e. the food supply within a country). The Food and Agricultural Organization (FAO) defines food balance sheets as:

A national account of the annual production of food, changes
in stocks, imports and exports, and distribution of food over
various uses within the country (FAO, 1980).

Food balance sheets do not measure the food actually ingested by the
population or provide information on food consumption in relation to regional, economic, demographic, seasonal, or socio-economic differences
within a country. Hence, food balance sheet data should not be used to
estimate nutritional inadequacies in a particular country or region of the
world (Dowler and Ok Seo, 1985). Nevertheless, the data can be used
to formulate agricultural policies concerned with the production, distribution, and consumption of foods, and as a basis for monitoring changes
and forecasting food consumption patterns. It can also be used to make
inter-country comparisons of food supplies.

Several different terms have been used to describe food balance sheets.
These include: national food accounts, food moving into consumption,
food consumption statistics, food disappearance data, and consumption
level estimates. The various terms reflect differences in the methods of
calculation, but all provide information on a country's available food
supply over a specified period. This may be a calendar year, the
agricultural year, or the crop year. The FAO has published food balance
sheets since 1949, covering the period 1934–1948, and up to the present.
The food balance sheets are compiled on an annual basis from data
supplied by about 200 countries.

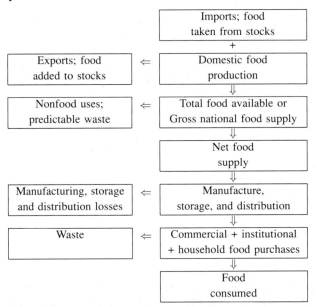

Figure 2.1: The derivation of food balance sheets. Adapted from
Nelson (1984) with permission.

	Energy (per person per day)				
	Total	Plant sources		Animal sources	
	Kcals	Kcals	Percent of total	Kcals	Percent of total
Developing Countries	2282	2075	90.9	207	9.1
Centrally Planned Countries	2721	2259	83.0	461	16.9
Developed Countries	3373	2336	69.3	1037	30.7

	Protein (per person per day)				
	Total	Plant sources		Animal sources	
	Grams	Grams	Percent of total	Grams	Percent of total
Developing Countries	57.8	45.4	78.5	12.4	21.5
Centrally Planned Countries	74.5	50.2	67.4	24.3	32.6
Developed Countries	98.5	43.3	44.1	55.1	55.9

Table 2.1: Estimates of the available food supply in developing countries, centrally planned countries of Eastern Europe and Asia, and developed countries, 1975–1977. From Food and Agriculture Organization of the United Nations (1980) with permission.

In general, the food supply is calculated from domestic food production plus imports and food taken from stocks. Exports and food added to stocks are then subtracted, to yield an estimate of total food available (the gross national food supply). Food diverted for non-human-food uses, such as animal feed, seed, and sugar in the brewing industry, together with an estimate for waste, is subtracted from the gross food supply. The result is a figure for the net amount of food available for human consumption in a country at the retail level (the net food supply) (Figure 2.1) (Campbell, 1981). An example of a national food balance sheet is given in Appendix A2.1.

Once the net food supply has been calculated, it is usually converted to a daily *per capita* basis using population estimates for that country. The FAO uses the United Nations Population Division midyear estimates of population size for its food balance sheet data (FAO, 1980; 1982) and to calculate *per capita* food availability. This is expressed in terms of grams *per capita* of individual food commodities, and energy and nutrient availability *per capita* (Table 2.1). To obtain estimates of the latter, *per capita* quantities of each food commodity are multiplied by the appropriate food composition values. No deduction is made for household food waste or for the loss of nutrients during food preparation. For FAO food balance sheets, regional FAO food composition tables are used.

The validity of food supply data is affected by errors which can be introduced at each stage in the calculation of the *per capita* food nutrient availability. In less developed countries, the method is said to result in an underestimate of per capita energy availability (Poleman, 1981).

In Canada, data on *per capita* food availability are prepared annually by Statistics Canada (1980; 1982) and termed 'food disappearance' data. They represent food available at the retail level. The data are mainly derived from farm surveys and reports from firms in the food industry engaged in production and marketing. Errors in Canadian food disappearance data arise from the use of inappropriate conversion factors to determine meat disappearance, absence of data for food items such as cake mixes, ready-to-serve meals, and fruit drink crystals, and imputation of data for some cereal products, fruit, and vegetables. Changes in the method of reporting and/or double counting may also produce errors (Campbell, 1981). *Per capita* nutrient disappearance data, calculated from the food disappearance data using the Health and Welfare Nutrient Data File (Health and Welfare, 1982), have been prepared annually by Statistics Canada since 1979 (Robbins and Barewal, 1981).

In the United States, annual estimates of the total amount of 260 different foods consumed by the U.S. civilian population at approximately the wholesale distribution level are compiled by the Economics, Statistics, and Co-operatives Service (ESCS) of the United States Department of Agriculture (USDA) (Manchester and Farrell, 1981). Sources of the data are similar to those used by Statistics Canada (1980). An estimate of wastage and losses is then applied to convert these wholesale estimates to quantities available for consumption at the retail level. Food composition values from recent revisions of the USDA Handbook No. 8 (USDA, 1976–1987) are then applied to the *per capita* food consumption data to calculate nutritive value data for energy and fifteen nutrients. In addition, the percentage of total nutrients contributed by twenty-four major food categories is computed. These data are published by the USDA in the 'National Food Situation'.

Limitations in the U.S. *per capita* food consumption data arise partly from incomplete measurement of food obtained from noncommercial gardens, sport fishing, and hunting (Manchester and Farrell, 1981). Flour consumption is measured but very little data are available for products such as bread, other bakery and cereal products, and soup. Limitations in the estimates of the nutrient content of the food supply also arise. Although only nutrients from the foods 'as eaten' are included, nevertheless some of these edible parts are not always eaten. Furthermore, the nutrient estimates also include food waste and nutrient losses that may occur in processing, marketing, cooking, and from plate waste. Hence, in general, the levels are probably an overestimate of the levels of nutrients in the U.S. food supply.

Some countries use food balance sheet data in place of national household food consumption surveys as a basis for estimating food consumption. This practice should be avoided because food balance sheets and household food consumption surveys have different objectives and yield different average *per capita* figures for daily energy and nutrient intakes. The size of the difference between the two methods is not necessarily constant between countries, or over time, and appears to depend in part on the gross national product (Dowler and Ok Seo, 1985).

2.1.2   Market databases

Commercial market databases report nationally projected unit and dollar sales of most packaged foods sold in grocery stores. These data can be used to analyse trends in consumer purchases of specific foods and commodity groups, down to the level of individual brands if desired (Schucker, 1982).

The United States Food and Drug Administration (USFDA) has a database of food label information, obtained by modifying the market database of the A.C. Nielson Company (Castle, 1981). This has been used to monitor trends in consumer purchases of nutritionally modified foods, such as fortified foods, or foods low in sodium, cholesterol, or 'calories'. Food label information can also be used to monitor food avoidance behavior by assessing changes in purchases of foods containing specific components, such as preservatives, artificial sweeteners, etc. Alternatively, the database of food label information can be used to measure the effect of product warning labels, such as those dealing with saccharin, on product sales.

2.1.3   Universal product codes and electronic scanning devices

The advent of universal product codes (UPC) in association with laser scanning devices will enable food purchases to be monitored at store checkout counters. The UPC codes appear on nearly all canned and packaged foods and even some fresh items that are repackaged in stores (Pearl, 1981). They are standard multi-digit numbers with a machine-readable code that represents product, size, manufacturer, and the nature of the contents. Information generated at store checkout counters could be used in the future to monitor food expenditure and purchases at the local, regional, and national levels. Future developments may include methods of recording food purchases at the household level, so that the data can be analyzed in socio-demographic detail.

2.2   Measuring food consumption at the household level

Household food consumption is the food and beverages available for consumption by the household, family group, or institution. It has been defined as:

> The total amount of food available for consumption in the household, generally excluding that eaten away from home unless taken from the home (Klaver et al., 1982).

The household food consumption methods described in this chapter do not provide information on the consumption of food by specific individuals within the household. Instead, food consumption *per capita* is calculated, irrespective of the age or sex structure of the household. Generally, no record is taken of edible food waste or food obtained outside the household food supply.

Information on the age and sex of persons in the household, their physiological state and activity level, number of meals eaten at home and away from home, income, and other socio-economic characteristics of the household members are collected, enabling food consumption *per capita* to be calculated in terms of income level, family size, region of the country, etc. Estimates of nutrient intake *per capita* are derived by multiplying the average food consumption data by the corresponding nutrient values for the edible portion of the food obtained from appropriate food composition tables.

Many of the technical problems of household surveys are similar to those of individual dietary surveys, and will be discussed in later sections (Chapters 4 and 5).

2.2.1   Food account method

A food account consists of a daily record, prepared by the householder, of all food entering the household, either purchased, received as gifts, or produced for household use during a specified period — usually seven days. Quantities of each food item are recorded in retail units (where applicable) and household measures. Records may also include brand names and retail price of the food items. The method assumes that there are no major changes in household inventories during the survey period (Burk and Pao, 1976). Generally, no account is taken of food and beverages consumed outside the home, or food discarded as plate waste, spoilage, or fed to pets. This method has been used since 1951 for the United Kingdom National Food Survey, with the additional application of a wastage factor equal to 10% of all edible portions of the foods consumed (Derry, 1984).

The respondent burden for the food account method is low, and it is relatively inexpensive. The diet does not appear to be altered by the recording process. The response rate is generally high, but there is some evidence that householders agreeing to participate are of above average socio-economic status (Young, 1981). The food accounts method can be used to collect data from a large sample, often during different months of the year to account for seasonal variation. As a result, information on the annual mean food consumption and selection patterns of a population can be obtained (Burk and Pao, 1976).

2.2.2 List-recall method

In this method the householder is asked by a trained interviewer to recall all foods used by the household on an 'as purchased' basis, and their quantity, price, or purchase value, over a specified period of time — usually the preceding one to seven days. A structured questionnaire containing a list of major food items likely to be consumed is generally used to assist in the recall. Frequently, no account is taken of food wasted, spoiled, or fed to pets. Quantities may be estimated by weight or household measures. Food models are sometimes used as memory aids. Information on the characteristics of each food (e.g. whether it is canned, fresh or frozen, enriched or unenriched) should be included as such information is essential for calculating the nutrient content of the foods used. Additional information on the age and sex of persons consuming the household food supply, the number of meals eaten both at home and away from home for each household member, income and other socio-economic characteristics of the household may also be obtained (Burk and Pao, 1976).

Only one interview, taking up to two and half hours, is required for this method, so that the field survey costs are lower than for other household methods, and the response rate is generally high. This method is currently used by the USDA for their National Food Consumption Survey (Section 2.3) (Hegsted, 1982).

2.2.3 Inventory method

The inventory method aims at recording acquisitions and changes in the food inventory of households during the survey period. It was formerly used for the United Kingdom National Food Survey. An inventory is prepared of the weight and type of all food commodities (i.e. 'larder stocks') in the household at the beginning and end of the survey period, which is generally one week (Burk and Pao, 1976). In addition, the types and weights of all food items brought into the home, whether purchased, home produced, as gifts, or as payment in kind, are also recorded daily during the survey period (Table 2.2) (Weiner and Lourie, 1969). A wastage factor of 10% of all edible portions of the foods consumed is often applied in this method. Alternatively, all foods items discarded during the survey period as a result of spoilage, plate-waste, or to be fed to pets, can be collected and weighed separately. The wastage weights

Name of householder: Street address: Town/city: Number in household:			1st visit date: 1st visit time: 2nd visit date: 2nd visit time:		
Commodity (Brand name)	Quantity 1st visit g / oz^a	Additional purchases, home production, or gifts g / oz^a	Quantity 2nd visit g / oz^a	LAB. USE ONLY	
				Total used	Food code
^{a} Draw a circle around units in which your quantities are measured					

Table 2.2: Data sheet for the inventory method. Modified from Weiner and Lourie (1969) with permission.

can then be subtracted from the inventory weights. From these data, the net amount of each commodity used by the household during the survey period can be calculated.

The number and age of persons consuming each meal are often recorded on a daily basis during the survey, allowing detailed information on the mean food consumption per person during the survey period to be calculated. Nevertheless, this method was abandoned by the United Kingdom National Food Survey in 1951 because it had too high a respondent burden. Furthermore, the response rate was adversely affected, and the normal pattern of food consumption was distorted. Existing larder stocks tended to be used in place of food items generally purchased during the week (Derry, 1984).

2.2.4 Household food record method

Food records are usually completed over at least a one-week period, either by the householder or a fieldworker. During this time, the amount of all foods consumed at each meal is recorded separately, either by weight or household measure, *before* subdivision into individual helpings (Burk and Pao, 1976). Detailed descriptions of all foods (including brand names) and their method of preparation are recorded. For composite dishes such as spaghetti bolognese, the amount of each raw ingredient used in the recipe and the final weight of the prepared composite dish should also be recorded. An example of a data sheet used for a weighed household food record is shown in Table 2.3. Sometimes, plate waste from each meal is collected and separated, and waste for individual food items weighed. Generally, however, kitchen and plate waste, and food fed to pets, is not

Family Name:			Date:			
Steet address:			Time:			
Town/city:			Name of meal:			
Number in household:						

| | | | | | LAB. USE ONLY | | |
Family members consuming the food (use code)	Description of food & method of cooking. One line per food.	Weight served g/oz[a]	Weight of waste g/oz[a]	Wt. of food g/oz[a]	Intake per 'person'[b]	Food Code

Meals eaten outside the Home: Describe foods and cooking methods. Estimate weights

[a] Draw a circle around units in which your quantities are measured
[b] Calculate from total 'man values' using the Rome Scale
Mother (M) age (...), Father (F) age (...), Son (S1) age (...), Son (S2) age (...),
Daughter (D1) age (...), Daughter (D2) age (...), Male visitor (MV1) age (...),
Female visitor (FV1) age (...)

Table 2.3: Data sheet for a weighed household food record. Modified from Weiner and Lourie (1969) with permission.

accounted for in this method. Instead, an arbitrary wastage factor of 10% of all edible portions of the foods consumed is applied, as noted for the inventory and food accounts methods.

Adjustments are sometimes made in this method for food eaten outside the home, and for the presence of nonhousehold members during the survey period. The number of family members and visitors eating each meal can be recorded, and a 'man value' assigned to each person, weighted according to their age and sex. If the Rome scale is used, males above fourteen years of age are assigned a value of 1.0; females above eleven years of age and boys eleven to fourteen years, a value of 0.90; children aged seven to ten years, a value of 0.75; children between four and six years, a value of 0.40; and children less than four years, a value of 0.15 (Møller Jensen et al., 1984). The amount of each food consumed by the entire household can then be divided by the corresponding total 'man value' to provide food intakes per 'person'. This approach produces a better estimate of the adequacy of the household food intake, particularly for families.

The weighed food record method is the most accurate of the household methods. Nevertheless, it has a high respondent burden, if the recording is performed by the householder. Consequently, the nonresponse rate may be high, resulting in a small and unrepresentative sample. Food consumption patterns may also be altered during the survey period, either to simplify the process of measuring the food, or to impress the interviewer. It is also an expensive method because the households should be visited frequently during the survey period to encourage compliance. This method was used for the earlier USDA food consumption surveys (Burk and Pao, 1976; Young, 1984).

The Food and Agricultural Organization has recommended this method for use in rural areas in less developed countries, where the variety of foods is often limited, home production is very important, and units for buying foods are not standardized (Pekkarinen, 1970). In these countries, the weighing and recording should be performed daily by field investigators, rather than by the householder.

2.2.5 Telephone survey

Until recently, the use of the telephone for household surveys in some countries has been hampered by the problem of unlisted telephone numbers producing an unknown bias in the sample (Schucker, 1982). This difficulty has been largely overcome in the United States, where it is now possible to include unlisted telephone numbers.

Telephone surveys have been used recently by the USFDA to collect consumer information on the purchase and use of certain products. In a recent survey on the use of protein supplements, telephone interviews were conducted online with a computer, thus eliminating paper and pencil recording. The final completion response rate in this survey was 87%, 6616 interviews being completed in five weeks (Schucker and Gunn, 1978). Telephone surveys may be used more frequently in the future, because they cost on average 40–50% of personal interviews.

2.2.6 Family food scale

Some investigators have used scalogram techniques, such as a Guttman scale, to measure the complexity and diversity of food patterns of families (Chassy et al., 1967), particularly in less developed countries (Beaudry-Darismé et al., 1972). The food scale is constructed from information on the frequency with which a range of food items or food groups is eaten. It is cumulative in the sense that a diet which includes food items within a given scale step position (or score) will also include the items in all the preceding steps. Thus, once the position of a respondent on the scale is determined, it is possible both to predict the food items consumed and to specify the dietary complexity and diversity. For example, a scale step position of four on a family food scale used in Haiti (Beaudry-Darismé et al., 1972) (Table 2.4), automatically indicates that the diet of the respondent included starchy foods, fats and oils, spices and condiments, and fruits and fruit juices. Starchy foods are the lowest item on this

Step	Item	% of Respondents
1	Starchy foods	100
2	Fats and oils, excluding dairy butter	98
3	Spices and condiments	97
4	Fruits and fruit juices	96
5	Milk, all types	93
6	Nondairy beverages	92
7	Fish, fresh and dried	89
8	Tomatoes, tomato juice and paste	57
9	Meats and canned fish	46
10	Lettuce, carrots and cabbage	20

Table 2.4: Family food scale used in Haiti. From Beaudry-Darismé et al. (1972). Reproduced by permission of Gordon and Breach Science Publishers Inc.

scale and were consumed by 100% of the respondents. Lettuce, carrots and cabbage are the highest item and were consumed by only 20% of the respondents. Hence, a single scale step indicates both *which* food groups, and *how many* food groups, are consumed (Harrison and Bond, 1984). Highly trained interviewers are not required, and information on a large number of subjects can be collected using this technique (Cassidy, 1981). The method can be used for individuals (Schorr et al., 1972; Harrison and Bond, 1984) as well as households.

Beaudry-Darismé et al. (1972) used this scale to examine the relationship between the complexity of the diet of one to five-year-old Haitian children and the prevalence of malnutrition. Their results suggested that complexity of the diet may be an index of overall food intake quality. In some cases the scale has also been used to predict nutrient intake patterns. For example, Schorr et al. (1972) found a positive correlation between dietary diversity, as measured by the Guttman scale, and intake of selected nutrients (e.g. calcium, iron, vitamins A and C).

2.3   National food consumption surveys

Several countries use household methods for their national food consumption surveys. Close attention must be paid to the sampling design of these surveys to ensure that a representative national sample is obtained which accounts for the influence on food intake of season, holidays, weekends, socio-economic status, and region.

Most national surveys utilize an arbitrary allowance (e.g. 10%) for food waste at the domestic level (i.e. plate and kitchen wastage, spoilage, and food fed to pets) (Ministry of Agriculture, Fisheries and Food, 1982). A food waste survey established in the United Kingdom in 1976 demonstrated that 4–6% of potential food energy was discarded, regardless of season (Wenlock et al., 1980). Comparable estimates of consumer food waste in the United States range from 7% to 35% (Adelson et al., 1963; Harrison et al., 1975; Gallo, 1980). The wide range is, in part, attributed to the differences in the definitions of waste, methodologies used, and the study group.

In Canada, household food consumption surveys (called family expenditure surveys), are conducted at approximately four-yearly intervals. They provide an estimate of the amount of food 'as purchased' or brought into the home for family use. No account is taken of food consumed away from home, or of food wastage. Both list-recall and food record procedures are used (Statistics Canada, 1981). Food purchases are converted into nutrient content using the Health and Welfare Nutrient Data File (1982).

The United Kingdom National Food Survey originally used the household inventory method. At first, only urban working class households were surveyed. In 1950, the survey was extended to cover all types of households, and in 1951, the household inventory method was replaced by the food accounts method (Derry, 1984). The surveys are conducted annually. Data are collected weekly, from a large sample of households, during different months of the year to account for seasonal variation. Information on the average quantity of food purchased per person per week, and on the average amount spent on each of over 150 standard food categories, is obtained. Estimates of 'nutrient intake' are also derived by multiplying the average consumption data for 200 separate foods by corresponding nutrient values obtained from the U.K. food composition tables (Paul and Southgate, 1978). Despite a relatively low respondent burden, response rate for the United Kingdom National Food Survey is only about 55% (Derry, 1984).

The first U.S. nationwide household food consumption surveys employed the food accounts method. In the 1930's, this method was changed to the list-recall method, which has been used at approximately ten-year intervals ever since. Householders are interviewed and asked to recall, from a detailed list, all foods used from the home food supplies during the preceding seven days. Hence the recall data include food that has been eaten, discarded, and fed to household pets. For each food item, information on the quantity (in pounds), form (e.g. fresh, frozen, canned, or dried), source (e.g. purchased, home-produced, or received as gift or pay), and details of the unit and price of all purchased food items is collected. In addition, information on socio-economic and demographic characteristics of the household, general shopping practices, number of meals and snacks consumed from household food supplies, expenses for foods bought and eaten away from home, and participation in food assistance programs is also obtained (NRC, 1984).

In recent U.S. household food consumption surveys, information on food intake of individual household members, as well as the household survey component, has been included. For the individual component, a twenty-four-hour dietary recall, followed by two-day food records, is collected from individual household members (Section 3.1.1). The quantities of foods consumed are recorded in household measures, number of units, or weight. Questions on eating patterns, intake of specific foods and dietary supplements, height and weight, and general health status are also asked. By including both household and individual components, the nutrient content of the household food supplies and the nutrient intakes of the individual household members can be estimated (NRC, 1984).

2.4 Summary

Food consumption at the national level is most frequently determined by using food balance sheets (also termed national food accounts, food disappearance data, food consumption level estimates, etc). These provide information on national *per capita* food availability, of varying quality, over a specified period, but give no information on food consumption at the individual level. Further, food balance sheets do not yield data on food consumption in relation to regional, economic, demographic, seasonal, or socio-economic differences within a country. Data take into account supply (production, imports, and existing stocks) and losses (exports, nonfood use, animal food, losses to pests, and production and manufacturing losses) prior to availability for domestic consumption, and are expressed in terms of grams *per capita* of individual food commodities. The latter, when multiplied by corresponding food composition values, provide estimates of *per capita* energy and nutrient availability. In industrialized countries, trends in consumer purchases of specific foods, commodity groups, or individual brands are also monitored at the national level, using commercial market databases. Future methods of measuring national food consumption may involve monitoring food purchases at store check-out counters, using universal product codes and electronic scanning devices.

Household food consumption methods measure all food and beverages available for consumption by a household, family group, or institution, during a specified time period. The following methods are used: food accounts, list-recall methods, inventory methods, food records, family food scales, and telephone surveys. All involve collecting information on demographic and socio-economic characteristics of the household, enabling data to be presented in terms of income level, family size, region of the country, etc. *Per capita* nutrient intake data are derived by multiplying the *per capita* food consumption data by the corresponding nutrient values obtained from appropriate food composition data. 'Man' values, weighted according to age and sex, are sometimes assigned to each family member, and used to calculate more precisely nutrient intake per person.

The household food consumption methods vary in their complexity and respondent burden. Generally, no account is taken of food and beverages consumed outside the home, or food wasted, spoiled, or fed to pets. In some cases, a wastage factor of all edible foods consumed is applied. Some industrialized countries have adopted household food consumption methods for their national food consumption surveys.

References

Adelson SF, Delaney I, Miller C, Noble IT. (1963). Discard of edible food in households. Journal of Home Economics 55: 633–639.

Beaudry-Darismé MN, Hayes-Blend LC, van Veen AG. (1972). The application of sociological research methods to food and nutrition problems on a Caribbean island. Ecology of Food and Nutrition 1: 103–119.

Burk MC, Pao EM. (1976). Methodology for large-scale surveys of household and individual diets. Home Economics Research Report No. 40. US Department of Agriculture, Washington, D.C.

Campbell JA. (1981). An assessment of data bases relating to nutritional aspects of food. Food and Nutrition Service, Marketing and Economics Branch, Agriculture Canada, Ottawa.

Cassidy CM. (1981). Collecting data on American Food Consumption patterns: An anthropological perspective. In: Assessing Changing Food Consumption Patterns. Committee on Food Consumption Patterns, Food and Nutrition Board, National Research Council. National Academy Press, Washington, D.C., pp. 135–154.

Castle OS. (1981). A.C. Nielsen Company Services In: Assessing Changing Food Consumption Patterns, Committee on Food Consumption Patterns, Food and Nutrition Board, National Research Council. National Academy Press, Washington D.C., pp. 72–85.

Chassy JP, Veen AG van, Young FW. (1967). The application of social science research methods to the study of food habits and food consumption in an industrializing area. American Journal of Clinical Nutrition 20: 56–64.

Derry B. (1984). Food Purchases — Strengths and weaknesses of the National Food Survey. In: The Dietary Assessment of Populations. Medical Research Council Scientific Report No. 4: 22–25.

Dowler EA, Ok Seo YI. (1985). Assessment of energy intake. Food Policy, August, 278–288.

FAO (Food and Agriculture Organization) (1979). Production Yearbook 1978. FAO Statistics Series No. 22. Food and Agriculture Organization, Rome.

FAO (Food and Agriculture Organization) (1980). Food Balance Sheets 1975–77. Average and Per Capita Food Supplies 1961–65, Average 1967–77. Food and Agriculture Organization, Rome.

FAO (Food and Agriculture Organization) (1982). Production Yearbook 1980. Volume 34. FAO Statistics Service No. 34. Food and Agriculture Organization, Rome.

Gallo AE. (1980). Consumer food waste in the United States. National Food Review Fall, 13–16.

Harrison GG, Rathje WL, Hughes WW. (1975). Food waste behavior in an urban population. Journal of Nutrition Education 7: 13–16.

Harrison KR, Bond JB. (1984). Guttman scalogram techniques as a method of dietary analysis. Journal of the Canadian Dietetic Association 45: 26–32.

Health and Welfare Canada (1982). Canadian Nutrient File. Bureau of Nutritional Sciences, Health and Welfare, Ottawa.

Hegsted DM. (1982). The classic approach — the USDA nationwide food consumption survey. American Journal of Clinical Nutrition 35: 1302–1305.

Klaver W, Knuiman JT, Staveren WA van. (1982). Proposed definitions for use in the methodology of food consumption studies. In: Hautvast JGAJ, Klaver W (eds) Euronut Report 1. The Diet Factor in Epdemiological Research, Wageningen, pp. 77–85.

Manchester AC, Farrell KR. (1981). Measurement and forecasting of food consumption by USDA. In: Assessing Changing Food Consumption Patterns. Committee on Food Consumption Patterns, Food and Nutrition Board, National Research Council. National Academy Press, Washington, D.C., pp. 51–71.

Ministry of Agriculture, Fisheries and Food (1982). Household Food Consumption and Expenditure: 1980. Her Majesty's Stationery Office, London.

Møller Jensen O, Wahrendorf J, Rosenqvist A, Geser A. (1984). The reliability of questionnaire-derived historical dietary information and temporal stability of food habits in individuals. American Journal of Epidemiology 120: 281–290.

NRC (National Research Council) (1984). National Survey Data on Food Consumption: Uses and Recommendations. National Academy Press, Washington, D.C.

Nelson M. (1984). Food production and sales. In: The Dietary Assessment of Populations. Medical Research Council Scientific Report No. 4: 16–21.

Paul AA, Southgate DAT. (1978). McCance and Widdowsons's The Composition of Foods. Fourth edition. Her Majesty's Stationery Office, London.

Pearl RB. (1981). Possible alternative methods for data collection on food consumption and expenditures. In: Assessing Changing Food Consumption Patterns. Committee on Food Consumption Patterns, Food and Nutrition Board, National Research Council. National Academy Press, Washington D.C., pp. 198–203.

Pekkarinen M. (1970). Methodology in the collection of food consumption data. World Review of Nutrition and Dietetics 12: 145–171.

Poleman, TT. (1981). A reappraisal of the extent of world hunger. Food Policy 6: 236–252.

Robbins L, Barewal S. (1981). The apparent nutritive value of food available for consumption in Canada, 1960–1975. Agriculture Canada, Information Service, Ottawa.

Schorr BC, Sanjur D, Erickson E. (1972). Teenage food habits. Journal of the American Dietetic Association 61: 415–420.

Schucker RE. (1982). Alternative approaches to classic food consumption measurement methods: telephone interviewing and market data bases. American Journal of Clinical Nutrition 35: 1306–1309.

Schucker RE, Gunn WJ. (1978). A national survey of the use of protein products in conjunction with weight reduction diets among American women. Food and Drug Administration, Center for Disease Control, Washington, D.C.

Statistics Canada (1980). Urban family food expenditure in 1978. Catalogue 62–548, Occasional, Ottawa.

Statistics Canada (1981). Family expenditure in Canada. Volume 2. Major Urban Centres: Sixteen Cities 1978. Catalogue 62–550, Ottawa.

Statistics Canada (1982). Apparent per capita food consumption in Canada. Part 1, 1981. Catalogue 32–299, Ottawa.

USDA (U.S. Department of Agriculture) (1976). Composition of foods — raw, processed and prepared. Agriculture Handbook No. 8–1: Dairy and egg products. Agriculture Research Station, U.S. Department of Agriculture, Washington, D.C.

USDA (U.S. Department of Agriculture) (1977). Composition of foods — raw, processed and prepared. Agriculture Handbook No. 8–2: Spices and herbs. Agriculture Research Station, U.S. Department of Agriculture, Washington, D.C.

USDA (U.S. Department of Agriculture) (1978). Composition of foods — raw, processed and prepared. Agriculture Handbook No. 8–3: Baby foods. Agriculture Research Station, U.S. Department of Agriculture, Washington, D.C.

USDA (U.S. Department of Agriculture) (1979). Composition of foods — raw, processed and prepared. Agriculture Handbook No. 8–4: Fats and oils. Agriculture Research Station, U.S. Department of Agriculture, Washington, D.C.

USDA (U.S. Department of Agriculture) (1979). Composition of foods — raw, processed and prepared. Agriculture Handbook No. 8–5: Poultry products. Agriculture Research Station, U.S. Department of Agriculture, Washington, D.C.

USDA (U.S. Department of Agriculture) (1980). Composition of foods — raw, processed and prepared. Agriculture Handbook No. 8–6: Soups, sauces, gravies. Agriculture Research Station, U.S. Department of Agriculture, Washington, D.C.

USDA (U.S. Department of Agriculture) (1980). Composition of foods — raw, processed and prepared. Agriculture Handbook No. 8–7: Sausages and luncheon meats. Agriculture Research Station, U.S. Department of Agriculture, Washington, D.C.

USDA (U.S. Department of Agriculture) (1981). Composition of foods — raw, processed and prepared. Agriculture Handbook No. 8–8: Breakfast cereals. Agriculture Research Station, U.S. Department of Agriculture, Washington, D.C.

USDA (U.S. Department of Agriculture) (1982). Composition of foods — raw, processed and prepared. Agriculture Handbook No. 8–9: Fruits and fruit juices. Agriculture Research Station, U.S. Department of Agriculture, Washington, D.C.

USDA (U.S. Department of Agriculture) (1983). Composition of foods — raw, processed and prepared. Agriculture Handbook No. 8–10: Pork products. Agriculture Research Station, U.S. Department of Agriculture, Washington, D.C.

USDA (U.S. Department of Agriculture) (1984). Composition of foods — raw, processed and prepared. Agriculture Handbook No. 8–11: Vegetable products. Agriculture Research Station, U.S. Department of Agriculture, Washington, D.C.

USDA (U.S. Department of Agriculture) (1984). Composition of foods — raw, processed and prepared. Agriculture Handbook No. 8–12: Nut and seed products. Agriculture Research Station, U.S. Department of Agriculture, Washington, D.C.

USDA (U.S. Department of Agriculture) (1986). Composition of foods — raw, processed and prepared. Agriculture Handbook No. 8–13: Beef products. Agriculture Research Station, U.S. Department of Agriculture, Washington, D.C.

USDA (U.S. Department of Agriculture) (1986). Composition of foods — raw, processed and prepared. Agriculture Handbook No. 8–14: Beverages. Agriculture Research Station, U.S. Department of Agriculture, Washington, D.C.

USDA (U.S. Department of Agriculture) (1987). Composition of foods — raw, processed and prepared. Agriculture Handbook No. 8–15: Finfish and shellfish products. Agriculture Research Station, U.S. Department of Agriculture, Washington, D.C.

Weiner JS, Lourie JA. (1969). Human Biology: A Guide to Field Methods. International Biological Programme. IBP Handbook No. 9. Blackwell Scientific Publications, Oxford – Edinburgh.

Wenlock RW, Buss DH, Derry BJ, Dixon EJ. (1980). Household food wastage in Britain. British Journal of Nutrition 43: 50–53.

Young CM. (1981). Dietary methodology. In: Assessing Changing Food Consumption Patterns. Committee on Food Consumption Patterns, Food and Nutrition Board, National Research Council. National Academy Press, Washington, D.C., pp. 89–118.

Chapter 3

Food consumption of individuals

This chapter describes the methods for measuring food consumption of individuals. Subsequent chapters discuss factors associated with the precision and validity of each of these methods (Chapters 5–7) and the assessment and evaluation of nutrient intakes (Chapters 4 and 8).

3.1 Methods

Methods used for measuring food consumption of individuals can be classified into two major groups. The first group, known as quantitative daily consumption methods, consist of recalls or records, designed to measure the quantity of the individual foods consumed over a one-day period. By increasing the number of measurement days for these methods, quantitative estimates of actual recent intakes, or, for longer time periods, usual intakes of individuals, can be obtained. Assessment of usual intake is particularly critical when relationships between diet and biological parameters are assessed.

The second group of methods includes the dietary history and the food frequency questionnaire. Both obtain retrospective information on the patterns of food use during a longer, less precisely defined time period. Such methods are most frequently used to assess usual intake of foods or specific classes of foods. With modification, they can provide data on usual nutrient intakes.

3.1.1 Twenty-four-hour recall method

In the twenty-four-hour recall method, subjects, their parents, or caretakers are asked by the nutritionist, who has been trained in interviewing techniques, to recall the subject's exact food intake during the previous twenty-four-hour period or preceding day. Detailed descriptions of all foods and beverages consumed, including cooking methods and brand names (if possible), are recorded by the interviewer. Vitamin and mineral supplement use is also noted. Quantities of foods consumed are usually estimated in household measures and entered on the data sheet

Name: Street address: Town/city:				Date: Day of the week:		
				LAB. USE ONLY		
Place Eaten	Time	Description of food or drink. Give brand name if applicable	Amount	Day/Meal code	Food code	Amount code

Additional questions:
Was intake unusual in any way?   Yes (...) No (...)
If yes, in what way?

Do you take vitamin or mineral supplements? Yes (...) No (...)
If yes, how many per day? (...) per week? (...)
If yes, what kind? (give brand if possible)
Multivitamin   Iron   Ascorbic acid
Other (list)

Table 3.1: Sample data sheet for a twenty-four-hour record. Modified from Weiner and Lourie (1969) with permission.

(Table 3.1). Food models of various types (Section 5.2.3) can be used as memory aids and/or to assist the respondent in assessing portion size of food items consumed (Burk and Pao, 1976). Methods for coding the completed twenty-four-hour recalls and potential sources of coding errors are discussed in Section 5.2.7

The interview protocol must be standardized and pretested prior to the study. Adherence to the interview protocol, and accuracy of food coding by the interviewers, should be checked periodically during the survey and the interviewers retrained if necessary (Section 5.2.2). Detailed suggestions on how to conduct the interview can be found in Sanjur (1982) and Hughes (1986), who stressed that leading questions and judgmental comments should be avoided. An indirect approach is recommended, enabling respondents to freely express their feelings so that answers are not biased.

The flat slope syndrome may be a problem in the twenty-four-hour recall method (Gersovitz et al., 1978). In this syndrome, individuals appear to overestimate low intakes and underestimate high intakes — sometimes referred to as 'talking a good diet'. This observed relationship may be an artifact of the statistical analysis and the result of regression towards the mean (NRC, 1986).

A single twenty-four-hour recall is most appropriate for assessing average intakes of foods and nutrients for large groups, except for persons with poor memories (e.g. some elderly persons), and young children (Young, 1981). This method was used in the Nutrition Canada National Survey (Health and Welfare Canada, 1973). It is not suitable for assessing usual food and/or nutrient intakes of individuals. When using a twenty-four-hour recall to characterize the average usual intake for a population group, the sample should be representative of the population under study, and all days of the week should be proportionately included in the survey. In this way, any day-of-the-week effects on food and/or nutrient intakes will be taken into account (Section 6.2). The respondent burden is small for a twenty-four-hour recall, so that compliance is generally high. The method is quick, relatively inexpensive, and can be used with illiterate individuals.

The success of the twenty-four-hour recall depends on: the subject's memory, the ability of the respondent to convey accurate estimates of portion sizes consumed, the degree of motivation of the respondent, and the persistence of the interviewer (Acheson et al., 1980).

3.1.2 Repeated twenty-four-hour recalls

Twenty-four-hour recalls can be repeated during different seasons of the year to estimate the average food intake of individuals over a longer time period (i.e. usual food intake). The number of twenty-four-hour recalls required to estimate the usual nutrient intake of individuals depends on the degree of precision needed, the nutrient under study, and the population group. Repeated twenty-four-hour recalls have been recommended as part of a system for measuring food consumption patterns in the United States (Food and Nutrition Board, National Research Council, 1981). The United States Committee on Food Consumption Patterns have recommended that four twenty-four-hour recalls on the same individual within a one-year sampling period be used to estimate the distribution of usual nutrient intakes among individuals. In general, if an adequate sampling procedure is designed to take into account the influence of weekends, seasons, and holidays on the pattern of food intake, the results can provide an estimate of national food consumption. Section 6.1.1 provides a more detailed discussion of the precision of twenty-four-hour recalls.

3.1.3 Estimated food records

The respondent is asked to record, at the time of consumption, all foods and beverages (including snacks) eaten for a specified time period. Detailed descriptions of all foods and beverages (including brand names) and their method of preparation and cooking are recorded. For composite dishes such as spaghetti bolognese, the amount of each raw ingredient used in the recipe, the final weight of the composite dish, and the amount consumed by the subject should be recorded, wherever possible.

Food portion size can be estimated by the respondent using a variety of procedures, each differing in level of precision. Standard household measuring cups and spoons are used wherever possible, supplemented by measurements with a ruler (for meat and cake) and counts (for eggs and bread slices). Portion size measures are usually converted into grams by the investigator before calculating nutrient intakes. Unfortunately, errors may arise as a result of the inability of the respondent to adequately quantify portion sizes consumed and as a result of difficulties associated with the conversion of volume estimates to quantities expressed in grams (Section 5.2.4). The information is recorded on a form similar to that shown in Table 2.3, except that household measures are used for food amounts. Usually, the subject, parent, or caretaker completes the food record, although in less developed countries a local field investigator may perform this task (Pekkarinen, 1970; Marr, 1971; Burk and Pao, 1976).

The number of days included in an estimated record varies; usually three, five, or seven days are used. Weekend days should be proportionately included in the dietary survey period for each subject, to account for potential day-of-the-week effects on food and nutrient intakes. No consensus has been reached regarding the number, spacing, and selection of record days required for characterizing either the actual or usual food and/or nutrient intakes of individuals by this method. This problem is discussed in more detail in Sections 6.1.2 and 6.2.

3.1.4 Weighed food records

Weighed food records are more frequently used in the United Kingdom and Europe because householders often use weighing scales for food preparation in these countries. A weighed food record is the most precise method available for estimating usual food and/or nutrient intakes of individuals. Such data are essential for diet counselling, and for statistical analysis involving correlation or regression with biological parameters.

In a weighed record, the subject, parent, or caretaker is instructed to weigh all foods and beverages consumed by the subject during a specified time period. Details of methods of food preparation, description of foods, and brand names (if known) should also be recorded. For composite dishes such as spaghetti bolognese, weights of all raw ingredients used in the recipe should be noted, as well as the weight of the portion consumed and the final weight of the composite dish. The method of recording is similar to that shown for a household food record (Table 2.3). Respondents may require assistance in recalling food items if specific details and/or weights have been unintentionally omitted. For occasional meals eaten away from home, respondents are generally requested to record descriptions of the amounts of food eaten. The nutritionist can then buy and weigh a duplicate portion of each recorded food item, where possible, to assess the probable weight consumed.

As for the estimated record, the number, spacing, and selection of days necessary to characterize the actual or usual nutrient intakes of an individual using the weighed method vary, depending on the nutrient of interest, study population, objective of the survey, etc. Again, weekend days should be proportionately included in the dietary survey period to account for any weekend effect on the nutrient intake.

Respondents must be motivated, numerate, and literate, if a dietary record method is selected. Respondents may change their usual eating pattern to simplify the measuring or weighing process, or, alternatively, to impress the investigator (Pekkarinen, 1970; Marr, 1971; Burk and Pao, 1976) (also see Section 7.1.3). Respondent burden for food records is higher than for the twenty-four-hour recall, so that individuals may be less willing to co-operate. Precision is greater in the weighed record compared to the estimated record method because the portion sizes are weighed. Misreading the weighing scale and/or recording errors, however, may still occur.

3.1.5 Dietary history

The dietary history method, first developed by Burke in 1947, attempts to estimate the usual food intakes of individuals over a relatively long period of time (Burke, 1947). It is an interview method made up initially of three components, and should be carried out by a nutritionist trained in interviewing techniques. The first component consists of a twenty-four-hour recall of actual intake, and collection of general information on the overall eating pattern of the subject, both at mealtimes and between meals. The general information obtained includes detailed descriptions of foods, their frequency of consumption, and usual portion sizes in common household measures. Typical questions might be: 'What do you usually eat for breakfast?'

The second component serves as a 'cross check' for the information on usual intake obtained from the first stage. It consists of a questionnaire on the frequency of consumption of specific food items, which is used to verify and clarify the information on the kinds and amounts of foods given as the usual intake in the first component. Questions asked may include: 'Do you like or dislike milk?'

The third component consists of a three-day food record using house-hold measures. This stage is the least helpful; it is merely another method of measuring recent food intake for a specified time period. Conse-quently, it is often abandoned.

Numerous modifications of the dietary history method exist. For ex-ample, portion size estimates can be made using a variety of techniques including common utensils, commercial plastic food models, standard measuring cups and spoons, photographs, or real foods. The time periods covered by the dietary history method may also vary. The maximum time period which can be used has not been firmly established. When shorter time frames (i.e. one month) are used, precision and validity are apparently higher than for longer periods (see Section 7.1.2). Measurements of food intake over one-year periods are probably unrealistic if seasonal variations in food intakes occur (Callmer et al., 1985).

Dutch investigators used a three-part dietary history questionnaire covering one month to record usual food consumption separately on weekdays, Saturdays, and Sundays (van Staveren et al., 1985). This approach takes into account the potential effect of weekends on nutrient intake. The portion size of foods most frequently consumed in this study were weighed by a dietitian in the home. A weighted daily average intake was then calculated from the data, using the following formula:

$$\text{Average daily intake} = \frac{(5 \times \text{workday}) + \text{Saturday} + \text{Sunday}}{7}$$

The dietary history method is very labor intensive, and unsuitable for large surveys. Moreover, the results obtained depend on the skill of the interviewers. In general, dietary history methods provide qualitative, not quantitative, data on usual food intake over a period of several weeks or months. If certain modifications to the method are made, however (van Staveren et al., 1985), quantitative data on usual food and nutrient intakes of individuals over one-month time periods can be obtained.

3.1.6   Food frequency questionnaire

A food frequency questionnaire is designed to obtain qualitative, descriptive information about usual food consumption patterns. It does not generally provide quantitative data on food or nutrient intakes. The questionnaire consists of two components: (a) a list of foods and (b) a set of frequency-of-use response categories (Table 3.2). The list of foods may focus on specific groups of foods, particular foods, or foods consumed periodically in association with special events/seasons, when it is designated a focused questionnaire (Anderson, 1986). Alternatively, the food list may be extensive to enable estimates of total food intake, and hence dietary diversity, to be made.

The aim of the food frequency questionnaire is to assess the frequency with which certain food items or food groups are consumed during a specified time period (e.g. daily, weekly, monthly, yearly). Specific combinations of foods included in a focused questionnaire can be used as predictors for intakes of certain nutrients or non-nutrients, provided that the dietary components are concentrated in a relatively small number of foods or specific food groups. Examples include the frequency of consumption of fresh fruits and fruit juices as predictors of vitamin C

For each food item, indicate with a check mark the category that best describe the frequency with which you usually eat that particular food item						
Food item	More than once per day	Once per day	3–6 times per week	Once or twice per week	Once per month or less	Never
Beef, hamburger	☐	☐	☐	☐	☐	☐
Pork, ham	☐	☐	☐	☐	☐	☐
Liver	☐	☐	☐	☐	☐	☐
Poultry	☐	☐	☐	☐	☐	☐
Eggs	☐	☐	☐	☐	☐	☐
Dried peas/beans	☐	☐	☐	☐	☐	☐
Nuts	☐	☐	☐	☐	☐	☐
etc.	☐	☐	☐	☐	☐	☐
Enter other foods not listed that are eaten regularly:						
1	☐	☐	☐			
2	☐	☐	☐			
3	☐	☐	☐			
4	☐	☐	☐			

Table 3.2: Abbreviated food frequency questionnaire. A few foods and food categories are shown as examples. A complete questionnaire might contain more than 100 items.

intake; green leafy vegetables and carrots as predictors of carotenoid intakes; and whole grain cereals, legumes, nuts, fruits, and vegetables as predictors of dietary fiber intakes. The method can also be used to assess the intake of artificial sweeteners, certain contaminants present in specific foods, alcohol, and condiments (Burk and Pao, 1976; Hunt, 1984; Anderson, 1986).

The food frequency questionnaires should relate to simple, defined food categories: open-ended questions should be avoided, as pre-formatted lists of food categories act as a memory prompt. The data for the food frequency method may be obtained by a standardized interview or self-administered questionnaire, both taking fifteen to thirty minutes to complete (see abbreviated example given in Table 3.2). The results generally represent usual intakes over an extended period of time and are easy to collect and process. The food frequency questionnaire imposes less burden on respondents than most of the other dietary assessment methods. It is often used by epidemiologists studying associations between dietary habits (both usual and past) and disease (Acheson and Doll, 1964; Hankin et al., 1970; Hirayama, 1981), although its use for estimating food intakes in the remote past has not been clearly established (Byers et al., 1983; van Staveren et al., 1986). Food frequency

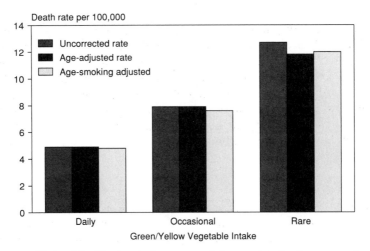

Figure 3.1: Death rate for cancer of the prostate by frequency of green-yellow vegetable intake. Redrawn from Hirayama (1981) by permission of Lawrence Erlbaum Associates Inc.

questionnaires can also be used in combination with more quantitative methods, providing additional or confirmatory data.

The data from a food frequency questionnaire are often used to rank subjects into broad categories of low, medium, and high intakes of certain foods, based on tertiles, for example. In epidemiological studies, such rankings are often compared with the prevalence and/or mortality statistics for a specific disease within the population studied. The example given in Figure 3.1 demonstrates an association between the death rate for cancer of the prostate and the frequency of consumption of green-yellow vegetables (Hirayama, 1981). Such data are very preliminary and only provide a guide for more extensive investigations. For example, several dietary components may be associated with the relationship presented in Figure 3.1, including dietary fiber, β-carotene, or vitamin C (Hunt, 1984).

Food scores can be calculated from food frequency data, based on the frequency of consumption of certain food groups. Canada's Food Guide (Health and Welfare Canada, 1983), or an equivalent standard, listing the optimum number of servings of the major food groups per person per day, can be used as a basis for the scores (Guthrie and Scheer, 1981). The scores can then be examined in relation to psychosocial influences (e.g. level of education, income), as well as vital statistics, season, geographic distribution, etc. An example of a 16-point dietary scoring system is given in Table 3.3.

Comparisons of the dietary patterns of different ethnic groups can also be made using a food scoring system. Figure 3.2 shows the percentage distribution of scores corresponding to the frequency of intakes of dairy

Food Group	Points per Serving	Maximum Possible Food Group Score
Milk and milk products (up to a maximum of 2)	2	4
Meat and meat alternatives [a] (up to a maximum of 2)	2	4
Fruit and vegetables (up to a maximum of 4)	1	4
Bread and cereals [b] (up to a maximum of 4)	1	4
Maximum total score		16

[a] Includes animal protein foods, legumes, and nuts.
[b] Includes enriched and whole grains.

Table 3.3: Sixteen-point dietary scoring system based on the U.S. four basic food groups. Adapted from Guthrie HA and Scheer JC. Validity of a dietary score for assessing nutrient adequacy. © The American Dietetic Association. Reproduced by permission from Journal of the American Dietetic Association, Vol. 78: 240–245, 1981.

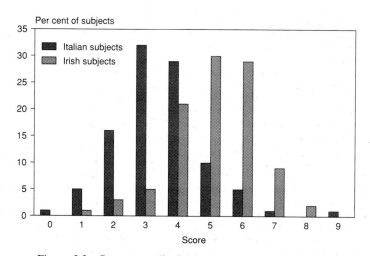

Figure 3.2: Percentage distribution of scores for dairy foods of 107 Irish and 145 Italian diets. Maximum possible score is nine. Categories recorded were: milk as beverage, cream, cereal milk, ice cream, butter in sandwiches, butter on bread, cheese in sandwiches, coffee milk, tea milk. From Stefanik and Trulson (1962). © Am. J. Clin. Nutr. American Society for Clinical Nutrition.

Food	Medium Serving	Serving			How Often?				
		S	M	L	D	W	M	Y	N
Apples, apple sauce, pears	(1) or 1/2 cup								
Bananas	1 medium								
Peaches, apricots (canned)	(1) or 1/2 cup								
Peaches, apricots (fresh)	1 medium								
Cantaloupe melon	1/4 medium								
Watermelon	1 slice								
Strawberries	1/2 cup								
Oranges	1 medium								
Orange juice	6-oz glass								
Grapefruit or grapefruit juice	1/2 or 6-oz glass								
etc.									

Table 3.4: An example of part of the self-administered semiquantitative food frequency questionnaire. Abbreviations: S M L = small, medium, and large relative to the medium serving; D W M Y N = daily, weekly, monthly, yearly, and never. Modified from Block G, Hartman AM, Dresser CM, Carroll MD, Gannon J, Gardner L. A data-based approach to diet questionnaire design and testing. American Journal of Epidemiology 124: 453–469, 1986.

foods in two groups of Americans of Irish and Italian origin (Stefanik and Trulson, 1962).

Sometimes, the food frequency questionnaire attempts to quantify usual portion sizes of the food items of interest, with or without the use of food models or photographs (Epstein et al., 1970; Jain et al., 1982).

This modification produces semiquantitative food frequency data. If this semiquantitative procedure is used, nutrient scores of each subject can be computed by multiplying the relative frequency that each food item is consumed (with, for example, once a day equal to one), by the nutrient content of the average portion size specified. The nutrient content is obtained from appropriate food composition data (Russel-Briefel et al., 1985).

Some investigators have used food records to calculate the weights of average portions of foods and derive a multiple regression equation to predict nutrient intake. With such information, only those foods in the multiple regression equation are included in any subsequent food frequency questionnaires (Hankin et al., 1970). A modification of this approach was adopted by Block et al. (1986) to derive a food list with portion sizes from the NHANES II dietary survey. Food items selected contributed significantly to the total population intake of energy and each of 17 nutrients. Portion sizes were estimated from observed portion size distributions in the NHANES II data. Medium serving sizes for each food were specified and the respondent indicated on the food frequency questionnaire whether his or her usual serving size was small, medium, or large (Table 3.4). A specialized food composition database was developed for use with this food frequency questionnaire, based on the frequency of consumption of specific food items from the NHANES II survey.

3.2 New developments in measuring food consumption

3.2.1 Telephone

In an extensive telephone-administered survey of low-income elderly persons, using a twenty-four-hour recall method (Posner et al., 1982), food portion size was estimated with the aid of two-dimensional food portion visual aids, which had been mailed to respondents. The telephone interviewing in this study was done by trained interviewers who were not nutritionists. Estimates of the mean intake and distributions of energy and eight nutrients were obtained.

Four telephone-assisted approaches were used to measure food consumed by college students in a dormitory dining hall cafeteria (Krantzler et al., 1982). For two of the variations, college students reported six-hour or twenty-four-hour recalls of food consumption by telephone to an interviewer. For the other two approaches, students telephoned results of written food records to either an interviewer or a recording device. Actual food consumption of the subjects was determined surreptitiously in the cafeteria, to validate the telephoned recall and record data. Results suggested that both twenty-four-hour telephone recall and seven-day telephoned food records are feasible and warrant further investigation.

3.2.2 Photographs

Elwood and Bird (1983) instructed subjects to photograph, at a specified distance and angle, all food items and leftovers, and to record descriptions of each foodstuff, including the method of preparation. Estimates of the weights of the food items consumed were obtained by viewing the photographs alongside previously prepared standard photographs of portions of foodstuffs of known weights.

The photographic method appears to be less demanding for the subject than the weighed record, and relatively easy and acceptable. Preliminary work suggests that nutrient intakes calculated from photographs and a weighed record are similar, provided that training for estimating weights from photographs is given (Bird and Elwood, 1983).

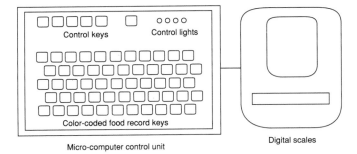

Figure 3.3: Diagram of a food-recording electronic device. Modified from Stockley et al. (1986a) with permission.

3.2.3 Electronic devices for recording food intakes

An electronic device has been developed by Stockley et al. (1986a; 1986b) for the quantitative collection of food intake data for individuals for periods of up to three weeks. The device consists of a digital balance with a capacity of 1 kg interfaced to a microcomputer with a keyboard (Figure 3.3). The latter has an upper bank of color-coded sequence control keys which register 'start', 'waste', 'no waste', 'mixed waste', and 'done' and 55 color-coded food record keys. The keyboard is fitted with a removable transparent keyboard overlay, to assist in the correct identification of the food keys. An incorrect food key entry can be cancelled using the 'error' function. The device is fully compatible with a more powerful computer. Consequently, at the end of the study period, the accumulated data on the weights and types of food consumed and time of consumption can be transferred to a host computer for calculation of the nutrient composition of the diet. The respondent burden is reduced when using the food-recording device because the subject does not have to read the balance or keep a written diary (Stockley et al., 1986b). Moreover, the memory capacity of the device is sufficient to store dietary data from surveys lasting up to three weeks. The device also eliminates the process of coding the food records, a task considered to be the most time-consuming part of a quantitative dietary study (Black, 1982).

A portable electronic set of tape-recording scales (PETRA) has been developed in the United Kingdom (Cherlyn Electronics, Cambridge, England). In this system, the respondent places an empty plate onto the PETRA digital recording scale, presses a switch in front of the machine, and describes the plate. The scale simultaneously records the spoken words and the weight in digitally coded form. The respondent then adds each food item separately onto the plate and, at the same time, dictates a description of the food into the microphone. At the end of the study, tapes are retrieved and read by the investigator using the PETRA Master Console. The latter plays back the description of the food and displays the decoded weight information. The system is simple to operate, and it

Desired Information	Preferred Approach
Actual nutrient intake over finite time period (e.g. in a balance study)	Chemical analysis of duplicate meals *or* calculated intake from weighed records
Estimate of 'usual' nutrient intake in free-living subjects Group average Proportion of the population 'at risk' Individual intake, for correlation or regression analysis	 One day intake with large number of subjects and adequate representation of days of week Replicate observations of intake *or* diet history Multiple replicate observations on each individual
Group or individual pattern of food use, proportion of population with particular pattern	Food frequency questionnaire
Average use of a particular food or food group for a group	Food frequency questionnaire *or* a one-day intake with large number of subjects and adequate representation of days of the week

Table 3.5: Selection of methodology to estimate either the usual nutrient intake or the pattern of food use of 'free-living' subjects. Modified after Beaton (1982) with permission.

is difficult for the subject to modify the coded food record. Consequently, the habitual food intake is more likely to be truthfully recorded compared to the conventional weighed food record (Bingham, 1987).

3.3 Selecting an appropriate method

There is no ideal method for assessing food or nutrient intakes, the choice depending primarily on the objectives of the study. None of the current methods are devoid of systematic errors (Chapter 5), or prevent alterations in the food habits of the subjects. Table 3.5 summarizes the most appropriate methods for assessing food or nutrient intakes in relation to the study objectives.

Actual nutrient intake of individuals

The actual nutrient intakes of an individual over a specified time period should be assessed using weighed food records (Section 3.1.4), completed for the duration of the time period. Nutrient intakes can then be calculated using food composition data. Alternatively, duplicate meals can be collected throughout the period for later chemical analysis (Section 4.5). Such data may be required for experimentally controlled studies.

Average usual nutrient intakes of a group

The average usual nutrient intakes of a large population group can be estimated by a single twenty-four-hour recall, or a single weighed or estimated food record, provided that in the design, all the days of the week are equally represented and the subjects are representative of the population under study. The size of the group necessary to characterize the average usual nutrient intake depends on the degree of precision required, and the day-to-day variation in the nutrient intakes (Anderson, 1986; NRC, 1986). Data on average usual nutrient intakes of a group can be used for international comparisons of the relationship of nutrient intakes to health and disease.

The proportion of the population 'at risk'

To determine the proportion of the population 'at risk' to inadequate intakes, the food consumption of each subject must be measured over more than one day. Hence, repeated twenty-four-hour recalls, or replicate weighed or estimated one-day food records are appropriate. The number of days included depends on the day-to-day variation of the nutrients of interest. Alternatively, a dietary history designed to obtain retrospective information on intakes over a longer period may be used. Data on the distribution of usual nutrient intakes of a population are essential for national food policy development and food fortification planning. Food patterns associated with inadequate nutrient intakes can also be identified using this approach, enabling food assistance programs to be designed and improvements in nutrition education to be made.

Usual nutrient intakes of individuals

Estimates of the usual nutrient intakes of individuals necessitate multiple replicates of daily food intake measurements on each individual, using either twenty-four-hour recalls or estimated or weighed food records. Again, the number of measurement days depends on the day-to-day variation of the nutrients of interest. Such data are essential for diet counselling and statistical analysis involving correlation or regression; they are the most difficult to collect (Beaton, 1982; Callmer et al., 1985).

Pattern of food use for a group and/or individual

The best method of assessing the pattern of food use for a group and/or individual involves using a food frequency questionnaire. The data for a group can be ranked into broad categories of low, medium, and high frequency of food use to assess the proportion of the population with a particular pattern of food use. Ranking is particularly useful in epidemiological studies for comparison with the prevalence and/or mortality statistics for a specific disease.

Average use of specified foods for a group

In population groups it is possible to estimate the average use of specified foods by means of a food frequency questionnaire. Alternatively, a twenty-four-hour recall or one-day food record can be used, as long as a large number of subjects are used and all the days of the week are adequately represented. Such data can be used for international comparisons of the relationship of patterns of food use to health and susceptibility to chronic disease, as discussed earlier.

Additional factors which should be considered when choosing a method for assessing the food consumption of individuals are the characteristics of the subjects within the study population, the respondent burden of the method, and the available resources. For instance, certain methods are unsuitable for elderly subjects with poor memories, for busy mothers with young children, or for illiterate subjects. Other methods require highly trained personnel and specialized laboratory and computing facilities, which may not be available. Generally, the more accurate methods are associated with higher costs, greater respondent burden, and lower response rates. Unfortunately, compromises often have to be made between the collection of precise data on usual nutrient intakes of individuals and a high response rate.

3.4 Summary

Details of the available methods for assessing food consumption of individuals, and their uses and limitations, are summarized in Table 3.6.

To characterize the average usual intake of a large group, a twenty-four-hour recall or one-day food record is appropriate, provided the sample is representative of the population under study, and all days of the week are equally represented. Depending on the number of measurement days, repeated twenty-four-hour recalls, or replicate weighed or estimated food records can also used to determine actual or usual nutrient intakes of an individual. The number, spacing, and days selected for the measurements depends on the day-to-day and, in some cases, on the seasonal variation in food consumption. The dietary history and the food frequency questionnaire can be used to assess usual food consumption patterns over a relatively long time period. With certain modifications, they can also be used to provide an estimate of usual intakes of nutrients.

New developments for measuring food consumption of individuals include telephone-assisted approaches, use of photographs to record both food items consumed and leftovers, and electronic devices for recording food intakes directly. All these developments aim to reduce respondent burden and hence increase compliance, reduce errors resulting from memory lapses, and in the case of electronic devices, to eliminate the tedious process of coding the food records.

Method and Procedures	Uses and Limitations
Twenty-four-hour Recall. Subject or caretaker recalls food intake of previous twenty-four hours in an interview. Quantities estimated in household measures using food models as memory aids and/or to assist in quantifying portion sizes. Nutrient intakes calculated using food composition data.	Useful for assessing average *usual* intakes of a large population, provided that the sample is truly representative and that the days of the week are adequately represented. Used for international comparisons of relationship of nutrient intakes to health and susceptibility to chronic disease. Inexpensive, easy, quick, with low respondent burden so that compliance is high. Large coverage possible; can be used with illiterate individuals. Element of surprise so less likely to modify eating pattern. Single twenty-four-hour recalls likely to omit foods consumed infrequently. Relies on memory and hence unsatisfactory for the elderly and young children. Multiple replicate twenty-four-hour recalls used to estimate *usual* intakes of individuals.
Estimated Food Record. Record of all food and beverages as eaten (including snacks), over periods from one to seven days. Quantities estimated in household measures. Nutrient intakes calculated using food composition data.	Used to assess *actual* or *usual* intakes of individuals, depending on number of measurement days. Data on *usual* intakes used for diet counselling and statistical analysis involving correlation and regression. Accuracy depends on conscientiousness of subject and ability to estimate quantities. Longer time frames result in a higher respondent burden and a lower co-operation. Subjects must be literate.
Weighed Food Record. All food consumed over defined period is weighed by the subject, caretaker, or assistant. Food samples may be saved individually, or as a composite, for nutrient analysis. Alternatively nutrient intakes calculated from food composition data.	Used to assess *actual* or *usual* intakes of individuals, depending on the number of measurement days. Accurate but time consuming. Condition must allow weighing. Subjects may change their usual eating pattern to simplify weighing or to impress investigator. Requires literate, motivated, and willing participants. Expensive.
Dietary History. Interview method consisting of a twenty-four-hour recall of *actual* intake, plus information on overall *usual* eating pattern, followed by a food frequency questionnaire to verify and clarify initial data. Usual portion sizes recorded in household measures. Nutrient intakes calculated using food composition data.	Used to describe *usual* food and/or nutrient intakes over a relatively long time period which can be used to estimate prevalence of inadequate intakes. Such information used for national food policy development, food fortification planning, and to identify food patterns associated with inadequate intakes. Labor intensive, time consuming and results depend on skill of interviewer.
Food Frequency Questionnaire. Uses comprehensive list or list of specific food items to record intakes over a given period (day, week, month, year). Record is obtained by interview, or self-administered questionnaire. Questionnaire can be semiquantitative when subjects asked to quantify usual portion sizes of food items, with or without the use of food models.	Designed to obtain qualitative, descriptive data on *usual* intakes of foods or classes of foods over a long time period. Useful in epidemiological studies for ranking subjects into broad categories of low, medium, and high intakes of specific foods, food components or nutrients, for comparison with the prevalence and/or mortality statistics of a specific disease. Can also identify food patterns associated with inadequate intakes of specific nutrients. Method is rapid with low respondent burden and high response rate but accuracy is lower than other methods.

Table 3.6: Uses and limitations of commonly used methods to assess the food consumption of individuals.

References

Acheson ED, Doll R. (1964). Dietary factors in carcinoma of the stomach: A study of 100 cases and 200 controls. Gut 5: 126–131.

Acheson KJ, Campbell IT, Edholm OG, Miller DS, Stock MJ. (1980). The measurement of food and energy intake in man — an evaluation of some techniques. American Journal of Clinical Nutrition 33: 1147–1154.

Anderson SA. (1986). Guidelines for Use of Dietary Intake Data. Life Sciences Research Office, Federation of American Societies for Experimental Biology, Bethesda, Maryland.

Beaton GH. (1982). What do we think we are measuring? In: Symposium on Dietary Data Collection, Analysis, and Significance. Massachusetts Agricultural Experimental Station, College of Food and Natural Resources, University of Massachusetts at Amherst, Research Bulletin No. 675, pp. 36–48.

Bingham SA. (1987). The dietary assessment of individuals; methods, accuracy, new techniques and recommendations. Nutrition Abstracts and Reviews (Series A) 57: 705–742.

Bird G, Elwood PC. (1983). The dietary intakes of subjects estimated from photographs compared with a weighed record. Human Nutrition: Applied Nutrition 37A: 470–473.

Black AE. (1982). The logistics of dietary surveys. Human Nutrition: Applied Nutrition 36A: 85–94.

Block G, Hartman AM, Dresser CM, Carroll MD, Gannon J, Gardner L. (1986). A data-based approach to diet questionnaire design and testing. American Journal of Epidemiology 124: 453–469.

Burk MC, Pao EM. (1976). Methodology for large-scale surveys of household and individual diets. Home Economics Research Report No. 40. Agriculture Research Service, U.S. Department of Agriculture, Washington, D.C.

Burke BS. (1947). The dietary history as a tool in research. Journal of the American Dietetic Association 23: 1041–1046.

Byers TE, Rosenthal RI, Marshall JR, Rzepka TF, Cummings KM, Graham S. (1983). Dietary history from the distant past: a methodological study. Nutrition and Cancer 5: 69–77.

Callmer E, Haraldsdottir J, Løker EB, Seppänen R, Solvoll K. (1985). Selecting a method for a dietary survey. Näringsforskning 2: 43–52.

Elwood PC, Bird G. (1983). A photographic method of diet evaluation. Human Nutrition: Applied Nutrition 37A: 474–477.

Epstein IM, Reshef A, Abrahamson JH, Bialik O. (1970). Validity of a short dietary questionnaire. Israel Journal of Medical Sciences 6: 589–597.

Food and Nutrition Board, National Research Council (1981). The proposed system. In: Assessing Changing Food Consumption Patterns. Committee on Food Consumption Patterns, Food and Nutrition Board, National Research Council. National Academy Press, Washington, D.C., pp. 13–18.

Gersovitz M, Madden JP, Smiciklas-Wright H. (1978). Validity of the 24-hr dietary recall and seven-day record for group comparisons. Journal of the American Dietetic Association 73: 48–55.

Guthrie HA, Scheer JC. (1981). Validity of a dietary score for assessing nutrient adequacy. Journal of the American Dietetic Association 78: 240–245.

Hankin JH, Messinger HB, Stallones RA. (1970). A short dietary method for epidemiological studies. IV: Evaluation of questionnaire. American Journal of Epidemiology 91: 562–567.

Health and Welfare Canada (1973). Nutrition Canada National Survey. Health and Welfare, Ottawa.

Health and Welfare Canada (1983). Canada's Food Guide Handbook (revised). Health Promotion Directorate, Health and Welfare, Ottawa.

Hirayama T. (1981). Diet and cancer. Nutrition and Cancer 1: 67–81.

Hughes BA. (1986). Nutrition interviewing and counselling in public health: the North Carolina experience. Topics in Clinical Nutrition 1: 43–50.

Hunt R. (1984). Questionnaires In: The Dietary Assessment of Populations. Medical Research Council Scientific Report No. 4: 9–13.

Jain MG, Harrison L, Howe GR, Miller AB. (1982). Evaluation of a self-administered dietary questionnaire for use in a cohort study. American Journal of Clinical Nutrition 36: 931–935.

Krantzler NJ, Mullen BJ, Schutz HG, Grivetti LE, Holden CA, Meiselman HL. (1982). Validity of telephoned diet recalls and records for assessment of individual food intake. American Journal of Clinical Nutrition 36: 1234–1242.

Marr JW. (1971). Individual dietary surveys: purposes and methods. World Reviews of Nutrition and Dietetics 13: 105–164.

NRC (National Research Council) (1986). Nutrient Adequacy: Assessment using Food Consumption Surveys. Subcommittee on Criteria for Dietary Evaluation, Coordinating Committee on Evaluation of Food Consumption Surveys. Food and Nutrition Board, Commission on Life Sciences. National Academy Press, Washington, D.C.

Pekkarinen M. (1970). Methodology in the collection of food consumption data. World Review of Nutrition and Dietetics 12: 145–171.

Posner BM, Borman CL, Morgan JL, Borden WS, Ohls JC. (1982). The validity of a telephone-administered 24-hr dietary recall methodology. American Journal of Clinical Nutrition 36: 546–553.

Russel-Briefel R, Caggiula AW, Kuller LH. (1985). A comparison of three dietary methods for estimating vitamin-A intake. American Journal of Epidemiology 122: 628–638.

Sanjur D. (1982). Food consumption survey: issues concerning the process of data collection. In: Social and Cultural Perspectives in Nutrition. Prentice-Hall Inc., Englewood Cliffs, New Jersey. pp. 169–194.

Staveren WA van, de Boer JO, Burema J. (1985). Validity and reproducibility of dietary history method estimating the usual food intake during one month. American Journal of Clinical Nutrition 42: 554–559.

Staveren WA van, West CE, Hoffmans MDAF, Bos P, Kardinaal AFM, Poppel GAFC van, Schipper HJ-A, Hautvast JGAJ, Hayes RB. (1986). Comparison of contemporaneous and retrospective estimates of food consumption made by a dietary history method. American Journal of Epidemiology 123: 884–893.

Stefanik PA, Trulson MF. (1962). Determining the frequency of intakes of foods in large group studies. American Journal of Clinical Nutrition 11: 335–343.

Stockley L, Chapman RI, Holley ML, Jones FA, Prescott EHA, Broadhurst AJ. (1986a). Description of a food recording electronic device for use in dietary surveys. Human Nutrition: Applied Nutrition 40A: 13–18.

Stockley L, Hurren CA, Chapman RI, Broadhurst AJ, Jones FA. (1986b). Energy, protein, and fat intake estimated using a food recording electronic device compared with a weighed diary. Human Nutrition: Applied Nutrition 40A: 19–23.

Weiner JS, Lourie JA. (1969). Human Biology: A Guide to Field Methods. International Biological Programme. IBP Handbook No. 9. Blackwell Scientific Publications, Oxford–Edinburgh.

Young CM. (1981). Dietary methodology. In: Assessing Changing Food Consumption Patterns. Committee on Food Consumption Patterns, Food and Nutrition Board, National Research Council. National Academy Press, Washington, D.C., pp. 89–118.

Chapter 4

Assessment of nutrient intakes from food consumption data

It is possible to calculate the nutrient intakes of individuals or population groups if quantitative methods have been used to collect the relevant food consumption data. Food composition values, representative of the average composition of a particular foodstuff on a year-round nationwide basis, are generally used for the calculation. The values are available as food composition tables, or from nutrient databases stored on a computer. This chapter discusses the uncertainties involved in this procedure and the associated assessment of the nutrient intakes of individuals and/or population groups.

Recognition of the potential sources of errors in the food composition values is important, as these errors affect the calculation of nutrient intakes whether food composition tables or nutrient databases are used. The errors may result from true random variability in the nutrient content of a food, or alternatively, the errors may be systematic. The extent of both random and systematic errors depends on the food item and the nutrient; systematic errors may produce consistent under- or overestimates of the nutrient content of individual food items, although the direction and magnitude of the error is often unknown (NRC, 1986).

In some instances, chemical analysis of individual food items or composite diets may be necessary to determine energy and nutrient intakes. This method is very time consuming and expensive, and consequently, it is generally used when precise information on nutrient intakes of individuals is required for metabolic studies, or when food composition values for specific nutrients are incomplete or nonexistent. Chemical analysis can also be used to validate nutrient intakes calculated from food composition tables or nutrient databases.

Food composition values generally indicate the total amount of the constituent in the food, rather than the amount absorbed. This is because the availability of most nutrients in individual food items has not been assessed. Hence intakes of most nutrients, calculated from

8-1 Dairy and egg products	8-13 Beef products
8-2 Spices and herbs	8-14 Beverages
8-3 Baby foods	8-15 Fish and shellfish
8-4 Fats and oils	8-16 Legumes
8-5 Poultry products	8-17 Lamb, veal, and game
8-6 Soups, sauces, and gravies	8-18 Bakery products
8-7 Sausages and luncheon meats	8-19 Sugars and sweets
8-8 Breakfast cereals	8-20 Cereal grains, flours, and pasta
8-9 Fruits and fruit juices	8-21 Fast foods
8-10 Pork and pork products	8-22 Mixed dishes
8-11 Vegetables and vegetable products	8-23 Miscellaneous foods
8-12 Nut and seed products	

Table 4.1: Major food groups of the revised USDA Handbook No. 8. Modified from Hepburn (1982). © Am. J. Clin. Nutr. American Society for Clinical Nutrition.

food consumption data, represent the maximum available to the body, and consequently, when nutrient intake data are evaluated, the potential bioavailability of the nutrients from the diets must always be considered.

4.1   Use of food composition tables

Nutrient values in food composition tables are based on a quantitative analysis of samples of each food. The data should be representative of the average composition of a particular foodstuff on a year-round, nationwide basis. Values can be expressed in terms of the nutrient content of the edible portion of the food per hundred grams and/or per common household measures. In some cases the tables also provide data on the nutrient content of edible portion of the food 'as purchased' (Watt et al., 1963). In some food composition tables, other items related to food composition such as dietary fiber, pH, and total solids are also included. The revisions of the USDA Handbook No. 8 contain, for most foods, values for nine minerals, eight vitamins, cholesterol, amino acids, fatty acids, some food constituents, and selected values for dietary fiber (USDA, 1976–87; Hepburn, 1982). The completed printed revisions of the USDA Handbook No. 8 will consist of over twenty food group sections, published separately, as well as sections on mixed dishes, fast foods, and miscellaneous items. These are listed in Table 4.1.

Only some food composition tables provide data on the number of samples used to derive the average energy or nutrient value, and a statistical parameter to describe the observed variation (e.g. USDA, 1976–1987). The mean, the number of observations, and the standard deviation or standard error should be given, provided that the distribution is not skewed (Southgate, 1974). The standard error is a measure of the variability of the mean nutrient value for a specific food item. It can be used to estimate the error resulting from the use of the average value for the nutrient content of a specific food, but does not differentiate between errors associated with sampling and/or methodology. The coefficient of variation (CV% = 100% × SD / mean), on the other hand, expresses the variability of the nutrient content in relation to the mean. As such, it can be used for comparing errors in estimating nutrient content between several foods, and subsequently for evaluating their effect on the estimates of nutrient intake (NRC, 1986).

For some countries (e.g. Cuba), the values for local foods in the composition tables are taken exclusively from tables of other countries. In contrast, Ethiopia, West Africa, and Zambia have food composition tables compiled predominantly from analyses of locally grown foods, although both the number of nutrients and samples analyzed for any one food are often small, and only the most common foods are included. Sometimes gaps in the local analytical data are filled by using values from other food tables (Périssé, 1982).

The Canadian (Health and Welfare Canada, 1988) and United States (USDA, 1976–1987) food composition tables, and some other regional tables are based on a compilation of food composition data from a variety of sources. For instance, for the United States, the most important sources of food composition data in recent years have been the food industry, published research, United States Department of Agriculture laboratories and contract research (Rizek et al., 1981). The Canadian food composition table entitled 'Nutrient Values of Some Common Foods' (Health and Welfare Canada, 1988) is based on the revised sections of the USDA Handbook No. 8 with certain adjustments for Canadian use (Verdier, 1987). In the United Kingdom, almost all the analyses for the fourth edition of McCance and Widdowson's 'The Composition of Foods' (Paul and Southgate, 1978) were undertaken at the laboratory of the Government Chemist. Since the preparation of the 1978 U.K. food composition tables, additional information has been published in scientific journals and as supplements to the tables, such as fractions of dietary fiber (e.g. noncellulosic polysaccharides, cellulose, and lignin) in selected foods (Paul and Southgate, 1979; Holland et al., 1988), individual free sugars (Southgate et al., 1978), details of the vitamin C content of several canned fruits and vegetables (Black et al., 1983), sampling details for meat (Paul and Southgate, 1977), nutrient composition of human milk (Department of Health and Social Security, 1977), and a supplement of the amino acid and fatty acid content of foods per 100 g (Paul et al., 1980). Food composition data for several trace elements (e.g. selenium, iodine, copper, zinc, fluoride, and chromium) (Thorn et al., 1978; Wenlock et al., 1979, 1982; Ministry of Agriculture, Fisheries and Food, 1981; Walters et al., 1983; Smart and Sherlock, 1985) and for immigrant foods (Tan et al., 1985) have also been published. New supplements are planned to update the food composition data for milk and milk products, potatoes, and folic acid (Paul et al., 1986).

4.2   Use of nutrient data banks

Nutrient data banks or computer-stored nutrient databases are food composition tables transferred to, and maintained on, a computer. Such data banks may be revised and updated readily.   They vary in size, comprehensiveness, currentness, the units used to express portion size and nutrient content, and in the source of the nutrient values (Butrum et al., 1976; Hoover and Pelican, 1984).   Food items in the nutrient data banks are usually identified by a numerical coding system, which varies in complexity.   Many commercially produced nutrient databases are available.   Some of the critical factors to be considered when selecting a database are the source of the information, the size and comprehensiveness of the database in relation to range of foods required, the number of nutrients listed, and the methods used to indicate missing and/or imputed data.   The competence of those involved with the database development, management, and documentation should also be considered (Hoover and Pelican, 1984).

The U.S. Nutrient Data Bank (USNDB) is one of the most comprehensive nutrient data banks available. It is maintained by the Nutrient Data Research Group of the USDA's Consumer Nutrition Center (Rizek et al., 1981).   Data from the revised editions of the USDA Handbook No. 8 (1976–1987) are included as they are released. Unlike the printed handbooks, blank spaces in the nutrient data bank have been filled where possible with imputed values (Hepburn, 1982). All the data submitted to the USNDB are carefully screened to ensure that the food is accurately identified and any conditions which may affect its nutritive value, such as sampling, treatment, processing, and method of nutrient analysis, are known.   The food identification code used by the USNDB is divided into two parts.   The first part of the code includes four levels to describe the food group (Table 4.1), major and minor food subgroups, and finally the individual food.   The second part describes the food in more detail and consists of qualifying terms (Table 4.2). These provide information on preserving technique, storage condition, etc.

The Bureau of Nutritional Sciences of Health and Welfare Canada produced the first issue of a national computerized nutrient database in 1981 (Health and Welfare Canada, 1982).   This contains data derived primarily from the revised sections of the USDA Handbook No. 8.   Some data based on chemical analysis of Canadian foods (e.g. meat) (Wood et al., 1988) and food products are also included. Certain adjustments have been made to some of the U.S. data to account for differences in the cuts of meats, their fat-to-lean ratio, and Canadian enrichment practices.   Portion sizes are reported in metric measurements (Verdier, 1987).   The nutrient database is revised

A.	Treatment applied
B.	Preserving technique
C.	Processing technique
D.	Cooking method
E.	Physical state
F.	Portion analyzed
G.	Packaging and storage conditions
H.	Grade, quality, appearance, size, and color
I.	Maturity and conditions of growth and production
J.	Special descriptors
L.	Category of varietal type
N–R.	Components of mixed dishes

Table 4.2: Categories of qualifying terms used in the U.S. Department of Agriculture Nutrient Data Bank.

annually. A computerized but abbreviated nutrient database, corresponding to the 1988 revision of the Canadian 'Nutrient Value of Some Common Foods' (Health and Welfare Canada, 1988), is also available.

A Canadian Hospital Nutrient Data Bank has been developed by Bell et al. (1979) at the Hospital for Sick Children in Toronto. The data bank is used for calculating nutrient intakes and diet counselling. The data bank was compiled from information on 2800 foods derived from the USDA Handbook No. 8, more than 600 commercial food products, and 360 recipes. For each food, values for 19 nutrients and 6 non-nutrients are included.

Certain food industries in the United States and Canada maintain their own nutrient data banks which contain data on their own products. They are used for product and recipe development, research, nutritional labelling, and quality control.

Several investigators have compared energy and nutrient values obtained from the same set of food records, using different computerized nutrient database systems but the same calculation procedures (Table 4.3) (Taylor et al., 1985). Results of these studies have emphasized the necessity for using a standardized model to check the quality of databases. Hoover and Perloff (1981) have developed such a diagnostic model. Included in the model are computing tasks to revalidate a nutrient database after updating; to validate recipe calculation procedures by calculating the nutrient content of a standard recipe; and to validate program computation using a reference dietary record.

Computer programs can also be used to compare all the nutrient values of the test nutrient database with corresponding values in the reference standard. Large discrepancies can be flagged. The validity of the computer program for calculating nutrient intakes can also be checked

Component	Database A Mean	Database A Range	Database B Mean	Database B Range	Database C Mean	Database C Range	Sig. of F
Energy (kcal)	1706	586–3771	1660	657–3520	1680	704–3802	ns
Protein (g)	75	24–268	72	24–187	74	30–233	ns
Fat (g)	72	9–145	70	20–152	73	15–154	ns
Carbohyd. (g)	195	59–371	191	69–352	187	62–381	ns
Calcium (mg)	1088	190–3026	966	206–1805	1023	154–2186	ns
Phosph. (mg)	1393	254–3481	1277	252–2217	1301	349–3204	ns
Iron (mg)	10.9	4.6–34.6	14.2	3.9–46.5	9.7	5.5–32.8	0.01
Vit. A (IU)	6040	604–17031	5890	750–17128	5052	585–17094	0.02
Thiamin (mg)	1.4	0.5–5.2	1.2	0.5–2.6	1.0	0.5–3.2	0.02
Riboflavin (mg)	2.2	0.4–4.6	1.9	0.5–3.4	1.8	0.4–3.8	0.01
Niacin (mg)	15.7	4.2–50.6	15.7	3.9–32.9	13.0	1.2–45.0	ns
Vit. C (mg)	89	0–228	103	0–229	93	1–215	0.02
Folic acid (μg)	184	54–438	202	54–409	143	27–280	0.01
Vit. E (mg)	6.6	0.8–45.0	8.3	0.3–47.5	4.9	1.4–11.1	ns
Vit. B-6 (mg)	1.1	0.1–3.17	1.3	0.4–3.1	1.2	0.4–4.5	0.03
Vit. B-12 (μg)	3.5	0–10.5	4.7	0.6–13.9	4.6	0.4–16.5	ns
Magnesium (mg)	237	14–494	253	83–482	243	71–579	ns
Vit. D (IU)	258	0–896	190	0–746	273	2–729	0.04
Zinc (mg)	6.6	1.9–18.7	10.7	3.7–30.3	9.7	4.4–34.8	< 0.001

Table 4.3: Energy and nutrient values derived by analysis of 24 uniformly coded records using three different computerized nutrient databases. From Taylor ML, Kozlowski BW, Baer MT. Energy and nutrient values from different computerized databases. © The American Dietetic Association. Reproduced by permission from Journal of the American Dietetic Association, Vol. 85: 1136–1138, 1985.

by comparing results with those based on hand calculation of nutrient intakes.

4.3 Sources of error in food composition values

Errors in food composition data included in food composition tables and nutrient databases may be random or systematic. All such errors, however, generate additional uncertainty in calculated nutrient intakes. The sources of error are considered in detail and summarized in Table 4.4.

4.3.1 Inadequate sampling protocols

When nutrient values for specific foods are required for a food composition table or nutrient data bank, protocols must be designed which will result in the collection of representative food samples for analysis. The protocol should take into account, where appropriate, such factors as seasonal and regional differences in the composition of the food, genetic

- Inadequate sampling protocols resulting in data for unrepresentative food samples being included in the food composition tables and/or nutrient databases;
- the use of inappropriate analytical methods for the analysis of the nutrients for the food composition data;
- errors in the analytical methods used in the analysis of the nutrients for the food composition data;
- the lack of standardized conversion factors for calculating energy and protein content of foods included in the food composition tables and/or nutrient databases;
- inconsistencies in terminology used to express certain nutrients;
- incorrect description of individual food items and/or source of nutrient values in food composition tables;
- inconsistencies resulting from genetic, environmental, food preparation, and processing factors.

Table 4.4: Sources of error in food composition tables.

variation, stage of ripeness, handling and storage procedures, variations resulting from the effects of fertilizer application, pest control, method of food preparation, processing, and production practices (Southgate, 1974; NRC, 1986). In this way, random errors resulting from true variability in the nutrient composition of individual food items can be eliminated. When standardized sampling protocols are not used, nutrient composition values may not reflect the average nutrient content of a food on a year-round, nationwide basis.

Systematic bias may also occur in some food composition data, particularly with nutrient-fortified, processed, and manufactured foods. In foods such as vitamin-C fortified fruit juices, for example, wide variations in vitamin C content occur. Hence, brand-specific nutrient composition data should be used for these food items, to prevent systematic bias.

4.3.2 Inappropriate analytical methods

Different analytical methods have been used for assaying nutrients during the compilation of food composition data tables. Some of these methods are very unsatisfactory, resulting in some cases in erroneous estimates of the nutrient content. The United States National Research Council (NRC, 1986) has summarized the state of development of nutrient analytical methods in foods. Methodologies for nutrients such as folacin, carotenoids, vitamin B-12, vitamin A, and vitamin C were classified as unsatisfactory, requiring further method development.

Certain new methods of nutrient analysis use high-performance liquid chromatography (HPLC) to separate and quantify the individual active and potentially active forms of the fat-soluble vitamins A, D, and E. Older procedures often underestimate the vitamin A content of the food because not all the active forms of this vitamin, or its precursors, are included in the analysis (Cooke, 1983). For instance, although there are approximately fifty carotenoids with vitamin A activity, current assay techniques cannot determine all the carotenoids in foods.

Microbiological assay techniques are frequently used for analysis of the B vitamins in foods. These are based on the use of a micro-organism which requires a specific B vitamin for its growth. Although these microbiological techniques are reasonably satisfactory for riboflavin and niacin, they are unsatisfactory for vitamin B-6 and folic acid. They are also not suitable for assaying vitamin B-12 in processed foods containing microbial growth inhibitors. Consequently, HPLC methods are currently being investigated for vitamin B-6 and folic acid. Although a protein-binding assay has recently been introduced for vitamin B-12, it is not very satisfactory, as it responds to vitamin B-12 isomers with no vitamin B-12 activity (NRC, 1986).

At present, there is no single assay that accurately measures all the biologically active isomers of folacin in foods. Early food composition tables may include folacin data which predate the use of ascorbic acid to prevent oxidation of labile folate during the assay. Hence these values underestimate the folacin content of foods.

Several procedures are available for the analysis of vitamin C in foodstuffs, some of which measure total vitamin C activity (i.e. ascorbic acid and dehydroascorbic acid). Others analyze only ascorbic acid (the reduced form of vitamin C) and thus may underestimate the total vitamin C content of a foodstuff. Acceptable methods are available for measuring both forms of vitamin C in fresh products. Unfortunately, none of the current methods differentiate between vitamin C and iso-ascorbate, a stereo-isomer of ascorbic acid which is being used increasingly by the food industry as an anti-oxidant. Iso-ascorbate, however, possesses little, if any, vitamin C activity (Cooke, 1983). Hence, vitamin C in processed foods may be consistently overestimated.

Numerous methods exist for the analysis of dietary fiber in foods, some of which are very unsatisfactory. Dietary fiber is made up of several different types of polysaccharides (pectins, hemicellulose, cellulose, algal polysaccharides, gums, and mucilages) and the nonpolysaccharide lignin. Cellulose and hemicelluloses compose the structural components of the plant cell wall, whereas pectins, gums, and mucilages are associated with the structure and metabolism of the plant cell.

Dietary fiber is defined by the Canadian Expert Committee on Dietary Fibre (Health and Welfare Canada, 1985) as:

> Endogenous components of plant material in the diet which are resistant to digestion by enzymes produced by man. They are predominantly nonstarch polysaccharides and lignin and may include, in addition, associated substances.

Cellulose + insoluble noncellulosic polysaccharides	Insoluble fiber[a]	Englyst fiber (nonstarch polysac-charides)	Southgate fiber[b] (unavailable carbo-hydrate)
Soluble noncellulosic polysaccharides	Soluble fiber		
Resistant starch Lignin			

Table 4.5: Relationship between the dietary fiber fractions. [a] Some methods of analysis also include lignin. [b] Fiber determined by the method of Southgate (1969) may differ from the sum of the fractions shown, because it can include starch which is not necessarily the same as the resistant starch measured by method of Englyst et al. (1982). Modified from Holland B, Unwin ID, Buss DH. (1988). Cereals and Cereal Products. The Third Supplement to McCance and Widdowson's 'The Composition of Foods'. 4th edition. Reproduced with permission of the Royal Society of Chemistry on behalf of the Controller of Her Majesty's Stationery Office.

This definition, modified from that of Trowell et al. (1976), includes the term 'endogenous' so that indigestible materials formed during food processing (e.g. products of the Maillard reaction) are excluded.

Southgate (1982) has defined dietary fiber in chemical terms as:

> The sum of lignin and the non-α-glucan (nonstarch) polysac-charides in foods.

A variety of methods can be used to analyze dietary fiber, the selection depending on whether information on total dietary fiber or some of its individual components is required. The relationships between the various forms and fractions of dietary fiber are summarized in Table 4.5.

The oldest method for fiber analysis in foods is the classical Weende procedure. It measures 'crude fiber', which consists primarily of cellu-lose and lignin. The method underestimates the true dietary fiber value, as 40% of the unavailable carbohydrates may be lost during the analy-sis (Williams and Olmstead, 1935). The neutral detergent fiber (NDF) method of van Soest (1967) measures the water-insoluble fibers (i.e. cel-lulose, the major hemicelluloses, and lignin), but not the water-soluble fibers (i.e. pectins, gums, mucilages), and some hemicelluloses. Erro-neously high fiber values may be reported for starchy materials such as flours and potatoes with this method; starch may not be rendered com-pletely soluble unless a modification of the NDF procedure (termed the enzymatic NDF procedure) is employed. The latter generally provides a good estimate of dietary fiber in cereal products, but underestimates the dietary fiber content of those foods containing a large amount of water-soluble fiber, such as oats, fruits, and most leafy and root vegetables (Lanza and Butrum, 1986). The acid detergent fiber (ADF) procedure, developed by Goering and van Soest (1970), measures primarily cellulose and lignin, although some pectin and hemicelluloses may also be included.

Food composition values for total dietary fiber, based on direct chemical analysis, are incomplete. So far, only dietary fiber values for certain foods are included in the revised USDA Handbooks No. 8. The U.K. food composition tables and supplements (Paul and Southgate, 1978; 1979; Holland et al., 1988) contain the most comprehensive source of dietary fiber values. The enzymatic procedure of Southgate (1969) was used for the dietary fiber values for cereals, cereal foods, and some vegetables and fruits in the 1978 U.K. food composition tables (Paul and Southgate, 1978). In this method, starch is first removed, sometimes incompletely, by enzymatic hydrolysis; the residue is then separated, using a series of extraction steps, into three fractions: cellulose, noncellulosic polysaccharides (hemicelluloses and pectins, gums, and mucilages), and lignin. Each fraction is then hydrolyzed by acid into its component sugars which are measured colorimetrically. The sum of the three fractions gives the total dietary fiber value. The remainder of the dietary fiber values for the U.K. food composition tables are based on an indirect method of measurement (Paul and Southgate, 1978).

More recently, alternative enzymatic gravimetric procedures have been developed for total dietary fiber which also include measurement of the soluble fraction. Large inconsistencies in dietary fiber values for the same food items occur when compared to values obtained by different methods of analysis. In general, total dietary fiber values derived from Southgate's method are higher for high-starch products such as cereals, legumes, and potatoes, perhaps associated with the incomplete removal of starch. Values are probably adequate for fruits and vegetables. The Association of Official Analytical Chemists recommends the enzymatic gravimetric method of Prosky et al. (1985) for the analysis of total dietary fiber in foods.

The various components of dietary fiber can be analyzed by gas chromatography (Englyst et al., 1982; Theander and Åman, 1982), following fractionation; HPLC may be used as an alternative method in the future (Thente, 1983). The third supplement to McCance and Widdowson's 'The Composition of Foods' (Holland et al., 1988) presents values for soluble (hemicelluloses) and insoluble (pectins, gum & mucilages) noncellulosic polysaccharides, lignin, cellulose, and resistant starch, as well as total dietary fiber values derived from the methods of Englyst et al. (1982) and Wenlock et al. (1985).

From this discussion, it is apparent that some dietary fiber methods are adequate only for certain foods. Therefore, details of the analytical

	Mean	SE	CV
Water (g)	735	0.420	0.18
Nitrogen (g)	2.89	0.0175	1.18
Fat (g)	68.2	0.259	1.20
Iron (mg)	7.6	0.201	8.36
Energy (kJ)	5590	95.3	0.54

Table 4.6: Mean values with their standard errors (SE) and coefficients of variation (CV) for energy and selected nutrients in ten replicate analyses of one sample of mashed potato. From Chan Chim Yuk AW, Wheeler EF, Leppington IM. Variations in the apparent nutrient content of foods: a study of sampling error. British Journal of Nutrition 34: 391–397, 1975. Reproduced by permission of Cambridge University Press.

methods used should always be included when the food composition data are compiled. In this way, the user can be alerted to any potential problems and biases in the published values.

4.3.3 Analytical errors

Analytical errors may occur during the determination of the nutrient content of any food (Chan Chim Yuk et al., 1975) leading to inaccuracies in the food composition data tables. Random sampling errors can be controlled by analysing homogeneous and finely ground samples. Nevertheless, they may be greater than the errors occurring during the analysis. Freeze drying followed by crushing is commonly used for sample homogenization, although other techniques should be used when analyzing fatty acids and certain vitamins: freeze drying modifies these nutrients (Cooke, 1983). As a check on the homogeneity of the ground sample, replicate aliquots should be analyzed and the coefficient of variation for each nutrient calculated (Table 4.6).

Accuracy of the analytical method can be controlled by including an aliquot of a reference material, of a similar matrix to the sample and certified for the nutrient of interest, with each batch of analysis. Such reference materials can be obtained from the U.S. National Bureau of Standards. To determine precision, aliquots from a homogeneous pooled sample should be repeatedly analyzed with each batch, and again the coefficient of variation of the analytical method estimated (Chan Chim Yuk et al., 1975). Food composition data should always include details on the accuracy and precision of the analytical methods used for each nutrient.

Food or Food Group	Protein (kcal/g)	Fat (kcal/g)	Carbo-hydrate (kcal/g)
Eggs, meat products, milk products			
Eggs	4.36	9.02	3.68
Meat	4.27	9.02	3.87
Milk and milk products	4.27	8.79	3.87
Fruits			
All (except lemons and limes)	3.36	8.37	3.60
Lemons and limes	3.36	8.37	2.48
Grain products			
Cornmeal (whole-ground)	2.73	8.37	4.03
Macaroni, spaghetti	3.91	8.37	4.12
Rice, white or polished	3.82	8.37	4.16
Wheat, 97–100% extraction	3.59	8.37	3.78
Wheat, 70–74% extraction	4.05	8.37	4.12
Legumes, nuts, sugars			
Peas, lima beans, cowpeas	3.47	8.37	4.07
Nuts	3.47	8.37	4.07
Cane or beet sugar			3.87
Vegetables			
Mushrooms	2.62	8.37	3.48
Potatoes and starchy roots	2.78	8.37	4.03
Most other vegetables	2.44	8.37	3.57

Table 4.7: Specific factors for calculating energy values of foods or food groups. Data from Merrill AL, Watts BK. (1973). Energy Value of Foods: basis and derivation. USDA, Agriculture Handbook No. 74, Washington, D.C.

4.3.4   Conversion factors

Energy

The absence of standard conversion factors in food composition tables leads to variations in the energy content of similar foods. The energy values of foods are calculated indirectly from the amounts of protein, fat, carbohydrate, and alcohol in the foods, using various energy conversion factors. The latter are all corrected to take into account the losses of energy occurring in digestion and absorption and through incomplete oxidation. Consequently, the calculated energy values represent the available or *metabolizable* energy content of foods. Many countries use the general conversion factors for calculating the energy value of all food items. These factors are: 17 kJ/g (4.0 kcal/g) for protein, 37 kJ/g (9.0 kcal/g) for fat, 17 kJ/g (4.0 kcal/g) for total carbohydrate, and 29 kJ/g (7.0 kcal/g) for alcohol. Other countries (e.g. the United States) use specific energy conversion factors for individual foods and

Food Type	Specific Factors for Different Classes of Food (kcal/100 g) (A)	Protein × 4.0 Fat × 9.0 Carbohydrate × 4.0 (kcal/100 g) (B)	Percentage Ratio Col.(B) ÷ Col.(A) × 100%
Beef	273	268	98
Salmon, canned	143	138	97
Eggs	162	158	98
Milk	68	69	101
Butter	716	733	102
Cornmeal, degermed	363	356	98
Oatmeal	390	396	102
Rice, brown	360	356	99
Wheat flour, patent	364	355	98
Beans, snap	35	42	120
Peas, dry seeds	339	349	103
Cabbage	24	29	120
Carrots	42	45	107
Potatoes	83	85	102
Turnips	32	35	109
Apples, raw	58	64	110
Lemons, raw	32	44	138
Peaches, canned	68	75	110
Sugar, cane or beet	385	398	103

Table 4.8: A comparison of the energy values (kcal/100 g) of the edible portion of selected foods using specific and general energy conversion factors (see text). Adapted from Périssé (1982) with permission.

food groups. These are based on the heat of combustion for the fat, protein, and carbohydrate content of specific foods as determined by Atwater and Bryant (1899), multiplied by the coefficient of apparent digestibility (Merrill and Watt, 1973). These specific conversion factors were recommended by FAO/WHO (1973) and a representative sample of such factors are shown in Table 4.7.

In the current U.K. food composition tables (Paul and Southgate, 1978), the energy conversion factor used for carbohydrate is 16 kJ/g (3.75 kcal/g). The latter is used because the free sugars (glucose, fructose, sucrose, lactose, maltose, and higher maltose homologs), dextrins, starch, and glycogen are all determined separately, by chemical analysis. Their sum represents the available carbohydrate content of the food, expressed as grams of monosaccharide. The Atwater and Bryant factors are used for protein, fat, and alcohol.

Table 4.8 compares the energy content of selected food items calculated using two of the methods described above. As can be seen, differences for the energy values are most marked for fruits and vegetables because in these foods much of the energy is provided by carbohydrate.

Food	Factor (per g N)
Cereals	
Wheat	
Wholemeal wheat products	5.83
Other wheat products	5.70
Bran	6.31
Rice	5.95
Barley, oats, rye	5.83
Soya	5.71
Nuts	
Peanuts, Brazil nuts	5.46
Almonds	5.18
All other nuts	5.30
Seeds	
Sesame, sunflower, pumpkin	5.30
Milk and milk products	6.38
Gelatin	5.55
All other foods	6.25

Table 4.9: Specific factors for converting nitrogen in foods to protein. Adapted from Paul AA, Southgate DAT (1978). McCance and Widdowson's 'The Composition of Foods'. 4th edition. Reproduced with the permission of the Controller of Her Majesty's Stationery Office.

Protein

Conventionally, the protein content of foods is calculated from the total nitrogen content using conversion factors. In some countries the factor of 6.25 is used indiscriminately to convert total nitrogen into protein, based on the assumption that all proteins, regardless of their source, contain 16% nitrogen. Most countries, however, apply specific nitrogen conversion factors recommended by the FAO/WHO Committee on Energy and Protein Requirements (FAO/WHO, 1973). These factors are dependent on the food or food group, and are derived from data of Jones (1941). Table 4.9 presents some of these specific nitrogen conversion factors.

Food composition tables of some countries (e.g. Ethiopia) use a conversion factor based on the amino-acid composition of the food to calculate the protein content (Ågren and Gibson, 1963). For some foods known to contain a large amount of nonprotein nitrogen in the form of urea, purine, or pyrimidine derivatives (e.g. mushrooms, beverages, and certain fish), corrections are applied to the total nitrogen content before the protein content is calculated.

4.3.5 Inconsistencies in terminology

Confusion may arise because of inconsistencies in the terminology for nutrients such as carbohydrate, vitamin A, vitamin D, vitamin E, niacin, and folic acid in food composition table data.

Carbohydrate

The treatment of carbohydrate in food composition tables is inconsistent. In some, the percentage of carbohydrate in foods is derived by difference using the following formula:

Percentage carbohydrate = 100 − (% water + % protein + % fat + % ash)

When this formula is used, unavailable complex carbohydrates, and any noncarbohydrate residue, as well as available sugar, dextrins, and starch, are included in the total carbohydrate. In contrast, in some older food tables, nitrogen-free-extract (sometimes termed 'available carbohydrate') is given and derived from the total carbohydrate value as shown below:

Nitrogen-free extract = total carbohydrate − crude fiber

In others, such as the United Kingdom (Paul and Southgate, 1978), the components of available carbohydrate are analyzed separately and expressed as the sum of the free sugars, dextrins, starch, and glycogen.

Vitamin A

The activity of vitamin A in foodstuffs should be expressed in terms of retinol equivalents (RE), in µg. The latter represent the sum of preformed vitamin A (retinol) and the vitamin A activity from the provitamin A carotenoids present (FAO/WHO, 1967). Retinol equivalents are calculated from the following equation:

$$RE\,(\mu g) = retinol\,(\mu g) + \frac{\beta\text{-carotene}\,(\mu g)}{6} + \frac{other\ provitamin\ A\ carotenoids\,(\mu g)}{12}$$

The divisor of six for β-carotene is based on a 33% absorption of β-carotene from diets, of which only 50% is subsequently converted to retinol. In practice, the efficiency of intestinal absorption of β-carotene varies among food groups, so different divisors should theoretically be used. For example, in the United Kingdom, the divisor of two is recommended for β-carotene in milk and milk products (Department of Health and Social Security, 1981). The other carotenoid isomers with vitamin A activity (e.g. α-carotene and cryptoxanthin) are assumed to provide half as much retinol as β-carotene, resulting in a factor of one twelfth.

There is little information on the type and proportions of carotenoid isomers in individual food items, or their biological potency, at the present time. The content of retinol, β-carotene, and other provitamin A carotenoids for certain food groups has been compiled by the FAO/WHO Expert Group (1972). These values can be used to derive total vitamin A activity, until more specific analyzed data for individual foodstuffs are available.

In older food composition tables, vitamin A activity is expressed in terms of international units (IU). These can be converted to retinol equivalents using the following expressions:

$$1 \text{ IU vitamin A activity} = 0.3\,\mu g \text{ retinol}$$

$$1 \text{ IU vitamin A activity} = 0.6\,\mu g \text{ β-carotene}$$

$$1 \text{ IU vitamin A activity} = 1.2\,\mu g \text{ other provitamin A carotenoids}$$

In some food composition data, carotene (usually as β-carotene) and retinol are listed separately (Paul and Southgate, 1978). For foods in which the provitamin A carotenoids are the predominant form of vitamin A, the calculation of retinol equivalents may have large associated errors, particularly if the measured carotenoids include non-provitamin A compounds.

Vitamin D

This vitamin should be expressed in terms of μg cholecalciferol.

$$1 \text{ IU vitamin D} = 0.025\,\mu g \text{ cholecalciferol}$$

In some older food composition data, vitamin D is expressed in terms of international units.

Vitamin E

The activity of vitamin E in foods should be expressed as milligrams of d-α-tocopherol equivalents (d-α-TE). This is the sum of α-tocopherol and the other tocopherols (tocols) (β-, γ-, and δ-tocopherol) and their four corresponding tocotrienols, after correcting for their biological activities relative to d-α-tocopherol. The conversion factors generally used are: β-tocopherol about 50%; γ-tocopherol 10%; δ-tocopherol 1%; α-tocotrienol 30%; β-tocotrienol 5%; γ-tocotrienol 1% (uncertain) (McClaughlin and Weihrauch, 1979; Bieri and McKenna, 1981). To convert international units to d-α-tocopherol equivalents, the IU value is divided by the IU equivalency, i.e. :

$$12 \text{ IU α-tocopherol} = \frac{12}{1.49} = 8 \text{ mg } d\text{-α-tocopherol equivalents.}$$

For mixed diets in which only the α-tocopherol content is given, the value in mg can be increased by 20% to allow for the presence of other vitamin E compounds, thus estimating d-α-TE (Bieri and McKenna, 1981).

Niacin

Niacin activity in foods is best expressed in terms of niacin equivalents, in mg. In some food composition data, niacin is quoted in terms of preformed niacin, in mg (Watt et al., 1963). Niacin equivalents include the contribution of niacin from tryptophan as well as preformed niacin. They are calculated on the following basis:

$$\text{niacin equivalents (mg)} = \text{niacin (mg)} + \frac{\text{tryptophan (mg)}}{60}$$

If the tryptophan intake is not known, it can be estimated by assuming that animal and vegetable protein contain 1.4% and 1% tryptophan respectively. The current U.K. food composition data includes information on both preformed niacin as well as the potential contribution of tryptophan to the niacin content, calculated using the conversion factor shown in the equation above. Large individual variation has been observed in the efficiency of conversion of tryptophan to niacin. When the tryptophan intake is low, less of the available tryptophan appears to be converted to niacin (Horwitt et al., 1981).

Folate

Folate in foods should be presented as total folacin, which should include folic acid and all related compounds which exhibit the biological activity of folic acid. At present, few methods accurately measure all the biologically active folacin isomers. Some food composition data present only values for free folate. The latter includes the various mono-, di-, and triglutamates, each with a comparatively high biological activity. Conjugated folates are excluded, although they often predominate over free folates in foods and are absorbed and utilized by the body to varying degrees. Hence, free-folate values will underestimate the total folacin activity in the foods (Poh Tan et al., 1984).

There is obviously an urgent need to standardize the terminology used for vitamin A, vitamin D, vitamin E, niacin, and folic acid. All published food composition data tables and nutrient databases should include information on the conversion factors and terminology used.

4.3.6 Incorrect description of individual food items and/or source of nutrient values

The system used to identify specific food items in food composition tables or nutrient data banks has also not been standardized. Sometimes descriptions of the foods in these sources of data are inadequate, making it difficult for the user to match precisely the food consumed with the appropriate food item or brand in the food composition data. Such errors produce biases in the calculated nutrient composition of the consumed food. It is essential to include information on both the common name of the food, with local synonyms, as well as scientific taxonomic names with variety, if known.   As well, details of the place and time of collection and number of samples collected should be recorded (Paul and Southgate, 1988). Additional details required for food composition data are itemized in Table 4.2. Food additive and contaminant levels vary with the manufacturer, making it essential to include brand names of manufactured foods in the food composition tables.

For composite dishes, such as coleslaw, nutrient values may be calculated by summing the nutrient composition data of the constituents. This procedure can yield acceptable estimates, provided that the nutrient values of all the ingredients are available.   In some cases, nutrient values are imputed by using the nutrient content of a similar food. This practice may introduce bias, as will assigning zero to the imputed value. Nutrient values for cooked composite dishes derived from specific recipes can be calculated from the raw ingredients using a computer program (Day, 1980) or using a calculation procedure outlined in detail by Paul and Southgate (1988). Nutrient values calculated from recipes, and/or imputed, should be identified in all food composition tables and nutrient data banks, and the procedures used for imputing missing values documented.

4.3.7   Inconsistencies resulting from to genetic, environmental, and food preparation and processing factors

Even if all the sources of error in food composition data discussed above are eliminated, discrepancies in nutrient composition values for similar food items will still occur among different sets of food composition data. These variations may arise from varietal and/or environmental factors, and (in some cases) from differences in methods of preparation and processing of the food. In some areas, such as New Zealand, Finland, and certain parts of the United States, the selenium content of foods is lower than elsewhere as a result of the low selenium levels in the soil. The iodine content of foods is also very variable because of differences in the content and availability of iodine in the soil, as well as the types and amounts of fertilizers used (Underwood, 1977).

National differences may arise from variations in the fortification or enrichment of selected foods with specific nutrients. For example, white flour in the United Kingdom is enriched with thiamin, niacin, iron, and calcium, whereas in Canada and the United States it is currently enriched with thiamin, riboflavin, niacin, and iron. Cow's milk is enriched with vitamin D in Canada and the United States but not in the United Kingdom.

The content of certain heat-labile and water-soluble nutrients in foods may be altered by differences in methods of preparation and processing. The content of thiamin and vitamin C in many foods varies with the cooking time and temperature used, the amount of water added, the pH in which food is prepared and the holding time before serving (Tucker et al., 1946; Eheart and Gott, 1965). These nutrient losses may result in large discrepancies between the actual thiamin and vitamin C content compared to the calculated values when food composition data of raw ingredients are used to compute nutrient values for cooked dishes. Data on nutrient retention during food preparation are limited, making it difficult to accurately estimate the nutrient values of a cooked composite dish (Hoover and Pelican, 1984).

The inconsistencies in food composition values arising from the factors discussed above emphasize the importance of using food composition values appropriate for the country, whenever possible.

4.4 International Network of Food Data Systems

In an effort to eliminate some of the potential sources of error and bias in food composition data, an International Network of Food Data Systems (INFOODS) has been established (Rand, 1985). This organization created a series of task forces to develop:

- standards and guidelines for the collection of food composition data;
- standardized terminology and nomenclature so that food composition data can be exchanged internationally;
- standards for data interchange;
- an international directory of existing databases;
- a detailed description of the needs of database users.

These new developments will assist in providing a more rigorous and accurate approach to the development of food composition databases. A publication describing the work of these task forces is now available (Rand et al., 1987).

4.5 Use of direct chemical analysis

Direct chemical analysis of representative samples of individual food items, meals, or prepared diet composites must be carried out if precise information on nutrient intakes of individuals is required for metabolic studies. This approach can also be used to validate food composition data obtained from tables or nutrient data banks (Gibson and Scythes, 1982).

Care must be taken to exclude adventitious contamination during sample collection, preparation, and analysis, particularly if trace elements are to be determined. Adequate storage and preliminary treatment of the sample are also essential to preserve the activity of certain vitamins (e.g. folic acid, thiamin, vitamin C, and riboflavin) (Cooke, 1983). The individual food items, meals, or composite diets must also be homogeneous, so that a representative aliquot can be removed for chemical analysis. Homogeneity can be checked by analyzing multiple aliquots of a single composite diet or food.

Three techniques are used for collecting meals or one-day diet composites for nutrient analysis (Pekkarinen, 1970):

Duplicate portions

This technique involves the collection of a duplicate portion of all foods and beverages consumed during a twenty-four-hour period. These are weighed, or estimated in household portions, by the respondent or a field worker. Several separate consecutive twenty-four-hour diet composites may be collected from each respondent. Alternatively, the daily diet composites may be combined into one single composite covering the whole survey period. The latter approach does not provide data on intra-subject variation in nutrient intakes (Section 6.2) and is not recommended. Diet composites are then homogenized using a blender and later chemically analyzed.

Aliquot sampling of foods

This procedure involves weighing all foods and beverages consumed by an individual during the survey period, and collecting daily aliquot samples of each item. These samples are then combined and subsequently analyzed. Care must be taken in this method to ensure that representative aliquots are taken both during the collection and the subsequent pooling and homogenization.

Equivalent food composites

These are used less frequently than the two methods described above. In this method, weights of all foods and beverages consumed by an individual during the survey period are again recorded. Subsequently, samples of raw foods, equivalent to the mean daily amounts of foods consumed by each individual in the survey, are chemically analyzed. Thus only the nutrient content of the uncooked food is determined and consequently the method is not suitable for estimating the intake of heat-labile and water-soluble vitamins.

Collection of duplicate food items or composite diets, followed by their direct chemical analyses, is not necessarily the most accurate method available for characterizing the usual nutrient intake of individuals; studies have shown that energy and nutrient intakes are consistently lower during the period of duplicate collections, compared to the other survey days (Gibson and Scythes, 1982; Kim et al., 1984). Nevertheless, this is the most appropriate method for assessing individual nutrient intakes for metabolic studies, provided that the amounts for the duplicate food items or composite diets are weighed.

Subject	No. of Samples	Calculated Energy (A) (kcal)	Calculated Energy (B) (kcal)	Analyzed Energy (C) (kcal)	(A-C)/C %	(B-C)/C %
1	7	2510	2460	2330	7.7	5.6
2	8	3070	3010	2800	9.6	7.5
3	10	2490	2450	2350	6.0	4.3
4	15	3370	3300	3120	8.0	5.8
5	6	2620	2540	2530	3.6	0.4
6	9	3020	2970	2970	1.7	0.0
7	6	3120	3060	2880	8.3	6.3
8	5	3690	3600	3470	6.3	3.8
9	10	3190	3150	2830	12.7	11.3
10	9	3800	3720	3640	4.4	2.2
11	6	3470	3390	3230	7.4	4.9
12	5	2630	2560	2590	1.5	-1.2
Mean					6.7	4.6

Table 4.10: Estimation of the energy content of diets determined from food composition data and nutrient conversion factors of Atwater and Bryant (1899) (Column A), food composition data and factors of Paul and Southgate (1978) (Column B), and by bomb calorimetry (Column C). From Acheson et al. (1980). © Am. J. Clin. Nutr. American Society for Clinical Nutrition.

4.6 Validation of calculated nutrient intakes

Several investigators have compared energy and nutrient intakes, calculated from food composition data, with results from direct chemical analysis of individual food items or composite diets. Acheson et al. (1980) examined discrepancies in the energy content of duplicate diets determined by direct bomb calorimetry, and from food composition data (Table 4.10). When the analyzed energy was expressed as metabolizable energy, mean errors in the calculated values ranged from approximately 5% to 7% of the calorimetry values, depending on the energy conversion factors used. The main sources of the discrepancies were the variable fat content of the composite dishes and differences in the water content of the analyzed duplicate food items, compared to the food composition table data.

Similar comparisons for the macronutrients (e.g. protein and carbohydrate) suggest that differences between the two methods can be within 10%, especially when the nutrient intake represents an average for a number of persons, or for a single person over a relatively long time period (e.g. four weeks) (Widdowson and McCance, 1943; Bingham and Cummings, 1985). In contrast, nutrients such as fat, iron, sodium, potassium, vitamin C, and vitamin A often show poorer agreement, the differences amounting to 20% or more (Bransby et al., 1948; Grant Whiting and Leverton, 1960; Stock and Wheeler, 1972; Bingham et al., 1982). Some of the differences arise from the sources of variation and bias in the nutrient composition data discussed in Section 4.3. Other more specific sources of

- The variable fat content of meat and made-up dishes
- differences in the water content
- trace metal contamination from knives and cooking utensils
- variability in the salt content of processed and home prepared foods
- large range in losses of heat labile and water soluble vitamins during different food preparation and cooking procedures

Table 4.11: Sources of discrepancies between analyzed and calculated nutrient contents arising during food preparation.

uncertainty, mainly arising during the food preparation stage, are shown in Table 4.11. In view of these discrepancies, perfect agreement between analyzed and calculated intakes should not be expected.

4.7 Assessment of available nutrient intakes

Nutrient intakes calculated from food composition data or determined by direct chemical analysis represent the maximum amount of that nutrient available to the body. For most nutrients, however, the amount actually absorbed and utilized by the body cells will probably be lower than the determined values, and depends on the chemical form of the nutrient, the nature of the food ingested, and the composition of the total diet. The level of the body stores of the nutrient and physiological status of the individual may also affect its absorption and utilization.

The term 'bioavailability' describes the absorption and utilization of nutrients. It is defined as:

> The proportion of a nutrient in food which is absorbed and utilized (O'Dell, 1983).

Factors known to affect the bioavailability of nutrients have been classified into two groups: extrinsic and intrinsic factors. Examples of these factors, particularly affecting the bioavailability of trace elements, are summarized in Table 4.12 (O'Dell, 1983).

At present, the major factors influencing bioavailability of most nutrients are not well established. Moreover, there is no consensus on the algorithms which should be used to predict bioavailability of nutrients in meals. Nevertheless, the dietary components which affect the bioavailability of iron are relatively well characterized. As a result, Monsen and co-workers (Monsen et al., 1978; Monsen and Balintfy, 1982) have developed an algorithm for estimating available iron from dietary iron intakes, provided that intakes of flesh foods, vitamin C, and total iron at *each meal* are known. In their model, 40% of the total iron found in meat, poultry, and fish is assumed to be heme iron. Absorption of heme

Extrinsic factors	Stability of the element species (e.g. CuS, $CuMoS_4$, and $Fe_4(P_2O_7)_3$)
	Absorption of diet components on large surfaces (e.g. fiber, silica, and $Ca_3(PO_4)_2$)
	State of oxidation of element; chemical form (e.g. Fe(II) vs. Fe(III); Cr(III) vs. Cr(VI); Mn(II) vs. Mn(VII))
	Competitive antagonism between ions (e.g. Cu-Zn; Cd-Zn; Fe-Zn; Mn-Fe)
	Chelation effects: positive or negative depending on relative solubilities and dissociation constants
Intrinsic factors	Species and genotype
	Age and sex
	Metabolic function: maintenance, growth, reproduction, lactation
	Nutritional status including adaptation to dietary intake
	Physiological stress
	Intestinal microflora and infection

Table 4.12: Factors affecting the bioavailability of trace elements in the diet. From O'Dell (1983). Reproduced by permission of the Federation of American Societies for Experimental Biology Journal.

iron can range from 15% in an iron-replete individual to 35% in a person with low or no iron stores. In the model of Monsen and Balintfy (1982), absorption of heme iron is assumed to be 23%, based on a reference individual with 500 mg body iron stores.

The amount of nonheme iron is calculated as the difference between total iron and heme iron intakes. Nonheme iron is absorbed at a lower rate, ranging from 2% in an iron-replete person consuming a meal low in enhancing factors to 20% in an iron-deplete individual consuming a meal high in enhancing factors. In the reference individual with 500 mg body iron stores, nonheme iron absorption is assumed to range from 3% to 8%, depending on the quantity of enhancing factors (ΣEF) present. The numerical value of ΣEF is calculated as the sum of the milligrams of ascorbic acid plus the grams of cooked meat, poultry, and fish at each meal or snack. When $\Sigma EF = 0$, the absorption of nonheme iron is assumed to be 3%; when $\Sigma EF > 75$, the absorption is assumed to remain stable at 8%. Table 4.13 shows the appropriate percent absorption for nonheme iron for various intermediate values of ΣEF calculated using the model of Monsen and Balintfy (1982). Total available iron intakes per day can be derived from the sum of available iron from each meal and snack. Gibson et al. (1988) have questioned the appropriateness of this model for children.

For other nutrients (e.g. calcium and zinc), the amount available for absorption can only be estimated from the proportion of plant- to animal-based foods in the diet. More work is required to develop algorithms

ΣEF	%	ΣEF	%	ΣEF	%	ΣEF	%	ΣEF	%
1	3.09	16	4.33	31	5.41	46	6.38	61	7.26
2	3.18	17	4.40	32	5.48	47	6.44	62	7.31
3	3.26	18	4.48	33	5.55	48	6.50	63	7.37
4	3.35	19	4.55	34	5.61	49	6.56	64	7.42
5	3.44	20	4.63	35	5.68	50	6.62	65	7.47
6	3.52	21	4.70	36	5.75	51	6.68	66	7.53
7	3.60	22	4.78	37	5.81	52	6.74	67	7.58
8	3.69	23	4.85	38	5.88	53	6.80	68	7.64
9	3.77	24	4.92	39	5.94	54	6.86	69	7.69
10	3.85	25	5.00	40	6.01	55	6.92	70	7.74
11	3.93	26	5.06	41	6.07	56	6.97	71	7.79
12	4.01	27	5.14	42	6.13	57	7.03	72	7.85
13	4.09	28	5.21	43	6.20	58	7.09	73	7.90
14	4.17	29	5.28	44	6.26	59	7.14	74	7.95
15	4.25	30	5.34	45	6.32	60	7.20	75	8.00

Table 4.13: Percent of bioavailable nonheme dietary iron for an individual with 500 mg body iron stores as a function of the total quantity of enhancing factors (ΣEF) present. From Monsen ER, Balintfy JL. Calculating dietary iron bioavailability: refinement and computerization. © The American Dietetic Association. Reproduced by permission from Journal of the American Dietetic Association, Vol. 80: 307–311, 1982.

for predicting the bioavailability of these nutrients in meals. The NRC Committee on Nutrient Adequacy (1986) emphasizes that variations in the bioavailability of iron, zinc, and folate probably have the greatest impact on the estimates of dietary intakes of these nutrients for *individuals*. For estimates of average nutrient intakes for a *group*, their impact may be small in relation to other sources of measurement error.

4.8 Summary

Energy and nutrient intakes can be calculated from quantitative food consumption data by using food composition data from tables, or data which have been transferred to and maintained on a computer (i.e. nutrient data banks). Food composition data are based on quantitative nutrient analysis of samples of each food, representative of the average composition of a particular foodstuff on a year-round, nationwide basis. Both random and systematic errors may occur in food composition data, depending on the food item and the nutrient. Such errors may include inadequacies in the sampling protocols and analytical methods, use of incorrect conversion factors for calculating energy and protein values, inconsistencies arising from differences in the terminology for certain nutrients and in methods of food preparation and processing, as well as genetic and environmental factors and incorrect descriptions of individual food items and/or sources of nutrient values. In an attempt to provide a more rigorous and accurate approach to the development of food composition databases, an international network of food data systems has been established.

When nutrient information for metabolic studies is required, or when values for specific nutrients are not available, direct chemical analysis of individual food items or composite diets must be performed. The latter can be prepared by three techniques: duplicate portions, aliquot sampling, and the equivalent composite method. Chemical analysis can also be used to validate energy and nutrient intakes calculated from food composition data. Perfect agreement between these two methods is unlikely because of variations in the fat content of meat and prepared dishes, differences in water content, adventitious trace element contamination from knives and cooking utensils, variability in salt content of processed and home prepared foods, as well as variable losses of heat-labile and water-soluble vitamins according to different food preparation and cooking procedures. Nutrient values derived from both food composition data and direct chemical analysis represent the maximum available to the body and not the amount actually absorbed and utilized.

References

Acheson KJ, Campbell IT, Edholm OG, Miller DS, Stock MJ. (1980). The measurement of food and energy intake in man — an evaluation of some techniques. American Journal of Clinical Nutrition 33: 1147–1154.

Ågren G, Gibson RS. (1963). Food Composition Tables for Use in Ethiopia. Children's Nutrition Unit Report No. 16. Swedish International Development Agency.

Atwater WO, Bryant AP. (1899). The availability and fuel value of food materials. Report of the Storrs Agricultural Experimental Station 1900: 73–110.

Bell L, Hatcher J, Chan L, Fraser D. (1979). Development of a computerized system for calculating nutrient intakes. Journal of the Canadian Dietetic Association 40: 30–36.

Bieri JG, McKenna MC. (1981). Expressing dietary values for fat-soluble vitamins: changes in concepts and terminology. American Journal of Clinical Nutrition 34: 289–295.

Bingham S, Cummings JH. (1985). Urine nitrogen as an independent validatory measure of dietary intake: a study of nitrogen balance in individuals consuming their normal diet. American Journal of Clinical Nutrition 42: 1276–1289.

Bingham S, Wiggins HS, Englyst H, Seppänen R, Helms P, Strand R, Burton R, Jørgensen IM, Poulsen L, Paerregaard A, Bjerrum L, James WP. (1982). Methods and validity of dietary assessments in four Scandinavian populations. Nutrition and Cancer 4: 23–33.

Black AE, Ashby DR, Day KC, Bates CJ, Paul AA. (1983). Analytical versus food table values for vitamin C in foods: the effect on calculated vitamin C intake of elderly subjects. Human Nutrition: Applied Nutrition 37A: 9–22.

Bransby ER, Daubney CG, King J. (1948). Comparison of nutrient values of individual diets found by calculation from food tables and by chemical analysis. British Journal of Nutrition 2: 232–236.

Butrum RV, Gebhardt SE. (1976). Nutrient Data Bank: Computer-based management of nutrient values in foods. Journal of American Oil Chemists Society 53: 727A–730A.

Chan Chim Yuk AW, Wheeler EF, Leppington IM. (1975). Variations in the apparent nutrient content of foods: a study of sampling error. British Journal of Nutrition 34: 391–397.

Cooke JR. (1983). Food composition tables — analytical problems in the collection of data. Human Nutrition: Applied Nutrition 37A: 441–447.

Day KC. (1980). 'Recipe', a computer program for calculating the nutrient contents of foods. Journal of Human Nutrition 34: 181–187.

Department of Health and Social Security (1977). The Composition of Mature Human Milk. Report on Health and Social Subjects No. 12. Her Majesty's Stationery Office, London.

Department of Health and Social Security (1981). Recommended Intakes of Nutrients for the United Kingdom. Fifth impression. Reports on Public Health and Medical Subjects No. 120. Her Majesty's Stationery Office, London.

Eheart MS, Gott C. (1965). Chlorophyll, ascorbic acid and pH changes in green vegetables by stir fry, microwave, and conventional methods. Food Technology 19: 867–870.

Englyst H, Wiggins HS, Cummings JH. (1982). Determination of the nonstarch polysaccharides in plant foods by gas-liquid chromatography of constituent sugars as alditol acetates. Analyst 107: 307–318.

FAO/WHO (Food and Agriculture Organization / World Health Organization) (1967). Requirements of Vitamin A, Thiamine, Riboflavin and Niacin. Report of a Joint FAO/WHO Expert Group. FAO Nutrition Meeting Report Series No. 41. WHO Technical Report Series No. 362. World Health Organization, Geneva.

FAO/WHO Expert Group (Food and Agriculture Organization / World Health Organization) (1972). Estimated distribution of sources of Vitamin A activity in various foods. In: Food Composition Table for Use in East Asia. Food and Agricultural Organization and National Institutes of Health, Bethesda, Maryland.

FAO/WHO (Food and Agriculture Organization / World Health Organization) (1973). Energy and Protein Requirements. WHO Technical Report Series No. 522. World Health Organization, Geneva.

Gibson RS, Scythes CA. (1982). Trace element intakes of women. British Journal of Nutrition 48: 241–248.

Gibson RS, Smit Vanderkooy PD, MacDonald AC. (1988). Serum ferritin and dietary iron parameters in a sample of Canadian preschool children. Journal of the Canadian Dietetic Association 49: 23–28.

Goering HK, Soest PJ van. (1970). Forage Fiber Analysis. US Department of Agriculture Handbook No. 379.

Grant Whiting M, Leverton RM. (1960). Reliability of dietary appraisal: comparisons between laboratory analysis and calculation from tables of food values. American Journal of Public Health 50: 815–823.

Health and Welfare Canada (1982). Canadian Nutrient File. Bureau of Nutritional Sciences, Health and Welfare, Ottawa.

Health and Welfare Canada (1985). Report of the Expert Advisory Committee on Dietary Fibre. Health and Welfare, Ottawa.

Health and Welfare Canada (1988). Nutrient Value of Some Common Foods. Health Services and Promotion Branch and Health Protection Branch, Health and Welfare, Ottawa.

Hepburn FN. (1982). The USDA National Nutrient Data Bank. American Journal of Clinical Nutrition 35: 1297–1301.

Holland B, Unwin ID, Buss DH. (1988). Cereals and Cereal Products. The Third Supplement to McCance and Widdowson's 'The Composition of Foods'. Fourth edition. The Royal Society of Chemistry and Ministry of Agriculture, Fisheries and Food. Unwin Brothers Ltd., Old Woking, Surrey.

Hoover LW, Perloff BP. (1981). Model for Review of Nutrient Data Base System Capabilities. University of Missouri, Columbia, Missouri.

Hoover LW, Pelican S. (1984). Nutrient data bases — considerations for educators. Journal of Nutrition Education 16: 58–62.

Horwitt MK, Harper AE, Henderson LM. (1981). Niacin-tryptophan relationships for evaluating niacin equivalents. American Journal of Clinical Nutrition 34: 423–427.

Jones DB. (1941). Factors for converting percentages of nitrogen in foods and feeds into percentages of protein. US Department of Agriculture, Circular 183.

Kim WW, Mertz W, Judd JT, Marshall MW, Kelsay JL, Prather ES. (1984). Effect of making duplicate food collections on nutrient intakes calculated from diet records. American Journal of Clinical Nutrition 40: 1333–1337.

Lanza E, Butrum RR. (1986). A critical review of food fiber analysis and data. Journal of the American Dietetic Association 86: 732–743.

McClaughlin PJ, Weihrauch JL. (1979). Vitamin E content of foods. Journal of the American Dietetic Association 75: 647–665.

Merrill AL, Watt BK. (1973). Energy Value of Foods: basis and derivation. US Department of Agriculture, Agriculture Handbook No. 74, Washington, D.C.

Ministry of Agriculture, Fisheries and Food (1981). Survey of copper and zinc in food. The Fifth Report of the Steering Group on Food Surveillance. The Working Party on the Monitoring of Foodstuffs for Heavy Metals. Food Surveillance Paper No. 5. Her Majesty's Stationery Office, London.

Monsen ER, Balintfy JL. (1982). Calculating dietary iron bioavailability: refinement and computerization. Journal of the American Dietetic Association 80: 307–311.

Monsen ER, Hallberg L, Layrisse M, Hegsted DM, Cook JD, Mertz W, Finch CA. (1978). Estimation of available dietary iron. American Journal of Clinical Nutrition 31: 134–141.

NRC (National Research Council) (1986). Nutrient Adequacy. Assessment using Food Consumption Surveys. Subcommittee on Criteria for Dietary Evaluation, Coordinating Committee on Evaluation of Food Consumption Surveys. Food and Nutrition Board, Commission on Life Sciences. National Academy Press, Washington, D.C.

O'Dell BL. (1983). Bioavailability of trace elements. Federation Proceedings 42: 1714–1715.

Paul AA, Southgate DAT. (1977). A study of the composition of retail meat: dissection into lean, separable fat and inedible portion. Journal of Human Nutrition 31: 259–272.

Paul AA, Southgate DAT. (1978). McCance and Widdowson's 'The Composition of Foods'. Fourth edition. Her Majesty's Stationery Office, London.

Paul AA, Southgate DAT. (1979). McCance and Widdowson's 'The Composition of Foods': dietary fibre in egg, meat, and fish dishes. Journal of Human Nutrition 33: 335–336.

Paul AA, Southgate DAT. (1988). Conversion into nutrients. In: Cameron ME, Staveren WA van (eds) Manual on Methodology for Food Consumption Studies. Oxford Medical Publications, Oxford University Press, Oxford, pp. 121–144.

Paul AA, Southgate DAT, Russell J. (1980). First Supplement to McCance and Widdowson's 'The Composition of Foods': Amino Acid Composition (mg per 100 g food) and Fatty Acid Composition (g per 100 g food). Her Majesty's Stationery Office, London.

Paul AA, Southgate DAT, Buss DH. (1986). McCance and Widdowson's 'The composition of foods': Supplementary information and review of new compositional data. Human Nutrition: Applied Nutrition 40A: 287–299.

Pekkarinen M. (1970). Methodology in the collection of food consumption data. World Review of Nutrition and Dietetics 12: 145–171.

Périssé J. (1982). The heterogeneity of food composition tables. In: Hautvast JGAJ, Klaver W (eds) The Diet Factor in Epidemiological Research. Euronut Report 1, Wageningen, pp. 100–105.

Poh Tan S, Wenlock RW, Buss DH. (1984). Folic acid content of the diet in various types of British households. Human Nutrition: Applied Nutrition 38A: 17–22.

Prosky L, Asp N-G, Furda I, DeVries JW, Schweizer TF, Harland BF. (1985). Determination of total dietary fiber in foods and food products: Collaborative study. Journal of the Association of Official Analytical Chemists 68: 677–679.

Rand WM. (1985). Food composition data: problems and plans. Journal of the American Dietetic Association 85: 1081–1083.

Rand WM, Windham CT, Wyse BW, Young VR (eds). (1987). Food Composition Data: a user's perspective. The United Nations University, Tokyo, Japan.

Rizek RL, Perloff BP, Posati LP. (1981). USDA's nutrient data bank. Food Technology in Australia 33: 112–114.

Smart GA, Sherlock JC. (1985). Chromium in foods and the diet. Food Additives and Contaminants 2: 139–147.

Soest PJ van. (1967). Development of a comprehensive system of feed analyses and its application to forages. Journal of Animal Science 26: 119–128.

Southgate DAT. (1969). Determination of carbohydrates in foods. II. Unavailable carbohydrates. Journal of the Science of Food and Agriculture 20: 331–335.

Southgate DAT. (1974). Guidelines for the Preparation of Tables of Food Composition. S.Karger, Basel, Switzerland.

Southgate DAT. (1982). The definitions, and terminology of dietary fiber. In: Vahouny GV, Kritchevsky D (eds) Dietary Fiber in Health and Disease. Plenum Press, New York, pp. 1–7.

Southgate DAT, Paul AA, Dean AC, Christie AA. (1978). Free sugars in foods. Journal of Human Nutrition 32: 335–347.

Stock AL, Wheeler EF. (1972). Evaluation of meals cooked by large-scale methods: a comparison of chemical analysis and calculation from food tables. British Journal of Nutrition 27: 439–448.

Tan SP, Wenlock RW, Buss DH. (1985). Second supplement to McCance and Widdowson's 'The Composition of Foods': Immigrant Foods. Her Majesty's Stationery Office, London.

Taylor ML, Kozlowski BW, Baer MT. (1985). Energy and nutrient values from different computerized data bases. Journal of the American Dietetic Association 85: 1136–1138.

Theander O, Åman P. (1982). Studies on dietary fiber: A method for the chemical characterization of total dietary fiber. Journal of the Science of Food and Agriculture 33: 340–344.

Thente K. (1983). HPLC analysis of component sugars in fiber polysaccharides from cereals. Developments in Food Science 5A: 477–482.

Thorn J, Robertson J, Buss DH. (1978). Trace nutrients. Selenium in British foods. British Journal of Nutrition 39: 391–396.

Trowell H, Southgate DAT, Wolever TMS, Leeds AR, Gassull MA, Jenkins DJA. (1976). Dietary fibre redefined. Lancet 1: 967.

Tucker RE, Hinman WF, Holliday EG. (1946). The retention of thiamin and riboflavin in beef cuts during braising, frying and broiling. Journal of the American Dietetic Association 22: 877–881.

Underwood EJ. (1977). Trace Elements in Human and Animal Nutrition. 4th edition. Academic Press, New York.

USDA (U.S. Department of Agriculture) (1976). Composition of foods — raw, processed and prepared. Agriculture Handbook No. 8–1: Dairy and egg products. Agriculture Research Service, U.S. Department of Agriculture, Washington, D.C.

USDA (U.S. Department of Agriculture) (1977). Composition of foods — raw, processed and prepared. Agriculture Handbook No. 8–2: Spices and herbs. Agriculture Research Service, U.S. Department of Agriculture, Washington, D.C.

USDA (U.S. Department of Agriculture) (1978). Composition of foods — raw, processed and prepared. Agriculture Handbook No. 8–3: Baby foods. Agriculture Research Service, U.S. Department of Agriculture, Washington, D.C.

USDA (U.S. Department of Agriculture) (1979). Composition of foods — raw, processed and prepared. Agriculture Handbook No. 8–4: Fats and oils. Agriculture Research Service, U.S. Department of Agriculture, Washington, D.C.

USDA (U.S. Department of Agriculture) (1979). Composition of foods — raw, processed and prepared. Agriculture Handbook No. 8–5. Poultry products: Agriculture Research Service, U.S. Department of Agriculture, Washington, D.C.

USDA (U.S. Department of Agriculture) (1980). Composition of foods — raw, processed and prepared. Agriculture Handbook No. 8–6: Soups, sauces, gravies. Agriculture Research Service, U.S. Department of Agriculture, Washington D.C.

USDA (U.S. Department of Agriculture) (1980). Composition of foods — raw, processed and prepared. Agriculture Handbook No. 8–7: Sausages and luncheon meats. Agriculture Research Service, U.S. Department of Agriculture, Washington D.C.

USDA (U.S. Department of Agriculture) (1981). Composition of foods — raw, processed and prepared. Agriculture Handbook No. 8–8: Breakfast cereals. Agriculture Research Service, U.S. Department of Agriculture, Washington D.C.

USDA (U.S. Department of Agriculture) (1982). Composition of foods — raw, processed and prepared. Agriculture Handbook No. 8–9: Fruits and fruit juices. Agriculture Research Service, U.S. Department of Agriculture, Washington, D.C.

USDA (U.S. Department of Agriculture) (1983). Composition of foods — raw, processed and prepared. Agriculture Handbook No. 8–10: Pork products. Agriculture Research Service, U.S. Department of Agriculture, Washington, D.C.

USDA (U.S. Department of Agriculture) (1984). Composition of foods — raw, processed and prepared. Agriculture Handbook No. 8–11: Vegetable products. Agriculture Research Station, U.S. Department of Agriculture, Washington, D.C.

USDA (U.S. Department of Agriculture) (1984). Composition of foods — raw, processed and prepared. Agriculture Handbook No. 8–12: Nut and seed products: Agriculture Research Station, U.S. Department of Agriculture, Washington, D.C.

USDA (U.S. Department of Agriculture) (1986). Composition of foods — raw, processed and prepared. Agriculture Handbook No. 8–13: Beef products. Agriculture Research Station, U.S. Department of Agriculture, Washington, D.C.

USDA (U.S. Department of Agriculture) (1986). Composition of foods — raw, processed and prepared. Agriculture Handbook No. 8–14: Beverages. Agriculture Research Station, U.S. Department of Agriculture, Washington, D.C.

USDA (U.S. Department of Agriculture) (1987). Composition of foods — raw, processed and prepared. Agriculture Handbook No. 8–15: Finfish and shellfish products. Agriculture Research Station, U.S. Department of Agriculture, Washington, D.C.

Verdier PC. (1987). The Canadian nutrient file: how Canadian are the data? Journal of the Canadian Dietetic Association 48: 21–23.

Walters CB, Sherlock JC, Evans WH, Read JI. (1983). Dietary intake of fluoride in the United Kingdom and fluoride content of some foodstuffs. Journal of the Science of Food and Agriculture 34: 523–528.

Watt BK, Merrill AL, Pecot RK, Adams CF, Orr ML, Miller DF. (1963). Composition of foods — Raw, processed and prepared. Agriculture Handbook No. 8., Agriculture Research Station, USDA U.S. Department of Agriculture, Washington, D.C.

Wenlock RW, Buss DH, Dixon EJ. (1982). Trace nutrients 2. Manganese in British food. British Journal of Nutrition 41: 381–390.

Wenlock RW, Buss DH, Moxon RE, Bunton NG. (1979). Trace nutrients 4. Iodine in British food. British Journal of Nutrition 47: 253–261.

Wenlock RW, Sivell LM, Agater IB. (1985). Dietary fibre fractions in cereal and cereal-containing products in Britain. Journal of Science of Food and Agriculture 36: 113–121.

Widdowson EM, McCance RA. (1943). Food tables: their scope and limitations. Lancet 1: 230–232.

Williams RD, Olmstead WH. (1935). A biochemical method for determining indigestible residue (crude fiber) in feces: lignin, cellulose and non-watersoluble hemicelluloses. Journal of Biological Chemistry 108: 653–666.

Wood DF, Stewart LM, Campbell CA. (1988). Nutrient composition of 21 retail cuts of Canadian beef. Journal of the Canadian Dietetic Association 49: 29–36.

Chapter 5

Measurement errors in dietary assessment

Random and/or systematic errors may occur during the measurement of food and/or nutrient intakes. The direction and extent of these errors vary with the method used and the population and nutrients studied. Both types of measurement error can be minimized by incorporating a variety of quality control procedures during each stage of the measurement process. Random errors affect the precision of the method (Chapter 6). They can be reduced by increasing the number of observations, but cannot be entirely eliminated. In contrast, systematic measurement errors cannot be minimized by extending the number of observations. They are important as they can introduce a significant bias into the results which cannot be removed by subsequent statistical analysis.

This chapter discusses the sources of random and systematic errors which occur during the collection and recording of food consumption data. Errors associated with the compilation of nutrient data and the nutrient analysis of food items are not considered here, but are discussed in Section 4.3.

5.1 Sources of measurement error

Many of the sources of both random and systematic error are similar in household and individual food consumption survey methods. The major errors in the collection and recording of the food consumption data are summarized in Table 5.1; the assessment and control of each type of error is then discussed in more detail below.

5.2 Assessment and control of measurement errors

Random and systematic measurement errors can be minimized by incorporating various quality control procedures into each stage of the dietary

- **Respondent biases** may lead respondents to overestimate facts such as income and age. Consumption of 'good' foods such as fruits and vegetables may also be over-reported, whereas the consumption of 'bad' foods, such as snack or 'fast' foods, and the use of alcohol and tobacco, may be under-reported. Overweight respondents may tend to under-report food intakes whereas underweight persons may over-report food intakes.

- **Interviewer biases** may occur if different interviewers probe for information to varying degrees, intentionally omit certain questions and/or record responses incorrectly.

- **Respondent memory lapses** may result in the unintentional omission or addition of foods in recall methods.

- **Incorrect estimation** of portion size occurs when respondents fail to quantify accurately the amount of food consumed. Alternatively, the respondent's concept of an average 'serving' size may deviate from the standard, or an interviewer may assume an answer such as an average serving size.

- **Supplement usage** may be omitted from the dietary record or recall, causing significant errors in the calculated nutrient intakes.

- **The 'flat slope syndrome'** is a bias that may be introduced by a tendency to overestimate low intakes and underestimate high intakes in recall methods. The observed relationship, however, may be an artifact of the statistical analysis and the result of regression towards the mean.

- **Coding and computation errors** arise when portion size estimates are converted from household measures into grams, or when food items are incorrectly coded (e.g. 2% milk is coded as whole milk). When computerized nutrient databases are used, the computer program and the associated database may be major sources of error.

Table 5.1: Major sources of error in the collection and recording of food consumption data.

assessment protocol. These can include training and retraining sessions for the interviewers and coders, standardization of interviewing techniques and questionnaires, pretesting of questionnaires, and administration of a pilot study prior to the survey. Each procedure in the method must be continuously checked to ensure compliance with standardized protocols.

Random errors, unlike systematic errors, can be minimized by increasing the number of observations. Random errors may occur across all subjects and all days. In contrast, systematic errors may exist for only certain respondents (e.g. obese or elderly subjects) and/or specific interviewers. The effects of systematic errors associated with specific interviewers can be minimized if it is ensured that the assignment of respondent to interviewer is random. In this way, subjects will not normally be questioned by the same interviewer on all occasions (Anderson, 1986).

5.2.1 Respondent biases

Respondent biases arise because the respondent may: misunderstand what the interviewer has requested; receive nonverbal cues to the 'right answers' from the interviewer; or have a need to give 'socially desirable' answers. Such biases may be random across days for an individual or, for persons with specific characteristics (e.g. obesity), be systematic. For example, if the study population is stratified by relative weight, and overweight persons in the population tend to under-report their food intake, then a systematic bias in the mean intakes for the overweight subgroup will occur (Anderson, 1986). Nonresponse may also bias the data if the sample loses its randomness.

Respondent bias in relation to the consumption of beer, wine, and distilled spirits was noted by the U.S. subcommittee on criteria for dietary evaluation (NRC, 1986). Reported intakes for adults in the United States National Food Consumption Survey and the United States National Health and Nutrition Examination Survey (NHANES) were under-reported compared to estimates of alcohol disappearance, prepared by the United States Bureau of Alcohol, Firearms and Tobacco Control (Pao et al., 1982).

Gersovitz et al. (1978) examined the potential bias resulting from poor response in their study of seven-day records completed by 65 elderly subjects. Demographic comparisons were made between those respondents who returned usable seven-day records and those who did not. Results indicated that the mean nutrient intakes calculated from the usable dietary records represented a selectively biased group of more highly educated respondents.

Very few studies have investigated other specific sources of respondent bias. Worsley et al. (1984) suggested that a social desirability response bias influenced responses to a dietary questionnaire (Table 5.2). Reported intakes of certain foods such as fresh fruits and vegetables and sweet foods were particularly susceptible to social approval needs and hence a potential source of systematic bias. They recommended the use of a social desirability scale in dietary surveys to identify and perhaps control for social desirability variables.

5.2.2 Interviewer biases

Interviewer biases include errors caused by incorrect questions, incorrect recording of responses, intentional omissions, biases associated with the interview setting, distractions, confidentiality and anonymity of the respondent, and the degree of rapport between interviewer and the respondent. Interviewer biases can be random across days and subjects, systematic for a specific interviewer, or exist as an interaction between certain interviewers and respondents only (Anderson, 1986).

Statement

I rarely eat snacks between meals. (T)
I always brush my teeth after every meal. (T)
I hardly ever eat candies or chocolate. (T)
I often watch TV or read a newspaper whilst eating a meal. (F)
There have been many occasions when I
        have not washed my hands before eating food. (F)
I never drink alcohol when I'm by myself. (T)
I often find myself eating food in a hurry. (F)
My table manners at home are as good as
        when I eat out in a restaurant. (T)
I try to avoid eating take-away foods. (T)
There have been few occasions when I
        have 'raided the refrigerator'. (F)
I usually eat everything on my plate. (T)
I have never been 'really drunk' in my life. (T)

Table 5.2: Statements used to assess attitudes to food and drink. The letters (T) or (F) after each statement indicate whether the true or false answer was the socially desirable response. From Worsley et al. (1984) with permission.

The most common approach to assess interviewer bias has been to compare nutrient intakes calculated from multiple interviews carried out independently on the same subjects during the same twenty-four-hour eating period, using different trained interviewers. Frank et al. (1984) utilized this method to investigate the effect of interviewer recording practices on calculated nutrient intakes. They examined the extent of agreement of food descriptors, food quantities, codes assigned, and calculated nutrient intakes. Their results indicated difficulties in quantifying selected food items such as meat and sweets. Significant differences in calculated intakes of energy, fat, and unsaturated fat resulting from differences in coding snack foods were also found. This multiple interview approach was also used successfully by the National Heart, Lung and Blood Institute for their Lipid Research Clinic Program (Beaton et al., 1979). They used a carefully standardized protocol and experimental design which enabled them to conclude that the interviewer had no effect on the calculated energy, protein, and lipid intakes of the subjects.

In order to minimize interviewer and respondent biases, the interviewer should be trained to anticipate and recognize potential sources of distortion and bias (Wakefield, 1966). Efforts should be made to minimize the nonresponse rate by training the interviewer to convey warmth, understanding, and trust. Value judgements by the interviewer should be avoided at all times (Hughes, 1986). When several interviewers are employed, the assignment of interviewers-respondents-days should be random to avoid systematic bias (Anderson, 1986).

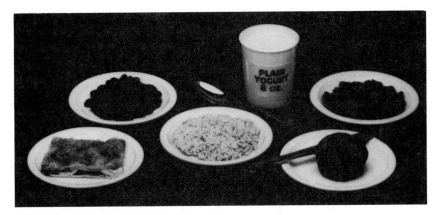

Figure 5.1: Food models for use as a memory aid in dietary assessment. Photograph courtesy of NASCO, 901 Janesville Ave., Fort Atkinson, Wisconsin, 53538.

5.2.3 Respondent memory lapses

Errors generated by memory lapses can be reduced by 'probing' questions and/or by using memory aids such as food models. Campbell and Dodds (1967) reported that probing increased reported dietary intakes of hospital patients, assessed by twenty-four-hour recalls, by 25% compared to those obtained without probing. Memory aids may consist of plastic or clay simulated foods, actual foods, natural-sized colored paintings or photographs (Figure 5.1).

Memory lapses will be minimized in recall methods if the time period between the actual food intake and its recall is short. Twenty-four hours is the time period most frequently selected for memory-based procedures. As a check on the recall ability of interviewees, duplicate recalls, collected independently by two trained interviewers for the same twenty-four-hour period, have been obtained (Frank et al., 1977). Such a procedure on children yielded errors ranging from 9% to 21%.

Generally, foods contributing to the main part of a meal are remembered better than condiments, salad dressings, etc. Guthrie (1984) reported that for one in six respondents, salad dressings were forgotten.

5.2.4 Incorrect estimations of portion size

The errors associated with the estimation of portion size of foods are probably the largest source of measurement error in many dietary survey methods. The respondent may be unable to accurately quantify the portion of food consumed, or the perceived average serving may differ from the standard average serving.

Unfortunately, few studies have attempted to quantify these sources of measurement error. Guthrie (1984) assessed the accuracy with which young adults could describe portion sizes of foods consumed, in terms

	n	Mean	Median	Range	Standard Measure
Slice of brown bread (g)	30	30	30	25–38	30
Butter/margarine (g)	60	4	4	2–12	5
Gouda cheese (g)	34	21	20	9–42	20
Teacup (mL)	8	136	128	110–175	125
Drinking-glass (mL)	19	184	173	85–300	150
Teaspoon of sugar (g)	43	5	4	2–13	3

Table 5.3: Variation in household measures and portion sizes. From van Staveren and Hulshof (1980).

of common household measures or weights. No food models were used in this study. The ability of the respondents to describe the amounts of food consumed was poor. For thirteen food items, from 6% to 75% of respondents estimated portion sizes that varied by more than 50% of their actual weight. Twenty-six percent of the respondents consistently over- or underestimated all food items in the meal. Reported intakes of orange juice and milk were closer to actual intakes than food items such as breakfast cereals and butter.

When appropriate, the use of short group training sessions for respondents using food models or household measures should be encouraged. Bolland et al. (1988) observed that such training sessions enhance the ability of respondents to estimate food portion sizes accurately.

Guthrie (1984) also compared the amount of food selected as a usual portion size by young adults, in relation to the U.S. standards of average portion size. The latter are derived from USDA Nationwide Food Consumption Survey data (Pao et al., 1982). Items such as butter on toast, sugar on cereal, milk as a beverage, and tossed salad corresponded closely with standards, whereas others such as dry cereals, orange juice, and fruit salad did not. Men tended to select larger portions than women.

Van Staveren and Hulshof (1980) measured the actual weights of portion sizes of certain foods (e.g. slice of bread, butter, gouda cheese) and the volumes of various household utensils (e.g. teacup, drinking-glass) used in 30 households, and compared the results with standard portion sizes. The results (Table 5.3) indicate the large inter-subject variation in portion sizes and emphasize the extensive errors that can be introduced if standard portion sizes are assumed. Even in institutional settings such as a school canteen, the actual weights of food served can vary by as much as 18% (Comstock and Symington, 1982).

Graduated food models have been developed to assist in quantifying portions of foods consumed in dietary methods based on recall (Moore et al., 1967). Their effect on accuracy, however, has not been extensively investigated. Moore et al. (1967) reported that graduated food models increased the extent of the agreement in estimated portion sizes of milk,

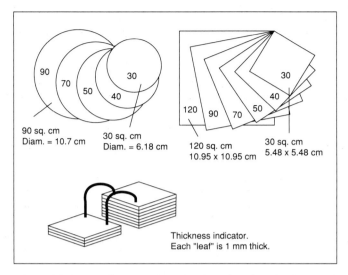

Figure 5.2: Models for use in the estimation of portion size developed by Health and Welfare Canada (1973).

rice, and kidney beans, when 30 couples were interviewed individually about their spouses' usual portion size, compared to the agreement found when only verbal descriptions in terms of household measures were used. More recently, Rutishauser (1982) noted that the coefficient of variation of the differences between actual and estimated weights of portion sizes by nutrition students ranged from 16% to 53% for household measures, but only 10% to 27% when food models and photographs were used.

The Nutrition Canada National Survey (Health and Welfare Canada, 1973) used a collection of *papier-maché,* wooden, or hardboard shapes of various volumes or surface areas as graduated food models. The surface area models were accompanied by thickness indicators made up of hardboard squares (Figure 5.2). These were used for the twenty-four-hour recalls to assist in assessing the overall size and thickness of foods such as cheese, cold meats, cakes, cookies, etc.

Graduated food models have also been used in several U.S. national food consumption surveys (NCHS, 1983.) The use of such models prevents the tendency to 'direct' response, a phenomenon observed when simulated plastic food models representing 'average' portion sizes are used (Samuelson, 1970).

To avoid errors associated with misconceptions of average portion sizes or servings of food, respondents should always be asked to measure and specify food portions by using household measures or, preferably, weights. If household measuring devices are used, they should be calibrated in each household (Nettleton et al., 1980). The practice of describing quantities of foods consumed in terms of standard servings should not be used for quantitative daily consumption methods. Such an approach, however, may be acceptable for a semiquantitative food frequency questionnaire. Hunter et al. (1988) suggest that specifying a standard portion size on the food frequency questionnaire may not introduce a large error in the estimation of food and nutrient intake. They noted that the contribution of the inter-subject variance to the total variance in portion size was smaller than the intra-subject variance. Consequently, additional questions on a food frequency questionnaire, to allow subjects to estimate individual 'usual' portion sizes, may not be justified. More studies are necessary, however, before any firm conclusions can be made.

5.2.5   Omission of information on nutrient supplement usage

Failure to collect data on the type, amount, and frequency of consumption of nutrient supplements will result in a systematic underestimate of intakes of certain nutrients. Unfortunately, this occurred during the 1977–1978 United States National Food Consumption Survey (NRC, 1984).

5.2.6   Tendency to overestimate low intakes and underestimate high intakes in recall methods

The flat slope syndrome in twenty-four-hour recalls has been has been demonstrated in more than three independent studies and among different age groups. The syndrome arises from the tendency for low dietary intakes to be overestimated and high intakes to be underestimated. Hence, the syndrome apparently produces a downward bias in the number of subjects with extremely low and extremely high intakes. The extent of the systematic error arising from the flat slope syndrome may vary with the age and sex of the study population (NRC, 1986), but the possible existence of the syndrome should be taken into account whenever nutrient intakes based on twenty-four-hour recall data are obtained.

Investigators have compared the ability of subjects to recall either a single meal (Gersovitz et al., 1978) or three meals (Linusson et al., 1974) after a twenty-four-hour period, with actual intakes obtained by unobtrusive weighing. Statistical analysis of the recall and actual intakes indicated a one-unit increase in the actual intake corresponded to significantly less than a one-unit increase in the recall intake (i.e. the slope was less than 1.0) (Figure 5.3).

The described syndrome may be partly a statistical artifact produced when regression analysis is used to examine the relationship between the actual intake (independent variable) and the reported intake (dependent variable). The numerical procedures are designed to minimize variation in the dependent variable and the result is an apparent downward bias in the number of subjects with extremely low and extremely high intakes.

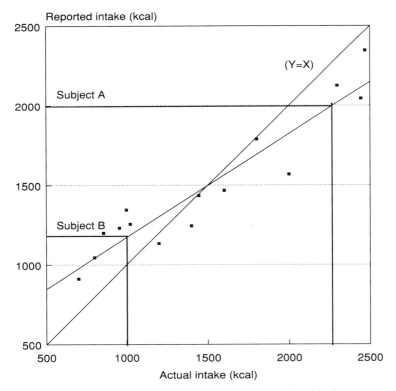

Figure 5.3: Hypothetical illustration of the relationship between the actual and reported dietary intakes. Individual observations are shown, along with the line Y = X and the regression line resulting from treating the actual intake as the independent variable. Points at the ends of the regression line appear to indicate under-reporting of intakes greater than the mean and over-reporting of intakes less than the mean. Adapted from Gersovitz M, Madden JP, Smiciklas-Wright H. Validity of the 24-hr dietary recall and seven-day record for group comparisons. © The American Dietetic Association. Reproduced by permission from Journal of the American Dietetic Association, Vol. 73: 48–55, 1978.

5.2.7 Coding errors

Duplicate coding of recalls or records by independent coders is used as a quality control for coding. Beaton et al. (1979) reported that coding errors arising exclusively from inadequate descriptions of foods, and not weight errors, resulted in coefficients of variation ranging from 3% for protein and 8% for total fat to 17% for the polyunsaturated:saturated fatty acid (P:S) ratio. Gross errors in coding can be reduced if 'coding rules' are established to deal with incomplete or ambiguous descriptors of the foods (Anderson, 1986), and large databases, with a comprehensive range of food items, are used (Dwyer and Suitor, 1984). The latter enable the

Sources of Error	24-hr. Recall	Dietary History	Estimated Record	Weighed Record
Omitting foods	+	+	±	±
Adding foods	+	+	−	−
Estimating food weights	+	+	+	−
Estimating frequency of food consumption	−	+	−	−
Day-to-day variation	+	−	+	+
Changes in diet	−	−	±	+
Coding errors	+	+	+	+

Table 5.4: Sources of error in techniques estimating food consumption. + error is likely; ± error is possible; − error is unlikely. Modified from Staveren WA van, Burema J. Food consumption surveys: frustrations and expectations. Näringsforskning 2: 38–42, 1985.

coder to select the appropriate food item more readily. Check digits can be included in the food code so that incorrect codes can be rapidly identified by the computer program. Detection of weight errors for food items during the coding can be facilitated by including a routine in the computer program which flags the subjects with the ten highest and ten lowest daily intakes of energy and selected nutrients such as protein, calcium, and iron. Checks can then be made for weight errors in the coded data for these selected subjects (Sabry et al., 1984).

Criteria for meal codes should be standardized and strictly adhered to throughout the study. Frank et al. (1984) noted that the use of quantity of food consumed for selecting meal codes, rather than time of consumption, led to some discrepancies in meal codes assignment by different interviewers.

5.3   Summary

This chapter has outlined the systematic and random errors that may occur during all stages of the collection and recording of food consumption data; the more important sources of error are summarized in Table 5.4.

Quality control procedures designed to minimize possible sources of measurement errors include training the interview and data coding staff, and developing standard interviewing techniques and questionnaires during the pilot survey. Sources of error arising from respondent memory lapses can be reduced by probing questions and/or by using visual aids such as food models. Graduated food models should be used to quantify portions of foods consumed when recall methods are used, rather than describing quantities of foods consumed in terms of standard serving sizes. Training respondents to estimate food portion sizes using food models or household measures will also improve the accuracy of recalled portion size estimates. Duplicate coding of recalls or records by independent coders can be used as a quality control for coding. When computerized nutrient databases are used, check digits can be included in the food code so that incorrect codes can be rapidly identified by the computer program. Systematic detection of wrongly coded weights of foods is more difficult.

References

Anderson SA. (1986). Guidelines for Use of Dietary Intake Data. Life Sciences Research Office, Federation of American Societies for Experimental Biology, Bethesda, Maryland.

Beaton GH, Milner J, Corey P, McGuire V, Cousins M, Stewart E, de Ramos M, Hewitt D, Grambsch PV, Kassim N, Little JA. (1979). Sources of variance in 24-hour dietary recall data: implications for nutrition study design and interpretation. American Journal of Clinical Nutrition 32: 2546–2559.

Bolland JE, Yuhas JA, Bolland TW. (1988). Estimation of food portion sizes: effectiveness of training. Journal of the American Dietetic Association 88: 817–821.

Campbell VA, Dodds ML. (1967). Collecting dietary information from groups of older people. Journal of the American Dietetic Association 51: 29–33.

Comstock EM, Symington LE. (1982). Distributions of serving sizes and plate waste in school lunches. Journal of the American Dietetic Association 81: 413–422.

Dwyer J, Suitor CW. (1984). Caveat emptor: assessing needs, evaluating computer options. Journal of the American Dietetic Association 84: 302–312.

Frank GC, Berenson GS, Schilling PE, Moore MC. (1977). Adapting the 24-hr recall for epidemiologic studies of school children. Journal of the American Dietetic Association 71: 26–31.

Frank GC, Hollatz AT, Webber LS, Berenson GS. (1984). Effect of interviewer recording practices on nutrient intake — Bogalusa Heart Study. Journal of the American Dietetic Association 84: 1432–1439.

Gersovitz M, Madden JP, Smiciklas-Wright H. (1978). Validity of the 24-hr dietary recall and seven-day record for group comparisons. Journal of the American Dietetic Association 73: 48–55.

Guthrie HA. (1984). Selection and quantification of typical food portions by young adults. Journal of the American Dietetic Association 84: 1440–1444.

Health and Welfare Canada (1973). Nutrition Canada National Survey. Health and Welfare, Ottawa.

Hughes BA. (1986). Nutrition interviewing and counseling in public health: the North Carolina experience. Topics in Clinical Nutrition 1: 43–50.

Hunter DJ, Sampson L, Stampfer MJ, Colditz GA, Rosner B, Willett WC. (1988). Variability in portion sizes of commonly consumed foods among a population of women in the United States. American Journal of Epidemiology 127: 1240–1249.

Linusson EEI, Sanjur D, Erickson EC. (1974). Validating the 24-hour recall as a dietary survey tool. Archivos Latinoamericanos de Nutrición 24: 277–281.

Moore MC, Judlin BC, Kennemur PM. (1967). Using graduated food models in taking dietary histories. Journal of the American Dietetic Association 51: 447–450.

NCHS (National Center for Health Statistics) (1983). Dietary Intake Source Data: United States, 1976–80. (Series 11, no. 231) (DHHS publication; no.(PHS) 83-1681), Washington, D.C.

NRC (National Research Council) (1984). National Survey Data on Food Consumption Uses and Recommendations. National Academy Press, Washington, D.C.

NRC (National Research Council) (1986). Nutrient Adequacy. Assessment using Food Consumption Surveys. Subcommittee on Criteria for Dietary Evaluation, Coordinating Committee on Evaluation of Food Consumption Surveys. Food and Nutrition Board, Commission on Life Sciences. National Academy Press, Washington, D.C.

Nettleton PA, Day KC, Nelson M. (1980). Dietary survey methods. 2. A comparison of nutrient intakes within families assessed by household measures and the semi-weighed method. Journal of Human Nutrition 34: 349–354.

Pao EM, Fleming KH, Guenther P, Mickle S. (1982). Foods commonly eaten by individuals. Amount per day and per eating occasion. Home Economics Research Report No. 44.

Rutishauser IHE. (1982). Food models, photographs or household measures? Proceedings of the Nutrition Society of Australia 7: 144.

Sabry JH, Gibson RS, Pen C. (1984). Nutrient Intake System. User's Guide for the Program. Department of Family Studies, University of Guelph.

Samuelson G. (1970). An epidemiological study of child health and nutrition in a northern Swedish county. 2. Methodological study of the recall technique. Nutrition and Metabolism 12: 321–340.

Staveren WA van, Burema J. (1985). Food consumption surveys: frustrations and expectations. Näringsforskning 2: 38–42.

Staveren WA van, Hulshof KFAM. (1980). De voedingsanamnese in het voedingsonderzoek, mogelijkheden en beperkingen. Voeding 41: 228–233.

Wakefield LM. (1966). The interview technique in research — source of bias. Journal of Home Economics 58: 640–642.

Worsley A, Baghurst KI, Leitch DR. (1984). Social desirability response bias and dietary inventory responses. Human Nutrition: Applied Nutrition 38A: 29–35.

Chapter 6

Precision in dietary assessment

A dietary assessment method is considered *precise* (reliable/reproducible) if it gives very similar results when used repeatedly in the same situation. The precision is a function of the measurement errors (discussed in Chapter 5) and uncertainty resulting from true variation in daily nutrient intakes (Hankin et al., 1967). Even if the measurement errors are minimized, uncertainty in the estimation of usual nutrient intakes remains. Consequently, although the dietary survey results from two separate occasions may disagree, the method may not be imprecise: the food intakes may indeed have changed. Therefore, only an estimate of precision can be made. True precision cannot be determined because replicate observations are impossible (Block, 1982).

For a group of individuals, true variability arises because dietary intakes differ among individuals (between- or inter-subject variation) and within one individual over time (within- or intra-subject variation) (Liu et al., 1978). Unlike measurement errors, no attempt should be made to minimize inter- and intra-subject variations because they characterize the true usual intake. Instead, the dietary assessment method should be designed in such a way that these two sources of variability can each be separated and estimated statistically using analysis of variance. In this way, the magnitude of the effect of inter-subject and intra-subject variation can be taken into account during the interpretation of the dietary data (Liu et al., 1978; Beaton et al., 1979; Sempos et al., 1985). Assessment of these two sources of variation is discussed in detail in Section 6.2.

If estimates of the inter- and intra-subject variation are obtained, they can be used to improve the design of a dietary assessment method to maximize the precision of the estimate of the usual intake of an individual or group. In this way, personnel, time, and budget can be used more effectively.

97

6.1   Estimation of precision in dietary assessment

In general, the precision of a dietary assessment method depends on
the time frame of the method, the population group under study, the
nutrient of interest, the technique used to measure the foods and quantities
consumed, and the inter- and intra-subject variance. Conventionally,
precision has been determined using a 'test-retest' design, in which the
same dietary method is repeated on the same subjects after a preselected
time interval. The selection of the latter depends on the time frame
of the dietary method selected. Care must be taken to avoid the
second measurement being influenced by the earlier one, as a result of
recollection of the first interview. The effects of season or changes in food
habits over time must also be minimized. Using the test-retest design,
the method has been considered precise if the nutrient intakes obtained
on the two separate occasions, by the same method, were similar. Lack
of agreement between the two sets of nutrient intake results, however,
does not necessarily reflect an imprecise method. The nutrient intake
may indeed have changed as a result of usual daily variations in food
intake (Räsänen, 1979; Block, 1982; Kim et al., 1984).

6.1.1   Precision of twenty-four-hour recalls

Several researchers have examined the precision of the twenty-four-hour
recall when used to estimate the mean nutrient intake of a group. In
general, results based on paired t-tests (Table 6.1) and/or correlation
analysis have suggested that this method can provide a relatively precise
estimate of the mean usual intakes of groups (Räsänen, 1979). However,
very few of these studies have measured the individual components of
variance as a basis for their conclusions.

In general, when single twenty-four-hour recalls are used, the number
of subjects required for estimation of the average usual intake of a group
is large. The number of subjects can be calculated, provided that the
inter-subject variation is known (Section 6.2). The number of subjects
needed will depend on the degree of precision required and the extent of
inter- and, for repeated recalls, intra-subject variability, which, in turn,
depends on the nature of the sample population and the nutrients of
interest.

Single twenty-four-hour recalls have been used to assess individual
intakes, presumably on the assumption that the intake over one twenty-
four-hour period adequately represents the habitual intake. This assumption is unlikely to be correct for individuals living in most industrialized
countries. Any estimate of an individual's usual intake, based on a single twenty-four-hour recall, has low precision because of relatively large
intra-subject variation in food intake. The precision can be improved
by obtaining several twenty-four-hour recalls for the same individual
(i.e. repeated twenty-four-hour recalls). Calculations can be performed

	Mean		Differences	
	Summer	Winter	Percentage	Significance
Energy (kcal)	2221	2256	−2	ns
Protein (g)	71	72	1	ns
Fat (g)	103	103	0	ns
Carbohydrate (g)	267	272	−2	ns
Calcium (mg)	1095	1080	1	ns
Iron (mg)	11.2	13.0	−14	**
Vitamin A (RE μg)	1004	1431	−30	*
Thiamin (mg)	1.3	1.4	−7	ns
Riboflavin (mg)	2.4	2.6	−8	ns
Niacin (mg)	11.7	12.0	−2	ns
Ascorbic acid (mg)	81	104	−22	**

Table 6.1: Comparison of mean daily intakes of energy and nutrients in two twenty-four-hour recalls (n = 158). Differences are expressed as percentages of the values obtained in the winter. Significant differences were observed for vitamin A ($0.01 < p < 0.05$ *), iron, and ascorbic acid ($0.001 < p < 0.01$ **), based on the results of the paired t-test. From Räsänen (1979). © Am. J. Clin. Nutr. American Society for Clinical Nutrition.

to determine the number of repeated twenty-four-hour recalls required to characterize the average intake of an individual, for a certain level of precision. For these calculations, the intra-subject variance must be known (Chalmers et al., 1952; Balogh et al., 1971; Liu et al., 1978; Beaton et al., 1979; Sempos et al., 1985). Measurement of inter- and intra-subject variation and details of these calculations are discussed more fully in Section 6.3.4.

6.1.2 Precision of food records

To minimize errors resulting from memory lapses and inadequate estimation of portion size, a weighed food record is often used. A seven-day weighed record is usually considered appropriate for the estimation of average intakes of individuals. However, respondent burden is high and problems with compliance may arise. Consequently, shorter periods, ranging from two to five days, are often used.

In general, studies of the precision of a seven-day weighed record have found good agreement between group mean values obtained for energy and most nutrients on two separate occasions, except when subjects have been on special diets. For example, Adelson (1960) found no significant differences between mean intakes derived from weighed records of thirty-nine professional men collected for two consecutive weeks. Average intakes for individuals, compared by paired difference tests, were also similar, with the exception of vitamin C. In a study of British bank

| | Correlation Coefficients Record 1 vs. 2 | |
	Pearson r	Intraclass r_I
Protein	0.56	0.56
Total fat	0.57	0.54
Saturated fat	0.57	0.56
Polyunsaturated fat	0.44	0.45
Cholesterol	0.54	0.53
Total carbohydrate	0.74	0.72
Sucrose	0.60	0.66
Crude fiber	0.65	0.65
Total vitamin A	0.47	0.56
Without supplements	0.34	0.41
Vitamin B-6	0.68	0.79
Without supplements	0.60	0.60
Vitamin C	0.67	0.70
Without supplements	0.63	0.68
Total calories	0.67	0.63

Table 6.2: Precision of seven-day weighed food records. Data obtained on two occasions one year apart from 173 female registered nurses, aged 34 to 59, residing in the Boston area, 1980–1981. Correlation coefficients were calculated on log transformed data to improve normality. From Willett WC, Sampson L, Stampfer MJ, Rosner B, Bain C, Witschi J, Hennekens CH, Speizer FE. Reproducibility and validity of a semiquantitative food frequency questionnaire. American Journal of Epidemiology 122: 51–65, 1985.

clerks, Heady (1961) compared the average weekly intakes of fifty men who completed two seven-day weighed records, one to nine months apart. Correlations ranging from 0.67 for protein to 0.84 for carbohydrate were reported. The bank clerks, however, were selected for the study because of their 'settled' diets.

In a more recent study of women living in the United States (Table 6.2), correlation coefficients between seven-day weighed records were generally lower (0.41 to 0.79), particularly for total vitamin A without supplements (intraclass r_I=0.41) and polyunsaturated fat (intraclass r_I=0.45) (Willett et al., 1985). Nevertheless, these studies suggest that the seven-day record can provide a relatively precise estimate of the usual nutrient intake of an individual.

The precision of two-day food records collected on two randomly selected days per sampling month over a two-year period was investigated by Sempos et al. (1985). The subjects were 151 middle-aged women. Precision in this study was based on analysis of variance estimates of the intra- and inter-subject variation and correlation analysis. Results

	1st Interview Mean	2nd Interview Mean	SD of Differences	Intraclass Correlation r_I
Energy (kcal)	2352	2327	434	0.86
Protein (g)	82	79	14	0.80
Fat (g)	101	103	26	0.81
Saturated fat (g)	45	46	9	0.89
Linoleic acid (g)	12	14	7	0.67
Carbohydrate (g)	256	248	46	0.87
Dietary fiber (g)	24	23	6	0.75
Alcohol (g)	12	12	8	0.91

Table 6.3: Precision of a dietary history based on interviews with forty-seven Dutch adults. Data were collected one month apart. From van Staveren et al. (1985). © Am. J. Clin. Nutr. American Society for Clinical Nutrition.

indicated that from one year to the next, the ratios of intra- to inter-subject variance were very similar. For all fifteen nutrients examined, intra-subject variation in the dietary intake was greater than inter-subject variation.

6.1.3 Precision of dietary histories

The precision of the dietary history for assessing usual mean intakes of individuals and/or groups depends on the time frame of the method, the time lag of the method, the technique of measuring amounts of foods consumed, and the population group. In general, this method yields good precision when used for a group, especially over a relatively short time frame. For example, van Staveren et al. (1985) concluded that their dietary history method, covering one month, provided precise estimates of group mean energy and nutrient intakes for an average weekday (Table 6.3). On an individual level, the high intraclass correlation coefficients (r_I) also indicated good overall agreement between the two dietary histories. For weekend days, precision was poorer, especially for saturated fat, carbohydrate, and linoleic acid, because of greater dietary variability at weekends.

In a case-control study on breast cancer in a group of Caucasian and Japanese-Hawaiian women, a dietary history questionnaire covering a typical week was repeated after three months (Hankin et al., 1983). Amounts of food consumed were estimated using photographs for each food shown in three serving sizes (small, medium, and large). Mean intakes of total fat, saturated fat, cholesterol, and animal protein for all subjects on the two occasions were not significantly different, as tested by the paired *t*-test. Furthermore, the extent of variability in nutrient intake, as measured by the standard deviation, was also similar in both interviews. Hence, the questionnaire yielded a reasonably precise

Question No.	No. of Possible Answers	Percentage of Number of Pairs of Answers				Total No. of Pairs of Answers
		Identical	Within One Grade of One Another	Separated by More than One Grade	Incomplete or Not Applicable	
2	5	39.6	46.0	14.2	0.0	63
3	5	58.2	30.7	9.3	1.8	3087
4	5	60.1	30.2	5.8	4.0	504
7	4	65.0	31.7	3.2	0.0	63
8	5	45.2	30.2	4.0	20.6	126

Table 6.4: Precision of the answers to questions in a food frequency questionnaire administered twice, with a three-month time lag. Subjects were ten cancer patients and fifty-three controls from the United Kingdom, all under the age of 75 years. From Acheson and Doll (1964) with permission.

estimate of the usual mean intake of total and saturated fat, cholesterol, and animal protein for the entire group. Nevertheless, when mean intakes for the two interviews were examined by ethnicity and case-control status, significant differences for the healthy Caucasian controls were found. These investigators suggested that a longer period was required to estimate the usual food intake of Caucasians, because of greater variability in their usual diets compared with Japanese-Hawaiian women.

Dutch investigators (van Beresteyn et al., 1987) evaluated, over a four-year period, the precision of a cross-check dietary history method covering one year. They noted that mean daily intakes of energy and most nutrients (total protein, vegetable and animal protein, total fat, saturated fat, mono- and polyunsaturated fat, carbohydrate, dietary fiber, calcium, phosphorus, cholesterol, iron, sodium) for the group of 246 women were very similar over each of the four years, with correlation coefficients ranging from 0.70 to 0.84. Vitamin A and vitamin C were exceptions, with lower correlation coefficients (0.63 and 0.67, respectively) attributed to variation in intakes of foods containing vitamins A and C.

6.1.4 Precision of food frequency questionnaires

Studies on the precision of food frequency questionnaires are limited. Acheson and Doll (1964) repeated a food frequency questionnaire after three months had elapsed. Respondents were asked to identify the frequency with which they consumed forty-eight foods and eight types of drinks using a five-point scale. After three months, 90% of the responses differed by less than one point from the original measurement, suggesting that the precision of the food frequency questionnaire for classifying the frequency of food use was good (Table 6.4).

	Correlation Coefficients Questionnaire 1 vs. 2	
	Pearson r	Intraclass r_I
Protein	0.54	0.52
Total fat	0.57	0.57
Saturated fat	0.55	0.55
Polyunsaturated fat	0.64	0.64
Cholesterol	0.64	0.63
Total carbohydrate	0.70	0.70
Sucrose	0.71	0.71
Crude fiber	0.67	0.64
Total vitamin A	0.57	0.58
Without supplements	0.52	0.49
Vitamin B-6	0.60	0.60
Without supplements	0.57	0.52
Vitamin C	0.59	0.58
Without supplements	0.62	0.59
Total calories	0.63	0.63

Table 6.5: Precision of a semiquantitative food frequency questionnaire. Data obtained on two occasions one year apart from 173 female registered nurses, aged 34 to 59, residing in the Boston area, 1980–1981. Correlation coefficients were calculated on log transformed data to improve normality. From Willett WC, Sampson L, Stampfer MJ, Rosner B, Bain C, Witschi J, Hennekens CH, Speizer FE. Reproducibility and validity of a semiquantitative food frequency questionnaire. American Journal of Epidemiology 122: 51–65, 1985.

Willett et al. (1985) evaluated the precision of a self-administered, semiquantitative food frequency questionnaire on 173 female registered nurses, after a time lapse of one year. Portion sizes of 99 foods were specified using household measures (e.g. slice of bread, 8-ounce (227 mL) glass of milk), where possible. Mean daily nutrient intakes were similar. Intraclass correlation coefficients (r_I) for nutrient intake scores, adjusted for total energy intake, ranged from 0.49 for total vitamin A (without supplements) to 0.71 for sucrose (Table 6.5).

6.2 Sources of true variability in nutrient intakes

If measurement errors are reduced, the precision of any method for assessing individual nutrient intakes of a group is a function of the overall true variability in nutrient intakes (Sempos et al., 1985). This variability is largely determined by the inter- (between) and intra- (within) subject variation. In dietary assessment procedures, no replicate observations are possible. Hence, as noted earlier, intra-subject variation cannot

	Mean	Coefficient of Variation			
		Total	Inter-	Intra-	Ratio
Energy (kcal/day)	2639	35.8	24.9	25.7	1.0
Protein (g/day)	98.2	46.1	29.1	35.7	1.2
Carbohydrate (g/day)	264.6	37.7	23.4	29.5	1.3
Fat (g/day)	113.9	41.7	28.1	30.8	1.1
Cholesterol (mg/day)	521.1	59.4	28.2	52.3	1.9
Calcium (mg/1000 kcal)	356.1	49.7	26.4	42.2	1.6
Iron (mg/1000 kcal)	5.99	27.6	12.7	24.5	1.9
Thiamin (mg/1000 kcal)	0.674	39.9	16.9	36.2	2.1
Riboflavin (mg/1000 kcal)	0.929	48.5	18.7	44.8	2.4
Vitamin C (mg/1000 kcal)	42.4	71.5	31.7	64.1	2.0
Crude fiber (g/1000 kcal)	1.43	50.5	23.6	44.7	1.9

Table 6.6: Estimated coefficients of variation for total, inter-subject and intra-subject variability, and the ratio of intra- to inter-subject coefficients of variation. Intra-subject variability is taken as the residual in the analysis of variance and includes both intra-subject variation and variability of the methodology. Data from a study of 30 Toronto male subjects using a twenty-four-hour dietary recall, repeated on six days. From Beaton et al. (1979; 1983). © Am. J. Clin. Nutr. American Society for Clinical Nutrition.

be distinguished statistically from the measurement errors described in Chapter 5. Nevertheless, if the quality control procedures outlined in Section 5.2 are used, some of the confounding effects of the measurement errors on intra-subject variability can be reduced, because measurement errors will be small in relation to intra-subject variability. As a result, intrasubject variability can be estimated, and inter-subject variability can be measured, using analysis of variance techniques.

Inter-subject variation

Subjects differ from each other in their true daily intake. The inter-subject variation is a measure of these difference and it varies with the nutrient. If inter-subject variation is large relative to intra-subject variation, subjects can be readily distinguished so that usual nutrient intakes of individuals can be characterized. Unfortunately, for most nutrients, inter-subject variation in nutrient intakes is usually smaller than intra-subject variation (Liu et al., 1978; Beaton et al., 1979; Gibson et al., 1985) (Table 6.6).

As a result, the mean intakes of a group can generally be assessed more precisely than individual intakes. To counteract the effect of inter-subject variation on group mean nutrient intakes, the sample size should be as large as possible, and representative of the group to be studied. For example, Table 6.7 shows that for any male study group with inter- and intra-subject variance comparable to the Toronto subjects, it would be necessary to include fifty or more subjects to be 95% certain that the

	Group Size, assuming one observation per individual					
	5	15	25	50	100	200
Energy (kcal/day)	± 32%	± 18%	± 14%	± 10%	± 7.2%	± 5.1%
Cholesterol (mg/day)	± 53%	± 31%	± 24%	± 17%	± 12%	± 8.4%

Table 6.7: Theoretical 95% confidence ranges for the percentage deviation of the group sample mean from the group usual intake, for groups of similar composition but different size. Data derived from a study of 30 Toronto male subjects using a twenty-four-hour dietary recall. From Beaton et al. (1979). © Am. J. Clin. Nutr. American Society for Clinical Nutrition.

observed group mean energy intake was within 10% of the true group mean.

Age and sex

Variation in nutrient intakes resulting from the age and sex differences of the subjects can contribute to the estimate of inter-subject variation. As a result, energy and nutrient intakes are generally presented separately by age and sex. Sex differences appear to be largely associated with differences in the amounts of food consumed, rather than the pattern of food consumption (Beaton et al., 1979). If nutrient intakes are expressed in terms of nutrient densities, differences between males and females tend to disappear (see example in Table 6.10 and Beaton et al., 1979). Moreover, the inter-subject variation is often reduced. This approach does not, however, reduce the intra-subject variation or the ratio of inter- to intra-subject variation (variance ratio) (Section 6.3.4).

Intra-subject variation

The true day-to-day variation in intake of the same subject is measured by the intra-subject variation: it cannot be estimated from a dietary history. Intra-subject variation, measured by analysis of variance, represents the sum of true variation in intake from day to day within the same person, plus all sources of random variation that remain in the data set. The extent to which intra-subject variation differs from person to person is unknown (Anderson, 1986). Consideration of intra-subject variation is particularly important if data on usual intakes of individuals are required for correlation with biochemical or clinical parameters. The effect of large intra-subject variation in a dietary component in relation to inter-subject variation is to mask significant correlations (Liu et al., 1978). This problem is particularly evident when a one-day diet record or recall is used to estimate usual intake of an individual. The theoretical reduction in the absolute value of the correlation coefficient can be calculated from the ratio of intra- to inter-subject variation (variance ratio) and the number of replicate observations (Table 6.8), provided that the sample size is large (i.e. > 100). For example, if the observed variance ratio is 2.0,

| Variance | Number of Replicates per Individual | | | | | |
Ratio	1	3	5	7	10	14
0.0	1.00	1.00	1.00	1.00	1.00	1.00
0.5	0.82	0.93	0.95	0.97	0.98	0.98
1.0	0.71	0.87	0.91	0.94	0.95	0.97
1.5	0.63	0.82	0.88	0.91	0.93	0.95
2.0	0.58	0.77	0.85	0.88	0.91	0.94
2.5	0.53	0.74	0.82	0.86	0.89	0.92
3.0	0.50	0.71	0.79	0.84	0.88	0.91
3.5	0.47	0.68	0.77	0.82	0.86	0.89
4.0	0.45	0.65	0.75	0.80	0.85	0.88
4.5	0.43	0.63	0.73	0.78	0.83	0.87
5.0	0.41	0.61	0.71	0.76	0.82	0.86

Table 6.8: Attenuation factors for simple correlation coefficients as determined by the number of replicate observations per individual and the variance ratio (the ratio of the intra- to inter-subject variances). Abstracted from a more complete data table given in Anderson SA. (1986). Guidelines for Use of Dietary Data. Life Sciences Research Office, Federation of American Societies for Experimental Biology.

as determined from three separate dietary intake measurements (such as three twenty-four-hour recalls) the correlation coefficient (r) between the estimated intake and some biochemical parameter is 77% of the true correlation. This figure represents the theoretical attenuation factor from Table 6.8. Hence, the calculated correlation coefficient can be corrected by dividing by 0.77 before testing the significance of the r value. With small sample sizes (i.e. < 100), however, this correction is not advised because the sampling error associated with the correlation coefficient may be too large. The complete data tables for attenuation factors for both simple correlation coefficients and simple linear regression coefficients are given in Appendix A6.1 and A6.2.

In summary, for individuals attenuation may: (a) reduce the absolute value of the correlation coefficient (discussed above); (b) reduce the significance of regression; or (c) result in misclassification of nutrient intakes of individuals into quintiles (Anderson, 1985). Such effects may have major implications in epidemiological studies of dietary risk factors and disease (Liu et al., 1978; Beaton et al., 1979; Sempos et al., 1985).

The effects of intra-subject variation on the estimate of the true usual mean nutrient intake of individuals can be minimized by increasing the number of days of the measurement on each individual. Table 6.9 shows that for male subjects comparable to the Californian group, it would be necessary to make weighed observations on at least five days to be 95% certain that the observed mean energy intake of an individual was within 25% of the true mean.

	Replicate Measures per Individual			
	1	2	5	'Infinite'
Energy	± 55%	± 39%	± 25%	± 10%
Protein	± 64%	± 45%	± 29%	± 12%

Table 6.9: Theoretical 95% confidence ranges for the percentage deviation of the observed mean intake of an individual from the true usual mean intake of the individual, for different numbers of replicate observations. Data calculated from fifteen-day weighed food intakes of eighteen healthy, male, Californian subjects, recorded on tape. From Todd et al. (1983). © Am. J. Clin. Nutr. American Society for Clinical Nutrition.

Measurement days should represent the population of days to be studied. For example, the days can be closely spaced to eliminate bias from seasonal changes, and selected such that weekend days as well as weekdays are proportionately included (Sempos et al., 1985). Nonadjacent days should be chosen rather than consecutive days because they yield greater statistical information (NRC, 1986). Minimizing intra-subject variation by increasing the number of measurement days does not affect the inter-subject variation; it simply enables the usual intake of individuals to be characterized more precisely.

The extent of intra-subject variation in a dietary assessment method depends, in part, on the diversity of food intake. For example, diets of persons in some less industrialized countries tend to be less varied than those of more industrialized countries, resulting in intakes with low intra-subject variability.

Both inter- and intra-subject variation depend on the nutrient of interest. Generally, for nutrients found in high concentrations in a few foods, such as vitamin A, vitamin D, sodium, cholesterol, and linoleic acid, inter- and intra-subject variation are high, making it more difficult to obtain precise estimates of the usual intakes of these nutrients. Conversely, inter- and intra-subject variation are lower for nutrients widely distributed in foods, such as carbohydrate and protein (Liu et al., 1978; Gibson et al., 1985) (Table 6.6).

Day-of-the-week effects

Group mean nutrient intakes (per day) and individual usual intakes (per day) may both vary with the day of the week. Beaton et al. (1979) demonstrated that women, not men, ate more food on Sundays than weekdays. Such sex differences have not been observed in other studies of the day-of-the-week effect. For example, van Staveren et al. (1982) demonstrated that both sexes had lower intakes of dietary fiber at

| | Fiber Intake (Mean ± SD) ||
	g/day	g/1000 kcal
Men (n=44)		
Weekdays	28.7 ± 8.5	10.7 ± 2.8
Weekends	24.5 ± 10.2	8.8 ± 3.7
Significance of differences	p < 0.01	p < 0.01
Women (n=56)		
Weekdays	21.9 ± 5.0	11.4 ± 2.7
Weekends	19.7 ± 6.7	9.6 ± 3.5
Significance of differences	p < 0.05	p < 0.01

Table 6.10: Comparison of the mean daily dietary fiber intakes of male and female subjects on weekdays (Monday to Friday) with weekends (Saturday and Sunday). Data from the intakes of 150 Dutch adults, calculated from seven-day estimated food records. From Staveren WA van, Hautvast JGAJ, Katan MB, Montfort MAJ van, Oosten-Van der Goes HGC van. Dietary fiber consumption in an adult Dutch population. A methodological study using a seven-day record. © The American Dietetic Association. Reproduced by permission from Journal of the American Dietetic Association, Vol. 80: 324–330, 1982.

weekends (Table 6.10). Not all nutrients exhibit a weekend effect: for those where there are large intra- and inter-subject fluctuations in daily intakes (e.g. cholesterol, vitamin A, and sodium), a weekend effect may not be evident (Gibson et al., 1985).

The weekend effect on nutrient intakes sometimes disappears when the latter are expressed in terms of nutrient densities (Beaton et al., 1979; Gibson et al., 1985). This finding suggests that food consumption patterns are comparable for weekdays and weekend days, but total energy intakes differ. This is not, however, always the case (Table 6.10).

Day-of-the-week effects on usual intakes of an individual or group can be accounted for by proportionately representing all days of the week in the study design (Beaton et al., 1979; Sempos et al., 1985).

Seasonal effects

The effects of the different seasons of the year on food or nutrient intake depend on the population group, its socio-economic status, and the country. In general, seasonal effects will probably be greater for food items rather than nutrient intakes.

Very few seasonal effects have been demonstrated for energy intakes in recent studies of preschool children (Räsänen, 1979) and adults in industrialized countries (Kim et al., 1984; Sempos et al., 1984; van Staveren et al., 1986), whereas marked effects have been noted in less industrialized countries (Ross et al., 1986). Intakes of nutrients such as vitamin A, vitamin C, iron, and in some cases fat, appear to show seasonal variation in both less developed and industrialized countries (Räsänen, 1979; Ross et al., 1986; van Staveren et al., 1986).

A seasonal effect can be taken into account by administering the survey over a long interval of time (e.g. one year), so as to include randomly selected days representative of all seasons of the year. If this is not done, investigators should beware of applying the results from one season over the whole year.

Training effects

Subjects may react to repeated interviews, showing a sequence or training effect which may alter reported nutrient intakes over time (Frank and Farris, 1984). This effect only occurs if subjects complete the recall or records on consecutive days. The presence or absence of a training effect on group mean or individual intakes can be assessed by completing the interviews or records on randomly selected days of the week and recording their order. Beaton et al. (1979) did not observe a training effect in their study involving highly trained, standardized interviewers.

The individual components of variance discussed above can all be estimated using analysis of variance (Section 6.3.4), provided that the initial design of the dietary assessment protocol allowed for their occurrence. The correct initial design is of the utmost importance.

6.3   Statistical assessment of precision

Until recently, very few studies of precision in dietary assessment methods have included any consideration of inter- and intra-subject variability. Instead, as noted earlier, precision of dietary methods has been assessed using the test-retest design, in which the same dietary method has been repeated on the same individuals after a preselected time interval.

The following section presents the statistical methods for assessing the extent of aggregate (group average) agreement (Section 6.3.1), and individual agreement (Sections 6.3.2 and 6.3.3), together with the analysis of variance for estimating sources of inter- and intra-subject variance (Section 6.3.4).

6.3.1   Paired tests on the mean or median intake

Paired *t*-tests or the nonparametric Wilcoxon's signed rank test for non-normally distributed data are commonly used to assess agreement between nutrient intakes on a group basis (Lee, 1980; Altman et al., 1983). No significant difference between the group mean or median intakes for the two sets of data is taken to indicate agreement (Table 6.1). The confounding effect of intra-subject variation on usual nutrient intakes is not taken into account when a paired *t*-test or the Wilcoxon's signed rank test is used. For instance, if intra-subject variation is large relative to inter-subject variation, the power of the *t*-test will be reduced. As a result, nonsignificant differences in group mean intakes may not necessarily indicate good precision but the confounding effect of large intra-subject variation.

6.3.2   Degree of misclassification

Assessment of the degree of misclassification is the simplest method of quantifying the extent of agreement on an individual basis (Lee, 1980). This approach is often used for food frequency questionnaires in which the data have been classified according to frequency of food use. The percentage of pairs with exact agreement or within a selected number of units is calculated (Table 6.4). Alternatively, if the food intake data collected are based on amounts in grams (e.g. semiquantitative food frequency questionnaire), the percentage of pairs agreeing within a defined amount (e.g. percentage agreeing within 10 g/week) of a specific food or food group can be determined. This approach, however, ignores the fact that a certain amount of agreement invariably occurs by chance alone.

6.3.3   Correlation analysis

Pearson's product moment correlation coefficients for normally distributed data or Spearman's nonparametric rank correlation coefficients are often calculated to assess agreement on an individual (within-pair) basis (Lee, 1980). High correlation coefficients for nutrient intakes calculated on the two separate occasions have been taken as indicative of good overall agreement between the two sets of nutrient data (Block, 1982). In fact, both parametric and nonparametric correlation coefficients quantify the extent of the linear trend relating the two sets of results, and not agreement. Instead, to measure the extent of overall agreement between the two sets of results, the intraclass correlation coefficient (r_I) should be used to correct for the number of chance expected agreements (Lee, 1980) (Tables 6.2 and 6.3; Section 7.3.2).

None of these correlation procedures takes into account the confounding effect of intra-subject variation on usual nutrient intakes. Its effect, if it is large relative to inter-subject variation, is to reduce the absolute value of the correlation coefficient relating pairs of individual nutrient intakes. Hence, the precision of the method may be incorrectly interpreted.

Caution must be used when correlation analysis is used to evaluate the extent of the agreement in a test-retest design for measuring precision. The correlation coefficients cannot be judged on a null hypothesis basis of no correlation because there is an *a priori* reason to believe that the methods are positively correlated (Altman et al., 1983).

6.3.4 Analysis of variance

The preferred statistical approach to estimate precision of any dietary method is to identify and estimate inter- and intra-subject variability using analysis of variance (Beaton et al., 1979; 1983). The variance ratio (the ratio of intra- (δ^2) to inter-subject (σ^2) variation) can then be calculated. It reflects the true usual intake and day-to-day variation in the nutrient intake (Sempos et al., 1985). Variance ratios depend critically on the nutrient, sample size, number of measurement days per subject, dietary methodology, and possibly the age, sex, and sociocultural group (NRC, 1986). Hence they should not used to compare different studies unless these factors are taken into consideration.

The NRC (1986) Report on Nutrient Adequacy presents a summary table of reported variance ratios for dietary studies of adults, compiled from the literature (Table 6.11). A ratio of 1.0 indicates that the intra-subject and inter-subject variances are equal. It will be seen that intra-subject variation is usually larger than inter-subject variation. Nutrients such as cholesterol, polyunsaturated fatty acids, and, in most cases, vitamin A have larger variance ratios than other dietary components. In general, energy intake appears to have the smallest variance ratio (approximately 1.0), with those for protein, carbohydrate, total fat, and saturated fats ranging approximately from 1.0 to 2.0. Use of nutrient supplements appears to reduce the variance ratios for the corresponding nutrients (Hunt et al., 1983; Sempos et al., 1985).

Once estimates of the inter- and intra-subject variability have been calculated using analysis of variance, they can be used in the following equations to estimate precision, based on the standard error of the mean. In practice, it is preferable to obtain estimates of the inter- and intra-subject variation before commencing the actual study. This can be achieved by conducting a pilot study, or by examining earlier survey data collected from a population comparable to the proposed study group. If such an approach is adopted, the intra- and inter-subject variance estimates can then be used to calculate either or both (a) the precision of the proposed dietary method to estimate the usual intake of a group, and (b) the precision of the proposed dietary method to estimate the usual intake of an individual (Cole and Black, 1984).

$$\text{(a) standard error of the group mean intake} = \sqrt{\frac{\sigma^2}{n} + \frac{\delta^2}{mn}}$$

$$\text{(b) standard error of the individual's mean intake} = \sqrt{\frac{\delta^2}{m}}$$

where: n = sample size, m = number of days measured, σ^2 = inter-subject variance, and δ^2 = intra-subject variance

Precision in dietary assessment

Nutrient	24-Hour Recall by Young Adults [a]	3-Day Record by Older Adults [b]	1-Day Recall by Women [c] Year 1	Year 2	7-Day Record by Men [d]	24-Hour Recall by Pregnant Women [e]
Males:						
Energy	1.1	1.0			0.8	
Protein	1.5	1.2			1.4	
Carbohydrate	1.6	2.1			0.6	
Fat	1.2	1.2			1.3	
SFA [f]	1.1	2.2			1.4	
PUFA [g]	2.8	3.5			1.9	
Cholesterol	3.4	5.6			1.9	
Vitamin A	[h]	1.6				
Vitamin C	3.5	2.3				
Thiamin	2.5	0.9				
Riboflavin	2.4	0.9				
Niacin equivalent	1.6	2.2				
Calcium	2.2	1.1				
Iron	1.7	1.8				
Females:						
Energy	1.4	0.8	1.6	1.6		1.1
Protein	1.5	1.3	2.1	2.1		1.4
Carbohydrate	1.4	1.2	NR [i]	NR		1.2
Fat	1.6	0.9	NR	NR		1.2
SFA [f]	1.4	1.7	NR	NR		NR
PUFA [g]	4.0	2.2	NR	NR		NR
Cholesterol	4.3	4.2	NR	NR		NR
Vitamin A	24.3	2.5	7.7	10.9		NR
Vitamin C	2.0	2.8	2.3	2.5		NR
Thiamin	4.4	1.6	3.3	3.9		NR
Riboflavin	2.2	1.8	3.0	3.3		NR
Niacin equivalent	4.0	2.5	NR	NR		NR
Calcium	0.9	1.7	1.1	1.2		1.0
Iron	2.5	1.5	2.7	2.5		NR

Table 6.11: Observed ratios of intra-subject to inter-subject variances. A ratio of 1.0 indicates that the intra-subject and inter-subject variances are equal. A ratio greater than 1.0 indicates that intra-subject variance is greater than inter-subject variance. The original papers contain additional data. Only those nutrient variables examined in two or more papers are included here. [a] From Beaton et al. (1979; 1983). [b] From Hunt et al. (1983). [c] From Sempos (1985). [d] From McGee et al. (1982). [e] From Rush and Kristal (1982). [f] Saturated fatty acids. [g] Polyunsaturated fatty acids. [h] None of the variance could be assigned to subjects. [i] NR = Not reported. Reproduced from Nutrient Adequacy: Assessment Using Food Consumption Surveys 1986, with permission of the National Academy Press, Washington, D.C.

Obviously, the experimental design will vary with the study objectives. Calculations can be made to improve the precision of the estimate of the usual intake of an individual or group by manipulating the sample size and the number of measurement days on each individual. Possible combinations range from many subjects and a few days to few subjects and many days depending on the degree of precision required and time, budget, and personnel constraints. Generally, it is more expensive and more time consuming to collect data from several measurement days on a smaller number of subjects than to study a larger sample for fewer measurement days (Cole and Black, 1984). Nevertheless, when comparisons of usual nutrient intakes between individuals are required, it is essential to measure intakes over multiple days. The U.S. subcommittee on criteria for dietary evaluation (NRC, 1986) recommended using independent days for replicating the measurements of one-day nutrient intakes to reduce any effect of autocorrelation between intakes on adjacent days.

Hence, once estimates of the inter- and intra-subject variability are known, the design of the dietary assessment protocol can be optimized. The true usual nutrient intakes of individuals or a group can be determined precisely, with the most efficient use of time, budget, and personnel.

6.4 Summary

Precision of dietary surveys refers to the extent to which a specific dietary method used repeatedly in the same situation gives similar results. In general, precision of a dietary assessment method depends on the time frame of the method, the population group under study, the nutrient of interest, the technique used to measure the foods and quantities consumed, and the inter- and intra-subject variance. True precision cannot be measured in dietary assessment because nutrient intakes vary daily. Instead, it is conventionally estimated using a test-retest design, followed by an assessment of the extent of the agreement between the nutrient intakes obtained on the two separate occasions, by the same method. Results of such tests suggest that the twenty-four-hour recall and dietary histories over a short time frame provide a relatively precise estimate of the average usual intake for most nutrients for a large group, but not for individuals. Weighed dietary records, especially those completed for seven days, yield more precise nutrient intakes on an individual basis, with the notable exception of vitamins A and C, and polyunsaturated fat. The precision of qualitative food frequency questionnaires for classifying individuals according to the frequency of use of certain foods/food groups is probably adequate; that of semiquantitative food frequency questionnaires depends on the nutrients under study.

Statistical methods to assess precision on a group average (aggregate) basis using a test-retest design include paired tests on the mean (paired t-tests), or median (Wilcoxon's signed rank test) intakes. For testing individual agreement, the simplest method is to calculate the percentage of misclassification, by comparing the number of pairs. For foods, this may be based on frequency of use, or amount (in grams), whereas for nutrients, scores (intakes per 1000 kcal) may be used. Alternatively, for individual agreement, correlation analysis can be performed, preferably using intraclass correlation to correct for the amount of chance-expected agreements. The preferred method of estimating precision in dietary assessment is to calculate the variance ratio (ratio of intra- to inter-subject variance), using analysis of variance. The variance ratio can only be calculated if the design of the dietary assessment enables inter- and intra-subject variation to be separated and estimated statistically. Variance ratios cannot be compared among different studies because they depend critically on the nutrient, sample size, number of measurement days per subject, dietary methodology, age, sex, and sociocultural group.

References

Acheson ED, Doll R. (1964). Dietary factors in carcinoma of the stomach: A study of 100 cases and 200 controls. Gut 5: 126–131.

Adelson S. (1960). Some problems in collecting dietary data for individuals. Journal of the American Dietetic Association 36: 453–461.

Altman DG, Gore SM, Gardner MJ, Pocock SJ. (1983). Statistical guidelines for contributors to medical journals. British Medical Journal 286: 1489–1495.

Anderson SA. (1986). Guidelines for Use of Dietary Data. Life Sciences Research Office, Federation of American Societies for Experimental Biology, Bethesda, Maryland.

Balogh M, Kahn HA, Medalie JH. (1971). Random repeat 24-hour dietary recalls. American Journal of Clinical Nutrition 24: 304–310.

Beaton GH, Milner J, Corey P, McGuire V, Cousins M, Stewart E, deRamos M, Hewitt D, Grambsch PV, Kassim N, Little JA. (1979). Sources of variance in 24-hour dietary recall data: implications for nutrition study design and interpretation. American Journal of Clinical Nutrition 32: 2546–2559.

Beaton GH, Milner J, McGuire V, Feather TE, Little JA. (1983). Sources of variance in a 24-hour dietary recall data; implications for nutrition study design and interpretation. Carbohydrate sources, vitamins, and minerals. American Journal of Clinical Nutrition 37: 986–995.

Beresteyn ECH van, Hof MA van't, Heiden-Winkeldermaat HJ van der, Ten Have-Witjes A, Neeter R. (1987). Evaluation of the usefulness of the cross-check dietary history method in longitudinal studies. Journal of Chronic Diseases 40: 1051–1058.

Block G. (1982). A review of validations of dietary assessment methods. American Journal of Epidemiology 115:492–505.

Chalmers FW, Clayton MM, Gates LO, Tucker RE, Wertz AW, Young CM, Foster WD. (1952). The dietary record — how many and which days? Journal of the American Dietetic Association 28: 711–717.

Cole T, Black A. (1984). Statistical aspects in the design of dietary surveys. In: The Dietary Assessment of Populations. Medical Research Council Scientific Report No. 4: 5–8.

Frank GC, Farris RP. (1984). Comparison of dietary intake by 2 computerized analysis systems. Journal of the American Dietetic Association 84: 818–820.

Gibson RS, Gibson IL, Kitching J. (1985). A study of inter- and intra-subject variability in seven-day weighed dietary intakes with particular emphasis on trace elements. Biological Trace Element Research 8: 79–91.

Hankin JH, Nomura AMY, Lee J. (1983). Reproducibility of a diet history questionnaire in a case-control study of breast cancer. American Journal of Clinical Nutrition 37: 981–985.

Hankin JH, Reynolds WE, Margan S. (1967). A short dietary method for epidemiologic studies. II Variability of measured nutrient intakes. American Journal of Clinical Nutrition 20: 935–945.

Heady JA. (1961). Diets of banks clerks. Development of a method of classifying the diets of individuals for use in epidemiologic studies. Journal of the Royal Statistical Society A124: 336–361.

Hunt WC, Leonard AG, Garry PJ, Goodwin JS. (1983). Components of variance in dietary data for an elderly population. Nutrition Research 3: 433–444.

Kim WW, Kelsay JL, Judd JT, Marshall MW, Mertz W, Prather ES. (1984). Evaluation of long-term dietary intakes of adults consuming self-selected diets. American Journal of Clinical Nutrition 40: 1327–1332.

Lee J. (1980). Alternate approaches for quantifying aggregate and individual agreements between two methods for assessing dietary intakes. American Journal of Clinical Nutrition 33: 956–958.

Liu K, Stamler J, Dyer A, McKeever J, McKeever P. (1978). Statistical methods to assess and minimize the role of intra-individual variability in obscuring relation ship between dietary lipids and serum cholesterol. Journal of Chronic Diseases 31: 399–418.

McGee D, Rhoads G, Hankin J, Yano K, Tillotson J. (1982). Within-person variability of nutrient intake in a group of Hawaiian men of Japanese ancestry. American Journal of Clinical Nutrition 36: 657–663.

NRC (National Research Council) (1986). Nutrient Adequacy. Assessment using Food Consumption Surveys. Subcommittee on Criteria for Dietary Evaluation, Coordinating Committee on Evaluation of Food Consumption Surveys. Food and Nutrition Board, Commission on Life Sciences. National Academy Press, Washington, D.C.

Räsänen L. (1979). Nutrition survey of Finnish rural children VI. Methodological study comparing the 24-hour recall and the dietary history interview. American Journal of Clinical Nutrition 32: 2560–2567.

Ross J, Gibson RS, Sabry JH. (1986). A study of seasonal trace element concentrations in selected households from the Wosera, Papua New Guinea. Tropical and Geographical Medicine 38: 246–254.

Rush F, Kristal AR. (1982). Methodologic studies during pregnancy: the reliability of the 24-hour dietary recall. American Journal of Clinical Nutrition 35: 1259–1268.

Sempos CT, Johnson NE, Smith EL, Gilligan C. (1984). A two-year dietary survey of middle-aged women: repeated dietary records as a measure of usual intake. Journal of the American Dietetic Association 84: 1008–1013.

Sempos CT, Johnson NE, Smith EL, Gilligan C. (1985). Effects of intraindividual and interindividual variation in repeated dietary records. American Journal of Epidemiology 121: 120–130.

Staveren WA van, de Boer JO, Burema J. (1985). Validity and reproducibility of a dietary history method estimating the usual food intake during one month. American Journal of Clinical Nutrition 42: 554–559.

Staveren WA van, Deurenberg P, Burema J, deGroot LCPGM, Hauvast JGAJ. (1986). Seasonal variation in food intake, pattern of physical activity and change in body weight in a group of young adult Dutch women consuming self-selected diets. International Journal of Obesity 10: 133–145.

Staveren WA van, Hautvast JGAJ, Katan MB, Montfort MAJ van, Oosten-Van der Goes HGC van. (1982). Dietary fiber consumption in an adult Dutch population. A methodological study using a seven-day record. Journal of the American Dietetic Association 80: 324–330.

Todd KS, Hudes M, Calloway DH. (1983). Food intake measurements: problems and approaches. American Journal of Clinical Nutrition 37: 139–146.

Willett WC, Sampson L, Stampfer MJ, Rosner B, Bain C, Witschi J, Hennekens CH, Speizer FE. (1985). Reproducibility and validity of a semiquantitative food frequency questionnaire. American Journal of Epidemiology 122: 51–65.

Chapter 7

Validity in dietary assessment methods

Validity describes the degree to which a dietary method measures what it purports to measure (Klaver et al., 1988). As discussed in Chapter 3, quantitative methods such as recalls or records are designed to measure actual or usual nutrient intakes at an individual or group level, depending on the number of measurements days, and/or the size of the study group. Others, such as the dietary history and food frequency questionnaire, provide retrospective information on food consumption patterns during a longer, less precisely defined time period. Such methods are most appropriate for measuring average use of foods, and sometimes nutrients, on both an individual and group basis.

Dietary methods designed to characterize usual intakes of individuals are the most difficult to validate because the 'truth' is never known with absolute certainty. Even if the actual food intake, monitored from the results of unobtrusive weighed observations, compares favorably with results obtained from food records maintained by the subjects during the same period, there is no guarantee that the records represent the usual food intake (Block, 1982). To detect any changes in usual intake during the study, observations of actual food intake both during, and either before or after, the study period should be compared. Such a procedure presents overwhelming practical difficulties, and consequently validity is generally determined in dietary methods covering relatively short time frames.

The errors that affect the validity of a dietary method are systematic errors; those associated with precision are random. At present, very little is known about the extent or direction of systematic errors associated with validity. They are also much more difficult to control than the measurement errors discussed in Chapter 5. Subjects may eat atypically during a dietary period, even though every effort is made to discourage this.

7.1   Measurement of relative validity

Because of the difficulties in measuring absolute validity of dietary intake data, researchers have adopted an approach which measures 'relative validity'. In this approach, the 'test' dietary method is evaluated against another 'reference' method. The selection of appropriate combinations of test and reference methods for relative validity studies depends on several factors:

Accuracy and precision

Both accuracy and precision must be high in the reference method selected. The method chosen must also be designed to measure similar parameters over the same time frame as the test method. For example, the relative validity of a single twenty-four-hour recall should not be assessed by comparison with a diet history or a seven-day weighed record. The latter two methods are designed to assess average nutrient intakes of individuals over a longer time frame than the twenty-four-hour recall. Moreover, a single twenty-four-hour recall is designed to assess the mean intake of a group, not the intake of an individual (Madden et al., 1976; Gersovitz et al., 1978).

Spacing of the test and reference methods

The spacing of the two methods must be carefully selected so that completion of the test method does not influence responses to the reference method. For example, the process of measuring and recording food intakes may sensitize participants with respect to food consumption so that they complete the second method more accurately than the first. However, too long a time interval between the two methods may introduce seasonal effects on food intake (Willett et al., 1985).

Errors

Errors in the two methods should be independent. This necessitates the reference procedure being different from the test method (Willett et al., 1985).

Other effects

The effects of season, day of the week, training, and the use of vitamin and mineral supplements should be taken into account during both the test and reference method (Sempos et al., 1985). These sources of variance are discussed in Section 6.2.

Methods of assessing relative validity using a variety of combinations of dietary methods are discussed below. For any combination, good agreement does not necessarily indicate validity: agreement may merely indicate similar errors in both methods. On the other hand, poor

	Mean Observed	Mean Recalled	Mean ± SE Difference	t-value	p-value
Energy (kcal)	2348	1896	452 ± 144	3.13	≤ 0.002
Protein (g)	82	66	16 ± 5.8	2.83	≤ 0.004

Table 7.1: Comparison of average observed with recalled energy and protein intakes of twenty-eight 10 to 12-year-old children attending a summer camp. From Carter RL, Sharbaugh CO, Stapell CA. Reliability and validity of the 24-hour recall. © The American Dietetic Association. Reproduced by permission from Journal of the American Dietetic Association, Vol. 79: 542–547, 1981.

agreement between the two methods suggests that at least one of the dietary methods is invalid (Mahalko et al., 1985).

7.1.1 Validity of twenty-four-hour recalls

The twenty-four-hour recall can be validated directly, in terms of the actual intake, more readily than other methods of dietary assessment because the time frame covered is short. Methods used include surreptitious observation, or weighing duplicate portions of the actual intake of foods recalled by the same subjects, over the same twenty-four-hour period or for one meal. This procedure has been employed in institutional settings such as congregate meal sites (Madden et al., 1976; Gersovitz et al., 1978), school lunch programs (Emmons and Hayes, 1973), college cafeterias (Krantzler et al., 1982), a metabolic unit (Greger and Etnyre, 1978), hospitals (Linusson et al., 1974), and summer camps (Carter et al., 1981).

In general, the twenty-four-hour recall tends to *underestimate* mean intakes in the elderly (Campbell and Dodds, 1967; Madden et al., 1976) and children (Carter et al., 1981) (Table 7.1). In some cases, the average results differed by as much as 30%. For other population groups, acceptable agreement for group mean intakes of energy and certain nutrients have been obtained (Greger and Etnyre, 1978; Stunkard and Waxman, 1981). For example, Greger and Etnyre observed no significant differences between actual intakes and the mean recalled intakes of energy, protein, calcium, and zinc for adolescent girls. In contrast, average recalls of vitamin A, thiamin, riboflavin, niacin, vitamin C, and iron were significantly less than actual intakes (Table 7.2).

Other researchers have assessed the relative validity of the twenty-four-hour recall method by comparison with a dietary history (Young et al., 1952; Balogh et al., 1971; Morgan et al., 1978; Räsänen, 1979) or a seven-day weighed record (Young et al., 1952). These methods of validation are not strictly appropriate because the test and reference methods do not measure intakes over the same time frame, nor are they designed to measure the same parameter.

	Actual Mean Daily Intake	Mean ($\pm$ SD) of Recalled Daily Intake	p-value
Energy (kcal)	2172	2000 ± 408	ns
Protein (g)	44	51 ± 13	ns
Vitamin A (IU)	7663	3377 ± 2278	< 0.001
Thiamin (mg)	2.3	1.4 ± 0.7	< 0.001
Riboflavin (mg)	2.7	1.6 ± 0.8	< 0.001
Niacin (mg)	29	16 ± 9	< 0.001
Ascorbic acid (mg)	116	78 ± 31	< 0.001
Calcium (mg)	391	418 ± 118	ns
Iron (mg)	25.5	14 ± 8	< 0.001
Zinc (mg)	6.7	8 ± 2	ns

Table 7.2: Comparison of actual observed intakes with recalled intakes. Data from seventeen female subjects, age 12.5 to 14.5 years. Statistical significance of the mean differences were assessed using the paired *t*-test; ns = not significant. From Greger and Etnyre (1978) by permission of the American Public Health Association.

7.1.2 Validity of dietary histories

Very few studies have measured the validity of the dietary history method by comparison with actual food intake. Bray et al. (1978), in a study of fifteen obese patients hospitalized in a metabolic unit, compared the actual food intake for one week with the results of three retrospective dietary histories, conducted subsequently at monthly intervals. Energy intakes were underestimated in the first dietary history, but by the third history, the correlation between actual and reported energy intakes had increased, attributed to improved reporting of alcohol intake.

The relative validity of the dietary history method has been most extensively assessed using the seven-day weighed or estimated food record as the reference method. In general, the dietary history produces *higher* estimates of group mean intakes than the seven-day record, especially if the estimated usual consumption for the dietary history has been assessed over a relatively long time period (six months to one year) (Young et al., 1952; Jain et al., 1980). Unfortunately, it is not possible to establish whether this bias arises from an underestimation of food intake by recording, or overestimation by the diet history. In cases where a shorter time frame for the dietary history has been used, smaller differences in mean intakes have been reported (Trulson and McCann, 1959; Dawber et al., 1962; Reshef and Epstein, 1972). Nevertheless, for those nutrients for which day-to-day variation in individual diets is notoriously high, notably vitamin A, cholesterol, and linoleic acid, poor agreement is usually observed, regardless of the time frame of the dietary history used (Mahalko et al., 1985) (Table 7.3).

	Dietary History	Food Record	% Diff.	Pearson's r	Intraclass r_I	% with Diff. < 20%	% in Same Tercile	% in Opposite Tercile
Energy (kcal)	1634	1745	−6	0.59†	0.58†	67	54	15
Carbohydrate (g)	194	200	−3	0.25	0.25‡	44	43	15
Protein (g)	72	73	−1	0.56†	0.56†	56	46	17
Fat (g)	65	74	−12*	0.74†	0.70†	46	59	11
Vitamin A (IU)	6147	6908	−11	0.22	0.21	30	41	19
Ascorbic acid (mg)	106	90	+18*	0.45†	0.39†	37	59	7
Niacin eq. (mg)	31	31	0	0.56†	0.57†	63	52	9
Riboflavin (mg)	1.6	1.7	−6	0.45†	0.45†	43	54	11
Thiamin (mg)	1.3	1.2	+8	0.47†	0.46†	48	52	11
Calcium (mg)	754	725	+4	0.69†	0.69†	48	50	7
Phosphorus (mg)	1221	1206	+1	0.68†	0.68†	57	56	4
Iron (mg)	13.8	13.7	+1	0.43†	0.44†	50	50	9
Zinc (mg)	10.5	10.2	+3	0.59†	0.59†	43	48	11
Potassium (g)	2.8	2.6	+8**	0.51†	0.49†	46	43	11
Sat. fatty acids (g)	25	27	−7*	0.75†	0.73†	48	59	7
Oleate (g)	23	27	−15*	0.76†	0.71†	43	56	6
Linoleate (g)	10	11	−9**	0.57†	0.54†	37	46	9
Cholesterol (mg)	260	315	−17*	0.42†	0.34†	17	35	20

Table 7.3: Comparison of the dietary history and seven-day food record results from fifty-four older United States adults aged 55 to 95 years. % difference = (dietary history − food record) ÷ dietary history × 100. * paired t-test indicates that differences are significant at $p < 0.05$; ** $p < 0.01$; significance of r or r_I: † $p < 0.01$; ‡ $p < 0.05$. From Mahalko et al. (1985). © Am. J. Clin. Nutr. American Society for Clinical Nutrition.

Recent interest in diet in relation to disease has prompted several studies of the validity of dietary history methods to determine dietary intakes over a long time span (Herbert and Miller, 1988). In such methods, there is a danger that long-term information may be distorted by the current intake, so that validity is reduced (Byers et al., 1983). For instance, Jain et al. (1980), in a prospective study of diet and cancer, showed that newly diagnosed cancer patients who were asked to recall their food intake six months ago underestimated the intakes which had been recorded at that time. The authors concluded that the recalled intakes in this study had been sufficiently influenced by the current intakes to distort the recall. Among the controls, however, there was little difference between reported and recalled intakes. Van Staveren et al. (1986a) also concluded, in their study of contemporaneous and retrospective estimates of food intake using a dietary history, that current food intake affected the reporting of past food intake. These studies emphasize the difficulties of obtaining unbiased estimates of retrospective food intakes, and such difficulties must be taken into account when interpreting the results of studies of diet and cancer (Herbert and Miller, 1988).

	Breakfast n=18 Mean ± SD	Lunch n=15 Mean ± SD	Dinner n=19 Mean ± SD
No. of foods per meal	5.14 ± 2.08	5.72 ± 1.97	6.34 ± 2.24
No. of foods agreeing	4.66 ± 1.99	5.00 ± 1.90	5.31 ± 2.04
Foods observed, not reported	0.48 ± 0.84	0.72 ± 0.94	0.99 ± 1.24
Foods reported, not observed	0.47 ± 0.81	0.63 ± 1.09	0.57 ± 0.89
Total food entries [a]	709	475	850
Total meal entries	138	83	134
Percent agreement	91%	87%	84%

Table 7.4: Assessment of the validity of seven-day food records obtained from students eating in a dormitory hall, by comparison with actual observed intakes. [a]Foods may be listed more than once. From Krantzler et al. (1982). © Am. J. Clin. Nutr. American Society for Clinical Nutrition.

7.1.3 Validity of food records

Attempts to validate directly the seven-day weighed food record have been made by comparing noon meals from each record with actual intakes, weighed surreptitiously during lunch at a congregate meal site for the elderly (Gersovitz et al., 1978). Although the record tended to underestimate the actual mean intakes, differences were only significant for energy and thiamin. Regression analysis showed that records from the first two days of record keeping were more valid for assessing group comparisons than those from the last three days, because of deterioration in accuracy of recording. Usable records during days five to seven were from the more highly educated respondents, resulting in a sample bias. These results question the apparent validity of the seven-day record to assess usual intakes of the elderly.

More recently, Krantzler et al. (1982) assessed the absolute validity of three- and seven-day food records by observing the actual food intake periodically for twenty-eight days. Respondents were university students eating meals in a dormitory dining hall. Validity was assessed by a food item agreement score, expressed as:

$$\frac{\text{Number of foods correctly identified} \times 100\%}{\text{Total number of foods reported}}$$

Intermittent duplicate diet collections have also been used to validate weighed and estimated food records (Gibson and Scythes, 1982; Sherlock, 1983; Holbrook et al., 1984; Kim et al., 1984). For example, in a recent U.S. study, 29 subjects consuming self-selected diets kept detailed weighed food records for one year and periodically made duplicate diet collections (Kim et al., 1984). The daily energy and nutrient intakes calculated from the one-year food records were significantly higher than

	Yearly Mean	Collection Mean	% Reduction
Energy (kcal)	2188	1905	12.9
Protein (g)	81	69	14.9
Fat (g)	89	78	12.9
Carbohydrate (g)	240	224	6.7
Crude fiber (g)	3.9	3.6	6.7
Calcium (mg)	813	724	10.9
Iron (mg)	14	12	12.9
Phosphorous (mg)	1318	1175	10.9
Potassium (g)	2630	2344	10.9

Table 7.5: Comparison of yearly mean energy and nutrient intakes with intakes during food collection periods. The observed percentage reduction in intake during the collection period is statistically significant for energy and all nutrients ($p < 0.05$). Data for thirteen male and sixteen female adults, aged 20 to 53 years. From Kim et al. (1984). © Am. J. Clin. Nutr. American Society for Clinical Nutrition.

those calculated from the records made during collection of the duplicate diets (Table 7.5). Gibson and Scythes (1982) also demonstrated a decrease in energy intake associated with the collection of duplicate diets for analysis. These results suggest that food intake changes during a duplicate diet collection period — sometimes resulting in a decrease in energy intake of as much as 20%. Hence duplicate diets are not an ideal method for validating food record methods (Stockley, 1985).

7.1.4 Validity of food frequency questionnaires

Studies of absolute validity of food frequency methods are limited, despite their increasing use in epidemiological studies. Mullen et al. (1984) tested the absolute validity of a food frequency questionnaire by comparison with actual food consumption determined at each meal for twenty-eight consecutive days. Respondents recorded food items and number of servings selected on a form apparently designed to measure food preferences. Forms were later checked for accuracy against returned trays by staff. The focus on food preferences served to de-emphasize food selection in an effort to prevent changes in usual food intake. Correlation analysis indicated that a large proportion of individuals could accurately estimate their food intake using the food frequency questionnaire.

Other studies have assessed relative validity and have used the same interview as the basis for their test and reference methods (Morgan et al., 1978), or a short time period (i.e. less than twenty-four hours between the two methods) (Balogh et al., 1968). Hence the methods were not independent of one another.

Willett et al. (1985) investigated the validity of a semiquantitative food frequency questionnaire designed to estimate food intake during

	Lowest Quintile on Food Record			Highest Quintile on Food Record		
	Quintile of questionnaire			Quintile of questionnaire		
	Lowest (%)	Lowest 2 (%)	Highest (%)	Highest (%)	Highest 2 (%)	Lowest (%)
Protein	44	68	0	47	71	9
Total fat	53	71	3	33	70	3
Saturated fat	47	88	3	47	82	0
Polyunsaturated fat	47	71	9	41	79	3
Cholesterol	53	76	6	50	68	6
Total carbohydrate	47	71	9	46	71	0
Sucrose	38	62	9	50	82	0
Crude fiber	41	69	3	41	79	3
Vitamin A	44	68	3	44	79	3
Vitamin B-6	47	88	0	74	88	3
Vitamin C	68	85	0	62	79	0
Mean	48	74	4	49	77	3

Table 7.6: Comparison of semiquantitative food frequency questionnaire scores with mean daily intakes derived from four one-week food records, based on joint classification by quintiles. Both intake scores adjusted for total energy intake. Data from 173 Boston area registered nurses aged 34 to 59 years. From Willett WC, Sampson L, Stampfer MJ, Rosner B, Bain C, Witschi J, Hennekens CH, Speizer FE. Reproducibility and validity of a semiquantitative food frequency questionnaire. American Journal of Epidemiology 122: 51–65, 1985.

a one-year period. They compared nutrient intake scores derived from the food frequency questionnaire with those estimated from four one-week weighed records. The degree to which subjects were classified into the same lowest or highest quintiles by the two dietary methods was also examined. Weighed food records were collected by the same subjects at three-monthly intervals, spaced to account for seasonal and short-term variability. Hence the two methods were independent and assessed food and nutrient intake over the same time frame. Nutrient intake results assessed by the two methods, with the exception of vitamin A and polyunsaturated fat, were strongly correlated, especially when expressed as nutrient densities. Overall agreement for the two dietary methods, for subjects within the lowest and highest quintiles for all the nutrients examined, was 48% and 49%, respectively. For the intermediate (second and fourth quintiles), and the center quintile, however, agreement was significantly lower. On average, only 3% of subjects were misclassified into extreme quintiles (Table 7.6).

Some investigators have noted considerable variability between methods for classifying individuals in terms of their vitamin A intakes (Mahalko et al., 1985). This is unfortunate in view of a possible relationship between low intakes of vitamin A, especially carotenoids, and increased risk of cancer (Bjelke, 1975; Hirayama, 1981).

Other investigators have attempted to validate a food frequency questionnaire using weighed or estimated food records (Abramson et al., 1963; Balogh et al., 1968; Hankin et al., 1975; Russell-Briefel et al., 1985). Such weighed or estimated records, however, do not usually examine food intakes within the same time frame and are therefore not appropriate reference methods for assessing relative validity of a food frequency questionnaire. In contrast, the dietary history method generally estimates food intake over a longer period of time and is therefore a more suitable reference method for comparison. Studies using this combination have shown relatively good agreement in food intakes determined by the two methods for a group, but not for individuals (Browe et al., 1966; Jain et al., 1982). Jain et al. (1982) noted that less than 50% of individuals were classified into the same tertile using the dietary history and food frequency methods, except for cholesterol and animal protein.

There have been several attempts to develop prediction equations based on seven-day weighed records and which could be used subsequently to validate food frequency questionnaires for specific population groups (Heady, 1961; Hankin et al., 1970). Hankin et al. (1970) developed a seven-day recall questionnaire for recording the frequencies of intake of twenty-three food items. Results from the questionnaire were then used in multiple-regression equations to determine which foodstuffs best predicted the intake of energy, protein, fat, carbohydrate, and sodium. A simple food frequency questionnaire was then developed based on these key foodstuffs and subsequently tested in the remaining population. The measured food frequencies derived from the subpopulation were then used as factors in the previously defined regression equations to calculate a predicted nutrient intake. These predicted nutrient intakes were compared with those determined by another seven-day period of measurements. Hankin et al. (1970) found, however, that the predicted intakes for all nutrients exceeded those measured subsequently. Figure 7.1 shows that the correlation was poor: foodstuffs isolated as good predictors initially were not the same foods which would eventually predict nutrient intakes. So far methods based on prediction equations have had limited success in terms of their predictive ability and generalizability to other population groups.

Relative validity of food frequency questionnaires and dietary histories (Kolonel at al., 1977; Jain et al., 1980; Marshall et al., 1980) has also been assessed by comparing the respondent's results with those collected from another person, such as a spouse or parent. Good agreement between spouses has been found. In general, however, the results of the spouse cannot be assumed to be any more accurate than those of the original respondent.

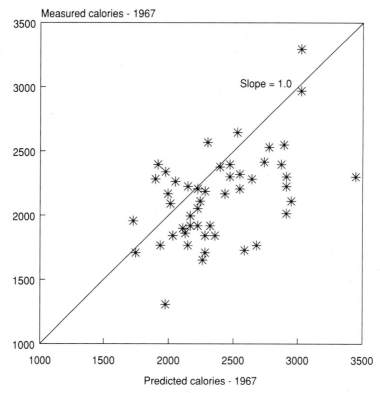

Figure 7.1: Comparison of 1967 measured calorie intakes with values predicted from 1967 questionnaires using 1965 regression equation. From Hankin JH, Messinger HB, Stallones RA. A short dietary method for epidemiological studies. IV: Evaluation of questionnaire. American Journal of Epidemiology 91: 562–567, 1970.

7.2   Use of biochemical markers to validate dietary data

As stated earlier, good agreement between the dietary intake results of the test and reference methods does not necessarily indicate validity. It may merely indicate similar errors in both methods. Recognition of this problem has prompted the development of more objective measures, independent of the measurement of food intake, to validate dietary intake data. In this approach, external variables such as biochemical indices or markers are used to validate dietary survey methods.

A biochemical marker is defined as: 'any biochemical index in an easily accessible sample that gives a predictive response to a given dietary component' (Bingham, 1984). Several have been proposed, although their accuracy as absolute standards for establishing the validity of dietary assessment methods requires further investigation.

7.2.1 Twenty-four-hour urinary nitrogen excretion

Isaksson (1980) was one of the first investigators to use nitrogen excretion levels in twenty-four-hour urine samples to validate a twenty-four-hour protein intake estimated by record or recall. This procedure was adopted because of the positive correlation observed between daily nitrogen intake and daily nitrogen excretion when dietary intake is kept constant, in metabolic studies of adults (Bingham, 1984). Nevertheless, there are several limitations to this approach:

Nitrogen balance

Subjects are assumed to be in nitrogen balance, a state in which no nitrogen is retained for growth or the repair of lost muscle tissue, and no nitrogen is lost as a result of starvation, or injury, etc. (Bingham and Cummings, 1983).

Extra-renal losses

Losses of nitrogen via the skin and feces are not measured directly and thus twenty-four-hour urinary nitrogen underestimates nitrogen output. To account for these extrarenal losses, 2 g of nitrogen are added to each twenty-four-hour nitrogen excretion in the urine. Hence the following relationship should apply if the subject is in nitrogen balance:

$$\frac{\text{Protein intake in 24 hours (g)}}{6.25} = \text{Nitrogen excretion in 24 hours (g)} + 2\ (g)$$

The use of a universal correction of 2 g is probably not appropriate because a large range in fecal nitrogen excretion exists among individuals. Moreover, intakes of protein and dietary fiber as well as exercise all affect the level of the external losses of nitrogen (Calloway et al., 1971; Cummings et al., 1981).

Complete twenty-four-hour urine collections

Complete twenty-four-hour urine samples are required. Creatinine excretion in the twenty-four-hour urine samples is often used to measure the completeness of urine collections (Webster and Garrow, 1985). This validation of the completeness of the urine collection is based on the assumption that creatinine excretion is constant from day to day in an individual. Several studies have questioned the constancy of creatinine excretion, some reporting the coefficient of variation in the twenty-four-hour output of creatinine to be as large as 25% (Webster and Garrow, 1985; Waterlow, 1986). This variation depends in part on the meat content of the diet.

British investigators have recently confirmed that 4-aminobenzoic acid (PABA) is a safe, reliable, exogenous marker to validate the completeness of urine collections (Bingham and Cummings, 1983). PABA can be easily

Subject	1	2	3	4	5	6	7	8	Mean
Dietary N (g)	13.2	21.7	21.2	15.8	15.7	11.7	12.7	14.0	—
Urinary N (g)	12.1	15.6	16.6	13.8	13.2	9.6	10.2	10.8	—
% Urine N / diet N	88	72	78	87	84	82	80	77	81 ± 5

Table 7.7: Comparison of nitrogen intake as assessed by eighteen days of observation and urinary nitrogen output after eight days of complete twenty-four-hour collections. From Bingham and Cummings (1985). © Am. J. Clin. Nutr. American Society for Clinical Nutrition.

administered in capsules and analyzed with a maximum inter-subject variation in excretion of only 15%. Over-collection of urine, however, cannot be detected by using PABA.

Intra-subject variation

Considerable daily variation in urinary nitrogen excretion exists. This variation may be large, necessitating repeated collections of consecutive twenty-four-hour urine samples if the method is used to validate protein intakes of individuals. For example, Bingham and Cummings (1985) reported that eight twenty-four-hour urine collections, verified for completeness, were necessary to estimate dietary nitrogen intakes of individuals to within 81 ± 5% (i.e. $\pm$SD), provided that a dietary method which assesses usual food intake is used (Table 7.7). The method cannot be used to validate dietary nitrogen intake on individuals using a single twenty-four-hour urine collection.

If validation of the group mean protein intake is needed, then only one twenty-four-hour urine sample, collected from each respondent on a preselected day, is required. Such an approach was used by van Staveren et al. (1985) to measure the validity of the nitrogen intake determined by a dietary history method. Twenty-four-hour urine samples were collected by each subject, on a preselected day, so that for the group as a whole urine collections for all days of the week were evenly represented. The mean urine nitrogen excretion of an average weekday was calculated, with the addition of a correction factor of 2 g for extrarenal nitrogen losses. The results suggested that there was no difference between mean excretion and mean intake of nitrogen for the group (Table 7.8). Hence the dietary history method had made a valid assessment of intake of foods containing protein, for the group as a whole.

The use of twenty-four-hour urinary nitrogen excretion to detect any changes in usual dietary intake during the assessment period has also been investigated. This can be achieved by comparing nitrogen in twenty-four-hour urine samples collected both during the dietary assessment period and at a time before or after the assessment is completed. This approach was used by Johnstone et al. (1981) and Bingham et al. (1982). The

	Total Group (n = 44)	Men (n = 22)	Women (n=22)
Nitrogen intake from dietary history (N_I)	13.3 ± 0.51	14.6 ± 0.77	11.9 ± 0.55
Nitrogen intake from nitrogen excretion in the urine (including 2 g allowance for extra-renal losses (N_E)	13.3 ± 0.46	14.4 ± 0.60	12.1 ± 0.63
(N_I) − (N_E)	0.0 ± 0.50	0.2 ± 0.94	-0.2 ± 0.57
95% confidence limits (N_I) − (N_E)	−1.1 and 1.1	−1.6 and 2.0	−1.5 and 1.1

Table 7.8: Comparison of nitrogen intake (g/day; mean ± SE) as assessed by a dietary history and daily urinary nitrogen excretion in young adults. From van Staveren et al. (1985). © Am. J. Clin. Nutr. American Society for Clinical Nutrition.

latter collected twenty-four-hour urine samples from their subjects on the last day of a four-day weighed duplicate diet collection, and on another occasion six weeks later. Samples were also analyzed for urinary sodium and potassium, as well as urinary nitrogen. No significant differences in these urinary components were observed between samples collected during and after the survey period, suggesting no change in dietary habits during the survey.

7.2.2 3-Methylhistidine excretion

The twenty-four-hour urinary excretion of 3-methylhistidine has been investigated as an index of meat consumption because it appears to show a linear dose response to meat intake (Elia et al., 1980; Jacobson et al., 1983). Recent studies, however, have emphasized large inter-subject differences in baseline excretion of 3-methylhistidine, even when no meat is fed, limiting its usefulness.

7.2.3 Urinary mineral excretion

Besides nitrogen, urinary excretion of certain electrolytes (e.g. sodium and potassium) for which the urine is the major excretory route has also been used as a biochemical marker of dietary intake (Holbrook et al., 1984; Caggiula et al., 1985).

Urinary sodium excretion is often used as a more reliable index of dietary sodium intake than calculation from food composition data. External losses of sodium via the feces and sweat are probably minimal in temperate climates. These losses may be increased by vigorous physical activity and/or diarrhea. Diurnal and day-to-day fluctuations in sodium excretion are larger than those for nitrogen, and consequently an even greater number of urine collections are required to characterize sodium

Fatty Acid or Ratio of Fatty Acids	Correlation Coefficient Observed	Correlation Coefficient Unattenuated
P/S	0.57	0.63
M/P	0.63	0.69
P	0.68	0.75
L/S	0.62	0.68
M/L	0.63	0.69
L	0.70	0.77

Table 7.9: Observed and unattenuated correlation coefficients between the fatty acid composition of the diet and of the adipose tissue. Subjects were fifty-nine adult Dutch women. P = polyunsaturated fatty acids, L = linoleic acid, M = mono-unsaturated fatty acids, S = saturated fatty acids. All correlation coefficients quoted are significant ($p < 0.05$). From Staveren WA van, Deurenberg P, Katan MB, Burema J, de Groot LCPGM, Hoffmans MDAF. Validity of the fatty acid composition of subcutaneous fat tissue microbiopsies as an estimate of the long-term average fatty acid composition of the diet of separate individuals. American Journal of Epidemiology 123: 455–463, 1986b.

excretion in an individual than nitrogen. Simpson et al. (1983) estimated that fifteen twenty-four-hour urine collections are required to characterize an individual's sodium output with 95% accuracy.

Urinary potassium has also been used as a biochemical marker of potassium intake. Fecal excretion of potassium is greater and more variable than sodium, thus limiting the usefulness of urinary potassium excretion as an index of potassium intake (Cummings et al., 1976). Only limited work has been done on other minerals which have urine as their main excretory route (e.g. selenium and chromium).

7.2.4   Fatty acid content of adipose tissue

The fatty acid composition of subcutaneous adipose tissue may indicate the type of fatty acids consumed (Beynen et al., 1980; Plakké et al., 1983).   Van Staveren et al. (1986b) reported highly significant correlations between the fatty acid composition of adipose tissue and the diet.   Dietary intakes were calculated from the mean of nineteen repeat twenty-four-hour recalls administered over a period of two and a half years, on 59 young adult women. Subcutaneous adipose tissue samples were taken from the buttock. These investigators also showed, using regression analysis, that the linoleic acid composition of the diet could be predicted from the linoleic acid composition of the adipose tissue (Figure 7.2).

Some investigators have taken subcutaneous fat samples from the outer upper arm in the deltoid area using a skin-biopsy punch (Smith et al., 1986).   This latter technique has been successfully employed in a major cross-sectional survey of lifestyle and coronary risk factors in Scotland (The Scottish Heart Health Study)

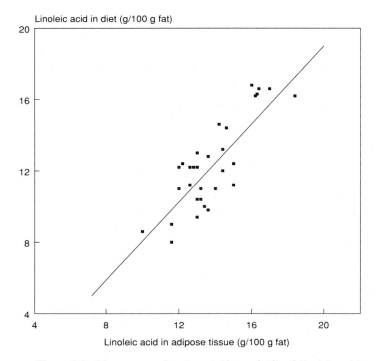

Figure 7.2: Linear regression (y = 1.10x − 3.12) of linoleic acid (g/100 g fat) in the diet of 32 Dutch female subjects, assessed with a twenty-four-hour recall repeated nineteen times during two and a half years, on the corresponding value in adipose tissue. From Staveren WA van, Deurenberg P, Katan MB, Burema J, de Groot LCPGM, Hoffmans MDAF. Validity of the fatty acid composition of subcutaneous fat tissue microbiopsies as an estimate of the long-term average fatty acid composition of the diet of separate individuals. American Journal of Epidemiology 123: 455–463, 1986b.

(Smith et al., 1985). The phospholipid fatty acid composition of human cheek (buccal epithelial) cells also appears promising as an noninvasive index of dietary lipid status. Human cheek cells appear to respond to differences in dietary lipid intakes of vegetarians and nonvegetarians (McMurchie et al., 1984a) and to manipulations in the dietary polyunsaturated:saturated fatty acid ratio (McMurchie et al., 1984b).

7.3   Statistical assessment of validity

The statistical methods for assessing validity are comparable to those used to assess precision (Section 6.3). They can be classified into: (a) those assessing the extent of agreement between the test and reference methods on an aggregate or group basis; and (b) those assessing individual (within-pair) agreement (Lee, 1980).

7.3.1 Assessment of aggregate agreement

For aggregate agreement, the mean and standard deviations for the intakes derived from the test and reference methods, are calculated. Then a paired *t*-test can be used to test whether the two means are statistically different at some predetermined probability level, provided that the data are 'normally' distributed (Tables 7.2, 7.3). If, however, the nutrient intake data are skewed, the median (50th percentile) and selected percentile points (e.g. 5th and 95th percentiles) should be used to quantify the average intakes and their variability. In such cases, the Wilcoxon's signed rank test is more appropriate than the paired *t*-test for testing for statistical differences (Snedecor and Cochran, 1980).

7.3.2 Assessment of individual agreement

The methods for quantifying individual agreement depend on whether the intake data are expressed in terms of frequencies or amounts. If frequencies have been calculated, the percentage of individuals (pairs) with exact agreement and/or within a selected number of units (Table 6.4; Sections 6.1.4 and 6.3.2) is often calculated. Alternatively, for intake data expressed in amounts (e.g. grams per day), the percentage of individuals (pairs) with agreement to within a certain amount can be given. Such an approach ignores the fact that a certain amount of individual agreement invariably occurs by chance alone. Hence, it is preferable to calculate a statistical index, the intraclass correlation coefficient r_I, that corrects for the amount of chance-expected agreements. A discussion of this statistical index can be found in Lee (1980). Tables 6.2 and 6.3 illustrate the use of intraclass correlation coefficients to assess the precision of seven-day weighed food records, and a dietary history method, respectively. Many studies have used the Pearson's product-moment correlation coefficient (r) instead of the intraclass correlation coefficient (r_I) to assess the extent of individual within-pair agreements (Table 6.2). The former is subject to certain limitations, and its use is discouraged (Lee, 1980). In some cases, regression analysis may be appropriate, particularly when validity is being assessed using biochemical markers (Figure 7.2).

7.4 Summary

Validity describes the degree to which a dietary method measures that which it purports to measure. Absolute validity is usually assessed in institutional settings by surreptitiously weighing or observing food items subsequently recalled by the subjects over the same time period. In general, the twenty-four-hour dietary recall tends to underestimate mean dietary intakes in the elderly and children, but produces valid mean intakes for other population groups. For most other dietary methods, relative, rather than absolute, validity is assessed by evaluating the 'test' dietary method against another reference method, chosen for its accuracy, precision, and ability to measure similar parameters over the same time frame. The appropriate methods for validating the dietary history are the seven-day weighed or estimated food record. Food records themselves have been validated, with limited success, by collecting intermittent duplicate diets. For food frequency questionnaires, dietary histories and weighed food records are used although the latter are not recommended because, in general, they do not examine food intakes within the same time frame. Prediction equations, based on seven-day weighed records, have been developed to validate food frequency questionnaires, but have not been successful.

Dietary intake data also can be validated by using biochemical markers such as twenty-four-hour urinary nitrogen excretion as a measure of protein intake, urinary excretion of sodium and potassium as measures sodium and potassium intakes, and the fatty acid composition of subcutaneous adipose tissue as a measure of fatty acid composition of the diet. Statistical methods used to measure validity include correlation and regression analysis, paired t-tests, and Wilcoxon's signed rank test.

References

Abramson JH, Slome C, Kosovosky C. (1963). Food frequency interviews as an epidemiological tool. American Journal of Public Health 53: 1093–1101.

Balogh M, Kahn HA, Medalie JH. (1971). Random repeat 24-hour dietary recalls. American Journal of Clinical Nutrition 24: 304–310.

Balogh M, Medalie JH, Smith H. (1968). The development of a dietary questionnaire for an ischaemic heart disease survey. Israel Journal of Medical Sciences 4: 195–203.

Beynen AC, Hermus RJ, Hantvast JG. (1980). A mathematical relationship between the fatty acid composition of the diet and that of the adipose tissue in man. American Journal of Clinical Nutrition 33: 81–85.

Bingham S. (1984). Biochemical markers of consumption. In: The Dietary Assessment of Populations. Medical Research Council Scientific Report No 4: 26–30.

Bingham S, Cummings JH. (1983). The use of 4-amino benzoic acid as a marker to validate the completeness of 24-hr urine collections in man. Clinical Science 64: 629–635.

Bingham SA, Cummings JH. (1985). Urine nitrogen as an independent validatory measure of dietary intake: a study of nitrogen balance in individuals consuming their normal diet. American Journal of Clinical Nutrition 42: 1276–1289.

Bingham S, Wiggins HW, Englyst H, Seppanen R, Helms P, Strand R, Bucton R, Jorgensen IM, Poulsen L, Paerrgaard A, Bjerrum L, James WPT. (1982). Methods and validity of the dietary assessments in four Scandinavian populations. Nutrition and Cancer 4: 23–33.

Bjelke E. (1975). Dietary vitamin A and human lung cancer. International Journal of Cancer 15: 561–565.

Block G. (1982). A review of validations of dietary assessment methods. American Journal of Epidemiology 115: 492–505.

Bray GA, Zachary B, Dahms WT, Atkinson RL, Oddie TH. (1978). Eating patterns of massively obese individuals. Journal of the American Dietetic Association 72: 24–27.

Browe JH, Gofstein RM, Morlley DM, McCarthy MC. (1966). Diet and heart disease in the cardiovascular health center. Journal of the American Dietetic Association 48: 95–100.

Byers TE, Rosenthal RI, Marshall JR, Rzepka TF, Cummings KM, Graham S. (1983). Dietary history from the distant past: a methodological study. Nutrition and Cancer 5: 69–77.

Caggiula AW, Wing RR, Nowalk MP, Milas NC, Lee S, Langford H. (1985). The measurement of sodium and potassium intake. American Journal of Clinical Nutrition 42: 391–398.

Calloway DH, Odell ACF, Margen S. (1971). Sweat and miscellaneous nitrogen losses in human balance studies. Journal of Nutrition 101: 775–786.

Campbell VA, Dodds ML. (1967). Collecting dietary information from groups of older people. Journal of the American Dietetic Association 51: 29–33.

Carter RL, Sharbaugh CO, Stapell CA. (1981). Reliability and validity of the 24-hour recall. Journal of the American Dietetic Association 79: 542–547.

Cummings JH, Hill MJ, Jenkins DJA, Pearson JR, Wiggins HS. (1976). Changes in faecal composition and colonic function due to cereal fiber. American Journal of Clinical Nutrition 29: 1468–1473.

Cummings JH, Stephen AM, Branch WJ. (1981). Implications of dietary fibre breakdown in the human colon. In: Banbury Report 7. Gastrointestinal Cancer: Endogenous Factors. Cold Spring Harbour Laboratory.

Dawber TR, Pearson G, Anderson P, Mann GV, Kannel WB, Shurtleff D, McNamara P. (1962). Dietary assessment in the epidemiologic study of coronary heart diesase: The Framingham Study 11. Reliability of measurement. American Journal of Clinical Nutrition 11:226–234.

Elia M, Carter A, Bacon S, Smith R. (1980). The effect of 3-methylhistidine in food on its urinary excretion in man. Clinical Science 59: 509–511.

Emmons L, Hayes M. (1973). Accuracy of 24-hr recalls of young children. Journal of the American Dietetic Association 162: 409–415.

Gersovitz M, Madden JP, Smiciklas-Wright H. (1978). Validity of the 24-hr dietary recall and seven-day record for group comparisons. Journal of the American Dietetic Association 73: 48–55.

Gibson RS, Scythes CA. (1982). Trace element intakes of women. British Journal of Nutrition 48: 241–248.

Greger JL, Etnyre GM. (1978). Validity of 24-hour dietary recalls by adolescent females. American Journal of Public Health 68: 70–72.

Hankin JH, Messinger HB, Stallones RA. (1970). A short dietary method for epidemiological studies. IV: Evaluation of questionnaire. American Journal of Epidemiology 91: 562–567.

Hankin JH, Rhoads GG, Glober GA. (1975). A dietary method for an epidemiological study of gastrointestinal cancer. American Journal of Clinical Nutrition 28: 1055–1060.

Heady JA. (1961). Diets of bank clerks: Development of a method of classifying the diets of individuals for use in epidemiological studies. Journal of the Royal Statistical Society A124: 336–361.

Herbert JR, Miller DR. (1988). Methodologic considerations for investigating the diet-cancer link. American Journal of Clinical Nutrition 47: 1068–1077.

Hirayama T. (1981). Diet and cancer. Nutrition and Cancer 1: 67–81.

Holbrook JT, Patterson KY, Bodner JE, Douglas LW, Veillon C, Kelsay JL, Mertz W, Smith JC. (1984). Sodium and potassium intake and balance in adults consuming self-selected diets. American Journal of Clinical Nutrition 40: 786–793.

Isaksson B. (1980). Urinary nitrogen output as a validity test in dietary surveys. American Journal of Clinical Nutrition 33: 4–6.

Jacobson EA, Newmark HL, McKeown-Eyssen G, Bruce WB. (1983). Excretion of 3-methyl histidine in urine as an estimate of meat consumption. Nutrition Reports International 27: 689–697.

Jain MG, Harrison L, Howe GR, Miller AB. (1982). Evaluation of a self-administered dietary questionnaire for use in a cohort study. American Journal of Clinical Nutrition 36: 931–935.

Jain MG, Howe GR, Johnson KC, Miller AB. (1980). Evaluation of a diet history questionnaire for epidemiologic studies. American Journal of Epidemiology 111: 212–219.

Johnstone FD, Campbell Brown M, Campbell D, MacGillivray I. (1981). Measurement of variables: data quality control. American Journal of Clinical Nutrition 34: 804–806.

Kim WW, Mertz W, Judd JT, Marshall MW, Kelsay JL, Prather ES. (1984). Effect of making duplicate food collections on nutrient intakes calculated from diet records. American Journal of Clinical Nutrition 40: 1333–1337.

Klaver W, Burema J, Staveren WA van, Knuiman JT. (1988). Definition of terms. In: Cameron ME, Staveren WA van (eds), Manual on Methodology for Food Consumption Studies. Oxford University Press, pp.11–23.

Kolonel LN, Hirohata T, Nomura AMY. (1977). Adequacy of survey data collected from substitute respondents. American Journal of Epidemiology 106: 476–484.

Krantzler NJ, Mullen BJ, Schutz HG, Grivetti LE, Holden CA, Meiselman HL. (1982). Validity of telephoned diet recalls and records for assessment of individual food intake. American Journal of Clinical Nutrition 36: 1234–1242.

Lee J. (1980). Alternate approaches for quantifying aggregate and individual agreements between two methods for assessing dietary intakes. American Journal of Clinical Nutrition 33: 956–964.

Linusson EEI, Sanjur D, Erickson EC. (1974). Validating the 24-hour recall as a dietary survey test. Archivos Latinoamericanos de Nutrición 24: 277–281.

Madden JP, Goodman SJ, Guthrie HA. (1976). Validity of the 24-hr recall: analysis of data obtained from elderly subjects. Journal of the American Dietetic Association 68: 143–147.

Mahalko JR, Johnson LK, Gallagher SK, Milne DB. (1985). Comparison of dietary histories and seven-day food records in a nutritional assessment of older adults. American Journal of Clinical Nutrition 42: 542–553.

Marshall J, Priore R, Haughey B, Rzepka T, Graham S. (1980). Spouse-subject interviews and the reliability of diet studies. American Journal of Epidemiology 112: 675–683.

McMurchie EJ, Potter JD, Rohan TE, Hetzel BS. (1984a). Human cheek cells: a noninvasive method for determining tissue lipid profiles in dietary and nutritional studies. Nutrition Reports International 29: 519–526.

McMurchie EJ, Margetts BM, Beilin LJ, Croft KD, Vandongen R, Armstrong BK. (1984b). Dietary-induced changes in the fatty acid composition of human cheek cell phospholipids: correlation with changes in the dietary polyunsaturated/saturated fat ratio. American Journal of Clinical Nutrition 39: 975–980.

Morgan RW, Jain M, Miller AB, Jain M, Miller AB, Choi NW, Matthews V, Munan L, Burch JD, Feather J, Howe GR, Kelly A. (1978). A comparison of dietary methods in epidemiologic studies. American Journal of Epidemiology 107: 488–498.

Mullen BJ, Krantzler NJ, Grivetti LE, Schutz HG, Meiselman HL. (1984). Validity of a food frequency questionnaire for the determination of individual food intake. American Journal of Clinical Nutrition 39: 136–142.

Plakké T, Berkel J, Beynen AC, Hermus RJJ, Katan MB. (1983). Relationship between the fatty acid composition of the diet and that of the subcutaneous adipose tissue in individual human subjects. Human Nutrition: Applied Nutrition 37A: 365–372.

Räsänen L. (1979). Nutrition survey of Finnish rural children. VI. Methodological study comparing the 24-hour recall and the dietary history interview. American Journal of Clinical Nutrition 32: 2560–2567.

Reshef A, Epstein LM. (1972). Reliability of a dietary questionnaire. American Journal of Clinical Nutrition 25: 91–95.

Russell-Briefel R, Caggiula AW, Kuller LH. (1985). A comparison of three dietary methods for estimating vitamin A intake. American Journal of Epidemiology 122: 628–636.

Sempos CT, Johnson NE, Smith EL, Gilligan C. (1985). Effects of intra-individual and inter-individual variation in repeated dietary records. American Journal of Epidemiology 121: 120–130.

Sherlock JC. (1983). Heavy metal intakes by critical groups. In: Proceedings of the International Conference on Heavy Metals in the Environment. CEP Consultants, Edinburgh, pp. 269–273.

Simpson FO, Paulin JM, Phelan EL. (1983). Repeated 24-hour urinary electrolyte estimations in the community. New Zealand Medical Journal 96: 910–911.

Smith WCS, Crombie IK, Irving JM, Kenicer MB, Tunstall-Pedoe H, Tavendale R. (1985). The Scottish Heart Health Study. European Heart Journal 6, Supplement 1, 105.

Smith WCS, Tavendale R, Tunstall-Pedoe H. (1986). Simplified subcutaneous fat biopsy for nutritional surveys. Human Nutrition: Clinical Nutrition 40C: 323–325.

Snedecor GW, Cochran WG. (1980). Statistical Methods. Seventh edition. Iowa State University Press, Ames, Iowa.

Staveren WA van, de Boer JO, Burema J. (1985). Validity and reproducibility of a dietary history method estimating the usual food intake during one month. American Journal of Clinical Nutrition 42: 554–559.

Staveren WA van, West CE, Hoffmans MDAF, Bos P, Kardinaal AFM, Poppel GAFC van, Schippper HJ-A, Hautvast JGAJ, Hayes RB. (1986a). Comparison of contemporaneous and retrospective estimates of food consumption made by a dietary history method. American Journal of Epidemiology 123: 884–893.

Staveren WA van, Deurenberg P, Katan MB, Burema J, de Groot LCPGM, Hoffmans MDAF. (1986b). Validity of the fatty acid composition of subcutaneous fat tissue microbiopsies as an estimate of the long-term average fatty acid composition of the diet of separate individuals. American Journal of Epidemiology 123: 455–463.

Stockley L. (1985). Changes in habitual food intake during weighed inventory surveys and duplicate diet collections. A short review. Ecology of Food and Nutrition 17: 263–269.

Stunkard AJ, Waxman M. (1981). Accuracy of self-reports of food intake. Journal of the American Dietetic Association 79: 547–551.

Trulson MF, McCann MB. (1959). Comparison of dietary survey methods. Journal of the American Dietetic Association 35: 672–676.

Waterlow JC. (1986). Observations on the variability of creatinine excretion. Human Nutrition: Clinical Nutrition 40C: 125–129.

Webster J, Garrow JS. (1985). Creatinine excretion over 24 hours as a measure of body composition or of completeness of urine collection. Human Nutrition: Clinical Nutrition 39C: 101–106.

Willett WC, Sampson L, Stampfer MJ, Rosner B, Bain C, Witschi J, Hennekens CH, Speizer FE. (1985). Reproducibility and validity of a semiquantitative food frequency questionnaire. American Journal of Epidemiology 122: 51–65.

Young CM, Hagan GC, Tucker RE. (1952). A comparison of dietary study methods. II. Dietary history vs seven-day records vs 24-hr recall. Journal of the American Dietetic Association 28: 218–221.

Chapter 8

Evaluation of nutrient intake data

Dietary intake data in nutritional assessment systems have been severely criticized because of the random and systematic errors which occur in measuring nutrient intakes and because of the frequent misinterpretation of the data. This is unfortunate because the careful evaluation of nutrient intake data from target populations and/or individuals can produce important information, provided that the limitations of the methods are clearly understood.

This chapter describes both the more conventional and some newer methods of evaluating nutrient intakes, both at the individual and at the population level. Most of the conventional methods involve direct comparison with tables of recommended nutrient intakes as a basis for assessing nutrient adequacy. These approaches have several limitations, often resulting in over- and under-estimations of nutritional problems. As a result, a probability approach has been developed to assess the risk of nutrient inadequacy in groups of individuals more reliably. Such an approach is preferable for identifying and targeting nutrition and food intervention programs at the more vulnerable groups. The probability approach can also be adapted to estimate the risk of individuals and/or population groups to excessive intakes of nutrients and/or food additives and contaminants, provided that the association between level of intake and risk of toxicity is known.

None of the methods described, however, provide information on the *nutritional status* of individuals and/or population groups. Such information can only be obtained when dietary intake data are combined with biochemical, anthropometric, and clinical indices.

8.1 Tables of recommended nutrient intakes

All the methods used to evaluate nutrient intake data depend on knowledge of the nutrient requirements for individuals in specified groups. Such data form the basis for the recommended nutrient intakes.

The first set of recommended nutrient intakes was produced by the Technical Commission on Nutrition, League of Nations (1938). These recommendations also formed the basis for the first Canadian Dietary Standard compiled by the Canadian Council on Nutrition in 1939 (Canadian Council on Nutrition, 1940). The United States Food and Nutrition Board prepared the first United States Recommended Dietary Allowances in 1941 (Food and Nutrition Board, 1943). Later, tables of recommended nutrient intakes were also developed by WHO/FAO and a number of individual countries.

The 1983 edition of the Canadian tables of recommended nutrient intakes contains recommendations for seventeen nutrients in the main summary table and recommendations for energy, sodium, potassium, and essential fatty acids within the text (Appendix A8.1 and A8.2) (Health and Welfare Canada, 1983). The ninth edition of the U.S. Recommended Dietary Allowances (Food and Nutrition Board, 1980) has recommendations for seventeen nutrients in the main summary table (Appendix A8.3 and A8.4), with additional tables for recommended energy intakes, and estimated safe and adequate daily dietary intakes of selected vitamins (vitamin K, biotin, pantothenic acid) and minerals (copper, manganese, fluoride, chromium, selenium, molybdenum, sodium, potassium, and chloride). The United Kingdom lists energy and nine nutrients in the main summary table (Appendix A8.5 and A8.6) (Department of Health and Social Security, 1981). Selected data from the Canadian (Health and Welfare Canada, 1983), United States (Food and Nutrition Board, 1980), United Kingdom (Department of Health and Social Security, 1981), and FAO/WHO (WHO, 1973; Passmore et al., 1974; FAO/WHO/UNU, 1985; FAO/WHO, in press) tables of recommended nutrient intakes are shown in Table 8.1. The WHO data for vitamin C, vitamin D, and calcium are derived from the 1974 WHO publication 'Handbook on Nutritional Requirements' (Passmore et al., 1974), whereas the values for magnesium and zinc are provisional estimates made by the WHO in 1973 (WHO, 1973). The FAO/WHO values for protein (and energy) in Table 8.1 are derived from a recent publication entitled 'Energy and Protein Requirements' (FAO/WHO/UNU, 1985), whereas the values for vitamin A, iron, folate, and vitamin B-12 are taken from an FAO/WHO report entitled 'Requirements of vitamin A, iron, folate and vitamin B-12' (FAO/WHO, in press). The number of nutrients included in the tables of recommended nutrient intakes varies among countries. All now include protein, calcium, iron, thiamin, riboflavin, niacin, vitamin C, and retinol. The West German tables include twenty-five nutrients, the highest number of all tables of recommended nutrient intakes (Deutsche Gesellschaft für Ernährung, 1975). The New Zealand nutrient intake tables define levels for both minimum safe intakes and adequate daily intakes for each nutrient (Nutrition Advisory Committee, 1983).

Nutrient	Canada	U.S.A.	U.K.	FAO/WHO
Protein (g)	61	56	72	52.5 [c]
Calcium (mg)	800	800	500	400–500
Phosphorus (mg)	800	800	–	–
Iron (mg)	8	10	10	8–23 [d]
Vitamin A (μg RE)	1000	1000	750	600 [e]
Vitamin D (μg)	2.5	5	2.5	2.5
Vitamin C (mg)	60	60	30	30
Folate (μg)	220 [a]	400 [a]	–	200 [a,e]
Vitamin E (mg)	9 [b]	10 [b]	–	–
Vitamin B-12 (μg)	2.0	3.0	–	1.0 [e]
Magnesium (mg)	250	350	–	–
Zinc (mg)	9	15	–	11 [f]
Iodine (μg)	160	150	–	–

Table 8.1: Selected recommended nutrient intakes for adult males. [a] as total folate; [b] as
d-α-tocopherol equivalents; [c] safe level of protein intake for 70 kg male; [d] basal requirement including variability; [e] safe level of intake; [f] assuming 20% available zinc content
of daily diet. Adapted from International Union of Nutritional Sciences (1983) with
permission of Nutrition Abstracts and Reviews, A (Human and Experimental); World
Health Organization (1973); Food and Agriculture Organization/World Health Organiza-
tion/United Nations University (1985); Food and Agriculture Organization/World Health
Organization (1988).

The way in which the recommended nutrient intakes are defined varies
among countries. The most recent versions of the Canadian (Health and
Welfare Canada, 1983) and United States (Food and Nutrition Board,
1980) tables of recommendations for nutrients use similar definitions:

> A recommended nutrient intake (RNI) is taken as the level
> of dietary intake thought to be sufficiently high to meet
> the requirements of almost all individuals in a group with
> specified characteristics. It takes into account individual
> variability. Of necessity, the RNI exceeds the requirement
> of almost all individuals (Health and Welfare Canada, 1983).

> Recommended Dietary Allowances (RDA) are the levels of
> intake of essential nutrients considered to be adequate to meet
> the known nutritional needs of practically all healthy persons
> (Food and Nutrition Board, 1980).

The definition used by the United Kingdom is as follows:

> A recommended dietary intake (RDI) is the average amount
> of the nutrient which should be provided per head in a group
> of people if the needs of practically all members of the group
> are met (Department of Health and Social Security, 1981).

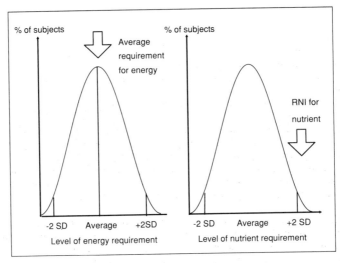

Figure 8.1: Comparison of the average requirement for energy and the recommended intake of a nutrient. It is assumed that in both cases individual requirements are normally distributed about the mean. From Health and Welfare Canada (1983). Reproduced with permission of the Minister of Supply and Services Canada.

Estimates of recommended nutrient intakes are derived from measurements of nutrient requirements on individuals of the same age and sex. These measurements generate a distribution of requirements because of individual variability for a specific nutrient, valid for a certain age and sex group. Data are available on the distribution of nutrient requirements for energy, protein, iron, and calcium; data for other nutrients are limited. The requirements are generally considered to follow a Gaussian distribution. The mean of this distribution represents the average requirement for that particular group of individuals and the standard deviation is a measure of the variability in the requirement. Recent committees in Canada and the United States have generally set the recommended nutrient intake at the average requirement (for a particular age and sex category) plus two standard deviations (Beaton, 1985). This means that the recommended nutrient intakes exceed the needs of all but 2% to 3% of individuals in the population (Figure 8.1). This conservative approach therefore accounts for inter-subject variability in nutrient requirements and is adopted because the risk to health is associated primarily with inadequate intakes (Beaton, 1985). When the standard deviation of the mean requirement is unknown, it is assumed to be 15% of the mean.

Recommended intakes for energy, however, are based on estimates of the average energy requirement for a group of comparable individuals (Figure 8.1). This approach has been adopted because excessive energy intake is injurious to health. Furthermore, the body's regulatory mechanisms maintain energy intakes near requirements over long periods. New estimates for energy requirements which include an estimate of the variance of energy requirements, based on the most precise data available, have been developed by the FAO/WHO/UNU (1985). Data on estimates of basal metabolic rate at all ages and the energy costs of various physical and discretionary activities are also included.

Some of the underlying principles used by the committees developing tables of recommended amounts of nutrients are similar. These are that recommended nutrient intakes:

- are always set for a particular group of individuals with specified characteristics, consuming a specified diet. This is because requirements for many nutrients are affected by age, sex, physical activity, body size, physiological state, and the nature of the diet. Such groupings, however, are not standardized and the number varies among countries. WHO (Passmore et al., 1974) have fourteen age/sex groupings, whereas Canada (Health and Welfare Canada, 1983), the United States (Food and Nutrition Board, 1980), and the United Kingdom (Department of Health and Social Security, 1981) have twenty-three, fifteen, and sixteen, respectively.
- refer to the average need over a reasonable period of time, although the latter has seldom been defined. Hence the suggested amounts do not have to be consumed every day, but omissions or shortfalls must be balanced by increased intake on other occasions.
- refer to levels of intake needed to maintain health in already healthy individuals. They do not allow for illnesses or stresses in life.
- are based on the typical dietary pattern of the country and may not be appropriate for persons following atypical diets.
- are calculated ignoring possible interactions involving nutrients and other dietary components, because these interactions cannot be adequately quantified at the present time.
- assume that requirements for energy and other nutrients are met.

The values for the recommended nutrient intakes for the same nutrient vary among countries. Table 8.2 illustrates the variations in recommended intakes for vitamin C for young men in selected countries (Buss, 1986). Some of these discrepancies arise from:

- differences in the sources and interpretation of the data on nutrient requirements;
- incomplete or nonexistent data for some nutrients and/or specific age groups;
- different age, sex, and physiological subgroupings;
- different criteria used to define adequacy. For example in both the United States and Canada, the vitamin C requirements have been set at a level sufficient to establish and maintain metabolic pools (Food and Nutrition Board, 1980; Health and Welfare Canada, 1983)

Argentina, Uruguay, Venezuela	30	United Kingdom	30
Bolivia, Colombia	40	German Democratic Republic	45
Spain	45	Mexico	50
United States of America	60	Federal Republic of Germany	75
Philippines, Portugal	75	Bulgaria	95

Table 8.2: Variations among the recommended intakes of vitamin C for young men in selected countries (mg/day). From International Union of Nutritional Sciences (1983). With permission of Nutrition Abstracts and Reviews, A (Human and Experimental).

whereas FAO/WHO (1970) used the maintenance of tissue levels as their criterion.

- differences in judgement by the committees setting the recommended nutrient intakes;
- differences in the characteristics of the diet.

The data used by the committees to estimate the requirements for the nutrients are derived from a number of sources. These may include metabolic studies; results of nutrient and food supplementation; epidemiological data linking food consumption or the food supply to relevant physiological variables; clinical trials; experience with parenteral and enteral nutrition; results of accidental or natural experiments such as the use of infant formulas; data on bioavailability, nutrient-nutrient and drug-nutrient interactions; and animal studies (Food and Nutrition Board, 1986). Such data provide information on minimum intakes of a nutrient associated with: the absence of any signs of a deficiency disease; curing clinical signs of deficiency; and the maintenance of functional integrity of systems or tissue saturation. For some nutrients and some age groups (e.g. adolescents and the elderly), the data on requirements are very limited. In such cases, requirements are often extrapolated from other age groups, or not defined at all.

In the future, multiple levels of nutrient requirements, each associated with a defined level of adequacy such as the prevention of clinical symptoms or the maintenance of tissue saturation, may be defined. With such a system, a multi-tiered population assessment will be possible (NRC, 1986). This approach has been adopted by a FAO/WHO report on requirements for vitamin A, iron, folate and vitamin B-12 (FAO/WHO, in press).

8.2   Evaluating nutrient intakes of individuals

None of the methods of evaluating nutrient intake data described below identify *actual* individuals in the population who have a specific nutrient deficiency. This can only be achieved if biochemical and clinical assessments are also carried out with the dietary investigation. Dietary data alone provide an estimate of the *risk* for nutrient inadequacies. The reliability of this risk estimate depends on the method used for the evaluation. None of the methods outlined below can accurately define an individual's degree of nutrient inadequacy at the present time. A probability approach to this problem is outlined in Section 8.4.

8.2.1 Nutrient adequacy ratio

The nutrient adequacy ratio (NAR) represents an index of adequacy for a nutrient based on the corresponding U.S. Recommended Daily Allowance (RDA) for that nutrient. The NAR is expressed as follows:

$$\text{NAR} = \frac{\text{Subject's daily intake of a nutrient}}{\text{RDA of that nutrient}}$$

The nutrients selected for the calculation of NAR's vary. Guthrie and Scheer (1981) calculated NAR's for twelve nutrients (protein, calcium, zinc, magnesium, iron, vitamins A, B-6, and B-12, ascorbic acid, thiamin, riboflavin, and folacin) in their study of twenty-four-hour dietary records recorded by 212 university students. Eleven nutrients (protein, calcium, iron, magnesium, phosphorus, vitamin A, thiamin, riboflavin, vitamins B-6, B-12, and C) were used by Krebs-Smith et al. (1987) in their study of the effects of variety in food choices on dietary quality, based on the USDA's 1977–1978 Nationwide Food Consumption Survey. For these studies, the NAR values are always truncated at 1.0, to prevent intakes in excess of the RDA for any nutrient from increasing the index. In this way, any false impressions of nutritional adequacy can be avoided. The NAR values for each of the selected nutrients are then averaged to yield a mean adequacy ratio (MAR) for each subject. The latter provides an index of the overall quality of the diet.

$$\text{MAR} = \frac{\text{Sum of the NARs for x nutrients}}{x}$$

Unfortunately, all the nutrients included in the MAR are assigned equal importance using this approach. Furthermore, the MAR does not identify which specific nutrients are inadequate in the diet or provide a means of evaluating the proportion of enery derived from protein, fat, and carbohydrate. (Crocetti and Guthrie, 1981).

8.2.2 Index of nutritional quality

This method, developed at Utah State University (Hansen, 1973), was designed to evaluate the adequacy of meals and diets of individuals and can therefore be used for individual counselling. The index of nutritional quality (INQ) for each nutrient represents the quality of a nutrient in a

Nutrient	Allowance per 1000 kcal	Nutrient	Allowance per 1000 kcal
Protein (g)	25	Sodium (mg)	1100
Fat (g)	39	Vitamin A (IU)	2000
Carbohydrate (g)	137.5	Thiamin (mg)	0.5
Sugar, added (g)	25	Riboflavin (mg)	0.6
Calcium (mg)	450	Vitamin B-6 (mg)	1
Iron (mg)	8	Vitamin B-12 (μg)	1.5
Magnesium (mg)	150	Vitamin C (mg)	30
Zinc (mg)	8	Folacin (μg)	200
Potassium (mg)	1875	Cholesterol (mg)	175

Table 8.3: Single-value nutrient allowances per 1000 kcal for heterogeneous populations one year of age and older. From Hansen RG, Wyse BW. Expression of nutrient allowances per 1,000 kilocalories. © The American Dietetic Association. Reproduced by permission from Journal of the American Dietetic Association, Vol. 76: 223–227, 1980.

food, meal, or diet relative to the recommended nutrient intake. It is expressed as:

$$\text{INQ} = \frac{\text{Amount of nutrient in 1000 kcal of food}}{\text{Allowance of the nutrient per 1000 kcal}}$$

An INQ value greater than 1.0 for any nutrient indicates that an amount of a particular food or a combination of foods that would satisfy the total energy requirement would also provide a sufficient amount of the nutrient. An INQ less than 1.0 indicates that for that nutrient, an excess of a particular food or groups of foods must be consumed to meet the recommended allowance. Thus the capacity of an individual's diet to provide both energy and nutrient needs can be evaluated.

The reference values for the nutrient allowances per 1000 kcal (with the exception of fat, carbohydrate, sugar, and cholesterol) are based on the United States Recommended Dietary Allowances (Food and Nutrition Board, 1980). These single-value nutrient allowances are designed to meet and in some cases exceed the needs of all age groups and physiological states in the population when the energy needs of each group are met (Table 8.3).

Table 8.4 compares the nutrient composition of skim milk per 1000 kcal with the single-value nutrient allowances, expressed as a ratio. High INQ values for calcium, riboflavin, vitamin B-12, and protein indicate that skim milk provides a rich source of these nutrients relative to energy. In some instances, however, the INQ value may be misleading. Whole milk, for example, has an INQ value for calcium which is lower (INQ = 4.0) than that of skim milk (INQ = 7.8), despite a similar calcium content per gram of fluid milk.

	Composition of Skim Milk per 1000 kcal (A)	Allowances per 1000 kcal (B)	INQ Ratio A : B
Energy (kcal)	1000	1000	1.0
Calcium (mg)	3514	450	7.8
Zinc (mg)	11.4	8	1.4
Riboflavin (mg)	4.0	0.6	6.7
Vitamin B-6 (mg)	1.1	1	1.1
Vitamin B-12 (μg)	10.9	1.5	7.2
Protein (g)	97	25	3.9
Fat (g)	5.7	39	0.1
Cholesterol (mg)	57	175	0.3
Sodium (mg)	1486	1100	1.3

Table 8.4: A comparison of the composition of skim milk with single-value nutrient allowances. From Wyse BW, Windham CT, Hansen RG. Nutrition intervention: Panacea or Pandora's box? © The American Dietetic Association. Reproduced by permission from Journal of the American Dietetic Association, Vol. 85: 1084–1090, 1985.

To meet nutritional needs, composite diets must have INQ values of 1.0 or more for all vitamins, minerals, and protein. For sodium and cholesterol, INQ should not greatly exceed 1.0 because moderate intakes of these nutrients are recommended.

8.2.3 Comparison of individual intakes with tables of recommended nutrient intakes

Nutrient intakes of individuals (and groups) are often evaluated by direct comparison with the corresponding recommended nutrient intakes for an individual of the same age, sex, and physiological state from a specific country. In cases where no tables of recommended intakes for a country are available, the FAO and/or WHO requirements are often used (FAO/WHO, 1970; WHO, 1973; Passmore et al., 1974; FAO/WHO/UNU, 1985; FAO/WHO, in press). When using this method for individuals, a nutrient intake below the recommended level does not necessarily mean that the intake is inadequate to meet the individual's own requirement. The recommended levels for the nutrient requirements (except for energy) exceed the actual requirements of most individuals because they are generally set at the mean requirement plus two standard deviations. On no account should individuals, or diets, be classified as 'deficient' or 'inadequate' in any nutrient just because the short-term nutrient intake appears to fall below the recommended intake. Nevertheless, the more the habitual intake of an individual falls below the recommended nutrient intake and the longer the duration of the low intake, the greater the risk of nutrient deficiency for that individual (also see discussion relating to evaluating intakes of populations in Sections 8.3 and 8.4).

8.2.4   Standard deviation score or Z score

The standard deviation or Z score is a measure of an individual's nutrient intake in relation to the distribution of corresponding nutrient intakes of the group. It is calculated as follows:

$$Z \text{ score} = \frac{\text{Individuals nutrient intake value} - \text{mean value for group}}{\text{SD value for that nutrient for the group}}$$

For example, a person with an intake one standard deviation above the group mean has a standard deviation score or Z score of +1.0. This method of evaluating individual intakes is particularly useful in longitudinal studies for monitoring nutrient intakes of individuals relative to the group. It does not, however, evaluate nutrient intakes in relation to the recommended nutrient intakes.

8.3   Evaluating the nutrient intakes of population groups

Three methods can be used for comparing the nutrient intakes of a group with recommended nutrient intakes (Anderson et al., 1982). These are described below. For two of the methods, the distribution of intakes among individuals is taken into account. In such cases, estimates of the usual nutrient intakes for the individuals must be obtained from nutrient intake data derived from multiple observations.

Mean nutrient intake as percentage of recommended nutrient intake

The mean nutrient intake of the group is expressed as a percentage of the corresponding recommended nutrient intake. This method thus assumes that the recommended nutrient intake applies to groups and not to individuals, and does not assess the distribution of intakes among individuals.

Recommended nutrient intake as the 'cutoff' value

In this method the recommended nutrient intake is used as the 'cutoff' value and the percentage of individuals with intakes below that value is calculated. Hence, the distribution of intakes among the individuals is taken into account. This approach is appropriate for comparing nutrient intakes across two groups in a population (Anderson, 1986). It assumes, however, that the recommended nutrient intake describes the requirement of *all* individuals. Consequently, the percentage of individuals with intakes below the recommended nutrient intake is generally a gross overestimate of the *actual* prevalence of intakes below individual requirements because the recommended nutrient intake is generally set at the mean requirement plus two standard deviations (Figure 8.1). As a result, the nutrient requirements of some individuals will always be below the recommended nutrient intake level. Furthermore, the percentage

% Population

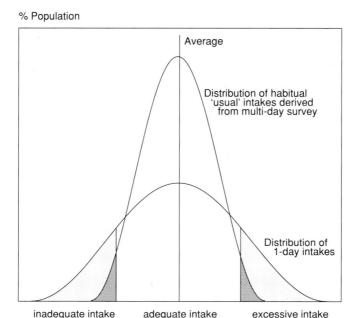

Figure 8.2: The effect of duration of observation or number of replicate observations on apparent distribution of nutrient intakes. Note the impact on the apparent prevalence of 'inadequate' or 'excess' intakes in the population. From Beaton (1982).

of individuals with intakes below the recommended nutrient intake will change according to the dietary methodology used. Figure 8.2 demonstrates the effects of using one day versus multiple days to characterize usual nutrient intakes of individuals on the apparent prevalence of inadequate intakes. Increasing the number of measurement days for each individual decreases the apparent prevalence of inadequate intakes. The extent of the bias in the prevalence estimate depends on the intra-subject variation in intake (Section 6.2) (Beaton, 1988). These results emphasize the importance of characterizing usual nutrient intakes for individuals by using multiple measurement days for each subject.

An arbitrary proportion of the recommended nutrient intake

In the third method, an arbitrary proportion of the recommended nutrient intake is used as the 'cutoff' value and the percentage of individuals with intakes below that value calculated. These individuals again are defined 'at risk'. The lower the cutoff point, the greater the likelihood that at-risk individuals actually have intakes below their individual requirements. No clearly defined rationale exists for the selection of the cutoff value. Two-thirds of the recommended nutrient intake has frequently been used. Using this cutoff rather than the recommended nutrient intake level

Number of individuals

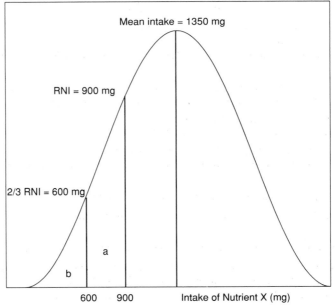

Figure 8.3: The hypothetical distribution of the intake of Nutrient X in a population. A total of (a + b) subjects have intakes below the recommended nutrient intake (RNI): only (b) subjects have intakes below two-thirds of the RNI.

reduces the tendency to overestimate the actual prevalence of inadequate intakes, i.e. the prevalence of intakes below individual requirements (Figure 8.3). Nevertheless, some misclassification of individuals will always occur, as shown in Figure 8.4 (Section 1.4.3). The magnitude and extent of this misclassification cannot be estimated because data on the sensitivity and specificity of the cutoff point are generally unknown (NRC, 1986).

8.4 Probability approach to evaluating nutrient intakes

The probability approach attempts to assess more reliably the risk of nutrient inadequacy both for an individual and a population. Beaton (1972) first used this method to evaluate iron intakes of Canadian women and found the predicted prevalence of inadequate iron intakes was consistent with the prevalence of suboptimal biochemical indices of iron status. It has since been applied to nutrients such as protein, vitamin A, vitamin C, thiamin, riboflavin, and calcium (Anderson et al., 1982; NRC, 1986).

The approach should not be applied to the interpretation of energy intakes because the intake and requirements for energy among non-obese

Number of individuals

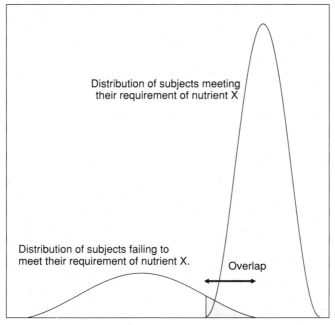

Figure 8.4: The distribution of people who truly fail to meet their requirement (inadequate) and those who truly meet it (adequate) for a hypothetical nutrient X. Reproduced from Nutrient Adequacy: Assessment using Food Consumption Surveys 1986, with permission of the National Academy Press, Washington, D.C.

individuals are highly correlated (NRC, 1986) and insufficient data on the extent of this correlation are available at the present time.

The method predicts the number of individuals within a group with nutrient intakes below their own requirements and hence provides an estimate of the population at risk, or the prevalence of inadequate intakes, for specific nutrients. For individuals, the method estimates the relative probability that the nutrient intake does not meet the individuals actual requirement. It is essential to note that this procedure does not identify with certainty which individuals are 'at risk' because of the absence of information about the actual requirements of each individual. In order to adopt this approach, the following information is required to evaluate the intakes:

- estimated average nutrient requirements for the particular age/sex group of individuals;
- the distribution of requirements for each nutrient among similar individuals. For most nutrients this is not precisely known. In the absence of such information, the distribution of requirements is assumed to be

	Class 1	Class 2	Class 3	Class 4	Class 5	Class 6
A. Individual's intake in terms of the distribution of requirements.	< −2 SD	−2 SD to −1 SD	−1 SD to mean	mean to +1 SD	+ 1 SD to +2 SD	> +2 SD
B. Individual's intake in terms of percentage of RNI.	< 54%	54% to 65.5%	65.5% to 77%	77% to 88.5%	88.5% to 100%	> 100%
C. Probability that individual intake doesn't meet requirement.	1.0	0.93	0.69	0.31	0.07	0.0

Table 8.5: Assignment of 'risk' or probability statements to six classes of observed intakes expressed as proportions of the Canadian Recommended Nutrient Intake. Assumptions in this model are: requirements are normally distributed with the coefficient of variation = 15%; the recommended intake is set at the average requirement + 2 SD. Modified after Beaton (1985). © Am. J. Clin. Nutr. American Society for Clinical Nutrition.

Gaussian with a coefficient of variation of 15% (about the estimated mean nutrient requirement) (Anderson et al., 1982).

- reliable data on the distribution of the usual nutrient intakes of those individuals being assessed, adjusted for intra-subject variation. The NRC (1986) report recommends the collection of nutrient intake data from two or more nonconsecutive days on each individual, depending on the nutrient.

- knowledge of the expected correlation between intake and requirements among individuals. For all nutrients, except energy, this is assumed to be very low.

- data on absorbed usual nutrient intakes. For some nutrients, notably calcium, iron, zinc, and folate, bioavailability is affected by the chemical form of the nutrient and the nature of the diet ingested.

In this approach, the nutrient intakes are classified into six classes defined by the recommended nutrient intake and the associated standard deviation units (Table 8.5, row A). The number of individuals with intakes of the nutrient within each class is determined. This number is then multiplied by the appropriate probability for each class (Table 8.5, row C) to give the number of individuals per class who were likely to have intakes below their own requirements. The sum of these numbers gives the total number of individuals in the population who are at risk for inadequate intakes for the nutrient. This sum can be expressed as a percentage of the total population to give a probability estimate for the population as a whole. For example, assume that in a population of n = 46, the numbers of individuals with usual intakes of vitamin C within

Nutrient	Sex	MI/RNI (%)	Proportion Below RNI (%)	Probability Estimate of Inadequacy (%)
Protein	M	207	2	2
	F	174	13	2
Vitamin C	M	597	2	0
	F	437	5	3
Thiamin	M	137	31	14
	F	118	44	24
Riboflavin	M	195	9	4
	F	169	24	8
Iron	M	136	24	12
	F	79	84	20
Calcium	M	150	24	11
	F	147	34	21

Table 8.6: Comparison of approaches to dietary assessment of nutrient inadequacy. MI = mean intake; RNI = recommended nutrient intakes. Reproduced with permission from Nutrition Research, Vol. 2. Anderson GH, Peterson RD, Beaton GH. Estimating nutrient deficiencies in a population from dietary records: the use of probability analyses. © 1982, Pergamon Press plc.

classes one to six, respectively, are 3, 5, 8, 9, 14, 7. When multiplied by the appropriate probabilities for each class (row C), the number of individuals per class likely to have vitamin C intakes below their own requirements becomes 3, 4.65, 5.52, 2.79, 0.98, 0. The sum of these numbers equals 16.9, and this represents the total number of individuals who are at risk for inadequate intakes for vitamin C. When expressed as a percentage, 37% of the total population are predicted to have intakes of vitamin C below their own requirements.

Anderson et al. (1982) used the probability approach to evaluate intakes of protein, vitamin C, thiamin, riboflavin, iron, and calcium calculated from seven-day food records collected from 83 Ontario school children. Table 8.6 shows that the probability approach usually results in fewer children with intakes below their own calculated requirements compared with the number of children with intakes below the recommended nutrient intake.

The absence of reliable estimates of the mean nutrient requirements and their variability for many nutrients, and the limitations of food composition data for certain nutrients, limit the general applicability of the probability approach to estimate the prevalence of inadequacy for every nutrient at the present time. Nevertheless, the United States Subcommittee on Dietary Evaluation (NRC, 1986) recommended the adoption of the probability approach to estimate the prevalence of inadequate intakes of most nutrients in future national nutrition surveys, with the exception of vitamin C, vitamin A, folate, and energy.

Theoretically, the approach also can be applied to assess excessive intakes of nutrients and/or food components such as food additives and contaminants. Information, comparable to that described above for establishing the prevalence of nutrient inadequacies, is required, as well as data on the distribution of excessive intakes. The latter, however, have not been adequately defined at the present time.

8.5 Summary

Most of the methods for evaluating nutrient intakes are based on comparisons with the estimates of recommended nutrient intakes, published in tables of recommended nutrient intakes. Such estimates are based on information on the nutrient requirements of individuals, derived from a variety of sources. Recommended nutrient intakes are set for a particular group of healthy individuals with specified characteristics, consuming a typical dietary pattern of the country. They refer to the average recommended intake for a nutrient consumed over a reasonable period of time and do not take into account possible interactions involving nutrients and other dietary components. Discrepancies among countries in the recommended nutrient intakes arise because of differences in the sources and interpretation of the nutrient requirement data, incomplete or nonexistent data for some nutrients and/or specific age groups, different age, sex, and physiological subgroupings, different criteria used to define adequacy, differences in judgement by the committees, and differences in the characteristics of the diets among countries.

Methods used to evaluate nutrient intakes of individuals include a nutrient adequacy ratio (NAR), an index of nutritional quality (INQ), comparison of individual intakes with corresponding recommended nutrient intakes, and a Z score. For population groups, the mean nutrient intakes can be expressed as percentages of the corresponding recommended nutrient intakes. Alternatively, the recommended nutrient intake, or an arbitrary proportion of the recommended nutrient intake, can be used as a cutoff value, and the percentage of individuals with intakes below the cutoff value calculated. This latter approach overestimates the actual proportion of individuals with intakes below their own requirements. More recently, a probability approach has been used. This method assesses more reliably the risk of nutrient inadequacy for an individual or, for a population, provides an estimate of the prevalence of inadequate intakes. To use this model, data on estimated average requirements and the distribution of requirements for the particular age/sex group are required, as well as reliable information on the distribution of the usual nutrient intakes of individuals. The probability approach can also be used to assess excessive intakes of nutrients and/or food components such as additives and contaminants, provided that the association between level of intake and risk of toxicity is known.

The methods outlined above only provide an estimate of the risk of a population and/or individual to nutrient inadequacies. They do not identify actual individuals in the population who are deficient in a nutrient, or define the severity of nutrient inadequacy. Such information can only be obtained when dietary intake data are combined with biochemical, anthropometric, and clinical indices.

References

Anderson SA (ed). (1986). Guidelines for Use of Dietary Intake Data. Life Sciences Research Office, Federation of American Societies for Experimental Biology, Bethesda, Maryland.

Anderson GH, Peterson RD, Beaton GH. (1982). Estimating nutrient deficiencies in a population from dietary records: the use of probability analyses. Nutrition Research 2: 409–415.

Beaton GH. (1972). The use of nutritional requirements and allowances. In: Proceedings of Western Hemisphere Nutrition Congress II. Futura Publishing Co. Inc., Mount Kisco, New York, pp. 356–363.

Beaton GH. (1982). What do we think we are measuring? In: Symposium on Dietary Data Collection, Analysis, and Significance. Massachusetts Agricultural Experimental Station, College of Food and Natural Resources, University of Massachusetts at Amherst, Research Bulletin No. 675, pp. 36–49.

Beaton GH. (1985). Uses and limits of the use of the Recommended Dietary Allowances for evaluating dietary intake data. American Journal of Clinical Nutrition 41: 155–164.

Beaton GH. (1988). Twelfth Boyd Orr Memorial Lecture. Nutrient Requirements and Population Data. Proceedings of the Nutrition Society 47: 63–78.

Buss DH. (1986). Symposium on nutrient recommendations for man — theory and practice. Variations in recommended nutrient intakes. Proceedings of the Nutrition Society 45: 345–350.

Canadian Council on Nutrition (1940). The Canadian Dietary Standard. National Health Review 8: 1–9.

Crocetti AF, Guthrie HA. (1981). Food consumption patterns and nutritional quality of U.S. diets: A preliminary report. Food Technology September 40–49.

Deutsche Gesellschaft für Ernährung (1975). Recommended Dietary Allowance of the Federal Republic of Germany (Empfehlungen für die Nahrstoffzufuhr). Umschau Verlag, Frankfurt/Main, West Germany.

Department of Health and Social Security (1981). Recommended Daily Amounts of Food Energy and Nutrients for Groups of People in the United Kingdom. Second impression. Report by the Committee on Medical Aspects of Food Policy. Report on Health and Social Subjects No.15. Her Majesty's Stationery Office, London.

FAO/WHO (Food and Agriculture Organization / World Health Organization) (1970). Requirements of Ascorbic Acid, Vitamin D, Vitamin B-12, Folate and Iron. Report of a Joint FAO/WHO Expert Group. WHO Technical Report Series No. 452. FAO Nutrition Meetings Report Series No. 47. World Health Organization, Geneva.

FAO/WHO (Food and Agriculture Organization / World Health Organization) (in press). Requirements of Vitamin A, Iron, Folate and Vitamin B-12. Report of a Joint FAO/WHO Expert Consultation. Rome (in press).

FAO/WHO/UNU (Food and Agriculture Organization / World Health Organization / United Nations University) (1985). Energy and Protein Requirements. WHO Technical Report Series No. 724. World Health Organization, Geneva.

Food and Nutrition Board (1943). Recommended Dietary Allowances. National Academy of Sciences, National Research Council Reprint and Circular Series No. 115, Washington, D.C.

Food and Nutrition Board, Committee on Dietary Allowances (1980). Recommended Dietary Allowances, Ninth edition. National Academy of Sciences, Washington, D.C.

Food and Nutrition Board, National Research Council – National Academy of Sciences (1986). Recommended Dietary Allowances: Scientific issues and process for the future. Journal of Nutrition 116: 482–488.

Guthrie HA, Scheer JC. (1981). Validity of a dietary score for assessing nutrient adequacy. Journal of the American Dietetic Association 78: 240–245.

Hansen RG. (1973). An index of food quality. Nutrition Reviews 31: 1–7.

Hansen RG and Wyse BW. (1980). Expression of nutrient allowances per 1,000 kilocalories. Journal of the American Dietetic Association 76: 223–227.

Harper AE.(1985). Origin of Recommended Dietary Allowances — an historic overview. American Journal of Clinical Nutrition 41: 140–148.

Health and Welfare Canada (1983). Recommended Nutrient Intakes for Canadians. Bureau of Nutritional Sciences, Health Protection Branch, Health and Welfare, Ottawa.

International Union of Nutritional Sciences (1983). Recommended Dietary Intakes around the World. A Report by Committee 1/5 of the International Union of Nutritional Sciences (1982). Nutrition Abstracts and Reviews 53: 1075–1118.

Krebs-Smith SM, Smiciklas-Wright H, Guthrie HA, Krebs-Smith J. (1987). The effects of variety in food choices on dietary quality. Journal of the American Dietetic Association 87: 897–903.

League of Nations (1938). Report by the Technical Commission on Nutrition as the work of its Third Session. Bulletin League of Nations Health Organization 7: 461–492.

NRC (National Research Council) (1986). Nutrient Adequacy. Assessment using Food Consumption Surveys. Subcommittee on Criteria for Dietary Evaluation, Coordinating Committee on Evaluation of Food Consumption Surveys. Food and Nutrition Board, Commission on Life Sciences. National Academy Press, Washington, D.C.

Nutrition Advisory Committee (1983). Recommendations for Selected Nutrient Intakes for New Zealanders.

Passmore R, Nicol BM, Rao MN. (1974). Handbook on Human Nutritional Requirements. World Health Organization Monograph Series No. 61, World Health Organization, Geneva.

WHO (World Health Organization) (1973). Trace Elements in Human Nutrition. WHO Technical Report Series No. 532. World Health Organization, Geneva.

Wretlind, A. (1982). Standards for nutritional adequacy of the diet. European and WHO/FAO viewpoints. American Journal of Clinical Nutrition 36: 366–375.

Wyse BW, Windham CT, Hansen RG. (1985). Nutrition intervention: Panacea or Pandora's box? Journal of the American Dietetic Association 85: 1084–1090.

Chapter 9

Anthropometric assessment

The term 'nutritional anthropometry' first appeared in 'Body measurements and Human Nutrition' (Brŏzek, 1956) and has been defined by Jelliffe (1966) as:

> measurements of the variations of the physical dimensions
> and the gross composition of the human body at different
> age levels and degrees of nutrition.

Subsequently, a number of publications made recommendations on specific body measurements for characterizing nutritional status, standardized measurement techniques, and suitable reference data (Jelliffe, 1966; WHO, 1968; Weiner and Lourie, 1969). Today, anthropometric measurements are widely used in the assessment of nutritional status, particularly when a chronic imbalance between intakes of protein and energy occurs. Such disturbances modify the patterns of physical growth and the relative proportions of body tissues such as fat, muscle, and total body water.

Anthropometric measurements are of two types: growth (Section 10.1) and body composition measurements. The latter can be further subdivided into measurements of body fat (Section 11.1) and fat-free mass (Section 11.2), the two major compartments of total body mass. Anthropometric indices can be derived directly from a single raw measurement (e.g. weight for age, height for age, and head circumference for age), or from a combination of raw measurements such as weight and height, skinfold thicknesses at various sites, and/or limb circumferences. Some combinations (e.g. triceps skinfold and mid-upper-arm circumference) are used to derive prediction equations to estimate mid-upper-arm muscle area and mid-upper-arm fat area. The latter give an indication of the muscle mass and total body fat content of the body, respectively. Alternatively, various anthropometric indices can be used in multiple-regression equations to predict body density and to calculate body fat and fat-free mass (Section 11.1.6). It should be noted that such prediction equations are more accurate for healthy lean subjects than malnourished or obese

155

subjects, because they were derived using measurements obtained from these populations (Heymsfield and Casper, 1987).

Selection of anthropometric indices for nutritional assessment systems depends on the factors discussed in detail in Section 1.3. Consideration of the sensitivity and specificity of anthropometric indices is especially critical. Sensitive indices exhibit large changes during nutritional deprivation, and after nutritional intervention, and correctly identify those individuals who are truly malnourished. Consequently, such anthropometric indices should be selected for nutritional assessment systems involving nutritional screening or surveillance. Similarly, anthropometric indices with high specificity are also desirable to identify healthy persons correctly, and, thus avoid giving nutritional intervention unnecessarily. Both the sensitivity and specificity of an anthropometric index will vary according to the severity and prevalence of the nutritional problem, as discussed in Section 1.3. These factors must also be considered when selecting an anthropometric index.

9.1   Advantages and limitations of anthropometric assessment

Anthropometric indices are of increasing importance in nutritional assessment as the measurement procedures have several advantages, which are listed in Table 9.1. Despite these advantages, nutritional anthropometry has several limitations. For example, it is a relatively insensitive method and it cannot detect disturbances in nutritional status over short periods of time or identify specific nutrient deficiencies. Furthermore, nutritional anthropometry is unable to distinguish disturbances in growth or body composition induced by nutrient (e.g. zinc) deficiencies from those caused by imbalances in protein and energy intake. Nevertheless, nutritional anthropometry can be used to monitor periodic changes in growth and/or body composition in individuals (e.g. hospital patients) and in population groups, after a nutrition intervention program.

Certain non-nutritional factors (such as disease, genetics, diurnal variation, and reduced energy expenditure) can reduce the specificity and sensitivity of anthropometric measurements (Section 1.3), although such effects generally can be excluded or taken into account by appropriate sampling and experimental design.

9.2   Sources of error in nutritional anthropometry

Errors may occur in nutritional anthropometry, all of which affect the precision, accuracy, and validity of the measurements/indices. The errors can be attributed to three major effects: measurement errors, alterations in the composition and physical properties of certain tissues, and use of invalid assumptions in the derivation of body composition from anthropometric measurements (Heymsfield and Casper, 1987).

Measurement errors, both random and systematic, may occur in nutritional anthropometry. They arise from: examiner error resulting from inadequate training, instrument error, and measurement difficulties (e.g. skinfold thicknesses) (Johnston, 1981; Himes, 1987). Some common sources of measurement errors in anthropometry have been summarized by Zerfas (1979) and are shown in Tables 9.2 and 9.3. Some of these measurement errors can be minimized by training personnel to use standardized, validated techniques, and instruments that are precise and correctly calibrated (Lohman et al., 1988). Furthermore, the precision and accuracy of each measurement technique should be firmly established, prior to use. The precision can be assessed by examiners repeating the measurements on the same subjects (a minimum of ten subjects is recommended) and calculating the inter- and intra-examiner coefficients of variation. Standardization procedures and calculation of the inter- and intra-examiner coefficients of variation for anthropometric measurements are given in WHO (1983). To improve precision, the measurements should be performed in triplicate and the mean reported. In the absence of an absolute reference standard, the accuracy of anthropometric measurements (defined as how close the measurements are to the true value) is estimated by comparing them with those made by the supervisor (WHO, 1983).

For longitudinal studies involving sequential anthropometric measurements on the same group of individuals (e.g. surveillance), it is preferable to have one person carrying out the same measurements throughout

---

- The procedures use simple, safe, noninvasive techniques which can be used at the bedside and are applicable to large sample sizes (Heymsfield and Casper, 1987).

- Equipment required is inexpensive, portable, and durable and can be made or purchased locally.

- Relatively unskilled personnel can perform measurement procedures.

- The methods are precise and accurate, provided that standardized techniques are used.

- Information is generated on past long-term nutritional history, which cannot be obtained with equal confidence using other techniques.

- The procedures can assist in the identification of mild to moderate malnutrition, as well as severe states of malnutrition.

- The methods may be used to evaluate changes in nutritional status over time and from one generation to the next, a phenomenon known as the secular trend (Johnston, 1981).

- Screening tests, to identify individuals at high risk to malnutrition, can be devised (Chen et al., 1980).

Table 9.1: The advantages of anthropometric assessment.

Measurements + Common Error	Proposed Solution
All measurements	
Inadequate instrument	select method appropriate to resources
Restless child	postpone measurement
	involve parent in procedure
	use culturally appropriate procedures
Reading	training and refresher exercises
	stressing accuracy
	intermittent revision by supervisor
Recording	record results immediately
	after measurement is taken
	have results checked by second person
Length	
Incorrect method for age	use only when subject is < 2 years old
Footwear or headwear	remove as local culture permits
not removed	(or make allowances)
Head not in correct plane	correct position of child before measuring
Child not straight along board	have assistant and child's parent present;
and/or feet not parallel	don't take the measurement while
with movable board	the child is struggling; settle child
Board not firmly against heels	correct pressure should be practised
Height	
Incorrect method for age	use only when subject is ≥ 2 years old
Footwear or headware not	remove as local culture permits
removed	(or make allowances)
Head not in correct plane,	correct technique with
subject not straight,	practice and regular retraining.
knees bent, or feet	Provide adequate assistance.
not flat on floor	Calm non-cooperative children
Board not firmly against head	Move head board to compress hair
Weight	
Room cold, no privacy	use appropriate clinic facilities
Scale not calibrated to zero	re-calibrate after every subject
Subject wearing heavy clothing	remove or make allowances for clothing
Subject moving or anxious	wait until subject is calm or remove
as a result of prior incident	cause of anxiety (e.g. scale too high)

Table 9.2: Common errors and possible solutions when measuring length, height, and weight. Modified from Zerfas AJ. (1979). In: Jelliffe DB, Jelliffe EFP (eds). Human Nutrition. A Comprehensive Treatise, Volume 2. Nutrition and Growth. Plenum Press.

the study to eliminate inter-examiner errors. This is particularly critical when increments in growth and body composition are calculated, because such increments, although generally small, are associated with two error terms, one on each measurement occasion. Changes in growth and body composition in individuals can then be correlated with factors such as age, the onset of disease, response to nutrition intervention, therapy,

Measurements + Common Error	Proposed Solution
Arm circumference	
Subject not standing in correct position	position subject correctly
Tape too thick, stretched, or creased	use correct instrument
Wrong arm	use left arm
Mid-arm point incorrectly marked	measure midpoint carefully
Arm not hanging loosely by side during measurement, examiner not comfortable or level with subject, tape around arm not at midpoint: too tight (causing skin contour indentation), too loose	correct techniques with training, supervision, and regular refresher courses. Take into account any cultural problems, such as wearing of arm band
Head circumference	
Occipital protuberance / supraorbital landmarks poorly defined	position tape correctly
Hair crushed inadequately, ears under tape or tension, and position poorly maintained at time of reading	correct technique with training, supervision, and regular refresher courses
Headwear not removed	remove as local culture permits
Triceps fatfold	
Wrong arm	use left arm
Mid-arm point or posterior plane incorrectly measured or marked	measure midpoint carefully
Arm not loose by side during measurement	
Finger-thumb pinch or caliper placement too deep (muscle) or too superficial (skin)	correct technique with training, supervision, and regular refresher courses
Caliper jaws not at marked site	
Reading done too early, pinch not maintained, caliper handle not fully released.	
Examiner not comfortable or level with subject	ensure examiner is level with subject for measurement

Table 9.3: Common errors and possible solutions when measuring mid-upper-arm circumference, head circumference, and triceps skinfold. Modified from Zerfas AJ. (1979). In: Jelliffe DB, Jelliffe EFP (eds). Human Nutrition. A Comprehensive Treatise, Volume 2. Nutrition and Growth. Plenum Press.

etc. Collection of longitudinal anthropometric measurements is more time consuming, expensive, and laborious than cross-sectional surveys, and, as a result, the sample size is generally smaller and the probability of systematic sampling bias is generally greater than in cross-sectional studies (Johnston, 1974).

For cross-sectional studies, examiners should be rotated among the subjects to reduce the effect of the bias of the individual examiners. Such surveys are particularly suitable for making comparisons between population groups, provided that probability sampling techniques have been used to ensure that the samples are representative of the populations from which they are drawn (Goldstein, 1974).

Alterations in the composition and/or physical properties of certain tissues may occur in both healthy and diseased subjects, resulting in inaccuracies in certain anthropometric measurements and/or indices. Even among healthy individuals, body weight may be affected by variations in tissue hydration with the menstrual cycle (Heymsfield and Casper, 1987), whereas skinfolds may be influenced by alterations in compressibility with age and site of the measurements (Himes et al., 1979). Generally, anthropometric measurements are not corrected to account for these effects. Errors also arise when the prediction equations, developed for healthy lean subjects, are applied to patients with certain diseases in which increases in total body water and alterations in the distribution of body fat occur (Section 11.1.6).

Invalid assumptions may lead to erroneous estimates of body composition when derived from anthropometric measurements, especially in protein-energy malnutrition, certain disease states, or obesity. For instance, use of skinfold thickness measurements to estimate total body fat assumes that: (a) the thickness of the subcutaneous adipose tissue reflects a constant proportion of the total body fat, and (b) the sites selected represent the average thickness of the subcutaneous adipose tissue. In fact, the relationship between subcutaneous and internal fat is nonlinear, and varies with body weight, age, and disease state. Very lean subjects have a smaller proportion of body fat deposited subcutaneously than obese subjects (Allen et al., 1956), and in malnourished persons there is probably a shift of fat storage from subcutaneous to deep visceral sites. Variations in the distribution of subcutaneous fat also occur with sex, race, and age (Robson et al., 1971; Durnin and Womersley, 1974).

Estimates of mid-upper-arm muscle area are used as an index of total body muscle and fat-free mass, regardless of age and health status, despite the known changes in the relationship between arm muscle and total skeletal muscle mass, and between arm muscle and fat-free mass, with age and certain disease states (Heymsfield and McManus, 1985).

9.3   Evaluation of anthropometric indices

The selection of appropriate reference data to allow comparison of the distributions of the anthropometric indices of the study group with those of an apparently healthy population, and to establish 'risk' categories or cutoff points, is a difficult problem. There is lack of agreement regarding the use of local versus international reference data. Some investigators advocate the use of local reference data derived from ethnically similar but privileged groups living in the same country, to minimize genetic influences (Goldstein and Tanner, 1980); others suggest that the advantages of one universal standard drawn from a well-defined and accurately sampled population outweigh the problems of genetic influence (Habicht et al., 1974; Graitcer and Gentry, 1981). The World Health Organization (WHO, 1983) has recommended the use of the United States National Center for Health Statistics (NCHS) growth percentiles (Hamill et al., 1979) as an international reference for comparisons of health and nutritional status among countries.

Several systems are available for classifying individuals as malnourished, based on anthropometric indices. All utilize at least one anthropometric index and one or more cutoff points based on appropriate reference data. The cutoff points may be expressed as percentiles, standard deviation scores, and, in some cases, as a percentage of the reference median, although the latter approach is not recommended (Dibley et al., 1987) (Section 13.1 and 13.2.2). Cutoff points are often established by reviewing anthropometric characteristics of individuals with clinically moderate and/or severe malnutrition or who subsequently die. In population studies, cutoff points may be combined with 'trigger levels' to define criteria for an intervention. For example, an intervention may only be initiated if at least 10% of the population have a specific anthropometric index (e.g. weight for age) below the established cutoff point (WHO, 1976). In this case 10% is the 'trigger level'.

Details of the techniques used to measure growth and body composition, together with the indices derived from these measurements, are discussed in Chapters 10 and 11. Sources of reference data available for comparison of both growth and body composition indices are presented in Chapter 12, whereas Chapter 13 includes a discussion of methods used for evaluation of anthropometric indices. Laboratory techniques used to measure body composition are discussed in Chapter 14.

References

Allen TH, Peng MT, Chen KP, Huang TF, Chang C, Fang HS. (1956). Prediction of total adiposity from skinfolds and the curvilinear relationship between external and internal adiposity. Metabolism 5: 346–352.

Brŏzek JF (ed). (1956). Body Measurements and Human Nutrition. Wayne State University Press, Detroit.

Chen LC, Chowdhury AKM, Huffman SL. (1980). Anthropometric assessment of energy-protein malnutrition and subsequent risk of mortality among preschool-aged children. American Journal of Clinical Nutrition 33: 1836–1845.

Dibley MJ, Goldsby JB, Staehling NW, Trowbridge FL. (1987). Development of normalized curves for the international growth reference: historical and technical considerations. American Journal of Clinical Nutrition 46: 736–748.

Durnin JVGA, Womersley J. (1974). Body fat assessed from total body density and its estimation from skinfold thickness: measurements on 481 men and women aged from 16 to 72 years. British Journal of Nutrition 32: 77–97.

Goldstein H. (1974). Some statistical considerations on the use of anthropometry to assess nutritional status. In: Roche AF, Falkner F (eds) Nutrition and Malnutrition: Identification and Measurement. Plenum Press, New York–London, pp. 221-230.

Goldstein H, Tanner JM. (1980). Ecological considerations in the creation and the use of child growth standards. Lancet 1: 582–585.

Graitcer PL, Gentry EM. (1981). Measuring children: one reference for all. Lancet 2: 297–299.

Habicht JP, Martorell R, Yarbrough C, Malina RM, Klein RE. (1974). Height and weight standards for preschool children. How relevant are ethnic differences in growth potential? Lancet I: 611–615.

Hamill PVV, Drizd TA, Johnson CL, Reed RB, Roche AF, Moore WM. (1979). Physical growth: National Center for Health Statistics Percentiles. American Journal of Clinical Nutrition 32: 607–629.

Heymsfield SB, Casper K. (1987). Anthropometric assessment of the adult hospitalized patient. Journal of Parenteral and Enteral Nutrition 11: 36S–41S.

Heymsfield SB, McManus CB. (1985). Tissue components of weight loss in cancer patients. Cancer 55: 238–249.

Himes JH. (1987). Purposeful assessment of nutritional status. In: Johnston FE (ed) Nutritional Anthropology. Alan R. Liss Inc., New York, pp. 85–99.

Himes JH, Roche AF, Siervogel RM. (1979). Compressibility of skinfolds and measurement of subcutaneous fat. American Journal of Clinical Nutrition 32: 1734–1740.

Jelliffe DB. (1966). The Assessment of the Nutritional Status of the Community. WHO Monograph No. 53. World Health Organization, Geneva.

Johnston FE. (1974). Cross-sectional versus longitudinal studies. In: Roche AF, Falkner (eds) Nutrition and Malnutrition: Identification and Measurement. Plenum Press, New York–London, pp. 287–308.

Johnston FE. (1981). Anthropometry and nutritional status. In: Assessing Changing Food Consumption Patterns. Committee on Food Consumption Patterns, Food and Nutrition Board, National Research Council. National Academy Press, Washington, D.C., pp. 252–264.

Lohman TG, Roche AF, Martorell R. (eds). (1988). Anthropometric Standardization Reference Manual. Human Kinetics Books, Champaign, Illinois.

Robson JRF, Bazin M, Soderstrom R. (1971). Ethnic differences in skin-fold thickness. American Journal of Clinical Nutrition 24: 864–868.

Weiner JS and Lourie JA. (1969). Human Biology: A Guide to Field Methods: International Biological Programme IBP Handbook, No. 9. Blackwell Scientific Publications, Oxford–Edinburgh.

WHO (World Health Organization) (1968). Nutritional Status of Populations. A Manual on Anthropometric Appraisal of Trends. WHO/Nutr/70. 129. World Health Organization, Geneva.

WHO (World Health Organization) (1976). Report on Methodology of Nutritional Surveillance. FAO/UNICEF/WHO Expert Committee. WHO Technical Report Series No. 593. World Health Organization, Geneva.

WHO (World Health Organization) (1983). Measuring Change in Nutritional Status. Guidelines for Assessing the Nutritional Impact of Supplementary Feeding Programmes for Vulnerable Groups. World Health Organization, Geneva.

Zerfas AJ. (1979). Anthropometric field methods: general. In: Jelliffe DB, Jelliffe EFP (eds) Human Nutrition. A Comprehensive Treatise. Volume 2. Nutrition and Growth. Plenum Press, New York, pp. 339–364.

Chapter 10

Anthropometric assessment of growth

The most widely used anthropometric measurements of growth are those of stature (height or length) and body weight. These measurements can be made quickly and easily, and, with care and training, accurately. Head circumference measurements are often taken in association with stature. Details of the standardized procedures for these growth measurements are summarized below, and are given in detail in Lohman et al. (1988). Indices such as head circumference for age, weight for age, weight for stature, and numerical weight:stature ratios are derived from these measurements. Some indices have been recommended by the World Health Organization (WHO, 1983) as primary measures of past or current nutritional status in children; in combination, these indices can distinguish between stunting and wasting. In hospital patients, anthropometric growth indices are used primarily to identify protein-energy malnutrition and obesity, and to monitor changes after nutrition intervention.

10.1 Growth measurements

Measurement of head circumference is important because it is closely related to brain size. It is often used with other measurements to detect pathological conditions associated with an unusually large (macrocephalic) or small (microcephalic) head. Recumbent length is measured in infants and children less than two years of age. Height is measured in older children and adults. Knee height measurements can also be used to estimate height in those persons with severe spinal curvature, or who are unable to stand. Weight in infants and young children can be measured using a suspended scale and a weighing sling, or a pediatric scale. For older children and adults, a beam balance with nondetachable weights is recommended. Elbow breadth is used as a measure of frame size, which is relatively independent of adiposity and age (Frisancho and Flegel, 1983). It should be measured with flat-bladed sliding calipers.

163

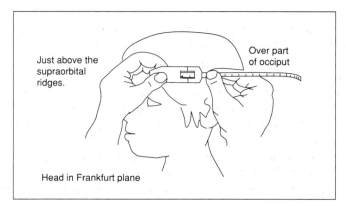

Figure 10.1: Measurement of head circumference.

10.1.1 Measurement of head circumference

For the measurement of head circumference, a narrow, flexible, and nonstretch tape made of fiberglass or steel about 0.6 cm wide should be used; alternatively a fiberglass insertion tape may be used. The subject stands relaxed with the left side facing the measurer, looking straight ahead so that the line of vision is perpendicular to the body and the Frankfurt plane of the head is in a horizontal position (Figure 10.4). The Frankfurt plane is a conceptual plane which passes through the external auditory meatus (the small flap of skin on the forward edge of the ear) and the tops of the lower bones of the eye sockets immediately below the eye. The tape is placed just above the supra-orbital ridges covering the most prominent part of the frontal bulge, and over the part of the occiput which gives the maximum circumference (Figure 10.1) (Weiner and Lourie, 1969). Care must be taken to ensure that the tape is at the same level on each side of the head and is pulled tightly to compress the hair. Measurements are made to the nearest millimeter.

10.1.2 Measurement of recumbent length

For infants and children less than two years of age, recumbent length is measured, generally with a wooden measuring board (Figure 10.2). Two examiners are required to correctly position the subject and ensure accurate and reliable measurements of length. The subject is placed, face upward, with the head towards the fixed end and the body parallel to the long axis of the board (Figure 10.3). The shoulder-blades should rest against the surface of the board. One examiner applies gentle traction to bring the crown of the child's head into contact with the fixed headboard and positions the head so that the Frankfurt plane is vertical. The second examiner holds the subject's feet, without shoes, toes pointing directly upward, and keeping the subject's knees straight, brings the movable

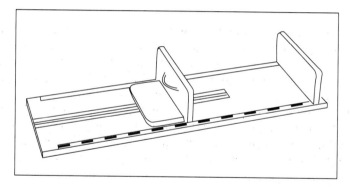

Figure 10.2: Device for the measurement of recumbent length.

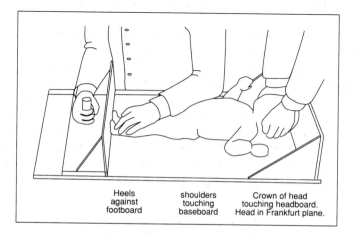

| Heels against footboard | shoulders touching baseboard | Crown of head touching headboard. Head in Frankfurt plane. |

Figure 10.3: Measurement of recumbent length. Reproduced from Robbins GE, Trowbridge FL. In: Nutrition Assessment: A Comprehensive Guide for Planning Intervention by M.D. Simko, C. Cowell, and J.A. Gilbride, p.75, with permission of Aspen Publishers, Inc., © 1984.

footboard to rest firmly against the heels (Figure 10.3). The reading is taken to the nearest millimeter. If the subject is restless, only the left leg should be positioned for the measurement (Tanner et al., 1966; Weiner and Lourie, 1969; Nutrition Canada, 1980). For field use, a portable infant length measuring scale can be used. This device is assembled from four separate plastic sections which lock together to form head and foot plates, with a strong, two-meter metal tape insert. Suppliers of measuring devices and scales are listed in Appendix A10.1.

10.1.3 Measurement of height

Children over two years of age and adults are generally measured in the standing position using a stadiometer or portable anthropometer. A

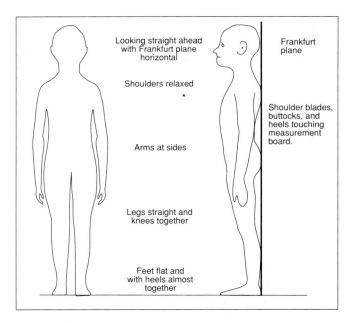

Figure 10.4: Positioning of subject for height measurement. Horizontal line is the Frankfurt plane, which should be in a horizontal position when height is measured. Reproduced from Robbins GE, Trowbridge FL. In: Nutrition Assessment: A Comprehensive Guide for Planning Intervention by M.D. Simko, C. Cowell, and J.A. Gilbride, p.77, with permission of Aspen Publishers, Inc., © 1984.

plastic instrument called the Accustat stadiometer is also available, which is less expensive than the conventional stadiometer for measuring stature (Roche et al., 1988). Alternatively, some form of right-angle headboard and a measuring rod or nonstretchable tape fixed to a vertical surface can be used. In the field, vertical surfaces are not always available. In such circumstances, modified tape measures such as the Microtoise, which measure up to two meters, can be used (Cameron, 1986). Platform scales with movable measuring rods are not suitable. Clothing should be minimal when measuring height so that posture can be clearly seen. Shoes and socks should not be worn.

When measuring height, the subject stands straight with the head positioned such that the Frankfurt plane is horizontal (Figure 10.4), feet together, knees straight, and heels, buttocks, and shoulder blades in contact with the vertical surface of the stadiometer, anthropometer, or wall. Arms should be hanging loosely at the sides with palms facing the thighs; the head is not necessarily in contact with the vertical surface. For younger subjects, it may be necessary to hold the heels to ensure that they do not leave the ground. Some investigators recommend applying gentle upward pressure to the mastoid processes to stretch

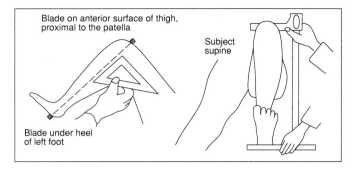

Figure 10.5: Measurement of knee height.

the spine and minimize effects produced by diurnal variation (Tanner et al., 1966). Subjects are asked to take a deep breath and stand tall to aid the straightening of the spine. Shoulders should be relaxed. The movable headboard is then gently lowered until it touches the crown of the head The height measurement is taken at maximum inspiration, with the examiner's eyes level with the headboard to avoid parallax errors. Height is recorded to the nearest millimeter. If the reading falls between two values, the lower reading is always recorded (Cameron, 1986). Successive measurements should agree within five millimeters (Weiner and Lourie, 1969; Nutrition Canada, 1980; Robbins and Trowbridge, 1984). The time at which the measurement is made should be noted because diurnal variations in height occur. In cases where large amounts of adipose tissue prevent the heels, buttocks, and shoulders from simultaneously touching the wall, subjects should simply be asked to stand erect (Chumlea et al., 1984).

The Microtoise consists of an 'L'-shaped device (the head-bar) to which is attached a spring-loaded coiled tape measure. In use, the head-bar is placed securely on the floor and the tape *fully* withdrawn. The free end of the tape is secured with a nail to a suitable vertical surface directly above the head-bar. The head-bar is then raised above the height of the subject, who is instructed to stand erect directly below the point of attachment, and is then positioned by the anthropometrist such that the Frankfurt plane of the head is horizontal. The head-bar is then lowered by a second person until it touches the crown of the head and compresses the hair: a direct reading of height to the nearest millimeter may then be obtained.

10.1.4 Measurement of knee height

Knee height is highly correlated with stature, and may be used to estimate height in persons with severe spinal curvature or who are unable to stand. Knee height is measured with a caliper consisting of an adjustable measuring stick with a blade attached to each end at a 90° angle (Figure 10.5).

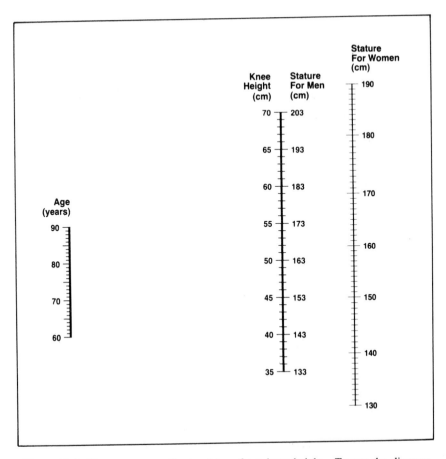

Figure 10.6: Nomogram to estimate stature from knee height. To use the diagram, locate the person's age on the column furthest to the left, and the knee height on the next column. Then lay a rule or straightedge so that it touches these two points. The estimated stature is indicated at the intersection of the straightedge and the stature column for the appropriate sex. Reproduced with permission of Ross Laboratories, Columbus, OH 43216. From Nutritional Assessment of the Elderly through Anthropometry. Figure 9, page 11, © 1984 Ross Laboratories.

Knee height is measured on the left leg, which is bent at the knee at a 90° angle, while the subject is in the supine position. One of the blades is positioned under the heel of the left foot and the other is placed over the anterior surface of the left thigh above the condyles of the femur and just proximal to the patella. The shaft of the caliper is held parallel to the shaft of the tibia and gentle pressure applied to the blades of the caliper. At least two successive measurements should be made which agree within five millimeters (Chumlea et al., 1985). A nomogram (Figure 10.6) or formulae (below) can be used to estimate stature from knee height in

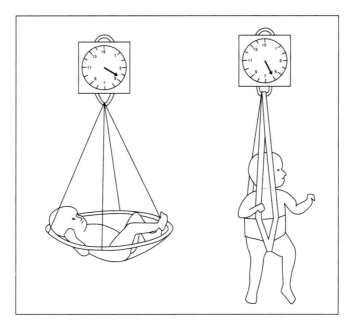

Figure 10.7: Measurement of weight in infants and children using a spring balance. The bowl for the baby is made from a metal or bamboo ring and netting.

men and women. Both of these methods are derived from Chumlea et al., 1984.

Male stature (cm) = (2.02 × knee height [cm]) − (0.04 × age [yr]) + 64.19

Female stature (cm) = (1.83 × knee height [cm]) − (0.24 × age [yr]) + 84.88

10.1.5 Measurement of weight in infants and children

In field surveys, a suspended scale and a weighing sling may be used for weighing infants and children less than two years of age (Figure 10.7). They should be weighed naked or with the minimum of clothing. After slipping the subject into the sling, the weight is recorded as soon as the indicator on the scale has stabilized (Jelliffe, 1966; Cameron, 1986). Alternatively, a pediatric scale (Figure 10.8a) with a pan may be used. Care must be taken to ensure that the infant is placed on the pan scale so the weight is distributed equally about the center of the pan. Once the infant is lying quietly, weight is recorded to the nearest 10 g. If there is no alternative, the mother and subject can be weighed together, and then the mother alone, using a beam balance. The subject's weight can then be calculated by subtraction.

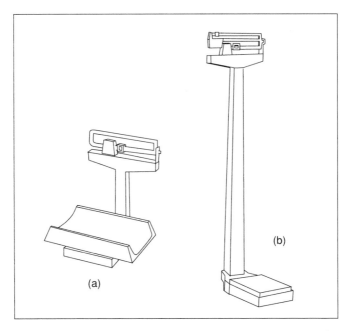

Figure 10.8: Measurement of weight using a pediatric scale (a) for an infant, and a beam balance (b) for a child or adult.

10.1.6 Measurement of weight in older children and adults

The measurement of weight in older children and adults should preferably be done after the bladder has been emptied, and before a meal. A beam balance with nondetachable weights should be used, where possible (Figure 10.8b). Unfortunately, beam balances tend to be heavy and bulky, and are therefore unsuitable for field use. In such cases, spring balance scales, although less accurate and reliable, are often used (Office of Population Censuses and Surveys, Social Survey Division, 1984). The balance should be placed on a hard flat surface, and checked for zero-balance before each measurement. The subject should stand unassisted, in the center of the platform, and be asked to look straight ahead, standing relaxed but still, preferably in the nude. If this is not possible, the subject should wear light underclothing and/or a paper examination gown. The weight of these garments should be recorded for later subtraction; standard corrections for clothing should not be used. The presence of visible edema should also be recorded. Body weight should be recorded to the nearest 0.1 kg (Weiner and Lourie, 1969; Nutrition Canada, 1980). Again, the time at which the measurement is made should be noted because diurnal variations in weight occur (Sumner and Whitacre, 1931). The balance should be calibrated with a set of weights regularly throughout the year, and whenever it is moved

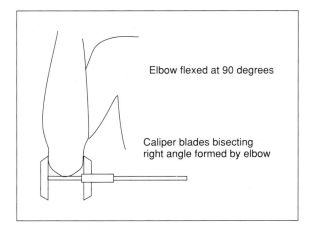

Figure 10.9: Measurement of elbow breadth.

to another location. Special equipment, such as a movable wheelchair balance beam scale or bed scales, is needed for weighing nonambulatory persons (Chumlea et al., 1984).

10.1.7 Measurement of elbow breadth

Elbow breadth is measured as the distance between the epicondyles of the humerus (Figure 10.9). For the measurement, the *right* arm is raised to the horizontal, and the elbow flexed to 90°, with the back of the hand facing the measurer. The measurer then stands in front of the subject and locates the lateral and medial epicondyles of the humerus. The blades of a flat-bladed sliding caliper are applied to the epicondyles, with the blades pointing upwards to bisect the right angle formed at the elbow. Care must be taken to ensure that the caliper is held at a slight angle to the epicondyles and that firm pressure is exerted to minimize the influence of soft tissue on the measurement. The latter is taken to the nearest millimeter (Lohman et al., 1988).

10.2 Indices derived from growth measurements

Indices are constructed from two or more raw anthropometric measurements and are simple numerical ratios such as weight/(height)^2, or combinations such as weight for age, height for age, and weight for height. These should not be written as weight/age, height/age, and weight/height to avoid confusion with the numerical ratios. Indices are an essential part of the interpretation of anthropometric measurements (WHO, 1986).

Age	Boys (cm)	Girls (cm)
Birth – 3 mo	5.9	5.7
3 mo – 6 mo	3.2	3.0
6 mo – 1 yr	3.2	3.1
1 yr – 2 yr	2.2	2.2
2 yr – 4 yr	1.7	2.1
4 yr – 6 yr	0.5	0.5
6 yr – 8 yr	1.0	1.1
8 yr – 10 yr	0.7	0.5
10 yr – 12 yr	0.6	0.9
12 yr – 14 yr	0.9	1.0
14 yr – 16 yr	0.8	0.6
16 yr – 18 yr	0.5	0.3
Total	21.2	21.0

Table 10.1: Mean increment in head circumference. From Nellhaus (1968). Reproduced by permission of Pediatrics Vol. 211, page 106 © 1968.

10.2.1 Head circumference for age

Head circumference for age can be used as an index of chronic protein-energy nutritional status during the first two years of life. Chronic malnutrition during the first few months of life, or intrauterine growth retardation, may decrease the number of brain cells and result in an abnormally low head circumference (Winick, 1969). Beyond age two years, growth in head circumference is so slow that its measurement is no longer useful (Nutrition Canada, 1980) (Table 10.1). Head circumference for age is not sensitive to less extreme malnutrition (Yarbrough et al., 1974). Certain non-nutritional factors (e.g. some diseases and pathological conditions), genetic variation, and cultural practices (such as binding of the head during infancy) may also influence head circumference.

10.2.2 Weight for age

Body weight represents the sum of protein, fat, water, and bone mineral mass, and does not provide any information on relative changes in these four chemical components. In normal adults, there is a tendency to increased fat deposition with age, concomitant with a reduction in muscle protein. Such changes are not evident in body weight measurements and can only be evaluated by determining body fat and/or fat-free mass. In persons with edema or ascites, an increase in total body water occurs, which may mask any body weight deficit resulting from losses of fat and/or muscle. Massive tumour growth may also mask losses of fat and muscle tissue which may occur during severe undernutrition. Conversely, in obese subjects, loss of muscle may be masked by residual fat (Heymsfield and Casper, 1987).

Weight for age in children from six months to seven years of age is an index of acute malnutrition, and is widely used to assess protein-energy malnutrition and overnutrition, especially in infancy when the measurement of length is difficult. Nevertheless, a major limitation of weight for age as an index of protein-energy malnutrition is that it does not take into account height differences; as a result, children with a low weight for age are not necessarily wasted. They may be genetically short, or their low weight for age may be associated with nutritional growth failure or 'stunting', a condition characterized by low height for age but a weight appropriate to their short stature. Consequently, the prevalence of malnutrition in small children may be overestimated if only weight for age is used.

To interpret a single measurement of weight in relation to the reference data, the exact age of the child must be known. In some countries, local calendars (Table 10.2) of special events can be constructed to assist in identifying the birth date of a child. Alternatively, for young children, age is sometimes assessed by counting deciduous teeth. This method is not appropriate for individuals because of the wide individual variation in the timing of deciduous eruption (Delgado et al., 1975).

10.2.3 Weight for height

Weight for height is a sensitive index of current nutritional status. It is relatively independent of age between one and ten years, enhancing its usefulness in areas where the ages of the children are uncertain. For ages less than one year, however, older infants at a given height tend to be heavier, so that age groupings with a narrow range should be used. Weight for height also appears to be relatively independent of ethnic group, particularly for children aged one to five years (Waterlow et al., 1977).

In contrast to weight for age, weight for height differentiates between nutritional stunting, when weight may be appropriate for height, and wasting, when weight is very low for height as a result of deficits in both tissue and fat mass. Wasting often develops very rapidly, but can be reversed quickly with appropriate intervention. Seasonal, geographical, and age differences in the prevalence of wasting occur, associated with fluctuations in the food supply or the prevalence of infectious diseases. The highest prevalence of wasting occurs during the postweaning period (i.e. from 12 to 23 months) (WHO, 1986).

Weight for height is also useful in evaluating the benefits of intervention programs, as this index is more sensitive to changes in nutritional

Major Event	Year	Month
Visit of Queen Elizabeth II (Baseline year)	1974	July
Isolated from capital by flooding New pump water supply installed	1975	Jan. June
Hurricane 'Bertha' Partial eclipse of the sun	1976	Feb. May
Opening of local sugar factory Independence celebrations	1977	Aug. Nov.
Earthquake with damage to church Election for President First pier built in harbour	1978	Jan. May Nov./Dec
Installation of radio station Hurricane 'Rose' Health Center opened in village	1979	Jan. March Dec.
New general store in village Sugar crop covered by volcanic ash	1980	Oct. Dec.
Cargo boat sinks in storm on reef	1981	Feb.

Table 10.2: A fictional example of a local calendar of the type used in establishing the approximate times of births and deaths, when these are uncertain.

status than height for age. The index is also frequently used in the nutritional assessment of hospital patients, to identify wasting.

Unfortunately, edema and obesity may complicate the interpretation of weight-for-height measurements. A further disadvantage of this index is that it classifies children with poor linear growth as 'normal'. Consequently, it is preferable in some cases to use a combination of weight for height and height for age (Section 10.2.4), as recommended by Waterlow et al. (1977).

10.2.4 Height for age

There are several lines of evidence that, within a given population, the heights of children at a given age reflect their nutritional status; these include:

- the trend in industrialized countries toward earlier maturity and increased height at all ages (including adulthood) over the last hundred

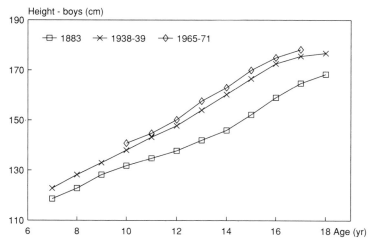

Figure 10.10: Secular trend in growth. Height of Swedish boys measured in 1883, 1938–1939 and 1965–1971. From Ljung et al. (1974). Reproduced by permission of the authors and Annals of Human Biology.

years; this trend is frequently referred to as 'the secular trend' (Tanner, 1976) (Figure 10.10) and appears to be the result of the improvement of diet which followed the industrial revolution;

• the existence of an association between the height of British children at all ages and the socio-economic status of their fathers (Goldstein, 1971; Tanner, 1976) (Figure 10.11); this association may no longer hold;

• the existence of a relationship between the height of African preschool children, and the socio-economic conditions affecting their families and their energy and nutrient intakes (Rea, 1971).

When considering individuals, the lines of evidence include:

• the reduction in the rate of growth during a period of undernutrition (Tanner, 1976);

• the rapid growth responses observed in children given dietary therapy or nutritional supplements (Ashworth, 1969; Lampl et al., 1978).

As a result of this evidence, height for age can be used as an index of the nutritional status of population groups as it estimates past or chronic nutritional status. It is particularly valuable as an index of 'stunting' of a child's full growth potential. Stunting is a slowing of skeletal growth and of stature, defined by Waterlow (1978) as "the end result of a reduced rate of linear growth". This condition results from extended periods of inadequate food intake and increased morbidity and is generally found in countries where economic conditions are poor. The prevalence of

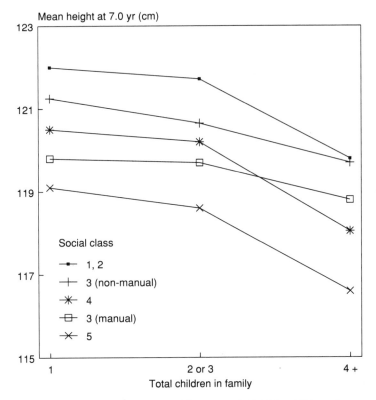

Figure 10.11: Height at 7.0 years of British children (sexes combined) according to number of children in the family and socio-economic level (1–5). Reproduced from Human Biology, Vol. 43, No. 1 (1971). H. Goldstein: Factors influencing the height of seven-year-old children: results from the National Child Development Study, pp. 92–111, by permission of the Wayne State University Press. © Wayne State University Press, 1971, Detroit, Michigan 48202.

stunting, unlike wasting, is highest during the second or third year of life (WHO, 1986).

The distribution of height measurements at a given age within most populations is usually narrow, so that accurate measuring techniques are essential. As a deficit in height takes some time to develop, assessment of nutritional status based on height for age alone may result in an underestimation of malnutrition in infants (Keller et al., 1976). The influence of possible genetic and ethnic differences must also be considered when evaluating height for age.

percentage usual weight	=	$\dfrac{\text{actual weight}}{\text{usual weight}} \times 100\%$
percentage weight loss	=	$\dfrac{\text{(usual weight} - \text{actual weight}}{\text{usual weight}} \times 100\%$
rate of change (kg/day)	=	$\dfrac{\text{BW}_p - \text{BW}_i}{\text{Day}_p - \text{Day}_i}$

Table 10.3: Calculation of percentage weight loss and rate of change. BW_p and BW_i indicate present and initial body weights on the respective days.

10.2.5 Weight changes

Alterations in body weight may reflect a change in protein, water, minerals, and/or body fat content. In healthy persons, daily variations in body weight are generally small (i.e. less than ± 0.5 kg). In conditions of acute or chronic illness, however, negative energy-nitrogen balance may occur as the body uses endogenous sources of energy (including protein) as fuel for metabolic reactions. Consequently, body weight declines. In conditions of total starvation, the maximal weight loss is approximately 30% of initial body weight, at which point death occurs. In chronic semistarvation, body weight may decrease to approximately 50% to 60% of ideal weight. When persistent positive energy balance occurs, there is an accumulation of adipose tissue, and body weight increases.

In general, absolute body weight can only be used to assess the severity of protein-energy malnutrition in patients with relatively uncomplicated, nonedematous forms of semistarvation (Heymsfield et al., 1984). In disease conditions in which edema, ascites, dehydration, diuresis, massive tumor growth, and organomegaly occur, or in obese patients undergoing rapid weight loss, body weight is a poor measure of body energy-nitrogen reserves. In such conditions, a relative increase in total body water, for example, may mask actual weight loss associated with changes in fat and skeletal muscle. Hence, it is always preferable to perform additional anthropometric measurements (e.g. skinfold thickness and mid-upper-arm circumference) to ascertain where the change in body weight occurred (Heymsfield et al., 1984).

To assess weight changes, current and usual weight of the patient must be known. From these two measurements, the percentage of usual weight, percentage weight loss, and rate of change can be calculated (Table 10.3). Percentage weight change can be evaluated using the guidelines of Blackburn et al. (1977) (Table 10.4). Marton et al. (1981) evaluated 91 patients with involuntary weight loss (> 5% of their usual body weight during the previous six months) in a prospective study. They

Time	Significant Weight Loss (%)	Severe Weight Loss (%)
1 week	1–2	> 2
1 month	5	> 5
3 months	7.5	> 7.5
6 months	10	> 10

Table 10.4: Evaluation of percentage weight changes. From GL Blackburn, BR Bistrain, BS Maini, HT Schlamm, MF Smith. Nutritional and metabolic assessment of the hospitalized patient. Journal of Parenteral and Enteral Nutrition 1: 11–22. © by Am. Soc. for Parenteral and Enteral Nutrition (1977).

estimated the prognosis of patients with weight loss; 25% of their patients had died and another 15% had deteriorated clinically one year after the initial visit. They also developed a diagnostic strategy for weight loss to distinguish patients with a physical cause of weight loss from patients with no physical cause of weight loss. Six attributes were identified as significant independent diagnostic predictors of weight loss, all of which were based on medical history and physical examination.

The patient's current weight should also be compared with appropriate age- and sex-specific reference data (Section 12.5). Marked trends in body weight with age have been documented in healthy adults in the NHANES I and the Nutrition Canada surveys, weight generally increasing through early adulthood and then decreasing with advancing age in the elderly.

10.2.6 Weight/height ratios

Weight/height ratios are frequently used for adults. They measure body weight corrected for height, with the underlying assumption that the ratios are highly correlated with obesity. Hence these ratios are frequently called obesity or body mass indices. They are employed in large-scale nutrition surveys and epidemiological studies as indirect measures of obesity, because measurements of weight and height are easy, quick, relatively noninvasive, and more precise than skinfold thickness measurements. Nevertheless, since obesity indices cannot be used to distinguish between excessive weight produced by adiposity, muscularity, or edema, a more direct measure of obesity, such as skinfold thickness, should also be employed when practical (Frisancho and Flegel, 1982).

There are two types of weight/height ratios: relative weight and power-type indices. Relative weight expresses the weight of a given subject as a percentage of the average weight of persons of the same height. Power-type indices express weight relative to some power function of

Weight/height ratio	=	$\dfrac{wt}{ht}$
Quetelet's index	=	$\dfrac{wt}{(ht)^2}$
Ponderal index	=	$\dfrac{ht}{\sqrt[3]{wt}}$
Benn's index	=	$\dfrac{wt}{(ht)^p}$

Table 10.5: Power-type indices for weight/height ratios.

height, or height relative to some power function of weight (Table 10.5). The numerical values of each of these indices depend on the units of measurement employed (e.g. meters and kilograms or inches and pounds). The power p in Benn's index is calculated to give an index that is apparently unrelated to height (Benn, 1971). It is derived from the weight/height ratio and the regression coefficients of weight on height for a specific age, sex, and population (Lee et al., 1981).

There is little agreement on the best power-type index for assessing obesity in adults or the basis on which a selection should be made. In general, any index of obesity should be highly correlated with weight and independent of height because there is no evidence that taller people are more or less likely to be obese. Several studies have compared the relative merits of these power indices, based on their correlation with measures of relative adiposity (e.g. Table 10.6), and the influence of height on the values of the indices (Billewicz et al., 1962; Khosla and Lowe, 1967; Lee et al., 1981; Frisancho and Flegel, 1982). For instance, Billewicz and colleagues (1962) found that all the indices correlated highly with relative adiposity, as estimated from body density measurements, whereas Keys et al. (1972) and Womersley and Durnin (1977) noted higher correlation coefficients between Quetelet's index, percentage fat (estimated by densitometry), and skinfold thickness, compared to other weight/height indices, but a relatively low correlation with height. Naturally, there are marked differences in the correlation between various power-type weight/height indices and height (Keys et al., 1972).

Obesity may be underestimated in short persons when assessed by the weight/height ratio (Billewicz et al., 1962), but overestimated by the Ponderal index because it has only a moderate correlation with weight and is markedly biased by height (Goldbourt and Medalie, 1974).

Variable	Triceps	Subscapular	Sum
Males (n = 5527)			
wt	0.58	0.67	0.68
wt/(ht)^2	0.61	0.75	0.75
wt/(ht)^3	0.57	0.72	0.71
wt/(ht)^p	0.61	0.74	0.74
Females (n = 8282)			
wt	0.62	0.68	0.71
wt/(ht)^2	0.64	0.73	0.75
wt/(ht)^3	0.62	0.71	0.73
wt/(ht)^p	0.63	0.72	0.74

Table 10.6: Age-adjusted correlation coefficients of weight and obesity indices for triceps, subscapular, and sum of skinfolds in white adults. Derived from data sets of the US Health and Nutrition Examination Survey I of 1971 to 1974. From Frisancho and Flegel (1982). © Am. J. Clin. Nutr. American Society for Clinical Nutrition.

The Ponderal index was used in the Nutrition Canada survey (Nutrition Canada, 1980). Some confusion may arise in its interpretation because the Ponderal index is negatively correlated with weight and so decreases with increasing obesity. For example, the risk categories developed for Nutrition Canada were: below 12.5 (high risk for obesity); 12.5 and above (low risk for obesity) (Nutrition Canada, 1980).

Lee et al. (1981) found that Benn's index was unbiased by height in five ethnic populations and, as a result, recommended the adoption of Benn's index for routine use in comparisons among populations (Lee et al., 1982; Lee and Kolonel, 1983). Benn's index can, however, only be used when the correct value for p for the sample population has been calculated.

Many investigators consider Quetelet's index to be the best body mass index for most *adult* population groups, as it is the least biased by height and easily calculated (Khosla and Lowe, 1967; Office of Population Censuses and Surveys, 1984; Garrow and Webster, 1985; Health and Welfare Canada, 1988a), although in children it is apparently more dependent on stature (Garn et al., 1986). Furthermore, in adults, Quetelet's index correlates with many health-related indices such as mortality risk (Waaler, 1984). Factors such as diet, smoking and levels of physical activity confound this latter relationship, so that it is not surprising that the range of acceptable values for Quetelet's index varies among communities; several have been proposed. Health and Welfare Canada (1988), who have adopted the term 'Body Mass Index' (BMI) for Quetelet's index, have recently recommended the range and classification for BMI shown in

Body Mass Index	Evaluation
Under 20	May be associated with health problems for some individuals.
20–25	'Ideal' index range associated with the lowest risk of illness for most people.
25–27	May be associated with health problems for some people.
Over 27	Associated with increased risk of health problems such as heart disease, high blood pressure, and diabetes.

Table 10.7: Classifications used for the Body Mass Index by Health and Welfare Canada (1988a).

Table 10.7 In the survey of heights and weights of adults in Great Britain (Office of Population Censuses and Surveys, 1984), values for Quetelet's index of < 20 were regarded as indicative of underweight, > 25 indicative of overweight, and > 30 as obese.

Health and Welfare Canada (1988b) have also produced a nomogram to facilitate calculation of Quetelet's index (Figure 10.12). Quetelet's index is not a valid index for those under twenty or over sixty-five years of age, or for those who are pregnant or lactating (Health and Welfare Canada, 1988b).

The precise relationship between Quetelet's index and percentage body fat is not clearly established, as only limited measurements of weight, height, and body fat of male and female adults exist (Garrow, 1983). Frisancho and Flegel (1982) recommend that, in addition to Quetelet's index, some measure of subcutaneous fat, such as a skinfold measurement, should also be included for the assessment of leanness or obesity. Other investigators have recommended measuring the waist-hip ratio (i.e. waist circumference divided by hip circumference) as a measure of fat distribution, together with Quetelet's index (Björntorp, 1987; Health and Welfare Canada, 1988a). The waist-hip ratio can be measured more precisely than skinfolds, and provides an index of both subcutaneous and intra-abdominal adipose tissue. Björntorp (1985) suggested that waist-hip ratios greater than 1.0 for men and 0.8 for women were indicative of increased risk of cardiovascular complications and related deaths. More research is needed before specific recommendations for classifying waist-hip ratios can be made (Health and Welfare Canada, 1988a). Note that Quetelet's index should not be used as an index of body fatness in individuals with a grossly abnormal relationship between leg and trunk length.

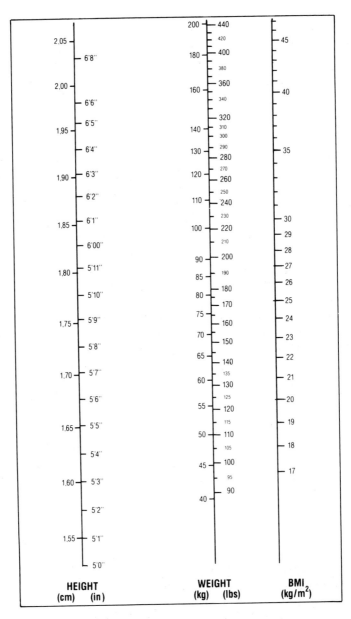

Figure 10.12: Nomogram to estimate the Body Mass Index. To use the nomogram, locate and mark the subject's height on line A and weight on line B. Lay a rule or straightedge so that it touches these two points. To locate the body mass index, extend the line to C. From Health and Welfare Canada (1988b). Canadian Guidelines for Healthy Weights. Report of an Expert Committee convened by Health Promotion Directorate, Health Services and Promotion Branch, with permission of Health and Welfare Canada.

10.3 Summary

Standardized techniques for measuring stature (height or length), knee height, head circumference, body weight, and elbow breadth in infants, children, and adults are available, and should always be used to ensure accurate and precise measurements. Indices can then be constructed from these raw measurements. Such indices include either simple numerical ratios (e.g. weight/(height)^2), or combinations such as weight for age, height for age, weight for height, and head circumference for age. The latter is closely related to brain size and is used as an index of protein-energy status during the first two years of life, provided that non-nutritional effects have been excluded. Weight for age assesses acute protein-energy malnutrition, but tends to overestimate malnutrition in children who are either genetically short, or 'stunted', because it does not take height differences into account. Consequently, weight for height should also be included; it differentiates between nutritional stunting, when weight may be appropriate for height, and wasting, when weight is very low for height. Furthermore, weight for height is relatively independent of age between one and ten years. The presence of edema, obesity, and/or poor linear growth may complicate the interpretation of this index, and, as a result, a combination of weight for height and height for age is often used. Height for age reflects past nutritional status in both children and adults, although genetic and ethnic influences must be taken into account.

Weight/height ratios are frequently called obesity or body mass indices. They measure body weight corrected for height, but cannot distinguish between excessive weight produced by adiposity, muscularity, or edema. Two types of weight/height ratios are used: relative weight, which expresses the weight of a given subject as a percentage of the average weight of persons of the same height, and power-type indices. The latter include weight/height ratio, Quetelet's index: weight/(height)^2; Ponderal index: height/$\sqrt[3]{\text{weight}}$; and Benn's index: weight/(height)^p. There is no agreement on which power-type index most adequately measures body mass, although in general Quetelet's index appears to be the best choice for nonpregnant adults from twenty to sixty-five years of age.

References

Ashworth A. (1969). Growth rates in children recovering from protein-calorie malnutrition. British Journal of Nutrition 23: 835–845.

Benn RT. (1971). Some mathematical properties of weight-for-height indices used as measures of adiposity. British Journal of Preventive and Social Medicine 25: 42–50.

Billewicz WZ, Kemsley WFF, Thomson AM. (1962). Indices of adiposity. British Journal of Preventive and Social Medicine 16: 183–188.

Björntorp P. (1985). Regional patterns of fat distribution: health implications. In: Health Implications of Obesity. A report on the US National Institutes of Health Consensus Development Conference. Bethesda, Maryland, pp. 35.

Björntorp P. (1987). Classification of obese patients and complications related to the distribution of surplus fat. American Journal of Clinical Nutrition 45: 1120–1125.

Blackburn GL, Bistrain BR, Maini BS, Schlamm HT, Smith MF. (1977). Nutritional and metabolic assessment of the hospitalized patient. Journal of Parenteral and Enteral Nutrition 1: 11–22.

Cameron N. (1986). The methods of auxological anthropometry. In: Falkner F, Tanner JM (eds), Human Growth, A Comprehensive Treatise. Volume 3: Methodology. Ecological, Genetic, and Nutritional Effects on Growth. Plenum Press, New York, pp. 3–46.

Chumlea WC, Roche AF, Mukherjee D. (1984). Nutritional Assessment of the Elderly through Anthropometry. Ross Laboratories, Columbus, Ohio.

Chumlea WC, Roche AF, Steinbaugh ML. (1985). Estimating stature from knee height for persons 60 to 90 years of age. Journal of the American Geriatrics Society 33: 116–120.

Delgado H, Habicht J-P, Yarbrough C, Lechtig A, Mortorell R, Malina RM, Klein RE. (1975). Nutritional status and the timing of deciduous tooth eruption. American Journal of Clinical Nutrition 28: 216–224.

Frisancho AR, Flegel PN. (1982). Relative merits of old and new indices of body mass with reference to skinfold thickness. American Journal of Clinical Nutrition 36: 697–699.

Frisancho AR, Flegel PN. (1983). Elbow breadth as a measure of frame size for United States males and females. American Journal of Clinical Nutrition 37: 311–314.

Garn SM, Leonard WR, Hawthorne VM. (1986). Three limitations of the body mass index. American Journal of Clinical Nutrition 44: 996–997.

Garrow JS. (1983). Indices of adiposity. Nutrition Abstracts and Reviews 53: 697–708.

Garrow JS, Webster J. (1985). Quetelet's index (W/H^2) as a measure of fatness. International Journal of Obesity 9: 147–153.

Goldbourt U, Medalie J. (1974). Weight height indices. British Journal of Preventive and Social Medicine 28: 110–112.

Goldstein H. (1971). Factors influencing the height of seven-year-old children: results from the National Child Development Study. Human Biology 43: 92–111.

Health and Welfare Canada (1988a). Promoting Healthy Weights: a discussion paper. Health Services and Promotion Branch, Health and Welfare, Ottawa.

Health and Welfare Canada (1988b). Canadian Guidelines for Healthy Weights. Report of an Expert Committee convened by Health Promotion Directorate, Health Services and Promotion Branch, Health and Welfare, Ottawa.

Heymsfield SB, Casper K. (1987). Anthropometric assessment of the adult hospitalized patient. Journal of Parenteral and Enteral Nutrition 11: 36S–41S.

Heymsfield SB, McManus CB, Seitz SB, Nixon DW, Smith Andrews J. (1984). Anthropometric assessment of adult protein-energy malnutrition. In: Wright RA, Heymsfield S (eds), Nutritional Assessment. Blackwell Scientific Publications, Boston, pp. 27–82.

Jelliffe DB. (1966). The Assessment of the Nutritional Status of the Community. WHO Monograph No. 53. World Health Organization, Geneva.

Keller W, Donoso G, De Maeyer EM. (1976). Anthropometry in nutritional surveillance: a review based on results of the WHO collaborative study on nutritional anthropometry. Nutrition Abstracts and Reviews 46: 591–609.

Keys A, Fidanza F, Karvonen MJ, Kimura N, Taylor HL. (1972). Indices of relative weight and obesity. Journal of Chronic Diseases 25: 329–343.

Khosla T, Lowe CR. (1967). Indices of obesity derived from body weight and height. British Journal of Preventive and Social Medicine 21: 122–128.

Lampl M, Johnston FE, Malcolm LA. (1978). The effect of protein supplementation on the growth and skeletal maturation of New Guinean school children. Annals of Human Biology 5: 219–227.

Lee J, Kolonel LN, Ward Hinds M. (1981). Relative merits of the weight-corrected-for-height indices. American Journal of Clinical Nutrition 34: 2521–2529.

Lee J, Kolonel LN, Ward Hinds M. (1982). Relative merits of old and new indices of body mass: a commentary. American Journal of Clinical Nutrition 36: 727–728.

Lee J, Kolonel LN. (1983). Body mass indices: a further commentary. American Journal of Clinical Nutrition 38: 660–661.

Ljung BO, Bergsten-Brucefors A, Lingren G. (1974). The secular trend in physical growth in Sweden. Annals of Human Biology 1: 245–256.

Lohman TG, Roche AF, Martorell R. (eds). (1988). Anthropometric Standardization Reference Manual. Human Kinetics Books, Champaign, Illinois.

Marton KI, Sox HC Jr., Krupp JR. (1981). Involuntary weight loss: diagnostic and prognostic significance. Annals of Internal Medicine 95: 568–574.

Nellhaus G. (1968). Head circumference from birth to eighteen years. Practical composite international and interracial graphs. Pediatrics 41: 106–114.

Nutrition Canada (1980). Anthropometry Report: Height, Weight and Body Dimensions. Bureau of Nutritional Sciences, Health Protection Branch, Health and Welfare, Ottawa.

Office of Population Censuses and Surveys, Social Survey Division (1984). The heights and weights of adults in Great Britain. Knight I (ed): Report of a survey carried out on behalf of the Department of Health and Social Security covering adults aged 16–64 years. Her Majesty's Stationery Office, London.

Rea JN. (1971). Social and economic influences on the growth of preschool children in Lagos. Human Biology 43: 46–63.

Robbins GE, Trowbridge FL. (1984). Anthropometric techniques and their application. In: Simko MD, Cowell C, Gilbride JA (eds), Nutrition Assessment. Aspen Corporation, Rockville, Maryland, pp. 69–92.

Roche AF, Guo S, Baumgartner RN, Falls RA. (1988). The measurement of stature. American Journal of Clinical Nutrition 47: 922.

Sumner EE, Whitacre J. (1931). Some factors affecting accuracy in the collection of data on the growth of weight in school children. Journal of Nutrition 4: 15–33.

Tanner JM, Whitehouse RH, Takish M. (1966). Standards from birth to maturity for height, weight, height velocity, and weight velocity: British children, 1965. Archives of Disease in Childhood 41: 454–472; 613–625.

Tanner JM. (1976). Growth as a monitor of nutritional status. Proceedings of the Nutrition Society 35: 315–322.

Waaler HTh. (1984). Height, weight and mortality. The Norwegian experience. Acta Medica Scandinavica, Supplement No. 679.

Waterlow JC. (1978). Observations on the assessment of protein-energy malnutrition with special reference to stunting. Extrait Courrier 28: 455–460.

Waterlow JC, Buzina R, Keller W, Lane JM, Nichaman MZ, Tanner JM. (1977). The presentation and use of height and weight data for comparing the nutritional status of groups of children under the age of 10 years. Bulletin of the World Health Organization 55: 489–498.

Weiner JS, Lourie JA. (1969). Human Biology: A Guide to Field Methods: International Biological Programme Handbook. IBP No. 9. Blackwell Scientific Publications, Oxford-Edinburgh.

WHO (World Health Organization) (1983). Measuring Change in Nutritional Status. Guidelines for assessing the nutritional impact of supplementary feeding programmes for vulnerable groups. World Health Organization, Geneva.

WHO (World Health Organization Working Group) (1986). Use and interpretation of anthropometric indicators of nutritional status. Bulletin of the World Health Organization 64: 929–941.

Winick M. (1969). Malnutrition and brain development. Journal of Pediatrics 74: 667–679.

Womersley J, Durnin JVGA. (1977). A comparison of the skinfold method with extent of 'overweight' and various weight-height relationships in the assessment of obesity. British Journal of Nutrition 38: 271–284.

Yarbrough C, Habicht J-P, Martorell R, Klein RE. (1974). Anthropometry as an index of nutritional status. In: Roche AF, Falkner R (eds), Nutrition and Malnutrition: Identification and Measurement. Plenum Press, New York–London, pp. 15–26.

Chapter 11

Anthropometric assessment of body composition

Most anthropometric methods used to assess body composition are based on a model in which the body consists of two chemically distinct compartments: fat and fat-free mass. The latter consists of the skeletal muscle, nonskeletal muscle and soft lean tissues, and the skeleton. Anthropometric techniques can indirectly assess these two body compartments, and variations in their amount and proportion can be used as indices of nutritional status. For example, fat is the main storage form of energy in the body and is sensitive to acute malnutrition. Alterations in body fat content provide indirect estimates of changes in energy balance. Body muscle, composed largely of protein, is a major component of the fat-free mass and serves as an index of the protein reserves of the body; these reserves become depleted during chronic undernutrition, resulting in muscle wasting.

Anthropometric measurements of body composition are relatively fast, noninvasive, and require the minimum of equipment compared to laboratory techniques. Details of the standardized procedures used for anthropometric body composition measurements, and the derivation of the more important indices, are summarized in this chapter and are given in detail in Lohman et al. (1988). Indices of body composition are used in clinical settings to identify hospital patients with chronic under- or overnutrition, and to monitor long-term changes in body composition during nutritional support. They are also used in public health to identify individuals who are vulnerable to under- or overnutrition, and/or to evaluate the effectiveness of nutrition intervention programs.

11.1 Assessment of body fat

The body fat content is the most variable component of the body, differing among individuals of the same sex, height, and weight. On average, the fat content of women is higher than that of men, representing 26.9% of

Fat Location	Reference Man		Reference Woman	
Essential fat (lipids of the bone marrow, central nervous systems, mammary glands, and other organs)	2.1		4.9	
Storage fat (depot)	8.2		10.4	
Subcutaneous		3.1		5.1
Inter-muscular		3.3		3.5
Intra-muscular		0.8		0.6
Fat of thoracic and abdominal cavity		1.0		1.2
Total fat	10.3		15.3	
Body weight	70.0		56.8	
Percentage fat	14.7%		26.9%	

Table 11.1: Distribution of body fat in reference man and women. Data in kilograms. Weights of reference man and woman for total fat and body weight from Behnke (1969). Other weights from Allen et al. (1956); Alexander (1964); Johnson et al. (1972); Wilmore and Brown (1974).

their total body weight compared to 14.7% for men. Table 11.1 presents data for the distribution of body fat in reference man and woman.

Body fat is deposited in two major types of storage site: one for essential lipids, and the other for general fat storage. Essential lipids are found in the bone marrow, central nervous system, mammary glands, and other organs, and are required for normal physiological functioning; fat from these sites makes up about 9% (4.9 kg) of body weight in reference woman and 3% (2.1 kg) in reference man. Storage fat consists of inter- and intramuscular fat, fat surrounding the organs and gastrointestinal tract, and subcutaneous fat (Lohman, 1981). The proportion of storage fat in males and females is relatively constant, and averages 12% of total body weight in males and 15% in females. One-third of the total body fat in reference man and woman is estimated to be subcutaneous fat (Allen et al., 1956).

Body fat can be measured either in absolute terms (the weight of total body fat, expressed in kilograms) or as a percentage of the total body weight (Roche et al., 1981). It can be assessed using one or more skinfold thickness measurements, either alone or in association with limb circumference measurements. Empirical equations exist which relate skinfold measurements to body fat. Estimates of initial body fat, together with the rate of change in body fat content, are recommended to assess the presence and severity of protein-energy malnutrition. A large and rapid loss of body fat is indicative of severe negative energy balance. Small changes in body fat (i.e. < 0.5 kg) cannot be measured accurately using anthropometry (Heymsfield et al., 1984). At present, the importance of percentage body fat and total body fat, in relation to particular disease states, is unknown.

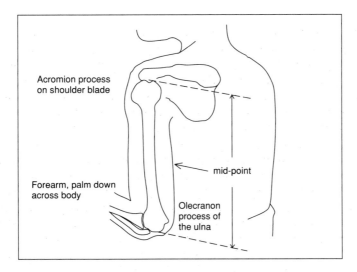

Figure 11.1: Location of the midpoint of the upper arm. Reproduced from Robbins GE, Trowbridge FL. In: Nutrition Assessment: A Comprehensive Guide for Planning Intervention by M.D. Simko, C. Cowell, and J.A. Gilbride, p. 87, with permission of Aspen Publishers, Inc., © 1984.

11.1.1 Measurement of skinfold thickness

Skinfold thickness measurements are said to provide an estimate of the size of the subcutaneous fat depot, which in turn provides an estimate of the total body fat (Durnin and Rahaman, 1967). Such estimates are based on two assumptions: (a) the thickness of the subcutaneous adipose tissue reflects a constant proportion of the total body fat, and (b) the skinfold sites selected for measurement, either singly or in combination, represent the average thickness of the entire subcutaneous adipose tissue (Lukaski, 1987). Neither of these assumptions is true. In fact, the relationship between subcutaneous and internal fat is nonlinear, and varies with body weight and age; very lean subjects have a smaller proportion of body fat deposited subcutaneously than obese subjects (Allen et al., 1956). Moreover, variations in the distribution of subcutaneous fat occur with sex, race, and age (Robson et al., 1971; Durnin and Womersley, 1974). The following sites are commonly used:

- Triceps skinfold — measured at the midpoint of the back of the upper left arm (Figure 11.1) (Weiner and Lourie, 1969).
- Biceps skinfold — measured as the thickness of a vertical fold on the front of the upper left arm, directly above the center of the cubital fossa, at the same level as the triceps skinfold (Weiner and Lourie, 1969).
- Subscapular skinfold — measured just below and laterally to the angle of the left shoulder blade, with the shoulder and left arm relaxed. Placing the subject's arm behind the back may assist in the identification

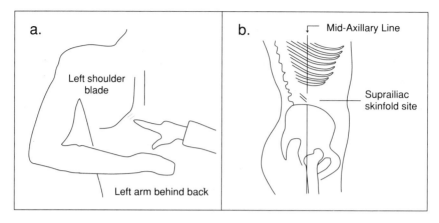

Figure 11.2: Location of the subscapular and suprailiac skinfold sites.

of the site. Skinfold is grasped at the marked site with the fingers on top, thumb below, and forefinger on the site at the lower tip of the scapular. The skinfold should angle 45° from horizontal, in the same direction as the inner border of the scapula (i.e. medially upward, and laterally downward) (Figure 11.2a) (Jetté, 1981; Lohman et al., 1988).

• Suprailiac skinfold—measured in the midaxillary line immediately superior to the iliac crest. The skinfold is picked up obliquely just posterior to the midaxillary line and parallel to the cleavage lines of the skin (Lohman et al., 1988). (Figure 11.2b).

• Midaxillary skinfold—the skinfold is picked up horizontally on the midaxillary line, at the level of the xiphoid process (Weiner and Lourie, 1969).

Skinfold thickness measurements are best made using precision skinfold thickness calipers; they measure the compressed double fold of fat plus skin. As a result of the compression, they always underestimate actual subcutaneous fat thickness. Three types of precision calipers can be used: Harpenden, Lange, and Holtain (Figure 11.3). The Lange is manufactured in the United States (Lange and Brŏzek, 1961), while both the Harpenden and Holtain calipers are manufactured in the United Kingdom. Some suppliers of this equipment are listed in Appendix A11.1. Low-cost plastic McGaw calipers are also available (Figure 11.3). All precision calipers are designed to exert a defined and constant pressure of 10 grams per square millimeter throughout the range of measured skinfolds, and to have a standard contact surface area or 'pinch' area of 20 to 40 mm^2 (Brŏzek and Henschel, 1963). They must be recalibrated at regular intervals using a calibration block.

The measurement technique is described in detail for the triceps skinfold, as the latter is the site most frequently used to obtain a single indirect measure of body fat; the technique used for the other skinfold

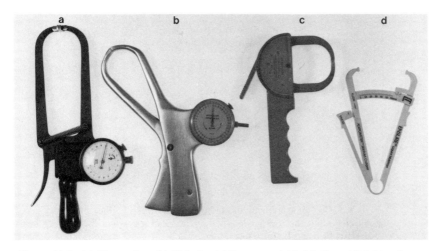

Figure 11.3: (a) Harpenden, (b) Holtain, (c) Lange, and (d) McGaw skinfold calipers.

sites is similar. For all the skinfold measurements, the subject stands erect with feet together and arms at the side.

The measurement of the triceps skinfold is performed at the midpoint of the upper left arm, between the acromion process and the tip of the olecranon, with the arm hanging relaxed (Figure 11.4). To mark the midpoint, the left arm is bent 90° at the elbow, and the forearm is placed palm down across the body. Then the tip of the acromion process of the shoulder blade at the outermost edge of the shoulder and the tip of the olecranon process of the ulna are located and marked. The distance between these two points is measured using a nonstretchable tape, and the midpoint is marked with a soft pen or indelible pencil, directly in line with the point of the elbow and acromium process. The left arm is then extended so that it is hanging loosely by the side. The examiner grasps a vertical fold of skin plus the underlying fat, 1 cm above the marked midpoint (Figure 11.1), in line with the tip of the olecranon process, using the thumb and forefinger. The skinfold is gently pulled away from the underlying muscle tissue, and then the caliper jaws applied at right angles, exactly at the marked midpoint. The skinfold remains held between the fingers while the measurement is taken. When using the Lange, Harpenden, or Holtain calipers, pressure must be applied to open the jaws before the instrument is placed on the skinfold; the jaws will then close under spring pressure. As the jaws compress the tissue, the caliper reading generally diminishes for 2 to 3 seconds, and then the measurements are taken. When the McGaw skinfold calipers are used, they must be closed manually on the skinfold, using the thumb and forefinger, until the lines on the calipers are aligned. Two readings should

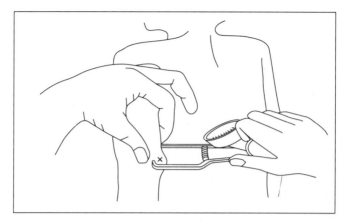

Figure 11.4: Measurement of the triceps skinfold in the upright position using the Harpenden caliper. Modified from Robbins GE, Trowbridge FL. In: Nutrition Assessment: A Comprehensive Guide for Planning Intervention by M.D. Simko, C. Cowell, and J.A. Gilbride, p. 90, with permission of Aspen Publishers, Inc., © 1984.

be taken in all cases; if differences are large, a third measurement is taken and the mean of the closest pair recorded (Jetté, 1981). Skinfolds should be recorded to 0.2 mm on the Harpenden and Holtain skinfold calipers, 0.5 mm on the Lange, and to the nearest 1.0 mm on the McGaw caliper. Duplicate skinfold measurements made with precision calipers should normally agree to within 1 mm. The McGaw calipers cannot be used to measure skinfolds on very obese subjects, because the measurement scale has an indicated maximum of 40 mm. Skinfold values obtained with the McGaw calipers are significantly lower than those made with the Lange Calipers, but the two sets of values correlate well (Burgert and Anderson, 1979).

Triceps skinfold measurements can also be made with the subject lying down. The subject lies on the right side with legs bent, the head supported by a pillow, and the right hand tucked under the pillow. The left arm rests along the trunk, with the palm down. The measurement is taken at the marked midpoint of the back of the upper left arm, as described above. The examiner should be careful to avoid parallax errors by bending down to read the calipers while taking the measurements (Chumlea et al., 1984).

Both intra-examiner and inter-examiner measurement errors can occur when measuring skinfolds, particularly for subjects with flabby, easily compressible tissue, or with very firm tissue which is not easily deformed (Lukaski, 1987). Intra-examiner measurement errors occur when an examiner fails to obtain identical results on repeated skinfolds on the same subject; such errors are a function of the skinfold site, the experience of the examiner, and the fatness of the subject (Lohman, 1981). For triceps skinfolds, intra-examiner measurement errors can be small, provided that training in standardized procedures is given; the errors in these circumstances typically range from 0.70 to 0.95 mm. Inter-examiner errors arise when two or more examiners measure the same subject and site; such errors are usually larger than intra-examiner errors, but can be reduced to not more than 2 mm by care and training (Burkinshaw et al., 1973). Both intra- and inter-examiner measurement errors may be larger if very large (> 15 mm) or small (< 5 mm) skinfolds are measured (Edwards et al., 1955).

11.1.2 Single skinfold measurements to assess body fat

Skinfold measurements at a single site are sometimes used to assess the total body fat or the percentage body fat. If this single measurement approach is used, it is critical to select the skinfold site which is most representative of the whole subcutaneous fat layer, because subcutaneous fat is not uniformly distributed about the body. Unfortunately, the most representative site is not the same for both sexes, nor is it the same for all age and ethnic groups. For example, Siervogel et al. (1982) concluded that the triceps skinfold was the most representative of the total subcutaneous layer for boys up to sixteen years of age, whereas for adult males both subscapular and midaxillary sites were equally representative. Hence, it is not surprising that there is no general agreement as to the best single skinfold site as an index of total body fat. The assessment is particularly difficult in adult females, for whom the distribution of subcutaneous fat is more variable than in males. Sloan et al. (1962) reported that the suprailiac skinfold was the best single index of total skinfold thickness for young women, whereas Siervogel et al. (1982) recommended the triceps skinfold.

Roche et al. (1981) emphasized that the most appropriate skinfold site also depends on whether total body fat or percentage body fat is the parameter of interest. They found that the triceps skinfold provided that the best estimate of percentage body fat in children and adult women, but not in adult men (Table 11.2). In contrast, the subscapular skinfold was recommended if total body fat in boys was to be estimated. For assessment of total body fat in girls and adults, no single skinfold measurement was regarded as adequate; instead, Quetelet's index was preferred.

The discussion above emphasizes the problems of using single skinfolds to assess total body fat or percentage body fat. In general, the triceps skinfold thickness has been the site most frequently selected for a single, indirect measure of body fat. This site, however, appears to be suitable for the assessment of percentage body fat in women and children only.

| | Correlation Coefficients | | | |
| | % Body fat | | Total body fat | |
	Men	Women	Men	Women
Weight	0.67	0.70	0.82	0.91
Relative weight	0.64	0.69	0.78	0.89
Weight/(height)^2	0.77	0.76	0.87	0.92
Weight/(height)^3	0.75	0.75	0.83	0.88
Triceps skinfold	0.70	0.77	0.73	0.80
Subscapular skinfold	0.75	0.71	0.79	0.80
Suprailiac skinfold	0.69	0.59	0.73	0.69

Table 11.2: Correlations between selected anthropometric variables and percentage body fat or total body fat in 276 adults aged 18 to 49 years. All correlations are significant ($p < 0.01$). From Roche et al. (1981). © Am. J. Clin. Nutr. American Society for Clinical Nutrition.

11.1.3 Multiple skinfold measurements to assess body fat

The optimum combination of skinfold measurement sites for assessing total body fat has not been extensively investigated. No single body region (for example, upper or lower trunk or limbs) appears to have skinfold sites which are consistently representative of the whole subcutaneous fat layer (Siervogel et al., 1982). In general, when studying both children and adults, investigators recommend taking one limb skinfold (left triceps) and one body skinfold measurement (left scapular) to account for the differing distribution of subcutaneous fat. As a result, Bowen and Custer (1984) compiled percentile curves for the sum of triceps and subscapular thickness, based on the NCHS reference data for adults.

Differential weightings rather than the simple sum or average of skinfolds may provide a better estimate of total body fat (Himes et al., 1980), but such an approach is not widely used. Roche (1984) suggests that the logarithm of the sum of skinfold thicknesses at various sites may be a 'useful' measure of subcutaneous fat thickness.

A combination of skinfold measurements can also provide information on the distribution of subcutaneous fat. Variations in the distribution may be associated with genetic differences among individuals or with particular disease states. For example, a relative excess of trunk subcutaneous fat has been associated with diabetes mellitus by some investigators (Feldman et al., 1969). Multiple skinfolds, rather than single skinfold measurements for estimating body fat, are particularly advisable for individuals undergoing rapid and pronounced weight gain. Changes in energy balance are known to alter the rate of fat accumulation differently between skinfold sites (Heymsfield et al., 1984).

11.1.4 Waist-hip circumference ratio

The waist-hip circumference ratio is a simple method for describing the distribution of both subcutaneous and intra-abdominal adipose tissue (Larsson et al., 1984; Jones et al., 1986), as discussed in Section 10.2.6. Subjects should fast overnight prior to the measurement and wear little clothing to ensure that the tape is correctly positioned. Subjects should stand erect with the abdomen relaxed, arms at the sides, feet together and with their weight equally divided over both legs. To perform the waist measurement, the lowest rib margin is first located and marked with a felt tip pen. The iliac crest is then palpated in the midaxillary line, and also marked. An elastic tape is then applied horizontally midway between the lowest rib margin and the iliac crest, and tied firmly so that it stays in position around the abdomen about the level of the umbilicus. The elastic tape thus defines the level of the waist circumference, which can then be measured by positioning a fiberglass tape over the elastic tape (Jones et al., 1986). Subjects are asked to breathe normally, and to breathe out gently at the time of the measurement to prevent them from contracting their muscles or from holding their breath. The reading is taken to the nearest millimeter.

For the hip circumference measurement, the subject should stand erect with arms at the side and feet together. The measurement should be taken at the point yielding the maximum circumference over the buttocks (Jones et al., 1986), with the tape held in a horizontal plane, touching the skin but not indenting the soft tissue (Lohman et al., 1988).

Changes of waist-hip circumference ratio with age and excessive weight are not yet known. Jones et al. (1986) measured waist-hip ratio in a semi-random, age-stratified sample of 4349 British Caucasian men aged twenty to sixty-four years. They noted that the ratio increased with age (curvilinearly) and excessive weight, both separately and in combination. Four percent of the sample had a waist-hip ratio greater than 1.0, the cutoff point associated with increased risk of mortality and morbidity (Björntorp, 1987), but an additional 12% had values between 0.95 and 0.99. Results of computer tomography scans in twenty-eight women (Section 14.7.4) showed a high degree of correlation between the waist-hip ratio and the proportion of fat situated intra-abdominally at the umbilical level (Ashwell et al., 1985).

11.1.5 Limb fat area

The calculated cross-sectional area of limb fat, derived from skinfold thickness and limb circumference measurements, may be used as an anthropometric index. It provides a better estimate of total body fat (i.e. fat weight) than a single skinfold thickness at the same site, because it is more highly correlated with total body fatness (Himes et al., 1980). In contrast, the estimation of *percentage* body fat from limb fat area is no better than the corresponding estimation by skinfold measurement, particularly in males (Himes et al., 1980). The advantage of using limb fat area to estimate body fat is not unexpected, since more fat is needed to cover a large limb with a given thickness of subcutaneous fat than to cover a smaller limb with the same thickness of fat. Subcutaneous fat, however, is not evenly distributed around the limbs or trunk. For example, triceps skinfolds are consistently larger than the corresponding biceps skinfold, and, as a result, either the sum or the average of these should theoretically be used for the calculation of mid-upper-arm fat area (Himes et al., 1980). In practice, current reference data are based only on triceps skinfold and mid-upper-arm circumference measurements. Reference data for mid-upper-arm fat area show little variation between one and seven years of age, so that mid-upper-arm fat area in adequately nourished children provides an age-independent assessment of total body fat for this age range (Gurney and Jelliffe, 1973).

The sites commonly selected for the calculation of limb fat area are the mid-upper-left arm, midthigh, and midcalf. Reference data compiled by the NCHS are only available for mid-upper-arm fat area (Frisancho, 1981; Bowen and Custer, 1984) (Section 12.9) and, as a result, this site is the one most frequently used in nutritional assessment.

Both skinfold thickness and the corresponding limb circumference should be measured by trained examiners using standard techniques. The calf and thigh skinfolds are taken on the lateral aspects of the left calf and thigh, at the point of their largest circumference. Measurements of circumferences for the calf, thigh, and arm are taken at the same level as the skinfolds, using the technique to be described for mid-upper-arm circumference (Section 11.2.1). The equation for calculating mid-upper-arm fat area is:

$$A = \frac{SKF \times C_1}{2} - \frac{\pi \times (SKF)^2}{4}$$

where A = mid-upper-arm fat area (mm^2), C_1 = mid-upper-arm circumference (mm), and SKF = triceps skinfold thickness (mm). Arm fat area calculated from this equation was reported to agree within 10% to values measured by computerized axial tomography in adults (Heymsfield et al., 1982).

Mid-upper-arm fat area can also be calculated in the field from nomograms developed by Gurney and Jelliffe (1973); a copy of these nomograms, one for children and one for adults, is given in the Appendix (A11.2 and A11.3), together with brief instructions for their use. It should be noted that the results obtained from the nomograms are less precise than those obtained by calculation.

The equation used for the calculation of mid-upper-arm fat area is based on several assumptions, each of which may result in inaccuracies. The equation assumes that the limb is cylindrical, with fat evenly distributed about its circumference, and also makes no allowance for variable skinfold compressibility. This compressibility probably varies with age, sex, site of the measurement, and among individuals and is a source of error in population studies when equal compressibility of skinfolds is assumed. A correction for skinfold compressibility may be advisable in future studies (Himes et al., 1979).

The determination of mid-upper-arm fat area as a measure of total body fat should not be used in patients with edema or ascites. Mid-upper-arm fat areas are also underestimated in obese persons. Furthermore, the appropriateness of this technique for severely undernourished hospital patients has not been adequately evaluated.

11.1.6 Calculation of body fat from skinfold measurements, via body density

Skinfold thickness measurements from multiple anatomical sites are also used to estimate body density. From body density, the percentage of body fat can be calculated using empirical equations from the literature. Total body fat (fat weight in kilograms) can then be determined by multiplying body weight by percentage fat (Lohman, 1981; Brodie, 1988). The method involves:

- Determination of appropriate skinfolds and other anthropometric measurements for the prediction of body density, the selection of the sites depending on the age, sex, and population group under investigation.
- Calculation of body density, using an appropriate regression equation.
- Calculation of percentage body fat from body density, using an empirical equation.
- Calculation of total body fat and/or the fat-free mass.

$$\text{Total body fat (kg)} = \frac{\text{body weight (kg)} \times \% \text{ body fat}}{100}$$

$$\text{Fat-free mass (kg)} = \text{body weight (kg)} - \text{body fat (kg)}$$

Several studies have investigated the best combination of skinfolds and other anthropometric measurements from which to derive a regression equation for the estimation of body density. Rarely have the studies recommended the same combination, particularly for young men (Durnin and Rahaman, 1967; Katch and McArdle, 1973). In general, a combination of skinfolds such as triceps, subscapular, suprailiac or thigh, and abdomen is preferred, as these sites are closely associated with body density in young adult men and women (Lohman, 1981).

Most of the established regression equations have been derived from small samples of specific population groups, homogeneous in terms of age, sex, and body fatness, and should not be applied to other age groups and populations (Sinning, 1978). For example, the regression equation developed by Sloan (1962), based on fifty college men, is applicable to studies of young men and male adolescents; the equation is not valid, however, for young women and middle-aged men. In general, population-specific regression equations apparently overestimate body fat for leaner groups and underestimate body fat in fatter groups (Sinning, 1978). These errors may largely be a statistical artefact of the regression procedure.

In view of these difficulties, generalized regression equations have been developed based on large, heterogeneous samples varying in age and degree of body fatness (Durnin and Womersley 1974; Jackson and Pollock, 1978; Jackson et al., 1980). These allow the calculation of body density for specified age/sex groups from selected skinfold thickness measurements and, sometimes, waist and forearm circumference measurements. In some equations, age is included as an independent variable. Logarithmic or quadratic transformations and/or curvilinear equations are used, because the relationship between skinfold fat and body density is curvilinear over a wide range of densities. For example, in more obese subjects relatively large increments in skinfold thickness are associated with only small changes in body density.

The failure of a single simple equation to relate skinfold measurements to body density for subjects of a wide age range is not surprising; the ratio of internal fat to subcutaneous fat, fat patterning, and bone density changes with age. The direction of these changes is controversial (Durnin and Womersley, 1974; Chien et al., 1975; Pollock et al., 1975). Differences in skinfold compressibility may be partly responsible for the necessity for different equations for the sexes (Durnin and Womersley, 1974; Heymsfield et al., 1979; Pollock and Jackson, 1984).

Two examples of these generalized regression equations for the calculation of body density are given below. A more extensive table of regression coefficients, suitable for a wide range of subjects of both sexes, appears in Appendix A11.4.

$$D \ (kg/m^3) = 1.1631 - (0.0632 \times \log_{10}(SK4 \ [mm]))$$

The above equation from Durnin and Womersley (1974) is valid for male subjects aged twenty to twenty-nine, and calculates the body density (D). SK4 represents the sum (in millimeters) of the skinfold measurements for the biceps, triceps, subscapular, and suprailiac skinfolds.

$$D = 1.10938 - 8.267 \times 10^{-4} \times SK3 + 1.6 \times 10^{-6} \times (SK3)^2 - 2.574 \times 10^{-4} \times AGE$$

This relationship, valid for adult male subjects aged eighteen to sixty-one of varying fatness, and taken from Jackson and Pollock (1978), uses SK3, the sum (expressed in millimeters) of the chest, abdomen, and thigh skinfolds, and the age in years to calculate the body density (kg/m^3). A similar equation was also developed for women (Jackson et al., 1980). The two equations take into account the potential change in ratio of internal to external fat and bone density with age and the nonlinear relationship between skinfold and body density. They appear to provide valid measurements of body density and percentage body fatness, even in formerly obese adults (Scherf et al., 1986). Nevertheless, some investigators question the validity of generalized regression equations and recommend the use of predictive equations applicable to the subjects under study (Norgan and Ferro-Luzzi, 1985).

The final stage in the calculation of the percentage of body fat (F) from multiple skinfold measurements is the selection of an equation relating fat content to body density (D). Several equations have been derived. All are based on the following assumptions: (a) the density of the fat-free mass is relatively constant; (b) the density of fat for normal persons does not vary among individuals; (c) the water content of the fat-free mass is constant; (d) the proportion of bone mineral (i.e. skeleton) to muscle in the fat-free body is constant. Different authors use different values for the density of fat and the fat-free mass.

$$\%F = \left\{ \frac{4.95}{D} - 4.50 \right\} \times 100\% \quad \text{(Siri, 1961)}$$

$$\%F = \left\{ \frac{4.570}{D} - 4.142 \right\} \times 100\% \quad \text{(Br\~ozek et al., 1963)}$$

$$\%F = \left\{ \frac{5.548}{D} - 5.044 \right\} \times 100\% \quad \text{(Rathburn and Pace, 1945)}$$

The Siri equation assumes that the density of fat is 0.900 g/cc and that the density of fat-free body is 1.100 g/cc. The equations of Brŏzek et al. (1963) and Rathburn and Pace (1945) are based on the concept of a reference man of a specified density and composition and avoid the requirement of estimating the density of fat-free mass. The equations of Siri (1961) and Brŏzek et al. (1963) yield similar absolute values for fat content except for very lean or obese subjects.

More research is needed to identify appropriate empirical equations for specific population groups. Studies have shown that the density of the fat-free body is not constant for all normal persons but varies in relation to obesity and muscular development, as well as age (Womersley et al., 1976). Not surprisingly, for patients with known abnormalities in mineral mass, variations in the density of the fat-free mass can be extreme (Werdein and Kyle, 1960). Even for healthy individuals, errors in body density ranging from 0.003 to 0.005 g/cc may arise from variations in bone density (Siri, 1956; Bakker and Struikenkamp, 1977). Such errors may result in a variation in percentage body fat of approximately 2%, whereas variations in the water content of the fat-free mass may produce a 2.7% error in percentage body fat (Werdein and Kyle, 1960).

It should be noted that the available empirical equations should not be used for undernourished individuals, as there is a decreasing correlation between skinfold thickness and total body fat content with increasing severity of undernutrition. This change in correlation may arise from a shift of fat storage from the regions represented by the subscapular and triceps skinfolds to other subcutaneous sites. Alternatively, a shift from subcutaneous to deep visceral sites may occur (Spurr et al., 1981). The empirical equations are also unsuitable for use with patients undergoing hyperalimentation with high-sodium fluids, with congestive heart failure, or with liver disease, as total body water content as a fraction of fat-free mass may be markedly increased. Consequently, large errors arise when the body fat content is calculated indirectly from skinfold measurements, via body density, especially in these patients (Heymsfield and Casper, 1987). Nevertheless, the method is sufficiently reliable to allow valid comparisons of changes in the body fat content of an individual to be made.

11.2   Assessment of fat-free mass

The fat-free mass is a mixture of water, protein, and minerals, with muscle serving as the major protein store. Assessment of muscle protein can therefore provide an index of the protein reserves of the body. Mid-upper-arm muscle circumference and mid-upper-arm muscle area are both correlated with measures of total muscle mass, and are therefore used to predict changes in total body muscle mass and hence protein nutritional status. Unfortunately, the ratios of mid-upper-arm muscle circumference/area to total skeletal muscle mass, and of mid-upper-arm muscle circumference/area to fat-free mass are not constant, but change with age and certain disease states (Heymsfield and McManus, 1985). As a result, these anthropometric indices do not provide accurate measures of changes in body protein and cannot be used to detect small changes. Arm muscle circumference and arm muscle area are both derived from the mid-upper-arm circumference and triceps skinfold measurements, taken on the left arm.

11.2.1   Mid-upper-arm circumference measurement

The arm contains subcutaneous fat and muscle; a decrease in mid-upper-arm circumference may therefore reflect either a reduction in muscle mass, a reduction in subcutaneous tissue, or both. In less industrialized countries, where the amount of subcutaneous fat is frequently small, changes in mid-upper-arm circumference tend to parallel changes in muscle mass and hence are particularly useful in the diagnosis of protein-energy malnutrition or starvation. Changes in mid-upper-arm circumference measurements can also be used to monitor progress during nutritional therapy (Hofvander and Eksmyr, 1969; Bray et al., 1978;

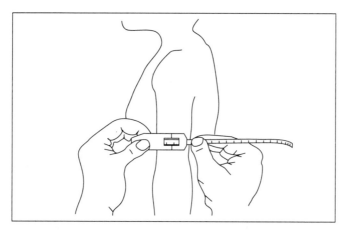

Figure 11.5: Use of insertion tape to measure mid-upper-arm circumference. Modified from Robbins GE, Trowbridge FL. In: Nutrition Assessment: A Comprehensive Guide for Planning Intervention by M.D. Simko, C. Cowell, and J.A. Gilbride, p. 88, with permission of Aspen Publishers, Inc., © 1984.

Harries et al., 1984), correlating positively with changes in weight. Arm circumference changes are easy to detect and require a minimal amount of time and equipment (Gurney and Jelliffe, 1973). Some investigators claim that mid-upper-arm circumference can differentiate normal children from those with protein-energy malnutrition as reliably as weight for age (Shakir and Morley, 1974).

Mid-upper-arm circumference measurements should be made using a flexible, nonstretch tape made of fiberglass or steel; alternatively, a fiberglass insertion tape can be used (Figure 11.5). The subject should stand erect and sideways to the measurer, with the head in the Frankfurt plane, arms relaxed and legs apart (Cameron, 1986). If the subject is wearing a sleeved garment, it should be removed or the sleeves rolled up. The measurement is taken at the midpoint of the upper left arm, between the acromion process and the tip of the olecranon (Figure 11.1). After locating the midpoint, the left arm is extended so that it is hanging loosely by the side, with the palm facing inwards. The tape is wrapped gently but firmly around the arm at the midpoint (Figure 11.5), care being taken to ensure that the arm is not squeezed. If necessary, mid-upper-arm circumference can be measured with subjects in the recumbent position. In this case, a sandbag is placed under the elbow to raise the arm slightly off the surface of the bed (Chumlea et al., 1984). Measurements are taken to the nearest millimeter. Precision of mid-upper-arm circumference measurements, both within and between examiners, can be high, even if the subjects are obese, when trained examiners are used (Harries et al., 1984). (es) Between the ages of six months and five years, mid-upper-arm circumference varies little (Burgess and Burgess, 1969), and

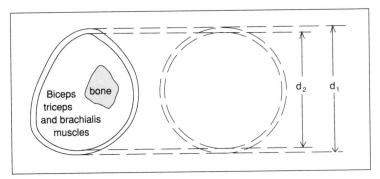

Figure 11.6: Calculation of mid-upper-arm muscle circumference. Let C_1 = mid-upper-arm circumference, TSK = triceps skinfold, d_1 = arm diameter and d_2 = muscle diameter. Then TSK = 2 × subcutaneous fat = $d_1 - d_2$ and $C_1 = \pi d_1$. But muscle circumference (C_2) = $\pi d_2 = \pi[d_1 - (d_1 - d_2)]$ = $\pi d_1 - \pi(d_1 - d_2)$. Hence $C_2 = C_1 - \pi \times$ TSK. From Jelliffe DB. The Assessment of the Nutritional Status of the Community. Geneva, World Health Organization (1966). WHO Monograph Series, No. 53, page 77, Figure 44, with permission.

as a result mid-upper-arm circumference measurements are frequently used in areas where the ages of the children are uncertain. However, children vary little in their mid-upper-arm circumference measurements at any given age within that range, and thus such measurements tend to form a narrow symmetrical distribution. The relative error associated with these measurements can therefore be rather large, particularly if untrained examiners or nonstandard techniques are used.

11.2.2 Mid-upper-arm muscle circumference

The muscle circumference of the mid-upper arm is derived from measurements of both mid-upper-arm circumference and triceps skinfold thickness, and represents the circumference of the inner circle of muscle mass surrounding a small central core of bone (Gurney and Jelliffe, 1973). Mid-upper-arm muscle circumference can be used to assess total body muscle mass, and is frequently used for this purpose in field surveys. It is also used in hospitals to assess protein-energy malnutrition, as the size of the muscle mass is an index of protein reserves. Mid-upper-arm muscle circumference is calculated using the following equation:

Mid-upper-arm muscle circ. (C_2) = mid-upper-arm circ. (C_1) − ($\pi \times$ TSK)

where TSK = triceps skinfold thickness (Figure 11.6). Note that this equation is only valid when all measurements are in the same units (preferably millimeters). A Nomogram for calculating mid-upper-arm muscle circumference can be found in the Appendix (A11.2). The equation and nomogram for the calculation of mid-upper-arm muscle circumference are based on the same assumptions as those described for mid-upper-arm fat area (Section 11.1.5). As variations in skinfold compressibility are ignored, and as the triceps skinfold of females is generally more compressible than that of males, female mid-upper-arm muscle circumferences may be underestimated (Clegg and Kent, 1967). As a further complication, the mid-upper-arm muscle circumference equation does not take into account inter-subject variation in the diameter of the humerus relative to mid-upper-arm circumference (Frisancho, 1981).

It is important to realize that mid-upper-arm muscle circumference is a one-dimensional measurement, whereas mid-upper-arm muscle area is two-dimensional, and mid-upper-arm muscle volume is three-dimensional. Consequently, if the volume of mid-upper-arm muscle declines as a result of protein-energy malnutrition or enlarges during nutritional support, the mid-upper-arm muscle circumference will undergo a proportionally smaller change than mid-upper-arm muscle area (Heymsfield et al., 1982). Hence arm muscle circumference is insensitive to small changes of muscle mass that might occur, for example, during an illness.

11.2.3 Mid-upper-arm muscle area

Mid-upper-arm muscle area is preferable to mid-upper-arm muscle circumference as an index of total body muscle mass because it more adequately reflects the true magnitude of muscle tissue changes (Frisancho, 1981). Studies of adults and children have consistently demonstrated higher correlations between mid-upper-arm muscle area and creatinine/height ratio (an index of body mass), compared to mid-upper-arm muscle circumference (Trowbridge et al., 1982). The following equation may be used to estimate mid-upper-arm muscle area:

$$\text{Arm muscle area} = \frac{(C - (\pi \times TSK))^2}{4\pi}$$

where C = mid-upper-arm circumference and TSK = triceps skinfold thickness (Frisancho, 1981). Consistent units, preferably millimeters, should be used throughout. The equation is based on the following assumptions:

- the mid-upper-arm cross-section is circular;
- the triceps skinfold is twice the average fat rim diameter;
- the mid-upper-arm muscle compartment is circular in cross-section;
- bone atrophies in proportion to muscle wastage during protein-energy malnutrition;
- the cross-sectional areas of neurovascular tissue and the humerus are relatively small and ignored.

The first three assumptions are those used in the calculations of mid-upper-arm fat area and muscle circumference. Nomograms may be used to calculate mid-upper-arm muscle area when high precision is not essential (Appendix A11.2 and A11.3) (Gurney and Jelliffe, 1973).

Heymsfield et al. (1982) examined the accuracy of the mid-upper-arm muscle area equation. They concluded that the equation overestimated mid-upper-arm muscle area by between 20% and 25% and, as a result, may underestimate the severity of muscle atrophy. The error can be corrected if the absolute mid-upper-arm muscle area values are expressed as a percentage of the median, because the latter contains the same overestimate. Alternatively, a revised equation which calculates absolute bone-free arm muscle area can be used (Heymsfield et al., 1982). This revised equation takes into account errors resulting from the noncircular nature of the muscle compartment and the inclusion of nonskeletal muscle tissue (e.g. neurovascular tissue and bone). It reduces the average error for a given subject to 7% to 8% for mid-upper-arm muscle area. Nevertheless, Heymsfield et al. (1982) caution that even the corrected mid-upper-arm muscle area equation is only an approximation (e.g. $\pm 8\%$) of actual mid-upper-arm muscle area. The revised equations have not been validated for use with elderly persons and are not appropriate for obese patients.

$$cAMA = \frac{(C_1 - (\pi \times TSK))^2}{4\pi} - 6.5 \qquad \text{for women}$$

$$cAMA = \frac{(C_1 - (\pi \times TSK))^2}{4\pi} - 10.0 \qquad \text{for men}$$

where $cAMA$ = corrected mid-upper-arm muscle area, C_1 = mid-upper-arm circumference, and TSK = triceps skinfold thickness. It should be noted that the equation assumes that the measurements have been made in centimeters, and not millimeters, for conformity with the original reference.

The estimated coefficient of variation for measurements of mid-upper-arm muscle area made by trained examiners is 7% (Heymsfield et al., 1982). Therefore, this index is not appropriate for detecting small changes in mid-upper-arm muscle area such as those which may follow short-term nutritional support or deprivation.

Heymsfield et al. (1982) also developed an equation to predict total body muscle mass from corrected mid-upper-arm muscle area, using estimates of muscle mass derived from urinary creatinine excretion (Section 16.1.1) (Forbes and Bruining, 1976). The error of this prediction ranges from 5% to 9%.

$$\text{Muscle mass (kg)} = \text{height (cm)} \times (0.0264 + [0.029 \times cAMA])$$

11.3 Summary

Indirect assessment of body fat and fat-free mass are made from selected anthropometric measurements taken by standardized techniques of skinfold thickness and circumference measurements. Skinfold thickness measured at one or more sites (e.g. triceps, biceps, subscapular, suprailiac, and the midaxillary skinfold thickness) provide estimates of the subcutaneous fat depot, and hence total body fat. No consensus exists on the best single, or combination of, skinfold site(s) to assess body fat. The most appropriate site(s) depend(s) on the age, sex, and race of the subject, and on whether an estimate of total body fat or percentage body fat is required. In general, a combination of skinfolds provides a more valid assessment of body fat content and distribution of subcutaneous fat. The latter can also be assessed from the waist-hip circumference ratio. Mid-upper-arm fat area, derived from triceps skinfold thickness and mid-upper-arm circumference measurements, also provides a better estimate of total body fat than a single skinfold at the same site. The mid-upper-arm fat area equation assumes that the limb is cylindrical, with fat evenly distributed about its circumference; no allowance is made for differences in skinfold compressibility. Such assumptions limit the accuracy of body fat estimates from mid-upper-arm fat areas. A combination of skinfold measurements can be used to estimate body density, which in turn can be used to derive the percentage of body fat using an empirical equation. Once the percentage of body fat is calculated, total body fat content and the fat-free mass can be derived. More research is necessary to identify appropriate empirical equations for specific population groups.

Mid-upper-arm circumference, either alone or combined with triceps skinfold thickness for calculating mid-upper-arm muscle circumference or muscle area, provides estimates of varying accuracy of the protein reserves of the body, and hence protein nutritional status. Mid-upper-arm muscle area is preferable to circumference, because it more adequately reflects the true magnitude of tissue changes. Nevertheless, the equation overestimates mid-upper-arm muscle area by 20% to 25%. Revised equations have been developed but are not validated for use with the elderly and are inappropriate for the obese. None of the anthropometric indices are sensitive enough to monitor small changes in body fat or fat-free mass which may arise after short-term nutritional support or deprivation.

References

Alexander ML. (1964). The postmortem estimation of total body fat, muscle and bone. Clinical Science 26: 193–202.

Allen TH, Peng MT, Chen KP, Huang TF, Chang C, Fang HS. (1956). Prediction of total adiposity from skinfolds and the curvilinear relationship between external and internal adiposity. Metabolism 5: 346–352.

Ashwell M, Cole TJ, Dixon AK. (1985). Obesity: new insight into the anthropometric classification of fat distribution shown by computed tomography. British Medical Journal 290: 1692–1694.

Bakker HK, Struikenkamp RS. (1977). Biological variability and lean body mass estimates. Human Biology 49: 187–202.

Behnke AR. (1969). New concepts of height-weight relationships. In: Wilson NL (ed). Obesity. FA Davis Co., Philadelphia, pp. 25–53.

Björntorp P. (1987). Classification of obese patients and complications related to the distribution of surplus fat. American Journal of Clinical Nutrition 45: 1120–1125.

Bowen PE, Custer PB. (1984). Reference values and age-related trends for arm muscle area, arm fat area and sum of skinfolds for United States adults. Journal of the American College of Nutrition 3: 357–376.

Bray GA, Greenway FL, Molitch ME, Dahms WT, Atkinson RL, Hamilton K. (1978). Use of anthropometric measures to assess weight loss. American Journal of Clinical Nutrition 31: 769–773.

Brodie DA. (1988). Techniques of measuring body composition. Part I. Sports Medicine 5: 11–40.

Brŏzek J, Grande F, Anderson JT, Keys A. (1963). Densitometric analysis of body composition: revision of some quantitative assumptions. Annals of the New York Academy of Sciences 110: 113–140.

Brŏzek JF, Henschel A (eds). (1963). Techniques for Measuring Body Composition. National Academy of Sciences, National Research Council, Washington, D.C.

Burgert SL, Anderson CF. (1979). A comparison of triceps skinfold values as measured by the plastic McGaw caliper and the Lange caliper. American Journal of Clinical Nutrition 32: 1531–1553.

Burgess HJL, Burgess AP. (1969). A modified standard for mid-upper-arm circumference in young children. Journal of Tropical Pediatrics 15: 189–192.

Burkinshaw L, Jones PRM, Krupowicz DW. (1973). Observer error in skinfold thickness measurements. Human Biology 45: 273–279.

Cameron N. (1986). The methods of auxological anthropometry. In: Falkner F, Tanner JM (eds). Human Growth. A Comprehensive Treatise. Volume 3. Methodology, Ecological, Genetic, and Nutritional Effects on Growth. Plenum Press, New York, pp. 3–46.

Chien S, Peng MT, Chen KP, Huang TF, Chang C, Fang HS. (1975). Longitudinal studies on adipose tissue and its distribution in human subjects. Journal of Applied Physiology 39: 825–830.

Chumlea WC, Roche AF, Mukherjee D. (1984). Nutritional Assessment of the Elderly through Anthropometry. Ross Laboratories, Columbus, Ohio.

Clegg EJ, Kent C. (1967). Skin-fold compressibility in young adults. Human Biology 39: 418–429.

Durnin JVGA, Rahaman MM. (1967). The assessment of the amount of fat in the human body from measurements of skinfold thickness. British Journal of Nutrition 21: 681–689.

Durnin JVGA, Womersley J. (1974). Body fat assessed from total body density and its estimation from skinfold thickness: measurements on 481 men and women aged from 16 to 72 years. British Journal of Nutrition 32: 77–97.

Edwards DAW, Hammond WH, Healy MJR, Tanner JM, Whitehouse RH. (1955). Design and accuracy of calipers for measuring subcutaneous tissue thickness. British Journal of Nutrition 9: 133–150.

Feldman R, Sender AJ, Siegelaub AB. (1969). Difference in diabetic and nondiabetic fat distribution patterns by skinfold measurements. Diabetes 18: 478–486.

Forbes GB, Bruining GJ. (1976). Urinary creatinine excretion and lean body mass. American Journal of Clinical Nutrition 29: 1359–1366.

Frisancho AR. (1981). New norms of upper limb fat muscle areas for assessment of nutritional status. American Journal of Clinical Nutrition 34: 2540–2545.

Gurney JM, Jelliffe DB. (1973). Arm anthropometry in nutritional assessment: nomogram for rapid calculation of muscle circumference and cross-sectional muscle and fat areas. American Journal of Clinical Nutrition 26: 912–915.

Harries AD, Jones LA, Heatley RV, Newcombe RG, Rhodes J. (1984). Precision of anthropometric measurements: the value of midarm circumference. Clinical Nutrition 2: 193–196.

Heymsfield SB, Casper K. (1987). Anthropometric assessment of the adult hospitalized patient. Journal of Parenteral and Enteral Nutrition 11: 36S–41S.

Heymsfield SB, McManus CB. (1985). Tissue components of weight loss in cancer patients. Cancer 55: 238–249.

Heymsfield SB, McManus CB, Smith J, Stevens V, Nixon DW. (1982). Anthropometric measurement of muscle mass: revised equations for calculating bone-free arm muscle area. American Journal of Clinical Nutrition 36: 680–690.

Heymsfield SB, Roche AF, Siervogel RM. (1979). Compressibility of skinfolds and the measurement of subcutaneous fat. American Journal of Clinical Nutrition 32: 1734–1740.

Heymsfield SB, McManus CB, Seitz SB, Nixon DW, Smith Andrews J. (1984). Anthropometric assessment of adult protein-energy malnutrition. In: Wright RA, Heymsfield B (eds). Nutritional Assessment of the Adult Hospitalized Patient. Blackwell Scientific Publications, Boston, pp. 27–82.

Himes JH, Roche AF, Siervogel RM. (1979). Compressibility of skinfolds and the measurement of subcutaneous fat. American Journal of Clinical Nutrition 32: 1734–1740.

Himes JH, Roche AF, Webb P. (1980). Fat areas as estimates of total body fat. American Journal of Clinical Nutrition 33: 2093–2100.

Hofvander Y, Eksmyr R. (1969). Changes in upper arm circumference and body weight in a 2-year follow-up of children in an applied nutrition programme in a representative Ethiopian highland village. Journal of Tropical Pediatrics 15: 251–252.

Jackson AS, Pollock ML. (1978). Generalized equations for predicting body density of men. British Journal of Nutrition 40: 497–504.

Jackson AS, Pollock ML, Ward A. (1980). Generalized equations for predicting body density of women. Medicine and Science in Sports and Exercise 12: 175–182.

Jelliffe DB. (1966). The Assessment of the Nutritional Status of the Community. WHO Monograph Series No. 53. World Health Organization, Geneva.

Jetté M. (1981). Guide for Anthropometric Classification of Canadian Adults for Use in Nutritional Assessment. Health and Welfare, Ottawa.

Johnson ER, Butterfield RM, Pyor WJ. (1972). Studies of fat distribution in the bovine carcass. 1: The partition of fatty tissues between depots. Australian Journal of Agricultural Research 23: 381–388.

Jones PRM, Hunt MJ, Brown TP, Norgan NG. (1986). Waist-hip circumference ratio and its relation to age and overweight in British men. Human Nutrition: Clinical Nutrition 40C: 239–247.

Katch FI, McArdle WD. (1973). Prediction of body density from simple anthropometric measurements in college-age men and women. Human Biology 45: 445–455.

Lange KO, Brözek J. (1961). A new model of skinfold caliper. American Journal of Physical Anthropology 19: 98–99 (abs).

Larsson B, Svardsudd B, Welin L, Wilhelmsen L, Björntorp P, Tibblin G. (1984). Abdominal adipose tissue distribution, obesity and risk of cardiovascular disease and death: 13-year follow-up of participants in the study of men born in 1913. British Medical Journal 288: 1401–1404.

Lohman TG. (1981). Skinfolds and body density and their relation to body fatness: A review. Human Biology 2: 181–225.

Lohman TG, Roche AF, Martorell R (eds). (1988). Anthropometric Standardization Reference Manual. Human Kinetics Books, Champagne, Illinois.

Lukaski HC. (1987). Methods for the assessment of human body composition: traditional and new. American Journal of Clinical Nutrition 46: 537–556.

Norgan NG, Ferro-Luzzi A. (1985). The estimation of body density in men: are general equations general? Annals of Human Biology 1: 1–15.

Pollock ML, Jackson AS. (1984). Research progress in validation of clinical methods of assessing body composition. Medicine and Science in Sports and Exercise 16: 606–613.

Pollock ML, Laughridge EE, Coleman B, Linnerud AC, Jackson A. (1975). Prediction of body density in young and middle-aged women. Journal of Applied Physiology 38: 745–749.

Rathbun EN, Pace N. (1945). Studies on body composition: I. The determination of total body fat by means of the body specific gravity. Journal of Biological Chemistry 158: 667–676.

Robson JRF, Bazin M, Soderstrom R. (1971). Ethnic differences in skin-fold thickness. American Journal of Clinical Nutrition 24: 864–868.

Roche AF. (1984). Anthropometric methods: New and old, what do they tell us. International Journal of Obesity. 8: 509–523.

Roche AF, Siervogel RM, Chumlea WC, Webb P. (1981). Grading body fatness from limited anthropometric data. American Journal of Clinical Nutrition 34: 2831–2838.

Scherf J, Franklin BA, Lucas CP, Stevenson D, Rubenfire M. (1986). Validity of skinfold thickness measures of formerly obese adults. American Journal of Clinical Nutrition 43: 128–135.

Shakir A, Morley D. (1974). Measuring malnutrition. Lancet 1: 758–759.

Siervogel RM, Roche AF, Himes JH, Chumlea WC, McCammon R. (1982). Subcutaneous fat distribution in males and females from 1 to 39 years of age. American Journal of Clinical Nutrition 36: 162–171.

Sinning WE. (1978). Anthropometric estimation of body density, fat and lean body mass in women gymnasts. Medicine and Science in Sports and Exercise 10: 243–249.

Siri WB. (1956). The gross composition of the body. In: Tobias CA, Lawrence JH (eds). Advances in Biological and Medical Physics. Volume 4. Academic Press, New York, pp. 239–280.

Siri WE. (1961). Body composition from fluid spaces and density: Analysis of methods. In: Techniques for Measuring Body Composition. National Academy of Sciences, National Research Council, Washington, D.C., pp. 223–244.

Sloan AW. (1962). Estimation of body fat in young men. Journal of Applied Physiology 17: 967–970.

Sloan AW, Burt JJ, Blyth CS. (1962). Estimation of body fat in young women. Journal of Applied Physiology 17: 967–970.

Spurr GB, Barac-Nieto M, Lotero H, Dahners HW. (1981). Comparisons of body fat estimated from total body water and skinfold thicknesses of undernourished men. American Journal of Clinical Nutrition 34: 1944–1953.

Trowbridge FL, Hiner CD, Robertson AD. (1982). Arm muscle indicators and creatinine excretion in children. American Journal of Clinical Nutrition 36: 691–696.

Weiner JS, Lourie JA. (1969). Human Biology: A Guide to Field Methods. International Biological Programme. IBP Handbook No. 9, Blackwell Scientific Publications, Oxford–Edinburgh.

Werdein EJ, Kyle LH. (1960). Estimation of the constancy of density of the fat-free body. Journal of Clinical Investigation 39: 626–629.

Wilmore JH, Brown CH. (1974). Physiological profiles of women distance runners. Medicine and Science in Sports and Exercise 6: 178–181.

Womersley J, Durnin JVGA, Boddy K, Mahaffy M. (1976). Influence of muscular development, obesity and age on the fat-free mass of adults. Journal of Applied Physiology 41: 223–229.

Chapter 12

Anthropometric reference data

Anthropometric reference data may be derived from two largely dissimilar sources: local and international. Local reference data should be compiled from measurements on well-nourished, healthy individuals, selected from a local elite group; the group should be ethnically and genetically representative of the population to be investigated. Such data may be preferred where ethnic and genetic factors influencing growth potential predominate, or where it is felt that international reference data, derived from populations with needlessly high energy intakes, are unrealistic. Where, however, ethnic and genetic differences are considered less important than the influences of nutrition, infection, parasitic disease, and environmental factors (Habicht et al., 1974; Graitcer and Gentry, 1981), international reference data may be preferred. Stephenson et al. (1983) showed that during the first five years of life, there is little difference between the growth curves for members of elite groups in less developed countries and those for infants and children of similar age in the industrialized nations.

The World Health Organization has recommended the National Center for Health Statistics (NCHS) reference growth data as an international standard for comparisons of health and nutritional status of children among countries. The NCHS data were selected because they met most of the criteria suggested by the International Union of Nutritional Sciences (IUNS, 1972) for ideal reference data. The sample was cross-sectional, data collection procedures were well-standardized and fully documented, raw data on individuals are available to any investigators, and the population examined appear to have attained their full growth potential. Furthermore, the sample was large and representative, including at least 200 well-nourished individuals in each age and sex group. In contrast, in less industrialized countries, well-nourished children are often few, and sometimes unrepresentative (Waterlow, 1976); as a result, appropriate 'local' reference data are rare.

At present, reference data are generally classified by age, sex, and (sometimes) race. Classification by additional variables (such as number

209

of siblings in a family and/or maturity level) may increase the sensitivity and specificity of the data for identifying individuals or groups at risk; this approach has not been extensively investigated.

Reference data enable comparisons to be made between the distribution of the anthropometric indices in the study group and the apparently healthy reference population. Also, the proportion of individuals with abnormal indices (compared to those in the reference population) can be determined. The comparison enables the extent and severity of malnutrition in the study group to be estimated. In surveillance studies, reference data allow trends over time, and the effectiveness of intervention programs, to be evaluated. Reference data can also be used in clinical settings to monitor growth of individuals and to identify those at risk to under- or overnutrition (screening), and to assess their response to treatment.

At present, comprehensive and contemporary sets of NCHS reference data are not available for all of the anthropometric indices of body composition. Percentile distributions, however, have been compiled by various investigators, using data from several U.S. national surveys. Bias exists in some of the data sets from which the distributions have been derived, which must be recognized when comparisons are made between the study and reference populations; consequently, details of the derivation of the reference data sets are included in the following discussion.

12.1   Distance growth reference data for children

Reference data for distance growth show stature and/or weight tabulated against age, allowing comparison with the stature or weight attained by an individual up to the time of observation (Tanner et al., 1966). The term 'distance growth' encompasses both stature and weight measurements. The reference data are usually compiled from cross-sectional sampling only — measurements taken once on children of varying ages. As a result, cross-sectional data are suitable for making comparisons with population groups which were also studied using cross-sectional surveys. Such reference data can additionally be used to identify individual *pre-adolescent* children with unusually low or high values for stature and/or weight and who may therefore be nutritionally at risk.

Cross-sectional distance growth data, however, give misleading assessments for individual children during adolescence, as a result of the distortion introduced by the adolescent growth spurt, which occurs in different children at markedly different ages. This is termed the *phase-difference* effect. To overcome this problem, distance growth charts based on mixed cross-sectional and longitudinal data have been compiled by Tanner and co-workers for both the United Kingdom (Tanner and Whitehouse, 1976) and the United States (Tanner and Davies, 1985). By using longitudinal growth data at adolescence to depict the shape of the curve, and cross-sectional data to obtain the absolute values for the beginning and end of the curves, distance reference data applicable to individual children during adolescence have been constructed. These reference data take into account the phase-difference effect and, therefore, are suitable for clinical use (Tanner and Whitehouse, 1976).

12.1.1   United States National Center for Health Statistics reference growth data for children

The United States NCHS percentile curves for assessing physical growth of children are based on a large, nationally representative probability sample. The data consist of accurate measurements made on children from birth to eighteen years of age and are mainly cross-sectional. Hence, they are not suitable for monitoring individuals during puberty. Percentile curves (5th, 10th, 25th, 50th, 75th, 90th, and 95th: both observed and smoothed), and means and standard deviations for weight, stature, and weight for stature for both males and females, are displayed as charts or tables (Hamill et al., 1979). Figure 12.1 shows the reference data for stature for age and weight for age for U.S. girls aged two to eighteen years and is typical of the NCHS reference growth data. The complete NCHS percentile curves are in Appendix A12.1 to A12.8.

The weight-for-stature percentiles apply only to prepubescent children, because weight for stature is nearly independent of age only between one year and puberty. The weight-for-stature percentiles are constructed from simultaneous measurements of weight and stature; the mean weight at a given height is then calculated (Figure 12.2) (Hamill et al., 1979). These curves are truncated at 90 cm, preventing their use for children shorter than 90 cm. Hence they cannot be used for young and underprivileged children (Dibley et al., 1987).

Tabulations of the polynomial equations describing the normalized growth reference curves for stature for age, weight for age, and weight for stature have also been prepared (Dibley et al., 1987) and are reproduced in Appendix A12.9 to A12.14. These equations allow calculation of the 3rd, 50th, and 97th percentiles for any individual for weight for age, height for age, and weight for stature (Dibley et al., 1987). Computer programs for mainframes and microcomputers, which use the normalized reference curves to calculate anthropometric indices for children from weight, height, sex, and age data, are available from the Center for Disease Control (Jordan, 1986).

The NCHS data are derived from several sources. The values for weight, length, and weight for length (Figure 12.6) from birth to thirty-six months are taken from longitudinal data collected by the Fels Research Institute, Yellow Springs, Ohio, between 1960 and 1975. The measurements were conducted on 720 white, predominantly middle-class,

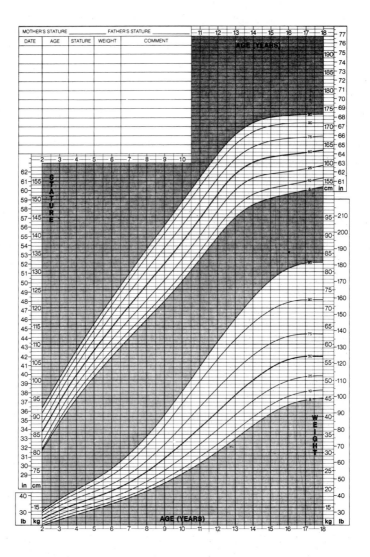

Figure 12.1: Reference data for stature for age and weight for age for U.S. girls aged two to eighteen years. Adapted from: Hamill PVV, Drizd TA, Johnson CL, Reed RB, Roche AF, Moore WM. (1979). Physical growth: National Center for Health Statistics percentiles. Am J Clin Nutr 32: 607–629. Data from the National Center For Health Statistics (NCHS), Hyattsville, Maryland. Reproduced with permission of Ross Laboratories.

infants and children. All weight data indicate nude body weight, and length data represent recumbent length without shoes. The majority of the infants were fed on proprietary formula-based products (DuRant and Linder, 1981). It must be emphasized that the birth-to-36-month charts

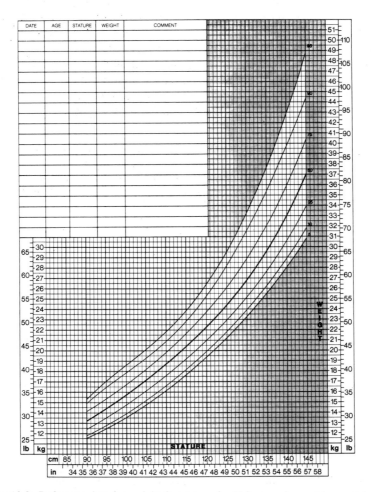

Figure 12.2: Reference data for weight for stature for U.S. prepubescent boys. Adapted from Hamill PVV, Drizd TA, Johnson CL, Reed RB, Roche AF, Moore WM. (1979). Physical growth: National Center for Health Statistics percentiles. Am J Clin Nutr 32: 607–629. Data from the National Center for Health Statistics (NCHS) Hyattsville, Maryland. Reproduced with permission of Ross Laboratories.

for recumbent length are not intended for comparison with standing height, as the recumbent length of a young child is greater than its standing height by approximately 1 to 2 cm, the difference changing with the age of the child (Eveleth and Tanner, 1976).

The data for children from two to eighteen years of age were compiled by NCHS from three sources: values collected during the Health Examination Survey (HES) Cycle I (1963–1965) for ages six to eleven; HES Cycle II (1966–1970) for ages twelve to seventeen; and the first National

Health and Nutrition Examination Survey NHANES I (1971–1974) for ages two to seventeen. Data include measurements on all ethnic, geographic, and income groups, using standardized techniques, and provide reliable population estimates of the attained growth of children in the United States for these ages.

Tanner and Davies (1985) have produced longitudinally based height distance charts for North American male and female children. These charts, unlike the cross-sectional NCHS reference data described above, are suitable for monitoring an individual child's progress throughout the growth period, including puberty. The prepubertal and adult percentiles for height attained were taken from the NCHS data described above and in Section 12.5.1, whereas the shape of the curves was taken from a review of longitudinal studies. Selected percentiles (5th, 50th, and 95th) for early and late maturers are also displayed on these growth charts (Figure 12.3). Details of their method of construction are given in Tanner and Davies (1985). Age standards for puberty stages (see Figure 12.3) are also presented.

12.1.2 Harvard reference growth data for children

The Harvard reference data are derived from a small cross-sectional sample of white, middle-class, American children from Boston and Iowa. The sample size at the extreme (3rd and 97th) percentiles is therefore very small. The charts were constructed in the 1930's and early 1940's from the combined data of Meredith from Iowa and Stuart from Boston (Stuart and Stevenson, 1975). The data provide weight-for-age, stature-for-age, and weight-for-stature percentiles for boys and girls, both separately and combined, from birth to thirty-six months; additionally, sex-specific weight-for-age and stature-for-age data are provided for children aged from two to eighteen years. Recumbent length was measured for children up to five years of age. In general, the 50th percentile values of the Harvard reference data are very similar to the NCHS values, although the average weight for boys appearing in the NCHS reference is slightly greater (Stephenson et al., 1983).

The WHO monograph on 'The Assessment of the Nutritional Status of the Community' (Jelliffe, 1966) used values derived from the Harvard reference data for weight, length, and weight for length, from birth to sixty months for the sexes combined, and weight for height data for the sexes separately for children from age six years.

12.1.3 United Kingdom growth reference data for children

Tanner et al. (1966) compiled smoothed percentile curves for children, using mixed cross-sectional and longitudinal data from a large but fairly homogeneous population living in London (England). The data

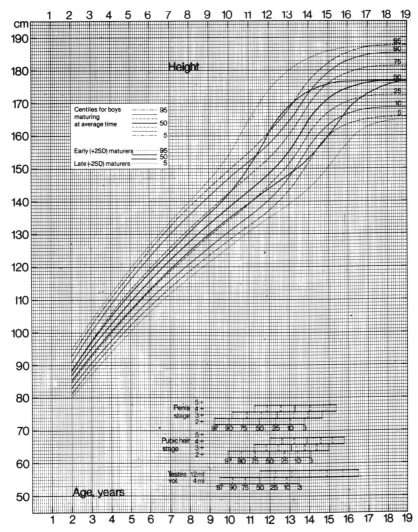

Figure 12.3: Reference data for height attained at a given age for U.S. boys aged two to nineteen years. From Tanner and Davies (1985). Reproduced with permission © Castlemead Publications 1984.

are probably still representative of the current situation in the United Kingdom.

Data for infants and children from birth to 5.5 years of age are based on about eighty children of each sex followed longitudinally, and are presented as weight for age and stature for age. Supine length was measured up to two years of age, and height thereafter. Data for children from 5.5 to 15.5 years of age are cross-sectional, compiled from approximately 1000 boys and 1000 girls for each year of age, selected from a random sample of London schools from a London County Council survey. The data for children from 16.5 years to twenty years of age are largely longitudinal, and were obtained from thirty children participating in the Harpenden Growth Study. The age scale for the distance charts is calibrated in tenths of a year, not in months. A copy of the decimal calendar is given in Appendix A12.15.

Seven percentiles for weight for age and height for age are presented, ranging from the 3rd to the 97th. These percentile curves were derived from the cross-sectional reference data and hence are appropriate only for comparing growth between population groups studied in cross-sectional surveys (Tanner et al., 1966). The longitudinal-type percentiles on these charts, suitable for following the growth of individuals, are indicated by grey-shaded bands.

In 1976, Tanner and Whitehouse revised their distance (and velocity) growth charts to emphasize the longitudinal-type percentiles appropriate for individuals, and to de-emphasize the curves based on the cross-sectional data (Figure 12.4). In addition, the limits for the ages at which successive stages of pubertal sexual development occur in a normal population have been added. It is noteworthy that on the revised charts, only the average child, whose growth spurt occurs at the average time, will actually follow the 50th percentile. Children of average weight or height but maturing early will rise above the 50th percentile and later rejoin it. Conversely, late-maturing children will fall below the 50th percentile and later rejoin it. The outside edges of the shaded areas of Figure 12.4, above the 97th and below the 3rd longitudinal percentiles, represent the limits of these percentiles in the cross-sectional data (Tanner et al., 1976). Copies of these growth reference data for length, height, and weight attained for boys and girls from both birth to five years and birth to nineteen years can be found in Tanner (1978).

12.1.4 Canadian reference growth data for children

The Canadian reference data were generated from the Nutrition Canada National Survey conducted between October 1970 and October 1972 (Nutrition Canada, 1980). The cross-sectional data, based on a nationally representative sample, are presented at six-monthly intervals from birth up to three years of age, and then at yearly intervals up to nineteen years of age. Seven percentiles are included in the published data, ranging from the 5th to the 95th, for weight, stature, weight for stature (up to 25 kg and .110 cm), sitting height, relative sitting height, height of anterior-superior iliac spine, relative leg length, and head circumference. Selected measurements are also classified by race. The Appendix contains percentile tables of stature and weight, and of weight for a

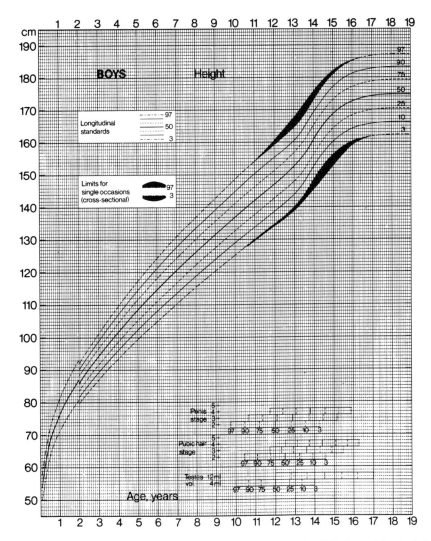

Figure 12.4: Reference data for height attained at a given age for U.K. boys. The shaded areas represent the 97th and 3rd percentile limits of cross-sectionally derived reference data. From Tanner and Whitehouse (1976). Reproduced with permission © Castlemead Publications 1984.

given height, for Canadian infants and children (0 to 19 years of age) and adults by sex (Appendix A12.16 to A12.21).

Cross-sectional measurements of height, weight, sitting height, and bi-cristal and bi-acromial diameters on Canadian children of French extraction were compiled by Demirjian et al. (1972). The sample consisted of 2722 boys aged from six to seventeen years of age and

2332 girls aged from six to sixteen years of age, from three socio-economically different areas of Montreal, Quebec. The mean ($\pm$ SD) and the 3rd, 10th, 25th, 50th, 75th, 90th, and 97th percentile values for weight for age, height for age, and weight for height are presented.

12.1.5   WHO reference growth data for children

The World Health Organization has recently produced two publications of percentiles for weight and height, recalculated from the NCHS data, for use as an international reference; the data are particularly intended for use in countries where no appropriate local reference data are available (WHO, 1978; 1983). The values listed in these two booklets differ, and are not identical with the NCHS percentiles.

The first of the above WHO publications ('The Growth Chart for International Use in Maternal and Child Health Care') (WHO, 1978) presents percentiles (3rd, 50th, and 97th) and the values for -3 SD and -4 SD, for weight for age and stature for age (but not weight for stature) in tabular form for male and females from birth to five years of age, at one-month intervals.

The second WHO publication (WHO, 1983) presents more extensive percentile tables for males and females from birth to thirty-six months, and from two to eighteen years of age, at one-month intervals. Percentile values included are: 3rd, 5th, 10th, 20th, 30th, 40th, 50th, 60th, 70th, 80th, 90th, 95th, and 97th, for weight for age, stature for age, and weight for stature (for prepubertal children). The median and ± 1, 2, and 3 SD are also given (see abbreviated example, Table 12.1); details of their derivation are given in Dibley et al. (1987). The authors of the WHO (1983) tables do not recommend using them for comparing the nutritional status of groups of children greater than ten years of age

Age	Percentiles					Standard Deviations (SD)						
(M)	3rd	20th	50th	80th	97th	-3 SD	-2 SD	-1 SD	Med.	+1 SD	+2 SD	+3 SD
0	2.5	2.9	3.3	3.7	4.2	2.0	2.4	2.9	3.3	3.8	4.3	4.8
6	6.0	7.0	7.8	8.7	9.7	4.9	5.9	6.9	7.8	8.8	9.8	10.8
12	8.2	9.3	10.2	11.1	12.2	7.1	8.1	9.1	10.2	11.3	12.4	13.5
18	9.3	10.5	11.5	12.5	13.8	7.9	9.1	10.3	11.5	12.7	13.9	15.2
24	10.1	11.5	12.6	13.7	15.0	8.6	9.9	11.3	12.6	13.9	15.2	16.5
30	10.9	12.4	13.7	14.8	16.2	9.3	10.8	12.2	13.7	15.0	16.4	17.7
36	11.8	13.4	14.7	15.9	17.5	10.0	11.6	13.1	14.7	16.2	17.7	19.1

Table 12.1: Weight (kg) by age of boys from birth to thirty-six months. Abstracted with permission from a more complete table of data in: Measuring Change in Nutritional Status: Guidelines for assessing the nutritional impact of supplementary feeding programmes for vulnerable groups. Page 75, table 22. Geneva, World Health Organization (1983).

because of the marked differences in the age of onset of puberty among populations.

Stephenson et al. (1983) have compared the Harvard, NCHS, and WHO references for weight, stature, and weight for stature for children from birth to five years of age. Differences between the three data sets for mean and median weights and statures were small.

12.2   Parent-allowed-for reference data

Tanner and colleagues (Tanner et al., 1970) have constructed distance reference data for height for ages two to nine years, which take into account the heights of the child's parents (Figure 12.5). Prior to about two years of age, the height of the child is not closely correlated to parental heights, while beyond nine years, the adolescent growth spurt produces complications. The reference data are only appropriate if the parents of the child have achieved their full height potential.

The data used to construct these reference data were for parents and children from the pooled data of the International Children's Centre Coordinated Longitudinal Growth Studies. The reference data are in the form of a regression line and associated theoretical percentiles. An average of mother's and father's height (midparent height) is used because there are no differences between the relationships of father with son and father with daughter, and mother with daughter and mother with son (Tanner, 1986). To use the reference data, the height percentile of the child is first obtained from the U.K. distance charts (Figure 12.4). The corresponding percentile is then located on the vertical axis of the parent-allowed-for reference data and the midparent height (in cm) on the horizontal axis. An imaginary line is then drawn across the reference data from the percentile on the vertical axis, and another, up from the horizontal axis at the midparent height. The point at which the lines cross is plotted, and its position interpreted in relation to the diagonal lines (marked in percentiles). The latter represent the regression equation standard.

12.3   Head circumference reference data

The National Center for Health Statistics has compiled percentile curves for the head circumference of children from birth to thirty-six months (Hamill et al., 1979). The percentile curves for boys are shown in Figure 12.6 and in Appendix A12.3; the data for girls are presented in Appendix A12.4. The measurements were taken on the same children who provided the length and weight data. Tables of head circumference percentiles were also calculated from the Nutrition Canada data for children up to and including age five years (Nutrition Canada, 1980).

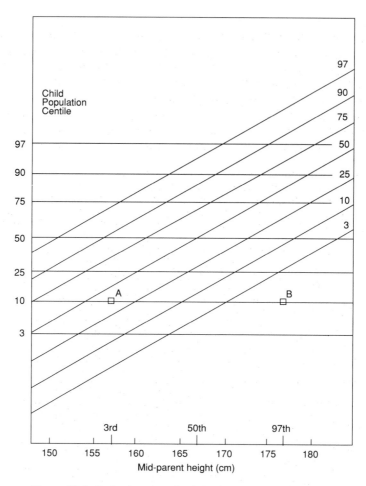

Figure 12.5: Reference data for height at ages two to nine years, allowing for midparent height. The height percentile of the child is obtained from the distance height percentile. A and B are two children both at the 10th percentile for the population, with midparent percentiles at 3rd and 97th. From Tanner JM. (1978). Fetus into Man: Physical Growth from Conception to Maturity. Reproduced by permission of the author, Harvard University Press, and Open Books Publishing Ltd.

A composite set of reference data for males and females from birth to eighteen years of age, compiled from data from the world literature since 1948, was produced by Nellhaus (1968). Measurements were made on 'full-term' infants, or, in the case of older children, on subjects apparently free from neurological disease or retardation. No distinction was made between serial measurements (made on the same individual) and cross-sectional data. Graphs were prepared from calculated grand means and standard deviations of each sex at birth, 1, 3, 6, 9, 12, 18, and 24 months

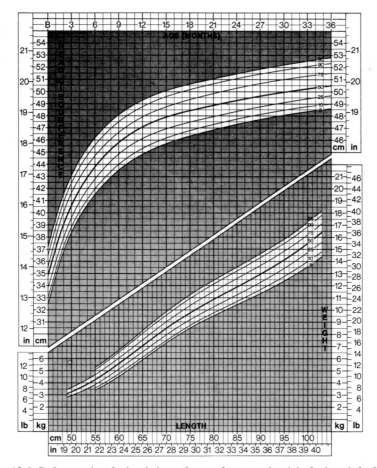

Figure 12.6: Reference data for head circumference for age and weight for length for U.S. boys aged zero to thirty-six months. Adapted from: Hamill PVV, Drizd TA, Johnson CL, Reed RB, Roche AF, Moore WM. (1979). Physical growth: National Center for Health Statistics percentiles. Am J Clin Nutr 32: 607–629. Data from the National Center for Health Statistics (NCHS), Hyattsville, Maryland. Reproduced with permission of Ross Laboratories.

of age, and at yearly intervals up to eighteen years of age. Curves for the mean ± 2 SD were presented. No differences in the data according to race, nation, or geographic location were found.

Mean and mean increments in head circumference measurements for U.K. children aged four weeks to three years, born in London in 1952–1954, are also available. Sex-specific distance curves and tables for the mean increments are given; the velocity curves are for boys and girls combined (Falkner, 1958). Head circumference percentiles for U.K. children are also presented by Forfar and Arneil (1978). The data are for males and females separately, from birth to sixteen years of age.

12.4   Growth velocity reference data

Growth velocity curves are derived from longitudinal studies (studies during which the same child is measured at regular intervals). They provide information on the rate of change of anthropometric variables with age (Figure 12.7); this rate of change is generally termed 'growth velocity'. Velocity curves can be used to establish the timing of the adolescent growth spurt, to detect abnormal changes in growth, and to evaluate individuals (rather than populations) in terms of changes in rates of growth and/or response to therapy. Recent changes in rates of growth can be identified much earlier using velocity growth charts than distance charts, as the latter reflect the past history of the child, including the effect of parental size (Tanner, 1976). Unlike distance curves, a child's percentile placement on the velocity growth curve may change markedly during growth, particularly during adolescence. This arises because velocity growth curves are much more sensitive than distance curves. For example, the range from the 25th to the 75th percentile for stature on the NCHS distance growth charts for ten-year-old boys is approximately 16 cm, compared to an increment range of only 1.5 cm on the velocity growth charts (Roche and Himes, 1980).

A high degree of precision is required for measurements in velocity studies, because two measurement errors may be included whenever growth increments are measured. Hence, measurement techniques should be standardized and preferably conducted by the same anthropometrist throughout the study. Increments measured over six months are the minimum interval which can be used to provide reliable data. For shorter intervals, measurement errors are too large in relation to the mean increments (Marshall, 1971). Growth velocity should be calculated over whole year periods, to minimize variation in growth rates (which are partly the result of seasonal variation). Height velocity, for example, may be faster in the spring than in the fall and winter (Marshall, 1971; Marshall and Swann, 1971). The following formula is used to calculate velocity:

$$\text{Velocity} = \frac{x_2 - x_1}{t_2 - t_1}$$

where x_2 and x_1 are values of the measurement on two occasions t_2 and t_1.

Growth increments during infancy should always be evaluated in relation to gestational age, body size, and weight for length at birth; premature and small-for-gestational-age infants tend to have larger increments than term infants. In the same way, incremental growth during pubescence should preferably be interpreted in relation to data on maturity levels (e.g. skeletal age); the latter influences the timing of the pubescent growth spurt (Baumgartner et al., 1986).

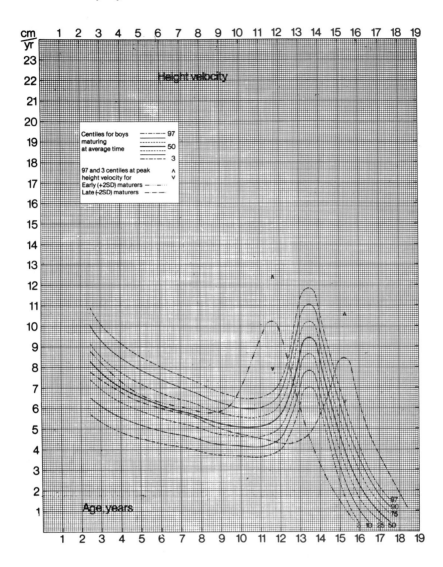

Figure 12.7: Height velocity for U.S. boys. Dotted line, 50th percentile for boys with growth spurt occurring 2 SD early; dashed line, 50th percentile for boys with growth spurt occurring 2 SD late. ∧ and ∨, the 97th and 3rd percentiles for peak velocities of early and late maturers, respectively. From Tanner and Davies (1985). Reproduced with permission © Castlemead Publications 1984.

12.4.1 United States growth velocity reference data

The Fels Research Institute have constructed curves from longitudinal data recorded between 1929 and 1978 from 818 Caucasian U.S. children. Measurements were recorded on approximately 200 children of each sex, at each increment, using standardized anthropometric techniques six times in the first year (birth, and 1, 3, 6, 9, and 12 months) and then six-monthly to eighteen years. Adjustments were made to the serial data for each child to remove errors associated with differences in the chronological ages at which examinations were made. No secular or seasonal effects were observed in the data. The charts are probably very similar to those obtained from a representative sample of the U.S. population (Roche and Himes, 1980).

Sex-specific increments were calculated during six-month intervals for weight, recumbent length, and head circumference from birth to three years, for weight from two to eighteen years, and for stature from thirty months to eighteen years. Seven percentiles — 3rd, 10th, 25th, 50th, 75th, 90th, and 97th — are presented for each age interval, except below 3.5 years for stature, both graphically (Roche and Himes, 1980) and as reference data tables (Baumgartner et al., 1986). The small sample of young children made it impossible to calculate extreme percentiles accurately. The percentiles for stature and weight, but not head circumference and length, are smoothed. To use the growth velocity charts, the observed increments must be plotted vertically above the age at the *end* of the increment. By using the reference data tables, measurements can be interpreted more precisely, enabling more subtle changes in growth to be detected.

The attained growth status of these children is very comparable to that shown by the NCHS cross-sectional distance reference data, at all ages. Hence, to evaluate both attained and incremental growth, a combination of the NCHS and Fels Institute reference data is recommended (Roche and Himes, 1980).

The U.S. infants studied by the Fels Institute tended to have more rapid rates of growth in weight, recumbent length, and head circumference, but more rapid decelerations in growth rate over the first one to two years, compared to the British infants (Section 12.4.2). Furthermore, the U.S. children had earlier and more pronounced pubescent growth spurts in weight and stature than British children (Baumgartner et al., 1986).

Tanner and Davies (1985) have constructed longitudinal reference data for height velocity for North American children, in which percentiles are given for early-, middle-, and late-maturing boys, as discussed in Section 12.1.1. Figure 12.7 presents such height velocity curves for U.S. boys; the comparable figure for female children is given in Tanner and Davies (1985).

A longitudinal growth study was carried out on 334 middle and upper-class U.S. children living in Denver, the majority being of Northern European extraction. Mean and median one-month increments in weight and height from birth to six months, then at nine and twelve months of age, followed by six-monthly intervals from one year to twenty-five years, are available (McCammon, 1970).

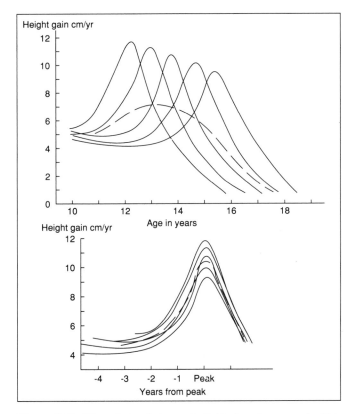

Figure 12.8: The relation between individual and mean velocities during the adolescent spurt: (above) the individual height velocity curves of five boys from the Harpenden Growth Study (solid lines) with the mean curve (dashed) constructed by averaging their values at each age; (below) the same curves all plotted according to their peak height velocity. From Tanner et al. (1966). Reproduced with permission of the authors and Archives of Disease in Childhood.

12.4.2 United Kingdom growth velocity reference data

The United Kingdom growth velocity reference data from birth to eleven to twelve years were compiled from a random sample of about eighty male and eighty female infants born between 1952 and 1954 in central London and followed longitudinally at the Child Study Centre in London. Measurements were made at three-monthly intervals up to age 5.5 years and then annually thereafter. During adolescence, data were based on the three-monthly measurements of forty-nine boys and forty-one girls participating in the Harpenden Growth study and followed throughout the whole of adolescence.

The data are presented as percentile curves (Figure 12.8) for the velocity of growth in height and weight from birth to maturity (i.e. zero to eighteen years), centered about the year of maximum or peak height velocity.

Data relate to increments calculated over the period of a whole year to eliminate seasonal differences in growth of children (Tanner, 1962). The velocity curves present 'individual-type' reference data during adolescence. The latter take into account the phase differences which occur among individuals resulting from variation in the time of onset of the adolescent growth spurt. Individual height velocity curves from ten to eighteen years for five boys from the Harpenden Growth Study are shown, each with their peak height velocity at a different age. The dashed line depicts the mean curve, obtained by averaging their values at each age. Such an approach clearly smooths out the adolescent growth spurt and does not take into account the phase differences between the individual curves (Tanner, 1986). The lower figure shows the same curves plotted according to their peak height velocity, a procedure often referred to as 'normalization' for the time of the adolescent growth spurt.

The unshaded percentiles at adolescence shown in Figure 12.9 represent the velocities for boys who have their peak height velocity at exactly the average time (i.e. 14.0 years in boys). These boys will follow one of the unshaded percentiles during their growth spurt. The shaded areas in Figure 12.9 represent the situation for early and late maturers. The arrowheads and diamonds, shown at ages 12.2 and 15.8 years, represent the 97th, 50th, and 3rd percentiles of boys with peak height velocities which are two standard deviations early or two standard deviations late. Data for an early- and a late-maturing boy, plotted every six months up to age fourteen years, are shown in Figure 12.9. All boys with normal growth velocity curves should lie within the shaded areas and have a velocity curve with a shape that approximates the percentile lines. Children whose growth velocity curves fall outside the shaded area should be investigated (Tanner, 1986). The age scale on the growth velocity curves is also calibrated in tenths of a year rather than months. Height velocity curves for girls and weight velocity curves for boys and girls are also available (Tanner and Whitehouse, 1976).

Longitudinal reference growth data were also compiled by the British Ministry of Health (1959) from data collected between 1949 and 1950. Infants included attended welfare clinics and were weighed monthly. After one year 10,039 infants were still being routinely measured. These data are particularly useful for comparison of velocity growth of U.K. infants because the sample size is larger than that of the data of Tanner et al. (1966).

12.5 Reference height and weight data for adults

Weight and height in adult years have been studied less intensively than during childhood. Reference data for height for adults may be used to estimate the degree of stunting during maturation; weight data provide information on subjects who are obese or underweight. The interpretation

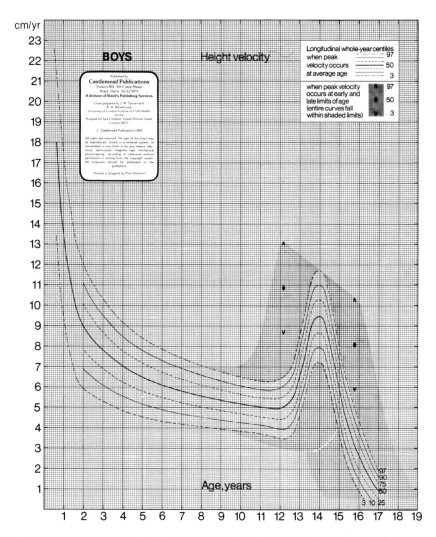

Figure 12.9: Height velocity for U.K. boys. Shaded area encloses all velocity curves within 3rd to 97th percentile limits for age and for peak velocity. 3rd, 50th, and 97th percentiles for early- and late-maturing boys are indicated by arrowhead and diamond symbols. From Tanner and Whitehouse (1976). Reproduced with permission © Castlemead Publications 1984.

of apparent age-related changes for such data may be confounded by the existence of secular trends in body size over successive generations. The adult reference data, with the exception of the Metropolitan Life Insurance tables, provide a reference base for observed weights and do not indicate 'desirable' weight (NCHS, 1979).

12.5.1   United States NCHS adult reference weight by height and age

Weight by height and age data for U.S. adults aged eighteen to seventy-four years are available. The measurements were taken on 13,645 civilian noninstitutionalized adults from a national probability sample selected for the NHANES I survey (1971–1974) (NCHS, 1979).

Height-weight tables are presented for men and women, with mean weight values (in pounds or kilograms) for each inch (or centimeter) of height ranging from 62 to 74 inches for men, and 57 to 68 inches for women, aged 18 to 74 and 18 to 24, 25 to 34, 35 to 44, 45 to 54, 55 to 64, and 65 to 74 years (Appendix A12.22). In addition, the sample size, estimated population in thousands, mean, standard deviation, standard error of the mean, and selected percentiles of weight by height for each sex-age group are presented. Tables comparing the NHANES I study (1971–1974) with those from the Health Examination Survey (HES) (1960–1962) are also given (NCHS, 1979). In general, adults in the NHANES I study were heavier than those in the HES survey. Mean weight increased consistently with age and height in both studies.

12.5.2   United States reference data of weight by frame size and height for adults

Frisancho (1984) has published reference data for weight, by frame size and height, for adults and the elderly developed from cross-sectional data collected by the NHANES I (1971–1974) and NHANES II (1976–1980) surveys, conducted by NCHS. The sample used for these reference data was representative of noninstitutionalized U.S. civilians aged twenty-five to seventy-four years.

The frame size categories — small, medium, and large — correspond to below the 15th, between the 15th and 85th, and above the 85th sex- and age-specific percentile of elbow breadth (Appendix A12.23). The latter measures skeletal breadth, and is used as an indicator of frame size which is relatively independent of adiposity and age (Frisancho and Flegel, 1983). Percentile distributions of weight for height were compiled for three categories of frame size for two age groups twenty-five to fifty-four years and fifty-five to seventy-four years (Appendix A12.24 and A12.25).

Age correction factors for each age, sex, and frame-specific group are also included to account for possible age-related changes in the measurements (Frisancho, 1984). The use of these age correction factors is illustrated by an example in Appendix A12.26.

12.5.3 Metropolitan Life Insurance height-weight tables for adults by frame size

The new Metropolitan height and weight tables (1983) are based on the 1979 Build Study and are derived from measurements on life insurance policyholders aged twenty-five to fifty-nine years from 1950 to 1971. The applicability of these tables to the general population, especially the elderly, is questionable (Frisancho, 1984; Simopoulos and Van Itallie, 1984). The subjects purchased life insurance policies from twenty-five life insurance companies in the United States and Canada and were followed until the policies were cancelled, death ensued, or until the end of the study. Consequently, mortality rates were derived from groups of people with varied follow-up periods. The average length of follow-up was 6.6 years. Ninety percent of the weights are actual weight measurements. Persons with major disease conditions at the time the policies were issued were not included in the study.

The Metropolitan Life Insurance height and weight tables show weight ranges for which people should have the greatest longevity (Appendix A12.27). They do not refer to weights that minimize illness or incidence of diseases. Weight is related to three frame sizes, small, medium, and large, based on elbow breadth. Categories of frame size were developed from the elbow breadth measurements such that 50% of the population falls within the medium frame and 25% each fall within the small and large frames. Weight of clothing, including shoes, for the 1983 tables was assumed to be 5 pounds for men and 3 pounds for women, whereas the height of heels for men and women was assumed to be 1 inch. The weights associated with the lowest mortality in the 1983 tables have increased and are closer to the average weights compared to those of the 1959 Metropolitan Life Insurance tables. Nevertheless, the 1983 Metropolitan Life Insurance range of weights still fall below the average weights of the NCHS reference data.

12.5.4 Canadian adult height and weight reference data

Age- and sex-specific reference data for adults aged twenty to seventy or more years compiled from the Nutrition Canada National Survey of 1970–1972 are available (Nutrition Canada, 1980). Age- and sex-specific percentiles are presented for: head circumference, weight, height, and weight for height, sitting height, anterior-superior iliac spine, relative sitting height, and leg length classified by three income groups and for Indians and Eskimos. Five groups of ten-year age intervals: 20–29, 30–39, 40–49, 50–59, 60–69 years, are used. Persons seventy years and older and pregnant women represent two additional groups. Percentile distributions are the same as those described for children (Section 12.1.4). Appendix A12.16 to A12.19 contain the stature and weight data for Canadian adults.

12.5.5 United Kingdom adult height and weight reference data

A survey of the heights and weights of a representative sample of the adult population of Great Britain, aged sixteen to sixty-four years, was conducted in 1980. Measurements were conducted in the subjects' homes using standardized methods (Rosenbaum et al., 1985). The final sample of 10,021 adults was based on a multistage design with minor biases for age and region. These biases were corrected later by poststratifying the sample at the data-processing stage. No nonresponse bias with respect to height existed, but some under-representation of overweight adults may have occurred.

Tables of the distribution of the mean ($\pm$ SEM), and median, for height (cm) for ten groups of four-year age intervals: 16–19, 20–24, 25–29, 30–34, 35–39, 40–44, 45–49, 50–54, 55–59, 60–64, for males and females separately, are available, together with the number of subjects. These data are also presented by social class, region, and height of parents. The average height was greatest in the age group twenty to twenty-four years for males, and thirty to thirty-four years for females. For all age groups, height tended to be related to social class.

The distribution for the mean $\pm$ SEM, and the median weights by sex, in 0.5-kg increments (range ≤ 45 kg to > 100 kg) for the ten groups are also given. As well, these data tables are also presented by social class and region. The average weight was greatest in age group forty-five to forty-nine years for males, after which it decreased. For females, the average weight was greatest in age group fifty-five to fifty-nine years; no decrease with age occurred. Tables of the percentage distribution of weight at each height for all ages, and for five groups of age intervals: 16–19, 20–29, 30–39, 40–49, 50–64 years, are also available (Rosenbaum et al., 1985; Office of Population Censuses and Surveys, 1984).

Quetelet's index (weight/height^2) was also calculated and its distribution for men and women presented using the following cutoff points: 20.0 or less = underweight; over 25 = overweight; over 30.0 = obesity. The percentage distribution of Quetelet's index, by cutoff point and age and sex, and by cutoff point and region and sex, for the ten groups of four-year age intervals are tabulated, together with the means $\pm$ SEM, by sex, and age group. Distributions of the Ponderal index (ht/$\sqrt[3]{\text{wt}}$) (by region and sex) and the average Ponderal index by social class within age groups are also given (Office of Population Censuses and Surveys, 1984).

12.6 Reference data for body composition

Marked racial differences in the amount and distribution of subcutaneous fat, and to a lesser degree muscle, occur (Robson et al., 1971). Native Americans, Afro-Americans, and Polynesians, for example, have more subcutaneous fat deposited on the trunk than the limbs (i.e. centripetal fat pattern) compared to Europeans (Norgan and Ferro-Luzzi, 1984). Such a fat pattern appears to be associated with a high incidence of coronary heart disease and diabetes (Vague, 1956). Secular changes have also been reported in some industrialized countries for selected indices of body composition (Bowen and Custer, 1984). Hence, international reference data for the assessment of indices of body composition should be used with these uncertainties in mind.

12.6.1 Jelliffe's reference triceps skinfold thickness data

The earliest reference data for triceps skinfold measurements for children aged zero to sixty months and five to fifteen years were compiled by Jelliffe (1966) from British data of Hammond (1955) and Tanner and Whitehouse (1962).

The data for triceps skinfolds for male adults reported by Jelliffe (1966) were compiled from NATO military personnel from Turkey, Greece, and Italy (Hertzberg et al., 1963) whereas those for adult women were derived from a study by the U.S. garment industry on volunteer, largely low-income women aged eighteen to seventy-five years (O'Brien and Shelton, 1941). Single, sex-specific reference data are presented for adults, and for selected age groups of children from birth to five years, and at yearly intervals thereafter up to fifteen years.

12.6.2 United States reference triceps skinfold thickness data

The NCHS (1981) have produced race-, sex-, and age-specific percentiles (5th, 10th, 15th, 25th, 50th, 75th, 85th, 90th, 95th) for triceps skinfold thickness for selected age groups from one to seventy-four years of age based on the NHANES I (1971–1974) data. Smoothed percentile curves for persons aged one to twenty years were also compiled from the National Health Examination Surveys (NHES) cycles II and III and the NHANES I data, as no major secular trends in skinfold data for the 25th to 75th percentile values were noted. Pooling the data resulted in a larger sample size for all age groups and more stable extreme percentile values. Values for the children were adjusted to account for the oversampling among lower socio-economic groups in the NHANES I survey design. Percentile values for these reference data are therefore representative of the childhood population of the United States (Owen, 1982).

Three additional sets of age- and sex-specific percentile distributions for triceps skinfold thickness of American adults have also been compiled from the NHANES I survey data (Bishop et al., 1981; Frisancho, 1981; Cronk and Roche, 1982). Discrepancies exist between these sets of data as the sample populations and age ranges included are not identical. Bishop et al. (1981) combined data for black and white adults aged eighteen to seventy-four years, whereas Frisancho (1981) used data from white subjects ranging in age from one to seventy-four years

(Appendix A12.28). Cronk and Roche (1982), in contrast, presented triceps reference data separated by race for subjects six to 50.9 years because they noted differences in triceps skinfold for white and black females, especially in the outlying percentiles. Cronk and Roche (1982) compiled race- and sex-specific percentiles for one-year intervals from six to seventeen years and three-year intervals for eighteen to 50.9 years. Of these additional data sets, that of Bishop et al. (1982) was adjusted to correct for the high rate of oversampling of persons of low socio-economic status in the NHANES I survey design.

In general, data from the NHANES I survey show that skinfold measurements for men are distributed over a narrower range than those for women. Furthermore, the mean skinfold thickness measurements for women exceed those for men, irrespective of age. Median and triceps skinfold thickness percentiles derived from the NHANES I survey data are greater in adult women than corresponding percentiles derived from the earlier United States Health Examination Survey (HES) between 1960 and 1962. These trends may be associated with secular and age-related variations (Frisancho, 1981; Bishop et al., 1981) (Figure 12.10) and emphasize the inadequacy of single sex-specific and/or outdated reference values to characterize the current triceps skinfold 'norm' for adult males and females.

Frisancho (1984) has also compiled percentile distributions of triceps skinfolds for U.S. adults aged twenty-five to seventy-four years, from data merged from NHANES I (1971–1974) and NHANES II (1976–1980) (Appendix A12.29 and A12.30). These data are presented in relation to frame size and height, since body composition is influenced by these factors as well as age and sex. Frame size was categorized into small, medium, and large, as discussed in Section 12.5.2. By using these reference data, investigators can distinguish a large-framed individual from a person who is truly obese, as indicated by excessive body weight and fat tissue. In the former, a large body weight is not associated with excessive fat tissue. Age correction factors are also included (Appendix A12.26) because the age groups covered are wide (25–54 and 55–74 years) and age-related changes in triceps skinfold measurements exist.

12.6.3   United Kingdom reference triceps skinfold thickness data

Tanner and Whitehouse (1962) compiled extensive cross-sectional data in the 1960's on triceps (and subscapular) measurements of British children. The data for children aged two to five years were from the longitudinal growth study of the Child Study Centre of the Institutes of Child Health and Education, and for children from five to sixteen years from the London County Council survey. The data for children aged one month to two years were derived from a longitudinal growth study in Belgium.

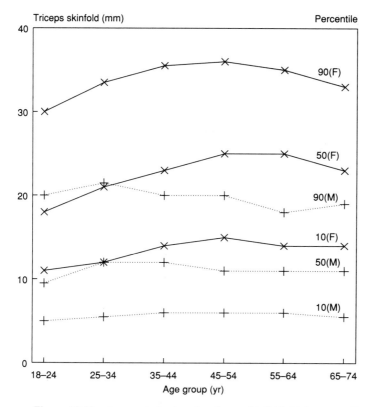

Figure 12.10: Apparent changes in triceps skinfold thicknesses of American adults with advancing age. The changes are much more marked in women than in men. Data from Bishop et al. (1981). © Am. J. Clin. Nutr. American Society for Clinical Nutrition.

Smoothed sex-specific percentile distributions from the 3rd to the 97th are available.

These reference data were revised in 1975 and are shown in Figure 12.11 (Tanner and Whitehouse, 1975). They are based exclusively on U.K. data derived at one month to one year on 200 children followed longitudinally in Infant Welfare clinics, for children one to five years from a random sample of West London children, and for five to nineteen years from an Inner London Education Authority (ILEA) survey. The latter consisted of 1000 children of each sex at each year of age. In general, all the percentiles are higher than those of the earlier U.K. charts.

12.6.4   Canadian reference triceps skinfold data

Triceps and subscapular skinfold measurements were taken during the Nutrition Canada Survey (1970–1972). Details of the sample are given in Section 12.5.4. At present only triceps skinfold percentile distributions

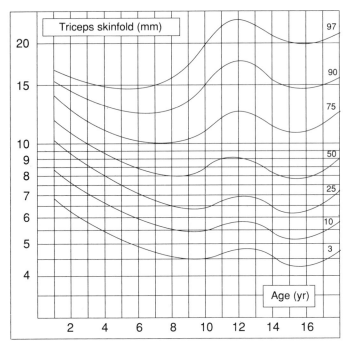

Figure 12.11: United Kingdom reference data for triceps skinfolds for boys. Redrawn from Tanner and Whitehouse (1975) with permission of the authors and Archives of Disease in Childhood.

are available for five groups of adult males and females in ten-year age intervals ranging from twenty to sixty-nine years with an additional group representing persons seventy years and older (Table 12.2) (Jetté, 1981). No Nutrition Canada triceps skinfold reference percentiles for children have been published.

Cross-sectional triceps and subscapular skinfold data on some third-generation French Canadian children were collected between 1969 and 1970 on 2722 boys aged six to seventeen years and 2332 girls aged six to sixteen years. All the measurements were taken by the same technician. Between 26 and 169 children were included at each six-month age interval, representing three socio-economic classes (Jenicek and Demirjian, 1972). Percentile distributions included were the 10th, 50th (median), and 90th.

12.7   Reference subscapular skinfold thickness data

Reference data for subscapular skinfolds are limited. Data for U.K. children and for U.S. children and adults are available.

Age	Percentiles						
(yrs)	5	10	25	50	75	90	95
Males							
20–29	3	4	7	10	16	21	28
30–39	4	6	7	10	16	19	23
40–49	5	6	8	11	14	17	19
50–59	4	5	8	11	14	16	20
60–69	5	6	7	10	14	20	21
70+	5	6	8	11	14	19	21
Females							
20–29	8	11	16	20	25	29	32
30–39	10	11	15	19	24	29	33
40–49	11	13	16	20	26	29	32
50–59	12	14	18	23	16	31	33
60–69	14	17	20	23	27	30	34
70+	11	13	17	21	25	30	31

Table 12.2: Percentiles for the triceps skinfold (mm) for Canadian adult males and females. From Jetté (1981) with permission.

12.7.1 United States reference subscapular skinfold thickness data

The NCHS (1981) have compiled race-, sex-, and age-specific percentiles (5th through the 95th), means and standard deviations, for subscapular skinfolds for selected groups aged one to seventy-four years based on the NHANES I (1971–1974) data (Appendix A12.31). Race-, age-, and sex-specific percentiles of subscapular skinfolds for persons aged two to eighteen years have also been developed from the pooled NHES II and III and the NHANES I data (NCHS, 1981).

Two additional sets of subscapular reference data for U.S. subjects, also derived from data of the NHANES I survey (1971–1974), are available. Age- and sex-specific percentile distributions for subscapular and sum of triceps and subscapular for adults (18 to 74 years) were developed by Bowen and Custer (1984). Data were not presented by race but were adjusted to correct for socio-economic bias. In contrast, Cronk and Roche (1982) compiled unadjusted, age-, and race-specific subscapular skinfold reference data for males only (6 to 50.9 years) from the NHANES I survey. Only data for males were used as subscapular skinfolds represent the most valid indicator of total body fat for boys six to eighteen years (Roche et al., 1981).

Frisancho (1984) has also compiled age- and sex-specific percentile distributions for the subscapular skinfolds of U.S. adults twenty-five to seventy-four years. These are based on the merged data from NHANES I and NHANES II and presented in relation to frame size and height (Appendix A12.32 and A12.33).

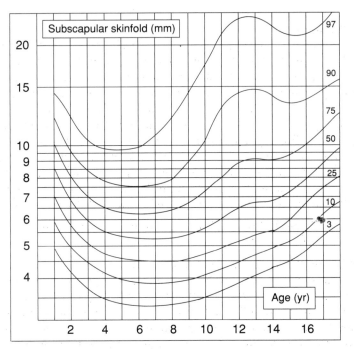

Figure 12.12: United Kingdom reference data for subscapular skin-folds for boys. Redrawn from Tanner and Whitehouse (1975) with permission of the authors and Archives of Disease in Childhood.

12.7.2 United Kingdom reference subscapular skinfold thickness data

Subscapular reference data were compiled for U.K. children aged five to sixteen years using the samples of children outlined in Section 12.6.3 (Figure 12.12) (Tanner and Whitehouse, 1962; 1975). The revised 1975 percentiles are higher than those of the earlier reference data (Tanner and Whitehouse, 1962), especially before school age.

12.7.3 Canadian reference subscapular skinfold thickness data

Subscapular reference data were also compiled from measurements on the French Canadian children described in Section 12.5.4. Subscapular skinfold values for the 1969–1970 data were consistently larger than those collected earlier, a secular trend also noted for triceps skinfold thickness measurements. Subscapular reference percentiles for children or adults, derived from the Nutrition Canada Survey, have yet to be published.

12.8 Reference mid-upper-arm circumference data

Mid-upper-arm circumference measurements are frequently used to screen for protein-energy malnutrition, when the amount of subcutaneous fat is likely to be small. In such circumstances, mid-upper-arm circumference tends to parallel changes in muscle mass. In apparently healthy population groups in industrialized countries, mid-upper-arm circumference is generally used together with triceps skinfold thickness to derive mid-upper-arm fat area or muscle circumference/area. Reference data for these derived parameters are discussed in Sections 12.9 and 12.10.

12.8.1 Jelliffe's reference mid-upper-arm circumference data

Sex- and age-specific mid-upper-arm circumference reference values for children were first compiled by Jelliffe (1966). These values were based on data from healthy Polish children aged from one to sixty months, and on United States data of O'Brien et al. (1941) for children aged six to seventeen years. A single value for both males and females between the ages two to four years was derived because differences between sexes at these times are small.

For adult men and women, Jelliffe (1966) used right arm circumference measurements from the same male and female subjects used for the triceps skinfold measurements (Section 12.6.1). Only one standard value is presented for adult males and another for females.

12.8.2 United States reference mid-upper-arm circumference data

The NCHS (1981) has compiled sex-, age-, and race-specific percentiles (5th through the 95th), means, and standard deviations for mid-upper-arm circumference for children and adolescents from the NHANES I data. Smoothed percentile curves were also derived for children aged two to eighteen years. For adults, age-, sex-, and race-specific percentiles, based on the NHANES I data, are also available (NCHS, 1981).

Two additional sets of mid-upper-arm circumference reference data have been compiled from data collected during the NHANES I survey (1971–1974) (Bishop et al., 1981; Frisancho, 1981). Both age- and sex-specific percentile distributions for similar adult age groups are given in Appendix A12.34. The origin of discrepancies between these data has been discussed in Section 12.6.2.

The mean mid-upper-arm circumference of men exceeds that of women at all ages and is, in general, less varied (Bishop et al., 1981). Both secular and age-related changes in mid-upper-arm circumference percentile distributions of U.S. men and women have been observed (Figure 12.13 and 12.14). Therefore, earlier U.S. reference data for mid-upper-arm circumference compiled by Frisancho (1974) from the Ten-State Nutrition Survey (1968–1970) should not be used.

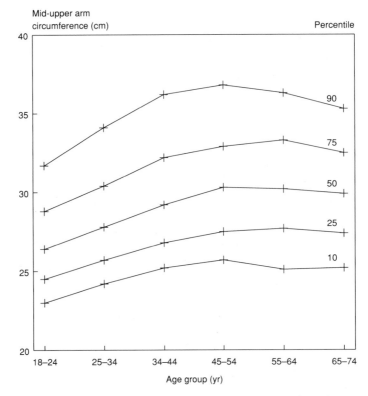

Figure 12.13: Apparent changes in the mid-upper-arm circumference of adult women with age. Data from Bishop et al. (1981). Very similar trends are apparent in the data of Jetté (1981) (Table 12.2). © Am. J. Clin. Nutr. American Society for Clinical Nutrition.

12.8.3   Canadian reference mid-upper-arm circumference data

Jetté (1981) has compiled sex- and age-specific percentiles for mid-upper-arm circumference data for Canadian adults (Table 12.3). No data are available for Canadian children.

12.9   Reference mid-upper-arm fat area data

Midarm fat area is derived from triceps skinfold thickness and mid-upper-arm circumference measurements. The index, not surprisingly, provides a better estimate of total body fat (i.e. fat weight) than a single skinfold thickness at the same site. The reference data for mid-upper-arm fat area varies little in children between one and seven years of age, thus providing an age-independent assessment of total body fat for adequately nourished children of this age group (Gurney and Jelliffe, 1973).

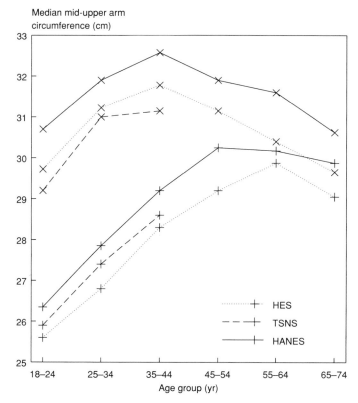

Figure 12.14: Comparison of the median mid-upper-arm circumference measurements from three surveys of the U.S. population: the NHANES of 1971–1974; the Ten-State Nutrition Survey (TSNS) of 1968–1970; and the HES of 1960–1962. Data from Bishop et al. (1981). © Am. J. Clin. Nutr. American Society for Clinical Nutrition.

12.9.1 United States reference mid-upper-arm fat area data

Two sets of percentile distributions for mid-upper-arm fat areas compiled from the NHANES I data collected by NCHS are currently available (Appendix A12.35). Frisancho (1981) published age- and sex-specific mid-upper-arm fat-area percentiles for white U.S. subjects aged one to seventy-four years, using the unadjusted data for triceps skinfold and mid-upper-arm circumference described in Sections 12.6.2 and 12.8.1. Bowen and Custer (1984) also produced sex- and age-specific percentiles for mid-upper-arm fat areas of adults aged eighteen to seventy-four years from NHANES I data (1971–1974). Their data were, however, adjusted to correct for socio-economic bias.

Secular changes in mid-upper-arm fat area have been demonstrated in females, but not in males (Bowen and Custer, 1984). Women from the United States showed a large apparent rise in mid-upper-arm fat area

Age	Percentiles						
(yrs)	5	10	25	50	75	90	95
Males							
20–29	25.5	26.0	27.3	30.2	32.5	35.3	35.8
30–39	26.8	27.2	28.7	31.3	33.2	35.2	37.1
40–49	26.6	28.3	29.8	31.3	33.1	34.0	35.3
50–59	26.7	27.2	29.3	30.9	32.6	33.9	36.0
60–69	25.8	27.2	29.0	30.8	32.5	34.9	36.2
70+	23.4	24.8	27.0	28.7	30.6	32.7	34.2
Females							
20–29	22.2	22.9	24.3	27.4	29.6	32.2	34.3
30–39	22.3	23.6	25.5	27.1	28.8	32.6	35.2
40–49	23.9	24.6	27.3	29.0	31.6	34.5	35.8
50–59	23.3	24.3	27.0	29.8	32.3	35.0	37.0
60–69	25.3	26.7	28.3	30.3	32.5	35.9	38.0
70+	23.1	24.8	27.3	29.7	32.3	34.4	38.4

Table 12.3: Percentiles for the mid-upper-arm circumference (cm) for Canadian adult males and females. From Jetté (1981) with permission.

with age between 1962 and 1972. Hence age- as well as sex-specific percentile distributions from contemporary U.S. reference data should be used to evaluate mid-upper-arm fat area values of persons from the United States.

12.10   Reference mid-upper-arm muscle-circumference and muscle-area data

Secular and age-related trends, as well as genetic differences, have been described for mid-upper-arm muscle circumference and arm muscle area indices, so contemporary and locally applicable reference data should be used if possible. Both indices are derived from measurements of the triceps skinfold thickness and mid-upper-arm circumference using the formulae given in Sections 11.2.2 and 11.2.3.

12.10.1   Jelliffe's reference mid-upper-arm muscle-circumference data

Arm muscle circumference sex-specific reference data for children aged six to sixty months have been calculated for selected ages from the reference data for triceps skinfold and mid-upper-arm circumference outlined in Sections 12.6.1 and 12.8.1. For children aged three to five years, triceps skinfold data were derived from measurements on U.K. children (Hammond, 1955), whereas the mid-upper-arm circumference reference data were compiled in 1941 from measurements on U.S. children (O'Brien et al., 1941). A single reference value for adult males of all ages, and a corresponding value for females, was calculated from the triceps skinfold and mid-upper-arm circumference data of Jelliffe (1966) (Sections 12.6.1 and 12.8.1).

12.10.2   United States reference mid-upper-arm muscle circumference and muscle area data

Some of the earliest U.S. reference data for mid-upper-arm muscle circumference and area were compiled from measurements taken on male and female white U.S. subjects up to forty-four years of age who participated in the Ten-State Nutrition Survey of 1968–1970 (Frisancho, 1974). The sample was also biased toward persons of low socio-economic status.

More recently, two sets of age- and sex-specific mid-upper-arm muscle circumference reference data (Bishop et al., 1981; Frisancho, 1981) and two sets of mid-upper-arm muscle area percentiles (Frisancho, 1981; Bowen and Custer, 1984) have been compiled from NHANES I triceps skinfold and mid-upper-arm circumference measurements described in Sections 12.6.2 and 12.8.2 (Appendix A12.36 and A12.37). Reference data from Frisancho (1981) are for white persons aged one to seventy-four years; reference data from Bowen and Custer (1984) are for adults aged eighteen to seventy-four years.

The distributions of the values for mid-upper-arm muscle circumference for adult males and females are similar and change with age. Arm muscle circumference and mid-upper-arm muscle area generally increase up to age sixty-five years in women and up to middle age in men and then steadily decrease. In women, mid-upper-arm muscle circumference and area steadily increase up to age sixty-five years and then stabilize or decline.

Arm muscle area percentiles for U.S. adults aged from twenty-five to seventy-four years, based on the merged NHANES I and II data, have also been compiled in relation to age, sex, height, and frame size (Frisancho 1984). In older persons, increased compressibility of fat may result in an overestimation of mid-upper-arm muscle area, whereas the trends in mid-upper-arm muscle area observed in the younger age groups may represent a combined increase in bone diameter and muscle area. Secular-related changes in mid-upper-arm muscle circumference and mid-upper-arm muscle area in both U.S. males and females have also been noted (Frisancho, 1974; Bowen and Custer, 1984).

Reference data for bone-free mid-upper-arm muscle area, calculated using the corrected equation of Heymsfield et al. (1982) (Section 11.2.3), have been compiled for three categories of frame size for U.S. male and female adults for two age groups, twenty-five to fifty-four and fifty-five to seventy-four years of age (Frisancho, 1984). Percentiles ranging from the 5th to the 95th are included.

Age	Percentiles						
(yrs)	5	10	25	50	75	90	95
Males							
20–29	23.24	23.71	24.90	26.31	29.15	29.98	30.64
30–39	23.57	24.87	26.28	27.43	29.24	30.47	30.88
40–49	24.43	25.08	26.14	27.90	29.38	29.91	30.45
50–59	24.11	24.57	25.94	27.33	28.63	29.93	30.90
60–69	22.95	23.95	25.47	27.40	28.67	29.87	31.47
70+	21.05	22.15	23.58	24.82	26.83	28.20	29.02
Females							
20–29	17.93	18.43	19.64	21.03	22.37	24.31	25.14
30–39	18.08	18.60	19.71	21.20	22.46	24.13	25.77
40–49	19.53	19.81	21.08	22.97	24.27	26.30	27.63
50–59	18.17	19.03	20.61	22.50	24.16	26.23	27.96
60–69	19.05	19.88	21.45	23.31	24.80	26.27	28.91
70 +	18.68	19.28	21.35	23.10	24.73	26.86	28.66

Table 12.4: Percentiles for mid-upper-arm muscle circumference (cm) for Canadian adult males and females. From Jetté (1981) with permission.

12.10.3   Canadian reference mid-upper-arm muscle circumference data

Jetté (1981) has compiled age- and sex-specific mid-upper-arm muscle circumference percentiles for Canadian adults aged twenty to seventy-nine years from the Nutrition Canada National Survey data (Table 12.4).

12.11   Summary

Sources of distance reference growth data for children in the United States include the NCHS (0–3; 2–18 years) and Harvard (0–3; 2–18 years) data; for Canada, the Nutrition Canada Survey data (0–18 years); and for the United Kingdom, the Tanner and Whitehouse (0–18 years) data. Percentiles of weight for age, stature for age, weight for stature (for the United States and Canada), and head circumference for age are available, ranging from the 5th to 95th percentiles for the U.S. and Canadian data, and from the 3rd to 97th percentiles for the U.K. data. The World Health Organization recommends the NCHS data as the international standard and has produced more extensive percentile tables for weight for age, stature for age, and weight for stature, together with the median and ± 1, 2, and 3 SD. Clinical longitudinal-type distance charts suitable for individuals are available for weight and height for age for the United Kingdom and height for age for the United States. Reference data for adults for weight and height for age are available for the United States (NCHS), Canada (Nutrition Canada Survey), and the United Kingdom

(Office of Population Censuses and Surveys). Some of the NCHS adult reference data and the Metropolitan Life Insurance tables include weight by frame size and height. The Metropolitan Life Insurance height-weight tables indicate a weight range commensurate with longevity.

Growth velocity reference data derived from longitudinal data have been compiled by the U.S. Fels Institute and by the United Kingdom London Child Study Centre. These reference data provide information on rate of growth, and weight (for United Kingdom only) and height velocity percentile curves for early- and late-maturers. Growth velocity reference data are more sensitive to growth abnormalities than distance growth data, provided accurate and precise measurements are taken.

Use of an international reference data set for body composition measurements is not appropriate. Reference data for selected body composition indices are available for the United States, United Kingdom, and Canada. For the United States, age-, sex-, and, sometimes, race-specific reference data, for triceps skinfold, subscapular skinfold, mid-upper-arm circumference, mid-upper-arm muscle circumference and area, and mid-upper-arm fat area are available for adults and, in some cases, for children. In Canada, reference data for triceps skinfold, mid-upper-arm circumference, and mid-upper-arm muscle circumference for adults only were compiled from the Nutrition Canada National Survey data. In the United Kingdom, reference data for triceps and subscapular skinfolds for children are available.

References

Baumgartner RN, Roche AF, Himes JH. (1986). Incremental growth tables: supplementary to previous charts. American Journal of Clinical Nutrition 43: 711–722.

Bishop CW, Bowen PE, Ritchey SJ. (1981). Norms for nutritional assessment of American adults by upper-arm anthropometry. American Journal of Clinical Nutrition 34: 2530–2539.

Bishop CW, Bowen PE, Ritchey SJ. (1982). Comparison of two newly developed sets of upper arm anthropometric norms for American adults. American Journal of Clinical Nutrition 36: 555–557.

Bowen PE, Custer PB. (1984). Reference values and age–related trends for arm muscle area, arm fat area, and sum of skinfolds for United States adults. Journal of the American College of Nutrition 3: 357–376.

Cronk CE, Roche AF. (1982). Race- and sex-specific reference data for triceps and subscapular skinfolds and weight stature. American Journal of Clinical Nutrition 35: 347–354.

Demirjian A, Jenicek M, Dubuc MB. (1972). Les normes staturo-pondérales de l'enfant urbain canadien français d'âge scolaire. Canadian Journal of Public Health 63: 14–30.

Dibley MJ, Goldsby JB, Staehling NW, Trowbridge FL. (1987). Development of normalized curves for the international growth reference: historical and technical considerations. American Journal of Clinical Nutrition 46: 736–748.

DuRant RH, Linder CW. (1981). An evaluation of five indexes of relative body weight for use with children. Journal of the American Dietetic Association 78: 35–41.

Eveleth PB, Tanner JM. (1976). Worldwide Variation in Human Growth. International Biological Programme No. 8, Cambridge University Press, Cambridge, pp. 262–272.

Falkner F. (1958). Some physical measurements in the first three years of life. Archives of Disease in Childhood 33: 1–9.

Forfar JO, Arneil GC. (eds). (1978). Textbook of Paediatrics. Second edition. Churchill Livingston, Edinburgh, pp. 156.

Frisancho AR. (1974). Triceps skinfold and upper arm muscle size norms for assessment of nutritional status. American Journal of Clinical Nutrition 27: 1052–1058.

Frisancho AR. (1981). New norms of upper limb fat and muscle areas for assessment of nutritional status. American Journal of Clinical Nutrition 34: 2540–2545.

Frisancho AR. (1984). New standards of weight and body composition by frame size and height for assessment of nutritional status of adults and the elderly. American Journal of Clinical Nutrition 40: 808–819.

Frisancho AR, Flegel PN. (1983). Elbow breadth as a measure of frame size for United States males and females. American Journal of Clinical Nutrition 37: 311–314.

Graitcer PL, Gentry EM. (1981). Measuring children: one reference for all. Lancet 2: 297–299.

Gurney JM, Jelliffe DB. (1973). Arm anthropometry in nutritional assessment: nomogram for rapid calculation of muscle circumference and cross-sectional muscle and fat areas. American Journal of Clinical Nutrition 26: 912–915.

Habicht JP, Martorell R, Yarbrough C, Malina RM, Klein RE. (1974). Height and weight standards for preschool children. How relevant are ethnic differences in growth potential? Lancet 1: 611–615.

Hamill PVV, Drizd TA, Johnson CL, Reed RB, Roche AF, Moore WM. (1979). Physical growth: National Center for Health Statistics percentiles. American Journal of Clinical Nutrition 32: 607–629.

Hammond WH. (1955). Measurement and interpretation of subcutaneous fat with norms for children and young adults males. British Journal of Preventive and Social Medicine 9: 201–211.

Hertzberg HTE, Churchill E, Dupertuis CW, White RM, Damon A. (1963). Anthropometric Survey of Turkey, Greece and Italy. Macmillan Company, New York.

Heymsfield SB, McManus C, Smith J, Stevens V, Nixon DW. (1982). Anthropometric measurement of muscle mass: revised equations for calculating bone-free arm muscle area. American Journal of Clinical Nutrition 36: 680–690.

IUNS (International Union of Nutritional Sciences) (1972). The creation of growth standards: a committee report. American Journal of Clinical Nutrition 25: 218–220.

Jelliffe DB. (1966). The Assessment of the Nutritional Status of the Community. WHO Monograph 53. World Health Organization, Geneva.

Jenicek M, Demirjian A. (1972). Triceps and subscapular skin-fold thickness in French-Canadian school-age children in Montreal. American Journal of Clinical Nutrition 25: 576–581.

Jetté M. (1981). Guide for Anthropometric Classification of Canadian Adults for use in Nutritional Assessment. Health and Welfare, Ottawa.

Jordan MD. (1986). Anthropometric Software Package, Tutorial Guide and Handbook. Version 3.0. Centers for Disease Control, Atlanta, Georgia.

Marshall WA. (1971). Evaluation of growth rate in height over periods of less than a year. Archives of Disease in Childhood 46: 414–420.

Marshall WA, Swan AV. (1971). Seasonal variation in growth rates of normal and blind children. Human Biology 43: 502–516.

McCammon RW. (1970). Human Growth and Development. Charles C Thomas, Springfield, Illinois.

Metropolitan Height and Weight Tables (1983). Statistical Bulletin, Metropolitan Life Insurance Company, New York 64: 1–9.

Ministry of Health (1959). Standards of normal weight in infancy. Reports of Public Health Medical Subjects. No. 99.

NCHS (National Center for Health Statistics) (1979). Weight by height and age for adults 18–74 years: United States, 1971–1974. (Vital and health statistics: Series 11, Data from the National Health Survey; no. 208) (DHEW publication; no. (PHS) 79–1656), Hyattsville, Maryland.

NCHS (National Center for Health Statistics) (1981). Basic data on anthropometric measurements and angular measurements of the hip and knee joints for selected age groups 1–74 years of age: United States, 1971–1975. (Vital and health statistics: Series 11, Data from the National Health Survey; no. 219) (DHHS publication; no.(PHS) 81-1669), Hyattsville, Maryland.

Nellhaus G. (1968). Head circumference from birth to eighteen years. Practical composite international and interracial graphs. Pediatrics 41: 106–114.

Norgan NG, Ferro-Luzzi A. (1984). Principal components as indicators of body fatness and subcutaneous fat patterning. Human Nutrition: Clinical Nutrition 39C: 45–53.

Nutrition Canada (1980). Anthropometry Report: Height, Weight and Body Dimensions. Bureau of Nutritional Sciences, Health Protection Branch, Health and Welfare, Ottawa.

O'Brien R, Girshik MA, Hunt EP. (1941). Body measurements of American boys and girls for garment and pattern construction. United States Department of Agriculture (Miscellaneous publication no. 366), Washington, D.C.

O'Brien R, Shelton WC. (1941). Women's Measurements for Garment and Pattern Construction. United States Department of Agriculture (Miscellaneous publication no. 454), Washington, D.C.

Office of Population Censuses and Surveys, Social Survey Division (1984). The heights and weights of adults in Great Britain. Knight I (ed). Report of a survey carried out on behalf of the Department of Health and Social Security covering adults aged 16-64 years. Her Majesty's Stationery Office, London.

Owen GM. (1982). Measurement, recording, and assessment of skinfold thickness in childhood and adolescence: report of a small meeting. American Journal of Clinical Nutrition 35: 629–638.

Robson JRK, Bazin M, Soderstrom R. (1971). Ethnic differences in skin–fold thickness. American Journal of Clinical Nutrition 24: 864–868.

Roche AF, Himes JH. (1980). Incremental growth charts. American Journal of Clinical Nutrition 33: 2041–2052.

Roche AF, Siervogel RM, Chumlea WC, Webb P. (1981). Grading body fatness from limited anthropometric data. American Journal of Clinical Nutrition 34: 2831–2838.

Rosenbaum S, Skinner RK, Knight IB, Garrow JS. (1985). A survey of heights and weights of adults in Great Britain, 1980. Annals of Human Biology 12: 115–127.

Simopoulos AP, Itallie TB van. (1984). Body weight, health, and longevity. Annals of Internal Medicine 100: 285–295.

Stephenson LS, Latham MC, Jansen A. (1983). A comparison of growth standards: Similarities between NCHS, Harvard, Denver and privileged African children and differences with Kenyan rural children. Cornell International Nutrition Monograph Series Number 12.

Stuart HAW, Stevenson SS. (1975). Physical growth and development. In: Nelson WE, Vaughan VC, McKay RJ (eds). Textbook of Pediatrics. Tenth edition. Saunders, Philadelphia, pp. 13–51.

Tanner JM. (1962). Growth at Adolescence. Second edition. Blackwell Scientific Publications, Oxford.

Tanner JM. (1976). Growth as a monitor of nutritional status. Proceedings of the Nutrition Society 35: 315–322.

Tanner JM. (1978). Fetus into Man. Physical Growth from Conception to Maturity. Harvard University Press, Cambridge, Massachusetts.

Tanner JM. (1986). Use and abuse of growth standards. In: Falkner F, Tanner JM (eds). Human Growth A Comprehensive Treatise. Second edition. Volume 3. Methodology, Ecological, Genetic, and Nutritional Effects on Growth. Plenum Press, New York–London, pp. 95–109.

Tanner JM, Davies PSW. (1985). Clinical longitudinal standards for height and height velocity for North American children. Pediatrics 107: 317–329.

Tanner JM, Goldstein H, Whitehouse RH. (1970). Standards for children's height at ages 2 to 9 years, allowing for height of parents. Archives of Disease in Childhood. 45: 755–762.

Tanner JM, Whitehouse RH. (1962). Standards for subcutaneous fat in British children. Percentiles for thickness of skinfolds over triceps and below scapula. British Medical Journal 1: 446–450.

Tanner JM, Whitehouse RH. (1975). Revised standards for triceps and subscapular skinfolds in British children. Archives of Disease in Childhood 50: 142–145.

Tanner JM, Whitehouse RH. (1976). Clinical longitudinal standards for height, weight, height velocity, and weight velocity, and the stages of puberty. Archives of Disease in Childhood 51: 170–179.

Tanner JM, Whitehouse RH, Takaishi M. (1966). Standards from birth to maturity for height, weight, height velocity, and weight velocity: British children, 1965. Archives of Disease in Childhood 41: 454–471; 613-625.

Vague J. (1956). The degree of masculine differentiation of obesities: a factor determining predisposition to diabetes, atherosclerosis, gout, and uric acid calculous disease. American Journal of Clinical Nutrition 4: 20–34.

Waterlow JC. (1976). Classification and definition of protein–energy malnutrition. In: Beaton GH, Bengoa JM (eds). Nutrition in Preventive Medicine. WHO Monograph No. 62. World Health Organization, Geneva, pp. 530–555.

WHO (World Health Organization) (1978). A Growth Chart for International Use in Maternal and Child Health Care. World Health Organization, Geneva.

WHO (World Health Organization) (1983). Measuring Change in Nutritional Status. Guidelines for Assessing the Nutritional Impact of Supplementary Feeding Programmes for Vulnerable Groups. World Health Organization, Geneva.

Chapter 13

Evaluation of anthropometric indices

Standardized methods of evaluating anthropometric indices are essential for assessing the nutritional status of population groups and identifying malnourished individuals. The methods selected will depend on the objectives of the study and the facilities available for data handling.

In population studies involving surveillance, or in cross-sectional nutrition surveys, the data should be presented as frequency distributions of the anthropometric indices. The World Health Organization (WHO, 1983) recommends comparison of these distributions with the corresponding NCHS reference data. In addition, the proportion of individuals in the sample with indices below or above predetermined *reference limits* drawn from the appropriate reference data can be determined. In some cases, *cutoff* points based on functional impairment and/or clinical signs of deficiency, and occasionally mortality risk, are used (Section 1.4). Cutoff points may be combined with *trigger* levels to set the level at which a predetermined intervention is initiated (or triggered).

To identify and classify malnourished individuals, the anthropometric indices can be compared with either predetermined reference limits or cutoff points which can classify an individual into one or more 'risk' categories indicative of the severity of malnutrition and/or mortality risk. Classification systems may also indicate the type of malnutrition.

Hence, to evaluate anthropometric indices at both the individual and population level, appropriate reference data for each index (discussed in Chapter 12) are generally required. Various methods of comparing anthropometric indices with the reference data are discussed in detail below, followed by a review of commonly used systems for identifying and classifying individuals at risk to malnutrition.

13.1 Evaluating indices in population studies

In population studies, the distribution of each anthropometric index can be compared using percentiles and/or standard deviation 'scores' derived from the reference data. In either case, the distribution of the index

247

Frequency

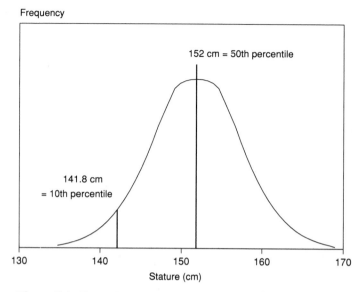

Figure 13.1: Frequency distribution for stature in 13-year old boys.

for the study population can then be tabulated or presented graphically. Such an approach highlights critical features of the distribution of the study population (WHO Working Group, 1986). Only in cases where the sample size drawn from the target population is very small should the mean or median value of the index by age and sex be compared with the corresponding mean or median value for the reference data (Keller et al., 1976). The latter comparison provides no information on the distribution of values within the sample.

13.1.1 Percentiles

A percentile refers to the position of the measurement value in relation to all (or 100%) of the measurements for the reference population, ranked in order of magnitude. Figure 13.1 is a cumulative frequency distribution of the heights of boys aged thirteen years, illustrating the use of percentiles. In this figure, a height of 152 cm represents the 50th percentile. This means that 50% of the boys have a height at or below this value, and 50% at or above this value. Similarly, 10% of the boys have a height at or below the 10th percentile which, in Figure 13.1, falls at 141.8 cm. For data with a Gaussian distribution (e.g. height for age), the 50th percentile corresponds to both the mean and the median; for skewed data (e.g. weight for age) the 50th percentile corresponds to the median.

For population studies, the number and percentage of individuals falling within specified percentiles of the reference data can be tabulated or presented as a histogram (Figure 13.2) (WHO, 1983). This procedure

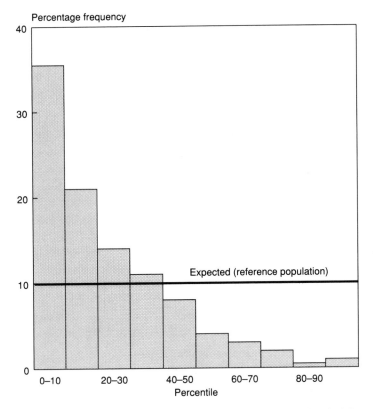

Figure 13.2: Percentage distribution of children by weight/height percentiles. Data taken from the 1974 Sahel nutrition studies based on measurements of 798 children. Reproduced from: Measuring Change in Nutritional Status: Guidelines for assessing the nutritional impact of supplementary feeding programmes for vulnerable groups. Geneva, World Health Organization, 1983: page 26, Figure 4, with permission.

is recommended for the evaluation of anthropometric measurements from relatively well-nourished populations from industrialized countries, as no errors are introduced if the data have a skewed distribution. Weight for age, weight for height, and many circumferential and skinfold indices have skewed distributions.

Percentiles are not recommended for evaluating anthropometric indices from less developed areas when reference data from industrialized countries, such as the NCHS data (Hamill et al., 1979), are used. In these circumstances, many of the study population may have indices below the extreme percentile of the reference population (i.e. below the 5th percentile), making it difficult to accurately classify large numbers of individuals (Waterlow et al., 1977).

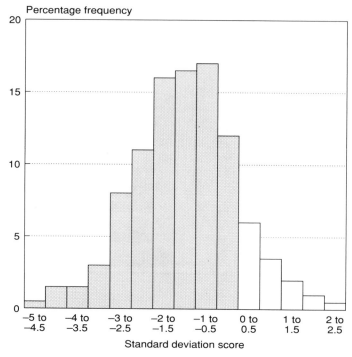

Figure 13.3: Frequency distribution of SD scores of height for age for 1395 children measured during the Sahel nutrition studies and who were aged 12 to 23.9 months. From: Measuring Change in Nutritional Status: Guidelines for assessing the nutritional impact of supplementary feeding programmes for vulnerable groups. Geneva, World Health Organization, 1983: page 26, Figure 4, with permission.

13.1.2 Standard deviation scores

The use of standard deviation (SD) scores is recommended by Waterlow et al. (1977) for evaluating anthropometric data from less industrialized countries. The method measures the deviation of the anthropometric measurement from the reference median in terms of standard deviations or Z scores. Standard deviation scores can be defined beyond the limits of the original reference data. Consequently, individuals with indices below the extreme percentiles of the reference data can be classified accurately. The number and proportion of subjects within a specified range of standard deviation scores for each age and sex group can be presented graphically (Figure 13.3), or as a table, as noted for percentiles.

The SD score, which is calculated for each subject within the sample, is a measure of an individual's value with respect to the distribution of the reference population. The score is calculated using the following formula, a modified version of the standard statistical Z-score transformation.

$$\text{SD score} = \frac{\text{Individual's value} - \text{median value of reference population}}{\text{Standard deviation value of reference population}}$$

The standard deviation values for the NCHS reference population are recommended for use in calculating SD scores and are published by WHO (1983). These reference standard deviations have been calculated by transforming the original NCHS reference data. Specific details of this process are given in Dibley et al. (1987). As the distributions of weight for age and weight for height are not symmetrical, standard deviations below and above the median differ and hence were calculated separately. In contrast, the distribution for height for age is symmetrical, so that a single set of age-specific standard deviations was calculated.

13.2 Evaluating indices in studies of individuals

The optimal system for identifying individuals 'at risk' to malnutrition is one for which no misclassification occurs. In this case, all the individuals designated as 'at risk' are actually malnourished (i.e. there are no false positives and sensitivity is 100%) (Section 1.3). Similarly, those individuals classified as 'not at risk' are truly unaffected (i.e. there are no false negatives and specificity is 100%). In practice, the classification schemes are *not* optimal; some misclassification always occurs so that some individuals identified as 'at risk' to malnutrition will not be truly malnourished (false positives), and others classified as 'not at risk' to malnutrition will in fact be malnourished (false negatives). Unfortunately, specificity and sensitivity data for the anthropometric indices selected are usually not known for the target population. Instead, values for sensitivity and specificity obtained elsewhere are often used and assumed to be appropriate for the target population (Habicht et al., 1979; Habicht et al., 1982).

Several systems are available for classifying individuals as 'at risk' to malnutrition. All utilize at least one anthropometric index and one or more *reference limits* drawn from appropriate reference data or *cutoff points* based on functional impairment and/or clinical signs of deficiency or mortality risk. In many systems, cutoff points are defined as a designated percentage of the median of the reference population. For some systems, both the severity and type of malnutrition are also defined.

Use of more than one classification system for the same population group will normally produce some contradictions, depending on the reference limits or the cutoff points selected. Figure 13.4 depicts the relation between the classifications 'low', 'normal', and 'high' for the indices weight for height, height for age, and weight for age, using the reference limits at two standard deviations above and below the median of the NCHS reference data (WHO, 1983). For the index height for

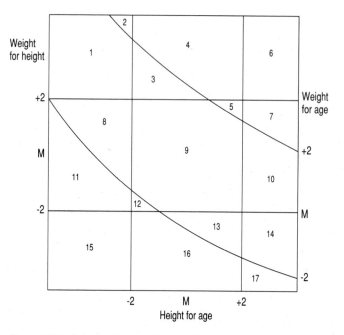

Figure 13.4: Relation between the classifications 'low', 'normal', and 'high' for the indices weight for height, height for age, and weight for age, with reference limits at two standard deviations above and below the median. Calculated from the data for eighteen-month-old boys in the NCHS reference population. From: Measuring Change in Nutritional Status: Guidelines for assessing the nutritional impact of supplementary feeding programmes for vulnerable groups. Geneva, World Health Organization, 1983: page 27, Figure 5 with permission.

age, for example (horizontal axis), children to the left of −2 SD will be classified as short, those to the right of +2 SD as tall, and those between the two reference limits as normal. Likewise, in terms of weight for height (indicated on the left vertical axis), children below −2 SD will be thin, those above +2 SD obese, and those between the two reference limits, normal. The reference limits for weight for age are shown running obliquely across those for weight for height and height for age. Hence children falling within the lower stippled area have weight-for-age values more than 2 SD below the median. The numbered areas shown in Figure 13.4 are seventeen different combinations of 'low', 'normal', and 'high' for the three indices, examples of which are shown in Table 13.1. From this table it is clear that if low weight for age is selected as the index, the children identified will be a mixed group in terms of their nutritional status. Some of the children (e.g. No. 11) will have low weight for age as a result of their very short stature, perhaps arising from a history of past malnutrition. In contrast, others (e.g. No. 17) will

Nos.	Combination of Indices	Nutritional Status
16 17 14	Low wt/ht + low wt/age + normal ht/age + low wt/age + high ht/age + normal wt/age + high ht/age	Currently underfed Currently underfed Currently underfed
11 9 7	Normal wt/ht + low wt/age + low ht/age + normal wt/age + normal ht/age + high wt/age + high ht/age	Short, normally nourished Normal Tall, normally nourished
1 2 4	High wt/ht + normal wt/age + low ht/age + high wt/age + low ht/age + high wt/age + normal ht/age	Currently overfed, short Obese Overfed, not necessarily obese

Table 13.1: The results of using various combinations of anthropometric indices and possible interpretations of the results. The numbers in the left hand column are taken from Figure 13.4. From: Measuring Change in Nutritional Status: Guidelines for assessing the nutritional impact of supplementary feeding programmes for vulnerable groups. Geneva, World Health Organization, 1983: page 27, text table, with permission.

indeed be currently malnourished with a low weight for age and weight for height, even though they have a high height for age.

At the present time, there is no universally accepted classification system for describing 'risk' of protein-energy malnutrition and overnutrition in terms of type, severity, or approximate duration. The results shown in Table 13.1, however, illustrate the importance of including height as one of the indices used to assess malnutrition.

13.2.1 Percentiles

Percentiles can also be used for classifying individuals. The percentile for a subject of known age and sex can be calculated exactly, if the numerical percentile values are available for the reference data. Alternatively, the percentile range within which the measurement of an individual falls can be read from graphs of the reference data. Depending on the reference data used, reference limits commonly used for designating individuals as 'at risk' to malnutrition are either below the 3rd or 5th percentiles or above the 97th or 95th percentiles.

13.2.2 Standard deviation scores

Standard deviation scores also can be calculated for individuals. For example, a child with a weight one standard deviation below the reference median for his age will have an SD score of -1.0, whereas a child with a weight two standard deviations above the reference median for his age has an SD score of $+2.0$.

Height in cm	−3 SD	−2 SD	−1 SD	Median	+1 SD	+2 SD	+3 SD
69	5.6	6.6	7.5	8.5	9.8	11.1	12.4

Table 13.2: A portion of a table showing weight (kg) for height in a reference population at different SD values. The data are for boys 69 cm in height. Note that the values below and above the median are different. From: Measuring Change in Nutritional Status: Guidelines for assessing the nutritional impact of supplementary feeding programmes for vulnerable groups. Geneva, World Health Organization, 1983: page 90, Table 27 with permission.

Exact values for the SD score of an individual can also be calculated using selected reference standard deviation values. For example, for a boy 69 cm tall, weighing 6.3 kg (Table 13.2) (i.e. with a weight below the reference population median), the SD score of the individual corresponds to:

$$\frac{\text{Weight of subject} - \text{median reference value of weight for height}}{\text{median reference value} - 1 \text{ SD below median reference value}}$$

$$\text{SD score of individual} = \frac{6.3 - 8.5}{8.5 - 7.5} = -2.2$$

The reference limits used with SD scores vary; often scores of below −2.0 are designated as indicating risk of severe protein-energy malnutrition, whereas scores above +2.0 are taken to indicate risk of obesity. Reference limits are comparable across all indices and at all ages, when based on the same standard deviation score values (e.g. −2.0 SD). For example, a reference limit of −2.0 SD represents the same *degree* of malnutrition, irrespective of the anthropometric index used (e.g. weight for age or weight for height) or the age of the child (Waterlow et al., 1977).

The use of percentiles and standard deviation scores to classify individuals is preferable to calculating the index value of the subject as a percentage of the reference median. Although this latter approach continues to be widely used (see below), it does not take into account the distribution of the data within the reference set or the variability in the relative width of the distributions of the weight-for-age, weight-for-height, and height-for-age indices (Waterlow et al., 1977). Such variability inhibits the universal use of a constant percentage of the reference median (e.g. 70%) across all ages and for all growth indices. For example, 60% of median weight for age represents a more severe state of malnutrition for younger compared to older children. Moreover, when the index weight for height is used, 60% of the median is inappropriate; such a deficit at any age is incompatible with life (Dibley et al., 1987).

13.2.3 Gomez classification

This is one of the earliest classification systems, and is still widely used; it is based on weight for age, and uses the Harvard reference

% Expected Weight for Age	Classification	Category of Nutritional Status
> 90%	Normal	Normal
76–90%	Mild malnutrition	1st degree malnutrition
61–75%	Moderate malnutrition	2nd degree malnutrition
≤ 60%	Severe malnutrition	3rd degree malnutrition

Table 13.3: The Gomez classification. Adapted from Gomez et al. (1956).

% Expected Weight for Age	Edema Present	Edema Absent
80–60%	Kwashiorkor	Underweight
< 60%	Marasmic-kwashiorkor	Marasmus

Table 13.4: The Wellcome classification. Adapted from the Wellcome Trust Working Party (1970).

data (Section 12.1.2). The observed weight of a child is expressed as a percentage of the expected weight of a child of that age, using the 50th percentile (median) of the Harvard reference data as the reference point. In this system, malnutrition is classified into first, second and third degrees, corresponding to 90% to 76%, 75% to 61%, and < 60% of the median of the Harvard weight-for-age reference data respectively (Table 13.3) (Gomez et al., 1955; 1956). Selection of the cutoff points was made by reviewing weight-for-age characteristics of children hospitalized with clinically severe malnutrition.

The Gomez classification does not differentiate between marasmus and kwashiorkor nor between wasting and stunting, because height is not taken into account. As a result, children with a very low weight for age are not necessarily malnourished; instead, their low body weight may be appropriate for their short stature. Other disadvantages of the Gomez classification arise from the frequent presence of edema in malnutrition, as edema may result in misleadingly high weights for age. A further disadvantage is that this system provides no estimate of the duration of malnutrition.

13.2.4 Wellcome classification

The Wellcome classification (Table 13.4) also uses weight for age as the index, but includes, in addition, the occurrence of edema to assist in distinguishing between marasmus and kwashiorkor. The child's weight for age is again expressed as a percentage of the expected weight for age, using the 50th percentile of the Harvard reference data as the reference. This system also depends (of course) on knowledge of the child's age and, like the Gomez classification, does not take into account height differences (Wellcome Trust Working Party, 1970).

13.2.5 Waterlow classification

The Waterlow classification system (Table 13.5) uses both height for age and weight for height as indices, and the 50th percentile of the Harvard reference data as the reference point. Both indices are again expressed as percentages of the corresponding reference medians as in the Gomez and Wellcome classifications. Four broad categories of malnutrition are defined: (a) normal; (b) wasting; (c) stunting and wasting; and (d) stunting only (Table 13.5). The reference limits selected for grades 1, 2, and 3 correspond approximately to 1, 2, and 3 standard deviations of height for age and weight for height of the Harvard reference data. Hence, by using this system, a distinction can be made between children who are thin (wasted), those who are short (stunted), and those who are both thin and short (wasted and stunted) (Waterlow, 1972; 1974). This distinction is important. Waterlow and Rutishauser (1974) suggest that children who are wasted or both stunted and wasted should receive the highest priority for nutrition intervention. Wasting is associated with impairment of mental development, which may be irreversible. Moreover, wasted children generally regain their normal body build with proper medical care and nutritional rehabilitation. In contrast, recovery in height, although possible under favorable conditions, takes much longer. Some investigators suggest that children who are stunted but not wasted have adapted to their chronic dietary restriction, resulting in limited linear growth (Trowbridge, 1979). More work is required, however, to clarify the short- and long-term risks associated with wasting and stunting (Nabarro and McNab, 1980).

Height for Age Degree of Stunting	Weight for Height Degree of Wasting			
Percent (Grade)	> 90% (0)	80–90% (1)	70–80% (2)	< 70% (3)
> 90% (Grade = 0) 95–90% (Grade = 1)	Normal		Wasting	
85–90% (Grade = 2) < 85% (Grade = 3)	Stunting		Stunting and wasting	

Table 13.5: The Waterlow classification. Adapted from Waterlow (1972).

13.3 Simple screening systems for malnutrition

All the methods of classification described in Section 13.2 depend on knowledge of the age of the child, accurate measurements of weight, and in some cases height, and the use of reference data for comparison. Hence their use may be limited in the field where low cost, portability of equipment, and use of trained, unskilled personnel are primary considerations. Consequently, simpler, quicker, but less precise methods of screening for malnutrition have been developed. Some of these alternative methods are described below.

13.3.1 Mid-upper-arm circumference

Mid-upper-arm circumference and mid-upper-arm circumference for age are used in screening for protein-energy malnutrition when weight and stature measurements are impossible and the precise age of the child is unknown. Arm circumference is relatively independent of age for children between one and five years (Burgess and Burgess, 1969) and easy to measure. Both mid-upper-arm circumference by itself and in relation to age are used to assess wasting, a condition resulting from acute malnutrition and amenable to nutrition intervention (McDowell and Savage King, 1982).

The mid-upper-arm circumference cutoff points used to distinguish between normal and malnourished children vary. Sometimes a single cutoff point is chosen (e.g. 13.5 cm) for children aged one to five years (Anderson, 1979; Trowbridge, 1979). Alternatively, a series of cutoff points, applicable to children aged from one to five years, can be used to classify degrees of malnutrition (Table 13.6).

When the index mid-upper-arm circumference for age is used instead of arm circumference alone, 85% or 80% of the reference median is commonly used a reference limit. The Polish mid-upper-arm circumference reference data of Wolanski (1974) have been used.

The validity of mid-upper-arm circumference indices in the assessment of nutritional status is disputed (Vijayaraghavan and Gowrinath Sastry, 1976; Trowbridge and Staehling, 1980; McDowell and Savage

Mid-Upper-Arm Circumference (cm)	Category
> 13.5	Normal
12.5–13.5	Possibly mildly malnourished
< 12.5	Malnourished

Table 13.6: Classification based on mid-upper-arm circumference. Adapted from Shakir and Morley (1974).

King, 1982). Some investigators claim that mid-upper-arm circumference differentiates normal children from those with protein-energy malnutrition in the same way as weight for age (Shakir and Morley, 1974; Shakir, 1975) and weight for length (McDowell and Savage King, 1982), whereas others contest this finding (Jelliffe and Jelliffe, 1969; Vijayaraghavan and Gowrinath Sastry, 1976; Margo, 1977). These discrepancies may, in part, result from regional differences in the patterns of malnutrition.

13.3.2 Mid-upper-arm circumference for height: QUAC stick

The Quaker arm circumference measuring stick (QUAC stick) was developed by a Quaker Service team in Nigeria as a rapid, cheap, and simple screening tool for nutritional assessment (Arnhold, 1969). A measuring stick is used to compare a child's mid-upper-arm circumference with two reference limits of the reference mid-upper-arm circumference data corresponding to the child's height. Local reference data for the height of rural West Nigerian children from birth to five years (Morley et al., 1968), and British reference data for the height of older children (Tanner et al., 1966) are used together with the Polish mid-upper-arm circumference reference data of Wolanski (1974). Reference limits commonly used are < 85% or < 80% of the reference median mid-upper-arm circumference for height. Children falling below the reference limit are classified as malnourished: grades of protein-energy malnutrition are not recognized. In general, 85% of the reference median mid-upper-arm circumference for height approximates to the 3rd percentile of the reference data (Arnhold, 1969). Children classified as malnourished using this reference limit have weight-for-age indices approximating 80% of the Harvard reference median (Sommer and Loewenstein, 1975).

The QUAC stick consists of a vertical stick on which are inscribed two scales, corresponding to 80% and 85% of the reference median mid-upper-arm circumference for height (Figure 13.5). In use, the mid-upper-arm circumference of the child is first measured, using the technique described in Section 11.2.1; the stick is then placed behind the child, and the 80% or 85% figure at the level of the top of the child's head read off. If the child's actual mid-upper-circumference is less than the indicated figure, the child is classed as malnourished; if, however, the child's actual mid-upper-arm circumference is greater than the indicated figure, the child is not classed as malnourished. Thus the stick gives an immediate indication of malnourishment, without requiring that the child's height be actually measured at all, and therefore eliminates the necessity for recording both height and mid-upper-arm circumference for subsequent comparison with reference data. Details of the construction of a QUAC stick are given in Arnhold (1969).

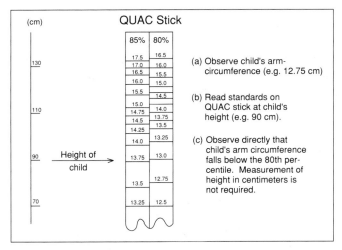

Figure 13.5: Diagram of a QUAC stick showing mid-upper-arm circumference values at 85% and 80% of the reference median for height. The markings on the stick are at positions appropriate to the height reference data, allowing direct nutritional classification. Modified from Arnhold R. The arm circumference as a public health index of protein-calorie malnutrition of early childhood. The QUAC stick: A field measure used by the Quaker Service team in Nigeria. Journal of Tropical Pediatrics 15: 243–247, (1969). With permission from Oxford University Press.

The QUAC stick was used by Sommer and Lowenstein (1975) in a community-based prospective study of mortality risk and nutritional status in over 8000 children in Bangladesh. After assessment of mid-upper-arm circumference for height using the QUAC stick, the children were followed prospectively over an eighteen-month period. The results suggested that the QUAC stick could be used to identify children at nutritional risk as well as families with children at a high risk of death.

13.3.3 Weight-for-height wall chart

A wall chart has been developed by Nabarro and McNab (1980) based on the index weight for height and three designated percentages of the corresponding median weight for height of the NCHS reference data. These are 70% to 80%, 80% to 90% and 90% to 110%. Wasted children are identified as those with a percentage weight for height less than 80% of the reference median.

The chart has the advantage of visually identifying the extent of wasting in a very simple manner. In addition, during nutritional rehabilitation, a target weight can be readily identified. The chart is fixed onto a smooth wall and the child positioned on a level floor against the chart at a point corresponding to the child's weight (Figure 13.6). The top of the child's head will be level with one of three color-coded bands on the chart,

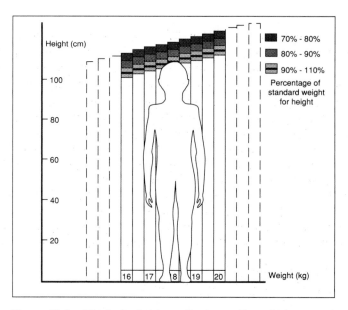

Figure 13.6: Weight-for-height wall chart. From Nabarro and McNab (1980) with permission.

equivalent to 70% to 80% (red), 80% to 90% (yellow) and 90% to 110% (green) expected weight for height and representing various degrees of malnutrition. The color should be read off the chart from the column marked with the child's weight and at a point level with the top of the child's head. (Figure 13.6). For small children, two persons may be required to position the child correctly for the measurement. To avoid misclassifying children with edema or ascites, a brief clinical examination should also be undertaken. The charts can be modified to include different colors, numbers of colors, and alternative reference limits, depending on the resources, needs, and the country.

13.4 Summary

In population studies, the distribution of the anthropometric indices can be compared using percentiles and/or standard deviation scores derived from appropriate reference data. Percentiles are recommended for evaluating anthropometric indices of persons from industrialized countries. Standard deviation scores are preferred for less developed countries because the study population often have indices below the extreme percentiles of the international reference data population (US NCHS). As well, the proportion of individuals with indices below predetermined reference limits can also be determined.

Several classification schemes, utilizing at least one anthropometric index with its associated reference limit(s) or cutoff point(s), are used to identify individuals 'at risk' to malnutrition, and, in some cases, identify the type and severity of malnutrition. The simplest use a single reference limit, drawn from a percentile or SD score of the reference data. Schemes such as the Gomez and the Wellcome classifications utilize weight for age for the anthropometric index and reference limits corresponding to specified percentages of the Harvard weight-for-age reference median. In addition, the Wellcome scheme includes the presence of edema to distinguish between marasmus and kwashiorkor. The Waterlow classification system uses two anthropometric indices: height for age and weight for height, together with risk categories designed to indicate the severity (based on the Harvard reference medians), as well as type of malnutrition. Alternative simpler classification schemes, developed for field survey use, include mid-upper-arm circumference, mid-upper-arm circumference for age, mid-upper-arm circumference for height (QUAC stick), and a weight-for-height wall chart. Most of these systems are independent of the age of the child, an advantage in studies in developing countries.

References

Anderson MA. (1979). Comparison of anthropometric measurements of nutritional status in preschool children in five developing countries. American Journal of Clinical Nutrition 32: 2339–2345.

Arnhold R. (1969). The arm circumference as a public health index of protein-calorie malnutrition of early childhood. The QUAC stick: A field measure used by the Quaker Service team in Nigeria. Journal of Tropical Pediatrics 15: 243–247.

Burgess HJL, Burgess AP. (1969). A modified standard for mid-upper-arm circumference in young children. Journal of Tropical Pediatrics 15: 189–192.

Dibley MJ, Goldsby JB, Staehling NW, Trowbridge FL. (1987). Development of normalized curves for the international growth reference: historical and technical considerations. American Journal of Clinical Nutrition 46: 736–748.

Gómez F, Galvan RR, Cravioto Muñoz J, Frenk S. (1955). Malnutrition in infancy and childhood with special reference to kwashiorkor. In: Levin S (ed). Advances in Pediatrics. Volume 7. Year Book Publishers, New York.

Gómez F, Galvan RR, Frenk S, Cravioto Muñoz J, Chávez R, Vázquez L. (1956). Mortality in second and third degree malnutrition. Journal of Tropical Pediatrics 2: 77–83.

Habicht J-P. Meyers LD, Brownie C. (1982). Indicators for identifying and counting the improperly nourished. American Journal of Clinical Nutrition 35: 1241–1254.

Habicht J-P, Yarbrough C, Martorell R. (1979). Anthropometric field methods: criteria for selection. In: Jelliffe DB, Jelliffe EFP (eds). Nutrition and Growth. Plenum Press, New York–London, pp. 365–387.

Hamill PVV, Drizd TA, Johnson CL, Reed RB, Roche AF, Moore WM. (1979). Physical growth: National Center for Health Statistics percentiles. American Journal of Clinical Nutrition 32: 607–629.

Healy MJR. (1986). Statistics of growth standards. In: Falkner F, Tanner JM (eds). Human Growth. A Comprehensive Treatise. Second edition. Volume 3. Methodology, Ecological, Genetic, and Nutritional Effects on Growth. Plenum Press, New York, pp. 47–58.

Jelliffe DB, Jelliffe EFP. (1969). The arm circumference as a public health index of protein-calorie malnutrition of early childhood. Journal of Tropical Pediatrics 15: 179–187.

Keller W, Donoso G, De Maeyer EM. (1976). Anthropometry in nutritional surveillance: a review based on results of the WHO collaborative study on nutritional anthropometry. Nutrition Abstracts and Reviews 46: 591–609.

Margo G. (1977). Assessing malnutrition with the midarm circumference. American Journal of Clinical Nutrition 30: 835–837.

McDowell I, Savage King F. (1982). Interpretation of arm circumference as an indicator of nutritional status. Archives of Disease in Childhood 57: 292–296.

Morley DC, Woodland M, Martin WI, Allen I. (1968). Heights and weights of West African village children from birth to the age of five. West African Medical Journal 17: 8–13.

Nabarro D, McNab S. (1980). A simple new technique for identifying thin children (The weight-for-height wall chart). Journal of Tropical Medicine and Hygiene 83: 21–33.

Shakir A. (1975). Arm circumference in the surveillance of protein-calorie malnutrition in Baghdad. American Journal of Clinical Nutrition 28: 661–665.

Shakir A, Morley D. (1974). Measuring malnutrition. Lancet 1: 758–759.

Sommer A, Loewenstein MS. (1975). Nutritional status and mortality: a prospective validation of the QUAC stick. American Journal of Clinical Nutrition 28: 287–292.

Tanner JM, Whitehouse RH, Takaishi M. (1966). Standards from birth to maturity for height, weight, height velocity, and weight velocity: British children, 1965. Archives of Disease in Childhood 41: 454–471; 613–625.

Trowbridge FL. (1979). Clinical and biochemical characteristics associated with anthropometric nutritional categories. American Journal of Clinical Nutrition 321: 758–766.

Trowbridge FL, Staehling N. (1980). Sensitivity and specificity of arm circumference indicators in identifying malnourished children. American Journal of Clinical Nutrition 33: 687–696.

Vijayaraghavan K, Gowrinath Sastry J. (1976). The efficacy of arm circumference as a substitute for weight in assessment of protein-calorie malnutrition. Annals of Human Biology 3: 229–233.

Waterlow JC. (1972). Classification and definition of protein calorie malnutrition. British Medical Journal 3: 566–569.

Waterlow JC. (1974). Some aspects of childhood malnutrition as a public health problem. British Medical Journal 4: 88–90.

Waterlow JC, Buzina R, Keller W, Lane JM, Nichaman MZ, Tanner JM. (1977). The presentation and use of height and weight data for comparing the nutritional status of groups of children under the age of 10 years. Bulletin of the World Health Organization 55: 489–498.

Waterlow JC, Rutishauser IHE. (1974). Malnutrition in man. In: Early Malnutrition and Mental Development. Symposia of the Swedish Nutrition Foundation, XII, Almqvist and Wiskell, Stockholm, pp. 13–26.

Wellcome Trust Working Party (1970). Classification of infantile malnutrition. Lancet 2: 302–303.

Wolanski NL. (1974). Biological reference systems in the assessment of nutritional status. In: Roche AF, Falkner F (eds). Nutrition and Malnutrition. Plenum Press, New York, pp. 231–269.

WHO (World Health Organization) (1983). Measuring Change in Nutritional Status, Guidelines for Assessing the Nutritional Impact of Supplementary Feeding Programmes for Vulnerable Groups. World Health Organization, Geneva.

WHO (World Health Organization) Working Group (1986). Use and interpretation of anthropometric indicators of nutritional status. Bulletin of the World Health Organization 64: 929–941.

Chapter 14

Laboratory assessment of body composition

Accurate methods for measuring specific components of body composition are necessary to assess the effects of nutritional deprivation and intervention on body composition. Such information is essential for establishing the appropriate prognosis and treatment of hospital patients. The methods currently use a two- or four-compartment model for body composition. The two-compartment model assumes that the total body mass is composed of two major chemical compartments: body fat and the fat-free mass, whereas the four-compartment model divides the body into four chemical groups: water, protein, minerals, and fat, all of which can now be determined *in vivo*.

The amount of body fat is very variable, but it has a relatively constant density of about $900 \, kg/m^3$ at $37°C$ (Allen et al., 1959) and a negligible water and potassium content. The fat-free mass consists of three components: total body protein, total body water, and bone minerals, with densities at $37°C$ of approximately 993, 1304, and $3000 \, kg/m^3$, respectively. The density of the fat-free mass depends on the proportions in which these three components occur. In healthy persons, the fat-free mass has a relatively constant composition, with a water content of 72% to 74% (Sheng and Huggins, 1979), a potassium content of about 60 to 70 mmol/kg in men and 50 to 60 mmol/kg in women (Womersley et al., 1976), and a protein content of about 20% (Garrow, 1982). On average, the density of the fat-free mass approximates $1100 \, kg/m^3$ at $37°C$ (Behnke et al., 1953). By measuring total body water, total body potassium, total body nitrogen, or body density, the proportion of the body composed of fat and the proportion composed of fat-free mass can be estimated.

Selection of a method to measure body composition depends on its precision and accuracy, the objective of the study, cost, convenience to the subject, equipment and technical expertise required, and the health of the subject (Lukaski, 1987). In normal healthy individuals,

Sex	Age (yr)	Water (g/kg)	Protein (g/kg)	Remainder (g/kg)	Density (kg/m^3)	Potassium (mmol/kg)
Male	25	728	195	77	1120	71.5
Male	35	775	165	60	1083	–
Female	42	733	192	75	1103	73.0
Male	46	674	234	92	1131	66.5
Male	48	730	206	64	1099	–
Male	60	704	238	58	1104	66.6
Mean		724	205	71	1106	69.4
SD		34	28	3	17	3.3

Table 14.1: The contribution of water and protein to the fat-free weights of six adults. From Garrow (1983) with permission of Nutrition Abstracts and Reviews, A (Human and Experimental).

all the body components except fat occur in relatively fixed proportions. In malnourished individuals and subjects with metabolic disturbances, the relative proportions of the body components may be altered. For instance, losses of protein and fat may occur, often in association with the rapid accumulation of water. Changes such as these invalidate the determination of fat and the fat-free mass in the two-compartment model. Therefore, in such circumstances, the four-compartment model must be used.

It is not possible to validate measurements of body composition with an absolute standard based on results of direct chemical analysis on the same subject. Instead, relative validity is estimated by comparing results with those obtained on the same subject using alternative, indirect methods. The following sections describe the individual procedures used to assess body composition and the assumptions of these methods.

14.1 Chemical analysis of cadavers

Studies of body composition by direct chemical analysis of human cadavers are limited. Most of the cadavers were analyzed between 1945 and 1968 and were adults of varying ages who had died as a result of illness; hence the values obtained may not be representative of an average healthy adult. Table 14.1 presents data on the contribution of water, protein, and potassium in the fat-free mass of six adult cadavers, compiled by Garrow (1983). The fat-free tissues of the cadavers were of a relatively constant composition, containing about 72% water, about 20% protein, and about 69 mmol/kg potassium. In contrast, the amount of fat was very variable, ranging from 4.3% to 27.9% of body weight in the six cadavers.

14.2   Total body potassium using ^{40}K

Potassium occurs almost exclusively as an intracellular cation, primarily in the muscle and viscera. Negligible amounts occur in extracellular fluid, bone, or other noncellular sites. Measurement of total body potassium is therefore used as an index of the fat-free mass in healthy subjects, on the assumption that the fat-free mass has a constant amount of potassium.

A constant fraction (0.012%) of potassium exists in the body as the isotope ^{40}K (half-life = 1.3×10^9 years). The latter emits a high-energy gamma ray of 1.46 MeV, allowing the amount of potassium in the body to be measured (Forbes et al., 1961). Once total body potassium has been determined from the ^{40}K measurements, the fat-free mass can be calculated, assuming a constant potassium content of the fat-free mass. Thus the determination of the fat-free mass and hence the total body fat and percentage body fat from total body potassium involves:

- Measurement of ^{40}K radiation from the subject using a whole body counter;
- Calculation of total body potassium (g) from ^{40}K data;
- Conversion of total body potassium (g) to mmol potassium:

$$\text{mmol K} = \frac{\text{Total body potassium (g)}}{\text{Atomic weight of potassium (39.098)}}$$

- Calculation of the fat-free mass (kg) from total body potassium assuming that the average potassium content of the fat-free mass = 69.4 mmol/kg (or an alternative factor);
- Calculation of total body fat (kg);

$$\text{Total body fat (kg)} = \text{Body weight (kg)} - \text{fat-free mass (kg)}$$

- Calculation of percentage body fat.

$$\% \text{ Body fat} = \frac{\text{Total body fat (kg)} \times 100}{\text{Body weight (kg)}}$$

The 1.46 MeV gamma ray of ^{40}K is counted with a whole body gamma spectrometer using either liquid/plastic scintillation counters or sodium iodide detectors. The latter are preferred because they have a good energy resolution and a low background rate. The isotope occurs in low concentrations so that the background counts from external radiation (cosmic rays and local sources of ionizing radiation) are usually large relative to the ^{40}K counts. Hence the whole body counter must be shielded from the background radiation with lead or steel shielding. The long counting times, necessary because of the low ^{40}K counts, may be a problem for ill patients. Calibration of the whole body counter is a major difficulty with this method because the ^{40}K count detected by the whole body counter is a function of both total body potassium and the geometric configuration of the subject. As a result, the whole body counter must be calibrated to allow for differences in the body build of the subjects being measured. This is achieved by using a phantom (usually a series of polyethylene bottles) arranged to simulate the proportions of the body and containing a known amount of potassium chloride solution (Garrow, 1983). A whole body counter has been developed by Cohn et al. (1969) at Brookhaven, New York, which overcomes some of the calibration difficulties. The system measures ^{40}K absolutely by determining attenuation factors for each subject which are then used to correct for inter-subject differences in body size and geometry and in gamma ray self-absorption. The attenuation factors are determined by counting the gamma rays emitted from a ^{137}Cs source positioned under the subject lying in the supine position. Accuracy and precision of this ^{40}K counting method are within 3%.

A decay product of atmospheric radon, ^{214}Bi, may also interfere with the ^{40}K method because it emits a gamma ray in the ^{40}K energy level. Background ^{214}Bi contamination can be reduced, however, by ensuring that the subjects shower and wash their hair and are supplied with clean clothing prior to undergoing whole-body counting (Lykken et al., 1983).

The potassium content of the fat-free mass was first derived from cadaver analysis (Table 14.1.). In fact, values lower than 69.4 mmol/kg are often used, particularly for women and older subjects, because the potassium concentration of fat-free tissue tends to decrease with age (Pierson et al., 1974). Womersley et al. (1976) use 68 mmol/kg for young men; 60 mmol/kg for older men fifty to fifty-nine years of age; 60 mmol/kg for young women; and 54 mmol/kg for older women. In contrast, Garrow et al. (1979) assume a value of 66 mmol/kg for men and 60 mmol/kg for women. The potassium concentration of the fat-free mass also appears to increase with muscular development and decline with obesity (Womersley et al., 1976). Although in obese subjects, some of the decrease may be explained by the lower proportion of muscle in the fat-free mass, Colt et al. (1981) suggest that the remainder arises from a measurement error resulting from absorption of the gamma rays by adipose tissue. Clearly, if appropriate constants for the potassium concentration of the fat-free mass of muscular, obese, and older individuals are not used, the estimates of fat-free mass derived from ^{40}K measurements will be in error. The latter may be as much as 20%.

Once the fat-free mass is determined, total body fat can be derived indirectly, as the difference between body weight and the fat-free mass. This indirect approach should not be used to derive total body fat for patients with a wasting disease such as cancer (Cohn et al., 1981a), because total body potassium measurements are low in these patients as a result of loss of muscle mass. Hence, total body fat derived indirectly as the difference between body weight and fat-free mass will always be overestimated in these patients.

14.3 Total body water using isotope dilution

Body fat contains no water. Instead, all the body water is present in the fat-free mass, which is assumed to contain 73.2% water on average (Pace and Rathburn, 1945). Hence, by measuring total body water (TBW), the fat-free mass can be estimated:

$$\text{Fat-free mass (kg)} = \frac{\text{Total body water (kg)}}{0.732}$$

Once the fat-free mass has been determined, total body fat and percentage body fat can be calculated by difference:

$$\text{Total body fat (kg)} = \text{Body weight (kg)} - \text{fat-free mass (kg)}$$

$$\% \text{ Body fat} = \frac{\text{Total body fat (kg)} \times 100}{\text{Body weight (kg)}}$$

Total body water can be measured in both healthy and diseased persons using an isotope dilution technique. Deuterium (^{2}H) and tritium (^{3}H) and the stable isotope of oxygen (^{18}O) can be used. Standardized conditions are necessary to measure total body water because fluid and/or food intake and exercise can all affect total body water. As a result, the measurements should be taken in the morning, after an overnight fast, with restriction of fluid intake, and after the bladder has been emptied. A tracer dose of sterile water labeled with an accurately weighed amount of ^{2}H, ^{3}H, or ^{18}O is administered either orally or intravenously to the subject and allowed to equilibrate. No food or water is permitted during equilibration, which may take two to six hours, depending on the isotope used, the sample form, and the health condition of the patient. Longer equilibration periods are necessary if urine samples are used, and for obese patients (Schoeller et al., 1980), or for those with edema, ascites, and shock (McMurrey et al., 1958). At the end of the equilibration period, a sample of serum, saliva, or urine is collected and total body water is calculated from the dilution observed. Saliva samples are preferable in field studies. Alternatively, if ^{18}O is used, breath samples can be collected and carbon dioxide analyzed for ^{18}O. Table 14.2 demonstrates the relatively small variations in total body water when calculated from isotopic enrichments of different physiological fluids and at different times postdose (Schoeller et al., 1985).

A	B	Isotope	N	$\dfrac{TBW_A}{TBW_B}$	SD	SEM
Saliva at 4 hr	Serum at 4 hr	^{18}O	33	1.006	±0.019	±0.003
Urine at 6 hr	Serum at 6 hr	^{18}O	11	1.012	±0.027	±0.008
Urine at 12 hr	Serum at 12 hr	^{18}O	14	1.006	±0.010	±0.003
Saliva at 3 hr	Saliva at 4 hr	^{18}O	20	0.997	±0.005	±0.001
Saliva at 3 hr	Saliva at 4 hr	^{2}H	43	0.996	±0.007	±0.001

Table 14.2: A demonstration of the relatively small variations in total body water, when calculated from isotopic enrichments of different physiological fluids and at different times postdose. From Schoeller et al. (1985). Reproduced with permission of Ross Laboratories, Columbus, OH 43216, from Report of the Sixth Ross Conference on Medical Research, page 26, © 1985 Ross Laboratories.

The calculation of total body water is based on the dilution principle (i.e. the extent to which the isotopic dose is diluted by the total body fluid).

$$\text{Total body water} = \frac{V_1 C_1}{C_2}$$

where V_1 = volume of dose; C_1 = concentration of administered isotope; and C_2 = concentration of isotope in serum/urine/breath sample. In the case of serum and breath samples, a correction may be necessary for urinary loss of the tracer.

Substances or tracers used to measure total body water should:

- be present only in body water;
- equilibrate rapidly and thoroughly with the body water;
- not be metabolized or excreted;
- be nontoxic in the amounts used; and
- not alter normal physiological processes or homeostatic mechanisms (Pinson, 1952).

Selection of the isotopic tracer depends on several factors. Tritium (^{3}H) is easy to measure by scintillation counting but involves radiation to the subject, making the technique unsuitable for children and women of childbearing age (Schoeller et al., 1980), or when repeated measurements over a short time period are necessary. The nonradioactive isotopes ^{2}H and ^{18}O must be measured by mass spectrometry. Sample preparation for ^{2}H is time consuming and tedious because the water sample must be converted to hydrogen gas. In contrast, ^{18}O can be readily analyzed, because the carbon dioxide expired by the subject is in isotopic equilibrium with body water (Lifson et al., 1949). Use of ^{2}H and ^{3}H produces an overestimate of total body water because the hydrogen label exchanges with some nonwater hydrogen in the body (Culebras and Moore, 1977). The stable isotope of oxygen (^{18}O) appears to be the isotope tracer of choice, but its use may be limited by the high cost and need for a mass spectrometer for the analysis.

The major limitations of the total body water method for estimating fat-free mass are the assumptions that the fat-free mass of an adult contains a constant percentage of water and that the total body water content is independent of the fat content of the body (Sheng and Huggins, 1979). Chemical analysis of human cadavers has shown that the actual total body water content of the fat-free mass body compartment can vary from 67% to 77% (Table 14.1). None of these cadavers was of a normal, healthy person, and the degree to which their illnesses may have affected total body water is unknown. Furthermore, the water content of the fat-free tissue has been shown to be higher in obese and pregnant subjects. Consequently, if the usual equation is applied in obese and pregnant individuals, fat-free mass will be overestimated, and body fat will be underestimated. In pregnant women, for example, the estimate of fat mass may be underestimated by as much as 1.0–2.0 kg (van Raaij et al., 1988). New equations have been developed for estimating body fat mass from total body water, which will result in more valid estimates of maternal body fat mass during pregnancy (van Raaij et al., 1988). These equations are shown in Table 14.3. Likewise, for patients with wasting disease, the hydration constant is also increased because of loss of body tissue and the accumulation of extracellular fluid, so the estimate of fat will be too low. Hence, measurement of total body water to estimate total body fat indirectly is not an appropriate method for obese persons and patients with wasting disease; the revised equations of van Raaij et al. (1988) should be used for pregnant women.

14.4   Other body fluid compartments using isotope dilution

The isotope dilution principle can be used to estimate the volume of various other body fluid compartments, which in turn can be used to derive estimates of the two components of fat-free mass (FFM): extracellular mass (ECM), and body cell mass (BCM). The ECM is defined as the component of fat-free mass which exists outside the cells. It consists of both fluid components (e.g. extracellular fluids, plasma volume) which are involved in transport, and solid components (e.g. skeleton, cartilage, tendons etc) which are involved in support; neither are metabolically active. The BCM represents the metabolically active, energy-exchanging mass of the body. Measurements of ECM and BCM are especially critical in malnourished patients. Although values for fat-free mass in these patients may remain unchanged, the composition of the fat-free mass is abnormal. Malnutrition results in a reduced body cell mass, concomitant with an expansion of the extracellular mass. These

Subject	Equation
Nonpregnant adult female	$W_{FM} = W_B - \dfrac{TBW}{0.724}$
No edema or leg edema only	
10 weeks gestation	$W_{FM} = W_B - \dfrac{TBW}{0.725}$
20 weeks gestation	$W_{FM} = W_B - \dfrac{TBW}{0.732}$
30 weeks gestation	$W_{FM} = W_B - \dfrac{TBW}{0.740}$
40 weeks gestation	$W_{FM} = W_B - \dfrac{TBW}{0.750}$
Generalized edema	
10 weeks gestation	$W_{FM} = W_B - \dfrac{TBW}{0.725}$
20 weeks gestation	$W_{FM} = W_B - \dfrac{TBW}{0.734}$
30 weeks gestation	$W_{FM} = W_B - \dfrac{TBW}{0.748}$
40 weeks gestation	$W_{FM} = W_B - \dfrac{TBW}{0.765}$

Table 14.3: Equations for estimating body fat mass (W_{FM}) during pregnancy from total body water (TBW) and body weight (W_B) The equations assume that the fraction of water in the fat-free mass is normally 0.724. From van Raaij et al. (1988). © Am J. Clin. Nutr. American Society for Clinical Nutrition.

changes are shown in Figure 14.1. Hence, any loss in body weight in such patients reflects a loss of body fat (Shizgal, 1987).

A dilution technique involving the simultaneous intravenous injection of ^{22}Na and tritiated water has been developed to measure body cell mass, extracellular mass, and body fat (Shizgal, 1985). Body fat is estimated indirectly from total body water, as described in Section 14.3. Body cell mass is derived from total exchangeable potassium (K_e), which in turn is determined indirectly from the relationship

$$K_e \text{ (kg)} = TBW \text{ (kg)} \times R - Na_e \text{ (kg)}$$

where TBW = total body water, in kilograms; R = the sum of the sodium and potassium content of a sample of whole blood, divided by its water content (R is a dimensionless constant less than unity); and Na_e = total exchangeable sodium, in kilograms (Shizgal et al., 1977). Total exchangeable potassium is not determined directly from ^{42}K because of

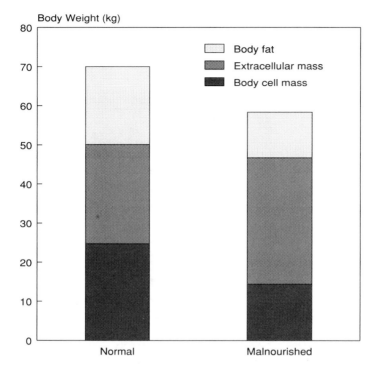

Figure 14.1: The mean body composition of 25 normally nourished healthy volunteers and 75 malnourished patients. From Shizgal HM. The effect of malnutrition on body composition. Surgery 152: 22–26, (1981) with permission.

the short half-life of this isotope (12.5 hours). The BCM is then estimated using the following relationship (Moore et al., 1963):

$$BCM \ (kg) = 8.33 \times K_e$$

Total exchangeable sodium (Na_e), measured using ^{22}Na, provides a measure of the fluid, but not the solid, component of the extracellular mass. The total extracellular mass can be calculated, however, from the difference between the FFM (determined via total body water), and the BCM:

$$ECM \ (kg) = FFM \ (kg) - BCM \ (kg)$$

Finally, body fat can be determined as the difference between body weight and the FFM as discussed earlier. The total radiation exposure from the injected isotopes using this dual isotope procedure is approximately 2.4 mSv (240 mrem) (Shizgal, 1987). This technique can be applied to patients with malnutrition and cancer to evaluate their response to nutritional therapy.

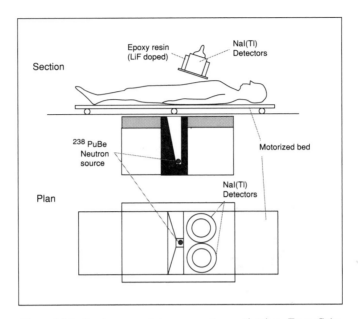

Figure 14.2: *In vivo* prompt gamma neutron activation. From Cohn et al. (1981b). Reproduced with permission of Ross Laboratories, Columbus, Ohio, from Report of the Second Ross Conference on Medical Research, page 99, © 1981 Ross Laboratories.

14.5   Total body nitrogen

Measurement of the nitrogen content of the body gives a measure of total body protein because the mass of nitrogen bears a fixed ratio to the mass of protein (1 g N : 6.25 g protein). A total-body neutron activation system has been developed to measure *in vivo* total body nitrogen. This technique is based on the conversion of a proportion of ^{14}N to an excited state of ^{15}N by bombarding the patient, in a supine position, with a low neutron flux from $^{238}PuBe$ sources or from a cyclotron or neutron generator. The resultant excited ^{15}N decays almost immediately to its ground state, emitting gamma rays at 10.83 MeV which are counted by sodium iodide detectors in a whole body counter (Figure 14.2). The detected gamma ray counts are then proportional to the absolute mass of total body nitrogen (McNeill et al., 1979; Beddoe and Hill, 1985).

The 10.83 MeV gamma ray is specific to nitrogen and is at an energy which is not affected by interference from other reactions. Extensive shielding, however, is necessary around the sodium iodide detectors to reduce the level of background radiation. Corrections to the gamma spectra are made for background counts and internal absorption of the emitted gamma rays. Until recently, calibration of the gamma spectrometer allowing counts to be converted to an absolute mass of total body nitrogen has been a major difficulty with this technique. Vartsky et al. (1979) have described a method in which hydrogen is used as an internal standard. Hydrogen is present in almost uniform concentrations in all soft tissues except bone and fat. By obtaining simultaneously an independent measurement of total body hydrogen, the ratio of nitrogen to hydrogen can be calculated. From the N:H ratio, and the known proportion of hydrogen to body weight, the mass of nitrogen can be derived. This approach also reduces the body shape effects. Protein is calculated from the total body nitrogen.

The accuracy of prompt gamma neutron activation for measuring total body nitrogen has been validated by comparing total body nitrogen in two human cadavers with results obtained on the same cadavers by direct chemical analysis of nitrogen (Knight et al., 1986). Close agreement between the two techniques was found. This study also confirmed the use of the ratio 6.25 for the relationship between total body protein and total body nitrogen.

Changes in total body protein of hospital patients with various diseases such as cancer, renal dysfunction, hypertension, chronic heart disease, rheumatoid arthritis, and anorexia nervosa, have been examined using prompt gamma neutron activation (Beddoe and Hill, 1985). Investigators have also used this technique to monitor body composition changes in critically ill patients with severe trauma or sepsis prior to, and following, intravenous feeding (Beddoe and Hill, 1985). Results indicate that substantial loss of body protein occurs in these critically ill patients, even when conventionally adequate nutritional support is given. Clearly, further research is required to identify nutritional intervention procedures which minimize loss of body protein. Prompt gamma neutron activation can also be used to simultaneously measure total body calcium, phosphorus, sodium, and chlorine (Cohn et al., 1984). The assessment of total body calcium by neutron activation analysis is discussed in Section 23.1.7.

14.6   Densitometry

14.6.1   Underwater weighing

The most widely used method of directly measuring whole body density is the determination of body volume according to Archimedes' principle, which allows the volume of an object submerged in water to be calculated from the apparent loss in weight. The percentage of body fat can then be calculated from the measured whole-body density using one of the empirical equations describing the relationship between fat content and body density (Rathburn and Pace, 1945; Keys and Brŏzek, 1953; Siri, 1961; Brŏzek et al., 1963). The assumptions on which these empirical equations are based are outlined in Section 11.1.6.

To measure body density, the volume of the subject is first determined. This is done by weighing the subject first in air and then when completely submerged in water in a large tank. The subject is instructed to squeeze out any air bubbles trapped inside the bathing suit, and to expel as much air as possible from the lungs before immersion. The underwater weight is recorded at the end of the forced expiration. Three readings are usually taken and the heaviest recorded corresponding to the most complete expiration. The body volume is then calculated from the apparent loss of weight in water (i.e. the difference between the weight of the person in air and his/her corresponding weight in water). Once total body mass and body volume have been determined, body density can be readily calculated, on the basis that density is mass per unit volume and the density of water is $1000 \, \text{kg/m}^3$ at $4°C$ (Brŏzek, 1961; Goldman and Buskirk, 1961).

$$\text{Body density} = \frac{\text{Body weight in air (kg)}}{\text{Volume of water displaced at } 4°C \text{ (l) [= apparent loss in weight (kg)]}}$$

Three corrections must be applied:

- underwater weighing is usually performed in water at $30°C$ instead of $4°C$. At this temperature, $1 \, \text{m}^3$ of water weighs $995.7 \, \text{kg}$ instead of $1000 \, \text{kg}$, and a water temperature correction factor must be applied;
- air trapped in the lungs also contributes to the amount of water displaced by the subject under water. Residual air in the lungs can be measured while the subject is in the tank or separately, using nitrogen washout, helium dilution, or oxygen dilution (Brodie, 1988). The residual air volume is then subtracted from the body volume;
- the volume of the air trapped in the gastrointestinal tract also contributes to the amount of water displaced. This volume never measured, and is often taken as $100 \, \text{mL}$; the intra-subject variability in gastrointestinal gas volume, however, can be quite large (0 to $500 \, \text{mL}$ in adults), reducing the precision of the method (Bedell et al., 1956).

The underwater weighing method can give very reproducible results for body density provided that the examiners and the subjects are well trained. For example, Durnin and Rahaman (1967) reported a standard deviation of $8 \, \text{kg/m}^3$ for serial measurements on three subjects over a one-year period. Lohman (1981) calculated the theoretical error for predicting body fat by densitometry to be 3% to 4%, attributed to variability in the water content of the fat-free mass and in the bone mineral density. The underwater weighing method is not suitable for children younger than eight years, the elderly, obese, or unhealthy persons.

Total body fat is derived from percentage body fat by multiplying body weight by percentage fat:

$$\text{Total body fat (kg)} = \frac{\text{Body weight (kg)} \times \% \text{ body fat}}{100}$$

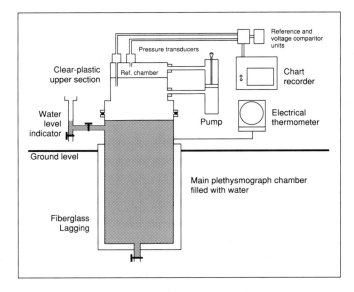

Figure 14.3: Measurement of body density using a plethysmograph. From Garrow JS, Stalley S, Diethelm R, Pittet PH, Hesp R, Halliday D. (1979). A new method for measuring the body density of obese adults. British Journal of Nutrition 42: 173–183. Reproduced with permission of Cambridge University Press.

The fat-free mass can then be calculated by subtracting the total body fat from the body weight:

$$\text{Fat-free mass (kg)} = \text{Body weight (kg)} - \text{total body fat (kg)}$$

14.6.2 Plethysmography

The use of a plethysmograph eliminates the necessity for totally immersing the subject in water, a disadvantage with the underwater weighing method (Section 14.6.1). For the measurement, the plethysmograph is first zeroed and filled with water (Figure 14.3). The subject is then weighed, and a weight of water equal to the weight of the subject is removed from the plethysmograph. The subject then stands with water up to the neck only and the head covered by a clear plastic dome. The volume of air surrounding the head of the subject, and in the lungs and gut, is then determined by measuring the pressure changes produced by a pump of known stroke volume (Garrow et al., 1979). This allows the total volume of the subject to be determined. The total time for the test, including three measurements on each subject, is about twenty minutes. The method has been used successfully to measure body density of obese adults (Garrow et al., 1979). Estimates of body fatness obtained compared favorably with those based on total body potassium.

14.7 Other laboratory methods for determining body composition

Several new, more direct methods are being developed to measure components of body composition, which do not rely on some of the assumptions discussed above. Some of these methods are discussed below.

14.7.1 Ultrasound

In the ultrasound technique, high-frequency sound waves emitted from an ultrasound source/meter penetrate the skin surface and pass through the adipose tissue until they reach the muscle tissue. At the adipose-muscle tissue interface, a proportion of the sound waves are reflected back as echoes that return to the ultrasound meter.

To use this technique, the measurement site is marked with a water-soluble transmission gel which provides acoustic contact without depression of the dermal surface. The high-resolution ultrasound source/meter is positioned so that the ultrasonic beam is perpendicular to the tissue interfaces at the marked site. A transducer receives the echoes and translates them into depth readings viewed on an oscilloscope screen. Subcutaneous fat thicknesses of 100 mm or more can be measured and density interfaces detected with an accuracy of 1 mm. The tissue is not compressed, eliminating errors associated with variations in compressibility of skinfolds (Fanelli and Kuczmarski, 1984).

The ultrasound technique can also be used to measure the thickness of muscle tissue as well as subcutaneous fat, enabling changes in body composition of hospital patients receiving nutritional support to be monitored. In general, studies of the validity of the ultrasound method suggest it provides a reasonable estimate of adipose tissue thickness in humans, compared to total electrical conductivity and skinfold caliper techniques (Booth et al., 1966; Fanelli and Kuczmarski, 1984). For obese persons, ultrasound may be superior to skinfold caliper techniques for measuring subcutaneous fat (Kuczmarski et al., 1987). Nevertheless, larger studies involving subjects with wide ranges in body fatness should be undertaken before the validity of this technique can be firmly established.

14.7.2 Total body electrical conductivity

The total body electrical conductivity (TOBEC) method is based on the change in electrical conductivity when the subject is placed in an electromagnetic field. The technique depends upon the differences in electrical conductivity and dielectric properties of the fat-free mass and fat of the body. For example, the fat-free mass, composed largely of electrolyte-containing water, will readily conduct an applied electric current, whereas fat is a poor conductor.

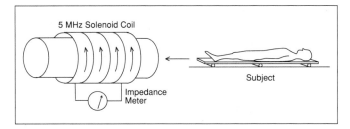

Figure 14.4: Measurement of body composition by total body electrical conductivity. From van Itallie et al. (1985). Reproduced with permission of Ross Laboratories, Columbus, Ohio, from Report of the Sixth Ross Conference on Medical Research, page 5, © 1985 Ross Laboratories.

For the measurement, the subject lies supine on a stretcher in a long uniform solenoid coil through which a 5 MHz current is passed for a few seconds (Figure 14.4). This induces an electromagnetic field in the space enclosed by the coil, which, in turn, induces a current in the subject, the magnitude depending on the conductivity of the subject. A secondary magnetic field is produced, which is then measured (van Itallie et al., 1982). A second measurement is taken when the coil is empty; the difference represents the measurement.

The method is claimed to be simple, safe, and fast and can be used on individuals who cannot be weighed underwater. The instrument, however, is expensive. Disturbances in electrolyte balance, such as edema, dehydration, and differences in body shape will influence the signal generated, although their effects have not been fully investigated (Harrison and van Itallie, 1982). Experimental data on humans comparing the estimates of fat-free mass by this method with alternative procedures such as ^{40}K and total body water are still limited.

14.7.3 Bioelectrical impedance

The bioelectrical impedance (BEI) method also depends upon the differences in electrical conductivity of fat-free mass and fat. The technique measures the impedance of a weak electrical current (800 μA; 50 KHz) passed between the right ankle and the right wrist of an individual. The impedance is proportional to the length of the conductor — a distance which is usually a function of the height of the subject — and indirectly proportional to the cross-sectional area; equivalently, the impedance is proportional to the square of the length of the conductor/subject, divided by its volume.

Subjects should avoid alcohol and vigorous exercise for twenty-four to forty-eight hours before testing, so that body fluids are not perturbed prior to the measurements. The measurements are taken on subjects approximately two hours after eating, and within thirty minutes of voiding. Subjects lie clothed, but without shoes and socks, in the supine position on a stretcher, with limbs not touching the body. Two current electrodes are placed on the dorsal surfaces of the right hand and foot, at the distal metacarpals and metatarsals respectively. Two detector electrodes are placed at the right pisiform prominence of the wrist and between the medial and lateral malleoli at the right ankle. A thin layer of electrode gel is applied to each electrode before it is placed on the skin. The resistive component of body impedance between the right wrist and right ankle is then measured to the nearest ohm. The lowest resistance (R) value for an individual is used to calculate the conductivity (ht^2/R), and hence to predict the fat-free mass. Bioelectrical impedance is safe and convenient, and the equipment is portable and relatively inexpensive. Studies to validate the relationship between conductivity and fat-free mass have reported errors in the derivation of body fat of 2.7% determined by BEI compared to values measured by densitometry (Lukaski et al., 1986). The precision of predicting fat-free body mass from BEI can be enhanced by using sex- and fatness-specific equations (Segal et al., 1988). Further research is needed to determine the sensitivity of BEI to detect body composition changes in patients undergoing nutritional therapy, and its validity in patients with water or electrolyte disturbances (Cohn, 1985). In over-hydration for example, resistance measurements will be higher, but lower in dehydration (Khaled et al., 1988). Predictive equations for assessing both total body water (Kushner and Schoeller, 1986) and total body fat (Khaled et al., 1988) from BEI have been developed, using total body water measured by isotope dilution and total body fat by underwater weighing as the reference methods. The applicability of these equations for a large heterogeneous population with a wide range of body fatness must be evaluated before their validity can be firmly established.

14.7.4 Computerized tomography

Computerized tomography (CT) is based on the relationship between the degree of attenuation of an X-ray beam and the density of the tissues through which the beam has passed. From this relationship, a two-dimensional radiographic image of the underlying anatomy of the scan area can be constructed.

The CT scanner is made up of two components: a collimated X-ray source and detectors, and a computer which processes the scan data and produces an X-ray image. The subject lies on a movable platform within the scanner gantry. The designated area to be scanned is a plane through the middle of the central aperture of the gantry, and parallel to the gantry. The X-ray beam is rotated around the subject, cutting a cross-sectional 'slice' through the patient. As the X-rays pass through the tissue, the beam undergoes attenuation, the intensity of which is recorded and stored in the scanner computer. The latter then processes the stored information by using a series of complex algorithms to reconstruct cross-sectional

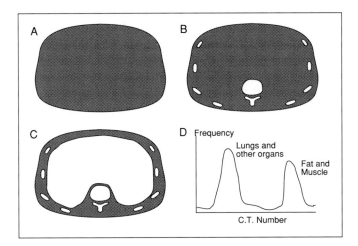

Figure 14.5: Body composition from a computerized tomography scan at the thorax level, showing three images resulting from different computer processing of the same scan. A: The air/skin interface. B: major skeletal elements. C: Adjusted to show the interface between the lungs and other organs and the surrounding muscle and fat. D: Histogram of the pixel density from scan C.

images (Figrue 14.5). The images consist of a matrix of picture elements, or pixels, each about 1 mm × 1 mm, arranged in rows and columns. The pixels vary in their degree of shading according to the magnitude of the X-ray beam attenuation, which in turn depends on the physical density of the scanned tissues. Tissues with a greater density cause a greater absorption of X-ray energy and consequently a higher attenuation value. The demarcation between tissues of differing density can be very good. The degree of pixel shading is scaled as the CT number, a measure of attenuation relative to that of water. Examples of the CT numbers and densities (D) are: fat: CT# = -70, D = 0.91 g/cc; muscle: CT# = 20, D = 1.05 g/cc; liver: CT# = 25, D = 1.06 g/cc; and water: CT# = 0, D = 1.0 g/cc.

The cross-sectional area of each of the tissues can be determined using specialized computer programs. The volume of tissues and organs (such as liver, kidney, and spleen) can also be assessed. When no sharp boundaries exist between structures, the pixels can be plotted as histograms separating them into fat-free and fat tissues (Heymsfield and Noel, 1981). As the volume represented by each pixel is known, the volume of the fat-free and fat tissue can then be calculated from the number of pixels forming each slice and the number of slices.

The method has several uses. It can be used to assess changes in the visceral organ mass in undernutrition and obesity; to measure regional muscle mass; to assess the distribution of subcutaneous versus internal fat; and to establish bone density in osteopenia (Heymsfield

Method and Procedures	Limitations
Total Body Potassium (TBK) TBK measured by counting radiation from naturally occurring ^{40}K in a whole body counter. FFM derived from assumption that average potassium concentration of FFM is constant.	Required equipment is expensive. Obese and elderly subjects have lower potassium concentrations, leading to overestimates of total body fat.
Total Body Water (TBW) Tracer dose of water, labeled with ^3H, ^2H or ^{18}O, is given orally or intravenously, and then equilibrated. Concentration of isotope measured in serum, urine, saliva, or breath (for ^{18}O). TBW calculated from dilution observed.	Involves radiation to the subject if ^3H is used. Water content of fat-free tissue is increased during obesity, pregnancy, and wasting disease leading to an underestimate of fat.
Neutron Activation Analysis Radioactive isotopes of N, P, Na, Cl, Ca are created by irradiating the subject. The radioactivity of the element is measured using a whole body counter.	Expensive. Subjects exposed to radioactivity. Elements are not uniformly activated, and thus sensitivity varies.
Underwater weighing Subject is weighed in air and then when totally submerged in water. Body volume calculated from the apparent loss of weight in water. Body density calculated from body mass and body volume measurements. Correction factors for water temperature, volume of air trapped in gastrointestinal tract. Preferable to measure residual lung volume.	Requires high degree of co-operation from subject. Not suitable for young children, the elderly, sick patients. Relatively expensive.

Table 14.4: Summary of laboratory techniques used to measure body composition and their limitations.

et al., 1987). Computerized tomography involves exposure to ionizing radiation, and hence is not recommended for pregnant women or children, for routine whole-body scans, or for multiple scans on the same person (Lukaski, 1987). The method is also very expensive.

14.8   Summary

Table 14.4 summarizes the characteristics of the various procedures used to assess body composition, together with their limitations. Selection of any method depends on the objectives of the study, cost, convenience, equipment and technical expertise available, the health of the subject, and the precision and accuracy required. Methods with the lowest cost are often the most imprecise. Methods based on the two-compartment

Method and Procedures	Limitations
Ultrasound High-frequency sound waves from an ultrasound meter pass through adipose tissue to adipose-muscle tissue interface. At interface, some sound waves reflected back as echoes, which are translated into depth readings via a transducer.	Validity of technique for subjects with wide range of body fatness unknown. Technique does not provide same degree of structure resolution possible with computerized tomography.
Total Body Electrical Conductivity (TOBEC) Subject lies supine in a solenoid coil through which a 5 MHz current is passed. The latter induces a current in the subject, which creates a secondary magnetic field. The conductivity value of the subject is obtained by subtracting the background value when the coil is empty. Conductivity value is proportional to body electrolyte content, and hence reflects amount of fat-free tissue.	Edema, ascites, dehydration, and electrolyte balance will alter conductivity and interfere with reading. Extent to which variation in body shape and size affects readings not yet known. Variations in bone mass may affect readings. Expensive method.
Bioelectrical Impedance (BEI) The impedance to a weak electrical current passed between the right ankle and right wrist of subject in supine position is measured. Impedance is proportional to the square of the length of the conductor — a function of the height of the subject — divided by the volume.	Edema, ascites, and dehydration will alter the resistance measurements and invalidate the method. Sensitivity of BEI to detect changes in body composition during nutrition intervention or physical training unknown.
Computerized Tomography (CT) Method measures attenuation of X-rays as they pass through tissues, the degree of attenuation being related to differences in physical density of the tissues. Image reconstructed from matrix of picture elements (pixels) which vary in their shading.	Exposure to ionizing radiation limits use of CT for whole body scans, multiple scans in same person, and scans of pregnant women or children. Expensive equipment which is not readily available. The CT does not provide information on chemical composition of the structures.

Table 14.4 (continued): Summary of laboratory techniques used to measure body composition, and their limitations.

model (i.e. body fat and fat-free mass) include total body water and total body potassium, densitometry, Total Body Electrical Conductivity, Bioelectrical Impedance. Such methods are not suitable for patients with chronic nutritional deprivation, because in such cases, the basic assumptions of the two-compartment model are invalid. In these patients, techniques utilizing the four-compartment model (i.e. water, protein, minerals, and fat) are more appropriate. These techniques include neutron activation analysis for protein and minerals and isotope dilution for total body water. Body fat can be calculated by subtracting the protein, minerals, and water from body weight.

References

Allen TH, Krzywicki HJ, Roberts JE. (1959). Density, fat, water and solids in freshly isolated tissues. Journal of Applied Physiology 14: 1005–1008.

Bedell GN, Marshall R, deBois AB, Harris JH. (1956). Measurement of the volume of gas in the gastrointestinal tract. Values in normal subjects and ambulatory patients. Journal of Clinical Investigation 35: 366–345.

Behnke AR, Osserman EF, Welham WW. (1953). Lean body mass: its clinical significance and estimation from excess fat and total body water determinations. Archives of Internal Medicine 91: 585–601.

Beddoe AH, Hill GL. (1985). Clinical measurement of body composition using *in vivo* neutron activation analysis. Journal of Parenteral and Enteral Nutrition 9: 504–520.

Booth RAD, Goddard BA, Paton A. (1966). Measurement of fat thickness in man: a comparison of ultrasound, Harpenden calipers, and electrical conductivity. British Journal of Nutrition 20: 719–725.

Brodie DA. (1988). Techniques of measuring body composition. Part I and Part II. Sports Medicine 5: 11–40; 74–98.

Brŏzek JF. (1961). The measurement of body composition. Historical perspective. In: Ashley Montague MF (ed), An Introduction to Physical Anthropology. Charles C Thomas, Springfield, Illinois, pp. 637–679.

Brŏzek JF, Grande F, Anderson JT, Keys A. (1963). Densitometric analysis of body composition: revision of some quantitative assumptions. Annals of the New York Academy of Sciences 110: 113–140.

Cohn SH. (1985). How valid are bioelectric impedance measurements in body composition studies? American Journal of Clinical Nutrition 42: 889–890.

Cohn SH, Dombrowski CS, Pate HR, Robertson JS. (1969). A whole body counter with an invariant response to radionucleide distribution and body size. Physics in Medicine and Biology 14: 645–658.

Cohn SH, Ellis KJ, Vartsky D, Sawitsky A, Gartenhaus W, Yasumura S, Vaswani AN. (1981a). Comparison of methods of estimating body fat in normal subjects and cancer patients. American Journal of Clinical Nutrition 34: 2839–2847.

Cohn SH, Satwitsky A, Vartsky D, Yasumura S, Zanzi I, Ellis KJ. (1981b). Body composition as measured by *in vivo* neutron activation analysis. In: Nutritional Assessment — Present Status, Future Directions and Prospects. Report of the Second Ross Conference on Medical Research. Ross Laboratories, Columbus, Ohio, pp. 99–102.

Cohn SH, Vaswani AN, Yasumura S, Yuens K and Ellis KJ. (1984). Improved models for determination of body fat by *in vivo* neutron activation. American Journal of Clinical Nutrition 40: 255–259.

Colt EW, Wang J, Stallone F, Itallie TB van, Pierson RN Jr (1981). A possible low intracellular potassium in obesity. American Journal of Clinical Nutrition 34: 367–372.

Culebras JM, Moore FD. (1977). Total body water and the exchangeable hydrogen. I. Theoretical calculation of nonaqueous exchangeable hydrogen in man. American Journal of Physiology 232: R54.

Durnin JVGA, Rahaman MM. (1967). The assessment of the amount of fat in the human body from measurements of skinfold thickness. British Journal of Nutrition 21: 681–689.

Fanelli MT, Kuczmarski RJ. (1984). Ultrasound as an approach to assessing body composition. American Journal of Clinical Nutrition 39: 703–709.

Forbes GB, Gallup J, Hursh JB. (1961). Estimation of total body fat from potassium-40 content. Science 133: 101–102.

Garrow JS, Stalley S, Diethelm R, Pittet PH , Hesp R, Halliday D. (1979). A new method for measuring the body density of obese adults. British Journal of Nutrition 42: 173–183.

Garrow JS. (1982). New approaches to body composition. American Journal of Clinical Nutrition 35: 1152–1158.

Garrow JS. (1983). Indices of adiposity. Nutrition Abstracts and Reviews 53: 697–708.

Goldman RF, Buskirk ER. (1961). Body volume measurement by underwater weighing: description of a method. In: Brŏzek J, Henschel A (eds). Techniques for Measuring Body Composition. National Academy of Sciences, Washington, D.C., pp. 78–89.

Harrison GG, Itallie TB van. (1982). Estimation of body composition: a new approach based on electromagnetic principles. American Journal of Clinical Nutrition 35: 1176–1179.

Heymsfield SB, Noel RA. (1981). Radiographic analysis of body composition by computerized axial tomography. In: Newel GR, Ellison NM (eds). Nutrition and Cancer: Etiology and Treatment. Progress in Cancer Research and Therapy. Volume 17. Raven Press, New York, pp. 161–172.

Heymsfield SB, Rolandelli R, Casper K, Settle RG, Koruda M. (1987). Application of electromagnetic and sound waves in nutritional assessment. Journal of Parenteral and Enteral Nutrition 11: 64S–69S.

Itallie TB van, Segal KR, Yang M-V, Funk RC. (1985). Clinical assessment of body fat content in adults: potential role of electrical impedance methods. In: Roche AF (ed), Body-Composition Assessments in Youth and Adults. Report of the Sixth Ross Conference on Medical Research, Ross Laboratories, Columbus, Ohio, pp. 5–8.

Keys A, Brŏzek J. (1953). Body fat in adult man. Physiological Reviews 33: 245–325.

Khaled MA, McCutcheon MJ, Reddy S, Pearman PL, Hunter GR, Weinsier RL. (1988). Electrical impedance in assessing human body composition: the BIA method. American Journal of Clinical Nutrition 47: 789–792.

Knight GS, Beddoe AH, Streat SJ, Hill GL. (1986). Body composition of two human cadavers by neutron activation and chemical analysis. American Journal of Physiology 250: E179–E185.

Kuczmarski RJ, Fanelli MT, Koch GG. (1987). Ultrasonic assessment of body composition in obese adults: overlooking the limitations of the skinfold caliper. American Journal of Clinical Nutrition 45: 717–724.

Kushner R, Schoeller DA. (1986). Estimation of total body water by bioelectrical impedance analysis. American Journal of Clinical Nutrition 44: 417–424.

Lifson N, Gordon GB, Visscher MB and Nier AO. (1949). The fate of utilized molecular oxygen and the source of the oxygen of respiratory carbon dioxide, studied with the aid of heavy oxygen. Journal of Biological Chemistry 180: 803–811.

Lohman TG. (1981). Skinfolds and body density and their relation to body fatness: A review. Human Biology 2: 181–225.

Lukaski HC. (1987). Methods for the assessment of human body composition: traditional and new. American Journal of Clinical Nutrition 46: 537–556.

Lukaski HC, Bolonchuk WW, Hall CA, Siders WA. (1986). Estimation of fat free mass in humans using the bioelectrical impedance method: a validation study. Journal of Applied Physiology 60: 1327–1332.

Lykken GI, Lukaski HC, Bolonchuk WW, Sandstead HH. (1983). Potential errors in body composition as estimated by whole body scintillation counting. Journal of Laboratory and Clinical Medicine 101: 651–658.

McMurrey JD, Boling EA, Davis JM, Parker HV, Magnus IC, Ball MR, Moore FD. (1958). Body composition: simultaneous determination of several aspects by the dilution principle. Metabolism 7: 651–667.

McNeill KG, Mernagh JR, Jeejeebhoy KN, Wolman SL, Harrison JE. (1979). *In vivo* measurements of body protein based on the determination of nitrogen by prompt γ analysis. American Journal of Clinical Nutrition 32: 1955–1961.

Moore FD, Olesen KH, McMurrey JD, Parker HV, Ball MR, Boyden CM (eds). (1963). The Body Cell Mass and Its Supporting Environment: Body Composition in Health and Disease. WB Saunders Co., Philadelphia.

Pace N, Rathburn EN. (1945). Studies on body composition. III. The body water and chemically combined nitrogen content in relation to fat content. Journal of Biological Chemistry 158: 685–691.

Pierson RN Jr, Lin DHY, Phillips RA. (1974). Total-body potassium in health: effects of age, sex, height, and fat. American Journal of Physiology 226: 206–212.

Pinson EA. (1952). Water exchanges and barriers as studied by the use of hydrogen isotopes. Physiology Reviews 32: 123–134.

Raaij JMA van, Peek MEM, Vermaat-Miedema SH, Schonk CM, Hautvast JGAJ. (1988). New equations for estimating body fat mass in pregnancy from body density or total body water. American Journal of Clinical Nutrition 48: 24–29.

Rathburn EN, Pace N. (1945). Studies on body composition: I. The determination of total body fat by means of the body specific gravity. Journal of Biological Chemistry 158: 667–676.

Schoeller DA, Santen E van, Peterson DW, Dietz W, Jaspan J, Klein PD. (1980). Total body water measurement in humans with ^{18}O and ^{2}H labeled water. American Journal of Clinical Nutrition 33: 2686–2693.

Schoeller DA, Kushner RF, Taylor P, Dietz WH, Bandini L. (1985). Measurement of total body water: isotope dilution technique. In: Roche AF (ed) Body-Composition Assessments in Youth and Adults. Report of the Sixth Ross Conference on Medical Research, Ross Laboratories, Columbus, Ohio, pp. 24–28.

Segal KR, Loan M van, Fitzgerald PI, Hodgdon JA, Itallie TB van. (1988). Lean body mass estimation by bioelectrical impedance analysis: a four-site cross-validation study. American Journal of Clinical Nutrition 47: 7–14.

Sheng HP, Huggins RA. (1979). A review of body composition studies with emphasis on total body water and fat. American Journal of Clinical Nutrition 32: 630–647.

Shizgal HM. (1981). The effect of malnutrition on body composition. Surgery 152: 22–26.

Shizgal HM. (1985). Body composition of patients with malnutrition and cancer. Cancer 55: 250–253.

Shizgal HM. (1987). Nutritional assessment with body composition measurements. Journal of Enteral and Parenteral Nutrition 11: 42S–47S.

Shizgal HM, Spanier AH, Humes J, Wood CD. (1977). Indirect measurement of total exchangeable potassium. American Journal of Physiology 233: F253–F259.

Siri WE. (1961). Body composition from fluid spaces and density. Analysis of methods. In: Techniques for Measuring Body Composition. National Academy of Sciences, National Research Council, Washington D.C., 223–244.

Vartsky D, Prestwich WV, Thomas BJ, Dabek JT, Chettle DR, Fremlin JH, Stammers K. (1979). The use of body hydrogen as an internal standard in the measurement of nitrogen *in vivo* by prompt neutron capture gamma-ray analysis. Journal of Radioanalytical Chemistry 48: 243–252.

Womersley J, Durnin JVGA, Boddy K, Mahaffy M. (1976). Influence of muscular development, obesity, and age on the fat-free mass of adults. Journal of Applied Physiology 41: 223–229.

Chapter 15

Laboratory assessment

Laboratory assessment is used primarily to detect subclinical deficiency states, and is becoming increasingly important with the growing emphasis on preventive medicine. It provides an objective means of assessing nutritional status, independent of emotional and other subjective factors. The procedures can be used to supplement other methods of nutritional assessment — for example, dietary, clinical, and anthropometric assessment — enabling specific nutritional problems to be identified. This chapter outlines the principles of the procedures involved in laboratory assessment; subsequent chapters assess the application of these methods to individual nutrients.

Theoretically, subclinical deficiency states can be identified by measuring the levels of a nutrient or its metabolite in a preselected biopsy material that reflects either the total body content of the nutrient or the size of the tissue store most sensitive to depletion. Such measurements are generally termed 'static biochemical tests'. In practice, for many nutrients the ideal biopsy material is not accessible for routine use, and/or the storage site most sensitive to depletion has not been identified. Furthermore, even if low nutrient levels in the biopsy material are detected, they may not necessarily reflect the presence of a pathological lesion (Mills, 1981); alternatively, the significance of these 'low' values to health may be unknown.

Alternative methods for identifying subclinical deficiency states, based on measurements of functional impairment, have also been developed. Such tests have greater biological significance than the static biochemical tests because they measure the extent of the functional consequences of a specific nutrient deficiency. Solomons and Allen (1983) define functional tests as:

> diagnostic tests to determine the sufficiency of host nutriture to permit cells, tissues, organs, anatomical systems, or the host to perform optimally the intended, nutrient-dependent biological function.

• Homeostatic regulation	• Recent dietary intake
• Diurnal variation	• Hemolysis — for serum/plasma
• Sample contamination	• Drugs
• Physiological state	• Disease states
• Infections	• Nutrient interactions
• Hormonal status	• Inflammatory stress
• Physical exercise	• Weight loss
• Age, sex, ethnic group	• Sampling and collection procedures
• Accuracy and precision of the analytical method	• Sensitivity and specificity of the analytical method

Table 15.1: Factors which may confound the interpretation of static biochemical tests.

Functional tests may include measuring changes in the activities of a specific enzyme(s) or in the concentrations of specific blood components dependent on a given nutrient; alternatively, the production of an abnormal metabolite may be measured. Other functional tests measure physiological or behavioral functions dependent on specific nutrients (e.g. taste acuity for zinc; cognitive function for iron) (Solomons and Allen, 1983). For some of the nutrients (e.g. niacin), functional tests are not available.

Unfortunately, static and functional tests are often affected by biological and technical factors other than depleted body stores of the nutrient, which may confound the interpretation of the results (Casey and Robinson, 1983). These factors are summarized in Table 15.1 and their effects on specific nutrients are discussed more fully in the following chapters. Frequently, the effects of these confounding factors can be minimized or eliminated by standardizing the sampling and collection procedures, and by an appropriate experimental design. For instance, in nutrition surveys the effects of diurnal variation on the concentration of nutrients such as zinc and iron in serum/plasma can be eliminated by collecting the blood samples from all subjects at a standardized time of the day. When factors such as age, sex, race, and physiological state influence laboratory indices, observations can be classified according to these variables. The influence of drugs, hormonal status, physical exercise, weight loss, physiological state, and presence of disease conditions on laboratory indices can also be considered, provided that such details are included in the survey questionnaire. For some nutrients — for example zinc, iron, and copper — circulating levels of the nutrient in the blood are altered by concurrent infection or inflammatory stress, and reflect a redistribution in body compartments rather than deficiency or excess (Solomons, 1985). In such cases, individuals with concurrent infections can be identified by a white blood cell count and can be subsequently excluded from the data analysis if appropriate (Pilch and Senti, 1984a).

In general, a combination of static biochemical and/or functional tests should be used, rather than a single test for each nutrient. Several concordant abnormal values are more reliable than a single aberrant value in diagnosing a deficiency state.

15.1 Static biochemical tests

The static biochemical tests have been classified into two major categories: measurement of a nutrient in biological fluids or tissues, and measurement of the urinary excretion rate of the nutrient (Sauberlich et al., 1974). These categories are discussed in detail below.

15.1.1 Measurement of a nutrient in biological fluids/tissues

Whole blood or some fraction of blood is the most frequently used biopsy material for static biochemical tests. Other body fluids and tissues, less widely used, include urine, hair, saliva, semen, amniotic fluid, fingernails, skin, and buccal mucosa. Ideally, as discussed above, the nutrient content of the biopsy material should reflect the level of the nutrient in a tissue most sensitive to a deficiency. Furthermore, the reduction in the nutrient content of the biopsy material should also reflect the presence of a metabolic lesion. In some cases, however, the level of the nutrient in the tissue may appear adequate, but the nutrient cannot be utilized because of a metabolic defect resulting in a deficiency state (Mills, 1981).

Blood

Samples of blood are readily accessible, require relatively noninvasive methods of collection, and are in general easily analyzed. Plasma/serum, however, carry newly absorbed nutrients and those being transported to tissues and hence, plasma/serum nutrient levels tend to reflect recent dietary intake and therefore provide an acute, rather than a long-term, index of nutrient status (Mertz, 1975). The effect of recent dietary intake on plasma/serum nutrient concentrations can be reduced by collecting fasting blood samples.

All blood samples must be collected and handled under controlled, standardized conditions to ensure accurate and precise analytical results. Factors such as fasting, fluctuations resulting from diurnal variation and meal consumption, use of oral contraceptive agents, medications, infection, inflammation, and stress may all confound the interpretation of the results (Pilch and Senti, 1984a; Smith et al., 1985).

Near-normal plasma/serum nutrient concentrations may be present even in the presence of severe depletion of body stores because some nutrient concentrations in plasma/serum are strongly homeostatically regulated. In such cases, alternative biochemical indices should be selected (Solomons, 1985).

The risk of errors arising from sample contamination is a particular problem in trace element analysis. Trace elements are present in low concentrations in biological tissues and fluids but are ubiquitous in the environment (Versieck, 1984). Artefacts in the trace element values for the blood and/or its components may result from inadequate control of external factors such as contamination during extraction, transfer, storage, and handling of the blood sample (Versieck et al., 1987). Venous occlusion, hemolysis, use of an inappropriate anticoagulant, collection-separation time, and element losses produced by adsorption on container surfaces or volatilization are additional confounding factors (Versieck, 1984; Smith et al., 1985; English et al., 1987).

Erythrocytes

The nutrient content of erythrocytes can only reflect chronic nutrient status because the erythrocyte half-life is quite long (120 days). The analysis of erythrocytes is technically difficult, and hence infrequently performed. Furthermore, if erythrocytes contain only a small percentage of the total body nutrient content, they are unlikely to be a valid index of nutrient status.

Leukocytes

Leukocytes or specific cell types such as lymphocytes or neutrophils can be used to monitor short-term changes in nutritional status because they have a relatively short half-life (Prasad and Cossack, 1982). As a result, these cell types may rapidly reflect a nutrient deficiency state, and hence are more sensitive biochemical indices than erythrocytes. Nevertheless, technical difficulties arise in isolating these cells in a highly purified form without introducing contamination from reagents during the isolation procedure (Milne et al., 1985). Moreover, if the centrifugal force used for washing and isolating the cell types is not standardized, the precision of the assay may be poor. Consequently, extreme care must be taken when separating these cell types. Furthermore, the relatively large blood sample required generally restricts the use of these indices to adults. Several methods are employed to express the nutrient content/concentration of cells such as leukocytes; these include nutrient per unit of protein, nutrient concentration per cell, nutrient per dry weight of cells and nutrient per unit of DNA (Elin, 1983).

Tissue stores

Liver and bone marrow, adipose tissue, and bone are the storage sites for iron, vitamin E, and calcium, respectively. Sampling of these biopsy

- The matrix and connective tissue papilla, with its blood and lymph vessels, are the source of elements that become incorporated into the hair during growth.

- Sweat from the eccrine sweat glands may contaminate the hair with elements derived from body tissues.

- Sebum from the sebaceous glands and fluids from the apocrine glands may also lead to endogenous contamination.

- The continuously desquamating epidermis, to which the hair is continually exposed, is probably only a minor source of trace elements.

- Exogenous materials that may modify the trace element composition of hair include: air, water, soap, shampoo, lacquers, dyes, and medications.

Table 15.2: Sources of trace elements in human hair. Modified after Hopps (1977).

materials is too invasive for population studies, and can only be used in research or clinical settings.

Hair

This biopsy material has been used for screening population groups and individuals at risk to certain trace element deficiencies, and to excessive exposure to heavy metals. In some circumstances, hair trace element content provides a retrospective, chronic index of trace element status during the period of hair growth. Analysis of trace element levels in hair has several advantages compared to that of blood or its components and urine: (a) trace elements are more concentrated in hair than in blood or urine, making analysis easier; results for the ultratrace elements such as chromium and manganese are more consistent; (b) trace element concentrations in hair are more stable and not subject to rapid fluctuations associated with diet, diurnal variation, etc.; and (c) hair samples are collected without trauma, require no special preservatives and can be stored without deterioration (Maugh, 1978; Katz, 1979; Chittleborough, 1980; Hambidge, 1982; Laker, 1982; Taylor, 1986). One of the problems with the use of scalp hair is its susceptibility to exogenous contaminants such as atmospheric pollutants, water, and sweat (Hopps, 1977). A wide variety of hair beauty treatments may also modify the trace element composition of hair (McKenzie, 1978). Therefore, standardized procedures are essential for hair sampling and washing prior to analysis (Katz, 1979). Hopps (1977) has summarized five possible sources of trace elements in human hair, which are shown in Table 15.2; unfortunately the relative importance of these sources remains uncertain.

Early studies of trace element concentrations in scalp hair used samples collected from barber shops (Schroeder and Nason, 1969; Petering et al., 1971; Eads and Lambdin, 1973). The currently recommended hair sampling method is to use the proximal 1.5–2.0 cm of hair, cut from the suboccipital portion of the scalp, minimizing the effects of abrasion of the hair shaft and exogenous contamination (Hambidge, 1982). Standardized washing procedures should always be adopted (Assarian and Oberleas, 1977). Several washing procedures have been investigated, including the use of nonionic or ionic detergents followed by rinsing in distilled, deionized water to remove absorbed detergent (Harrison et al., 1969; Petering et al., 1971; Salmela et al., 1981; Kumpulainen et al., 1982). Various organic solvents such as hexane-methanol, acetone (Hambidge et al., 1972a; Salmela et al., 1981; Kumpulainen et al., 1982), and ether (Petering et al., 1971) have also been recommended, either alone or in combination with a detergent. A metal-chelating agent, ethylenediamine-tetraacetate (edTA), has also been included in some hair-washing procedures (Hammer et al., 1971), especially those which are designed to remove adsorbed zinc and copper (McKenzie, 1978). Use of EDTA is not generally recommended because of the risk of removing endogenous minerals from the hair shaft (Sorenson et al., 1973; Hilderbrand and White, 1974).

Confounding factors which may affect trace element concentrations in hair include hair color, hair beauty treatments, age, sex, pregnancy, smoking, water supplies, the presence of certain disease states, season, and rate of hair growth (Hambidge et al., 1972b; Creason et al., 1975; McKenzie, 1978; Hambidge, 1982; Taylor, 1986). Selenium in antidandruff shampoos, for example, significantly increases hair selenium content and the selenium cannot be removed by standardized hair-washing procedures (Davies, 1982). For other trace elements, results have been equivocal. Some (Hilderbrand and White, 1974), but not all (Gibson and Gibson, 1984), investigators have observed marked changes in hair trace element concentrations after hair cosmetic treatments. Similarly, relationships between hair color and trace element content have been inconsistent. Creason et al. (1975) reported that only iron was related to hair color in adults, whereas other investigators have noted higher manganese and iron concentrations in dark versus blond scalp hair samples, and higher iron, nickel, copper, and zinc in red hair compared to brown (Sky-Peck and Joseph, 1983).

Some investigators suggest that rate of hair growth influences hair trace element concentrations. Scalp hair normally grows at the rate of 1 cm per month, but in some cases of severe protein-energy malnutrition (Erten et al., 1978) and zinc deficiency states (e.g. acrodermatitis enteropathica) (Hambidge et al., 1977), hair growth is impaired. In such cases, hair zinc concentrations may be normal, or even high. No significant differences, however, were observed in the trace element concentrations of scalp and pubic hair samples (DeAntonio et al., 1982), despite marked differences in the rate of hair growth at the two anatomical sites (Hopps, 1977). These results suggest that the relative rate of hair growth is not a significant factor in controlling hair trace element levels. To date, human hair trace element concentrations have been correlated most frequently with plasma/serum (McBean et al., 1971; Hambidge, 1982). More data on other tissues are urgently required for interpreting the significance of hair trace element concentrations.

Fingernails and toenails

Nails have recently been investigated as biopsy materials for trace element analysis (Bank et al., 1981; van Noord et al., 1987). Like hair, nails are also easy to sample and store but have a slower rate of growth, ranging from 0.025 mm/day for toenails to 0.1 mm/day for fingernails. Nails are formed by proliferating cells in the germinal layer of the nail matrix, which are converted during growth into the horny lamellae. The elemental composition of nails is influenced by age, sex, geographical location, and possibly by certain disease states (e.g. Wilson's disease, arthritis, cystic fibrosis and Alzheimer's disease) (Takagi et al., 1988; Vance et al., 1988). Environmental contamination is a potential problem limiting the use of nails as a biopsy material for trace element analysis. Bank et al. (1981) recommend cleaning fingernails with a scrubbing brush and a mild detergent, followed by mechanical scraping to remove any remaining soft tissue, before clipping. Nails should then be washed in aqueous detergents rather than organic solvents and dried under vacuum prior to analysis.

Measurement of the elemental composition of nails may provide a long-term index of nutritional status for some elements — for example, selenium (Morris et al., 1983) — but more investigations are needed before any definitive recommendations can be made.

15.1.2 Measurement of urinary excretion rate of the nutrient or its metabolite

Urine specimens can be used for the biochemical assessment of some minerals, water-soluble B-complex vitamins, vitamin C, and protein, provided that renal function is normal. Urine cannot be used to assess vitamins A, D, E, and K, as metabolites are not excreted in proportion to the amount of these vitamins consumed, absorbed, and metabolized (Hodges, 1981).

Urinary excretion assessment methods almost always reflect recent dietary intake (i.e. *acute* status), rather than the *chronic* nutritional status. The methods depend on the existence of a renal conservation mechanism that reduces the urinary excretion of the nutrient and/or metabolite when body stores of the nutrient are depleted. Unfortunately, for some nutrients (e.g. ascorbic acid and phosphorus), urinary excretion of the nutrient is reduced *before* body stores are depleted. In other circumstances, such as infections and/or the use of antibiotics, and in conditions which produce negative balance, increases in urinary excretion may occur despite depletion of body nutrient stores.

For measurement of a nutrient and/or a corresponding metabolite in urine, it is essential to collect a clean, properly preserved urine sample, preferably over a complete twenty-four-hour period (Solomons, 1985). To monitor the completeness of a twenty-four-hour urine collection, urinary creatinine excretion can be measured. This approach assumes that daily urinary creatinine excretion is constant for a given individual, the amount being related to muscle mass. In fact, it is highly variable within an individual (Waterlow, 1985; Webster and Garrow, 1985). Estimates of the within-subject coefficient of variation in sequential daily urine collections range from 1% to 36% (Jackson, 1966; Webster and Garrow, 1985). Hence, creatinine determinations will only detect gross errors in twenty-four-hour urine collections (Bingham and Cummings, 1985). As a result, another marker, para-aminobenzoic acid (PABA), has been used to assess completeness of urine collection (Bingham and Cummings, 1983). This substance is taken with meals, is harmless, easy to measure, and is rapidly and completely excreted in urine. Studies have shown that any urine collection containing less than 85% of the administered dose is probably incomplete (Bingham and Cummings, 1983), suggesting that PABA is a useful marker for monitoring the completeness of urine collection.

Twenty-four-hour urine samples are difficult to collect in noninstitutionalized population groups. Instead, first-voided fasting morning urine specimens are often used as they are not affected by recent dietary intake. In population studies, it may only be feasible to collect nonfasting casual urine samples. These are not recommended, because concentrations of nutrients and/or metabolites in such samples are affected by liquid consumption, recent dietary intake, physical activity, etc. When first-voided or casual urine specimens are collected, urinary excretion is expressed as a ratio of the nutrient to urinary creatinine (e.g. mg nutrient per g creatinine), to correct for both diurnal variation and fluctuations in urine volume.

15.2 Functional tests

Functional tests may involve measuring the production of an abnormal metabolite, or changes in the activities of certain enzymes/blood components, dependent on a specific nutrient. Alternatively, tests may measure physiological or behavioral functions dependent on specific nutrients. A complete classification of the functional tests is given in Solomons and Allen (1983). Some important examples of functional tests are given below:

- Measurement of abnormal metabolic products in blood or urine arising from suboptimal intakes of the nutrient (e.g. increased excretion of xanthurenic acid in vitamin B-6 deficiency);
- Measurement of changes in blood components or enzyme activities that are dependent on a given nutrient (e.g. whole blood hemoglobin for iron assessment; erythrocyte glutathione peroxidase activity for selenium; erythrocyte glutathione reductase activity for riboflavin; erythrocyte transketolase activity for thiamin);
- *In vitro* tests of *in vivo* functions (e.g. leukocyte chemotaxis for protein-energy, zinc and iron; d-uridine suppression test for vitamin B-12 and folate);
- Induced responses and load tests *in vivo* (e.g. delayed cutaneous hypersensitivity for the assessment of protein-energy and zinc; relative-dose-response for vitamin A; histidine load test for folate; tryptophan load test for vitamin B-6);
- Spontaneous *in vivo* responses (e.g. dark adaptation and taste acuity for vitamin A and zinc; muscle function for protein-energy)
- Growth or developmental responses (e.g. sexual maturation for zinc; growth velocity for protein-energy, zinc, iodine, etc.; cognitive performance for iron).

15.2.1 Abnormal metabolic products in blood or urine

Many vitamins and minerals act as coenzymes or prosthetic groups for enzyme systems. During deficiency, the activities of these enzymes may be reduced, resulting in the accumulation of abnormal metabolic products in the blood and/or urine. Hence, measurement of these abnormal metabolic products may provide a sensitive and specific index of nutrient depletion. For example, vitamin B-6, as pyridoxal phosphate, is a coenzyme for kynureninase in the tryptophan-niacin pathway. In vitamin B-6 deficiency, the activity of kynureninase is reduced, leading to increased formation and excretion of xanthurenic and other tryptophan metabolites such as kynurenic acid and 3-hydroxykynurenine (Brown, 1981). Usually, urinary xanthurenic acid is determined because it is easily measured.

15.2.2 Changes in enzyme activities or blood components

These are the preferred biochemical methods of nutritional assessment because they are generally the most sensitive and specific. The methods involve measuring a change in the activity of an enzyme that is dependent on a given nutrient, and for which a specific metabolic defect has been identified (e.g. lysyl oxidase for copper, aspartate aminotransferase for vitamin B-6, glutathione reductase for riboflavin, transketolase for thiamin). In some cases (e.g. vitamin B-6, riboflavin, and thiamin), the activity of the enzyme which requires the vitamin as the coenzyme is measured with and without the addition of saturating amounts of the coenzyme added *in vitro*. The *in vitro* stimulation of the enzyme by the coenzyme represents a direct measure of unsaturation of the enzyme with the coenzyme, and therefore a measure of deficiency.

The tissue selected for the enzyme assay should be particularly sensitive to the pathological lesion. Unfortunately, in practice, such pathologically sensitive tissues may be inaccessible or unknown (Mills, 1981). Ideally, the assay selected should: (a) reflect the amount of the nutrient available to the body; (b) respond rapidly to changes in supply of the nutrient; and (c) relate to the pathology of deficiency or excess (Casey and Robinson, 1983). Measurement of the copper-containing enzyme lysyl oxidase is an example of an assay which fulfills these criteria. Connective tissue defects occur during the early stages of the copper deficiency syndrome which are attributed to depressed activity of lysyl oxidase. The decreased enzyme activity inhibits cross-linking of collagen and elastin.

Many nutrients have more than one functional role, so that the activities of several enzymes may be affected during the development of a deficiency, thereby providing additional information on the severity of the deficiency state. In the case of copper deficiency, for example, erythrocyte Cu,Zn-superoxide dismutase activity is depressed during marginal copper deficiency, whereas a reduction in plasma ceruloplasmin occurs only in more severe deficiency states (L'Abbé and Fischer, 1984).

Instead of measuring the activity of an enzyme, changes in blood components that are related to the intake of a nutrient can be measured. For example, serum levels of the transport proteins thyroxine pre-albumin and retinol-binding protein are a better measure of the availability of iodine, and vitamin A, respectively, than levels of the corresponding nutrients in the blood (Casey and Robinson, 1983).

15.2.3   *In vitro* tests of *in vivo* functions

These tests involve replicating *in vitro* a corresponding function *in vivo*. For these tests, tissues/cells must be isolated and maintained under physiological conditions. Tests related to host-defense and immunocompetence are probably the most widely used assays of this type. They appear to provide a useful, functional, and quantitative index of nutritional status.

The immune system consists of two lymphoid components, thymus-dependent (T) lymphocytes arising in the thymus, and B-lymphocytes originating in the bone marrow. T-lymphocytes are the main effecters of cell-mediated immunity whereas B-lymphocytes are responsible for humoral immunity. During protein-energy malnutrition, both the proportion and absolute number of T-cells in the peripheral blood may be reduced (Chandra, 1974). An *in vitro* test has been developed to measure total T-lymphocytes. Details of this test are given in Section 16.5.2. Lymphocyte function is assessed by the *in vitro* responses of lymphocytes to selected mitogens (Section 16.5.3). Standardized techniques must be used for the tests, after isolating the lymphocytes from whole blood (Chandra and Scrimshaw, 1980). A control group should also be included where possible, because genetic factors regulate many aspects of the immune response.

Other *in vitro* tests include the erythrocyte hemolysis test, and the d-uridine (dU) suppression tests. In the former, the rate of hemolysis of red blood cells is measured; the rate correlates inversely with serum tocopherol levels (Section 18.3.6) (Binder and Spiro, 1967). Unfortunately this test is not very specific, as other nutrients, such as selenium, influence the rate of red blood cell hemolysis. The dU suppression test is used to diagnose marginal deficiencies of vitamin B-12 and/or folic acid (Section 22.2.2). In this test, bone marrow cells are incubated with nonradioactive deoxyuridine, which suppresses their ability to incorporate radioactive thymidine into DNA. This suppression is subnormal in patients with vitamin B-12 or folate deficiency (Herbert et al., 1973; Wickramasinghe and Saunders, 1975). Peripheral blood lymphocytes and whole blood can also be used for the dU suppression test (Wickramasinghe and Longland, 1974).

15.2.4 Load tests and induced responses *in vivo*

These functional tests, conducted on the subject *in vivo*, include many well-established load and tolerance tests. Such tests are used for individuals with a suspected deficiency of a nutrient; they are not suitable for survey studies. They are generally employed to assess the status of water-soluble vitamins (e.g. tryptophan load test for pyridoxine, histidine load test for folic acid, vitamin C load test, valine load test for vitamin B-12) and minerals (e.g. magnesium, zinc, and selenium) (Caddell et al., 1975; Robberecht and Deelstra, 1984; Fickel et al., 1986).

In a load test, a loading dose of the nutrient or an associated compound is administered orally, intramuscularly, or intravenously. After the load, a timed sample of the urine is collected and the excretion level of the nutrient or a metabolite is determined. In a deficiency state, when tissues are not saturated with the nutrient, excretion of the nutrient or a metabolite will be low because net retention is high. When calculating percentage excretion in load tests, the basal intake of the nutrient (i.e. the contribution from the diet) must be allowed for by means of a correction for the baseline urinary excretion of the nutrient (Robberecht and Deelstra, 1984).

Tolerance tests, sometimes referred to as plasma appearance tests, are used to assess nutritional status of nutrients such as zinc and manganese. In these tests, the concentration of the nutrient is measured both in fasting plasma and in plasma after an oral pharmacological dose of the nutrient. The response is enhanced in cases of nutrient depletion because intestinal absorption of the nutrient is assumed to increase in a nutrient deficiency state (Fickel et al., 1986).

Isotope dilution methods are used to estimate the body pool size of a nutrient. For the test, the nutrient, labeled with a radioactive or stable isotope, is administered orally or injected intravenously. After an equilibration period, the body pool size of the nutrient is determined from the dilution of the tracer isotope in a sample of plasma or whole blood (Section 14.3).

Examples of other functional *in vivo* physiological load tests include the relative-dose-response for vitamin A (Section 18.1.4), and, for chromium, changes in an oral glucose tolerance test after chromium supplementation (Section 24.1.6).

Delayed cutaneous hypersensitivity (DCH) to known recall antigens is the most common test of immunocompetence in hospital patients. It involves injecting a battery of specific antigens intradermally in the forearm and noting the induced response at selected time intervals (Section 16.5.4). This test, like the *in vitro* test of immune function described in Sections 15.2.3 and 16.5.3, is not specific enough to detect individual nutrient deficiencies because decreases in immune function are associated with protein-energy malnutrition and deficiencies of other nutrients (e.g. zinc, selenium, and iron). Moreover, in the case of the DCH test, many other non-nutritional confounding factors affect skin test reactivity. These factors include technical problems with the method *per se*, the presence of certain disease states and/or concurrent infections, hormones, age, race, drugs, circulation problems, and electrolyte imbalances (Miller, 1978; Bates et al., 1979; Twomey et al., 1982).

15.2.5 Spontaneous *in vivo* responses

The first functional tests to use a spontaneous physiological response *in vivo* involved dark adaptation and capillary fragility. A deficit in dark adaptation, resulting in night-blindness, was first described in association with vitamin A deficiency, and more recently, in some cases of zinc deficiency. The classical method of assessing night blindness is formal dark adaptometry. This method is very time-consuming (Solomons and Allen, 1983). It has recently has been superseded by a new, interactive, rapid dark adaptation test, the results of which correlate with those of the classical method (Section 18.1.5). Capillary fragility has been used as a functional test of vitamin C deficiency since 1913 (Hess, 1913) because frank petechial hemorrhages occur in overt vitamin C deficiency. The test, however, is not very specific to vitamin C deficiency states (Section 19.6); static biochemical tests are preferred to assess vitamin C status.

Abnormalities in taste function are sometimes associated with suboptimal zinc status in children (Hambidge et al., 1972b; Gibson et al., 1989) and certain disease states in which secondary zinc deficiency may occur (e.g. patients with Crohn's disease, celiac sprue, cystic fibrosis, chronic renal disease) (Watson et al., 1983; Henkin, 1984). A few studies have also demonstrated the recovery of taste function with repletion of body zinc stores (Henkin et al., 1975). Taste acuity can be assessed using the forced drop method which measures both the detection and recognition thresholds (Buzina et al., 1980; Henkin, 1984), or by measuring recognition thresholds only (Desor and Maller, 1975) (Section 24.5.9). Many other factors affect taste function, and taste acuity alone should not be used to assess zinc status.

Other tests based on spontaneous physiological responses *in vivo* include assessment of the contraction-relaxation characteristics and endurance of skeletal muscle (Section 16.4). The reduction in protein stores and muscle catabolism which occurs during protein-energy malnutrition alters muscle contractility, relaxation rate, and endurance, and may provide a sensitive index of protein status (Russell and Jeejeebhoy, 1983).

15.2.6 Growth or developmental responses

This category of physiological tests assesses the functional performance of the individual in areas such as growth, lactation, sexual maturation, and cognition. Such indices are not specific for any nutrient and are preferably used in association with other, more specific, laboratory indices. Growth velocity, for example, has frequently been used as a functional index of nutritional status of infants and young children and is discussed in Chapter 10.

Assessment of cognitive function requires rigorous methodology. A relationship between cognitive function and nutrient deficiency can only be established by: (a) documenting clinically important differences in cognitive function between deficient subjects and healthy controls, and (b) demonstrating improvement in cognitive function after supplementation. The subjects should be matched and the design should involve a double-blind randomized supplementation trial (Lozoff and Brittenham, 1986). So far, very few studies have met all these criteria.

Measures of cognitive function used in relation to iron deficiency include IQ-test performance in older children (Seshadri et al., 1982; Palti et al., 1983), and the Bayley Scales of Infant Development for infants (Bayley, 1969). The latter scales are well standardized and include three components: Mental Scale, Motor Scale, and Infant Behavior Record.

15.3 Selection of laboratory tests

Rigorous protocols must be followed for the sampling, transportation, preservation, and analysis of the biological tissues and/or fluids. This is

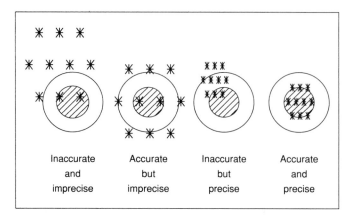

Figure 15.1: Differences between precision and accuracy. Modified from Pi-Sunyer and Woo. In: Nutrition Assessment: A Comprehensive Guide for Planning intervention by M.D. Simko, C. Cowell, and J.A. Gilbride, p. 140, with permission of Aspen Publishers, Inc., © 1984.

particularly important for samples collected under field conditions and for trace element analysis.

Laboratory tests vary with respect to their precision, accuracy, analytical specificity, analytical sensitivity, predictive value, and validity. All techniques may be subject to both random and systematic measurement errors, and hence personnel should be trained to use standardized and validated techniques which are continuously monitored by appropriate quality control procedures.

Precision

Repeated measurements on a single sample or individual can be used to assess precision. The coefficient of variation, as determined by the ratio of the standard deviation (SD) to the mean of the replicates, $SD/\bar{x}$, is the best quantitative measure of the precision. The level of precision attainable depends on the procedure, whereas the precision required depends on the projected application of the data. It is possible for a method to be precise but not accurate, as shown in Figure 15.1.

Accuracy

The difference between the reported and the true amount of the nutrient/metabolite present in the sample determines the accuracy of a method. For methods involving direct analysis of nutrients in tissues or fluids, a recovery test is generally performed. This involves the addition of known amounts of nutrient to the sample. These spiked samples are then analyzed together with unspiked aliquots to assess whether the analytical value accounts for close to 100% of the added nutrient. As an additional test for accuracy, an aliquot of a reference material of a similar matrix as the sample, certified for the nutrient of interest, should be included with each batch of analyses (Section 4.3.3). Such certified reference materials can be obtained from the United States National Bureau of Standards, the United States Center for Disease Control (for serum vitamin A and C), or the International Atomic Energy Agency. A reference material for erythrocyte enzymes for vitamin B-6, riboflavin, and thiamin has been developed by the Wolfson Research Laboratory in Birmingham, England. If suitable reference materials are not available, independent aliquots, from a homogeneous pooled test sample, should be analyzed by independent laboratories using different methods. Figure 15.1 highlights the differences between precision and accuracy.

Analytical sensitivity

For any analytical method, the analytical sensitivity refers to the smallest single result which can be distinguished from zero. Thus, unfortunately, the term 'sensitivity' is used in nutritional assessment methodology in two different ways (Section 1.3). To clarify the distinction, the term 'analytical sensitivity' should always be used in relation to an analytical method. Recognition of the analytical sensitivity of a biochemical method is particularly important when the nutrient is present in low concentrations (e.g. the ultratrace elements Cr, Mn, and Ni). Routine procedures should be capable of analyzing the nutrient of interest at a level which is five times greater than the detection limit (Wolf, 1982). The latter has been defined as a number equal to three times the standard deviation of the precision of the measurement at the blank value (Wolf, 1982). The definition of sensitivity given in Section 1.3 is also applicable to laboratory indices.

Analytical specificity

The ability of an analytical method to measure only the substance of interest is referred to as the 'analytical specificity'. Specific methods do not generate false-positive results and have few or no interferences. Analytical specificity is improved in the analysis of minerals or trace elements by removing organic material by dry ashing or wet digestion, prior to analysis. The definition of specificity given in Section 1.3 is also applicable to laboratory indices. 'Analytical specificity' should be used only in relation to an analytical method.

Predictive value

The predictive value refers to the ability of a laboratory test, when used as an index, to predict correctly the presence or absence of a nutrient deficiency or disease. Sensitivity, specificity, and prevalence affect the predictive value of a laboratory index, as discussed in Section 1.3. Sometimes, laboratory and/or anthropometric measurements are combined to form a multi-parameter index to enhance the predictive value of a test.

Validity

It follows from the definition of validity given in Section 1.3 that a laboratory test, when used as an index, can be considered valid if it correctly reflects the nutritional parameter of interest. Thus, for example, if the objective is to assess the total body content of a nutrient, and the laboratory index correctly reflects the total body content, the index is said to be valid. Unfortunately, the action of certain drugs and hormones on enzyme activity, and/or nutrient metabolism, may affect the validity of a laboratory index. For example, an increase in the concentration of a nutrient may occur in the tissues, concomitant with a fall in blood levels. Such discrepancies may decrease the validity of indices.

15.4   Evaluation of laboratory indices

Laboratory indices, both static and functional, are generally evaluated using the two techniques described in Section 1.4, for individuals and population groups. This involves comparing the observed values with reference values which have been derived from a reference sample and/or cutoff points based on data from subjects with clinical, and/or functional manifestations of the nutrient deficiency.

15.4.1   Reference values

Theoretically, to define reference values, only healthy persons should be included in the reference sample group. Hence, extensive medical history data must also be collected when defining a reference sample group, so that nonhealthy subjects can be excluded. For example, in the NHANES II survey on iron status (Pilch and Senti, 1984b), values for the reference sample were derived by excluding persons with conditions known to affect iron status (e.g. pregnant women and those who had been pregnant in the preceding year; persons with white blood cell count $< 3.4 \times 10^9$/L or $> 11.5 \times 10^9$/L; protoporphyrin values $> 70\,\mu$g/dL RBC; transferrin saturation $< 16\%$; or mean corpuscular volume < 80.0 or > 96.0 fL).

The most frequently used method for comparing the observed values of a biochemical index with the distribution of the reference values is to use percentiles. This approach was discussed in detail in relation to anthropometric indices (Section 13.1.1). As an example, Table 15.3 shows selected percentiles for two indices of iron status for males (all races) aged twenty to sixty-four years drawn from a reference sample derived from the NHANES II data (Pilch and Senti, 1984b). Percentiles

Age	Hemoglobin Percentiles (g/dL)						
(yr)	5	10	25	50	75	90	95
Males							
20–44	13.7	14.0	14.6	15.3	15.9	16.5	16.8
45–64	13.5	13.8	14.4	15.1	15.8	16.4	16.8
Age	Transferrin Saturation Percentiles (%)						
(yr)	5	10	25	50	75	90	95
Males							
20–44	16.6	18.4	23.3	29.1	35.9	43.7	48.5
45–64	15.2	17.6	21.8	27.8	34.2	39.7	44.4

Table 15.3: Hemoglobin (g/dL) and transferrin saturation (%) selected percentiles for male subjects (all races) between twenty and sixty-four years old. Percentiles are for the NHANES II 'reference population'. A more complete data set, including information for females and children, is given in the Appendix. Abstracted from comprehensive tables which include additional information on the SD, SEM, and the number of subjects studied in each age range. From Pilch and Senti (1984b).

were also used to define the reference limits (Section 1.4.2) for the iron indices in this survey. For instance, for the following biochemical iron indices for children aged one to fourteen years, 'normal' values, or those above the reference limit, were defined as: > 10th percentile for hemoglobin, > 5th percentile for mean cell volume, < 90th percentile for erythrocyte protoporphyrin, and > 10th percentile for transferrin saturation.

No data are available from national nutrition surveys for the distribution of reference values for physiological functional indices of nutritional status (e.g. relative dose response for vitamin A). Such tests are not feasible in large-scale nutrition surveys. Consequently, physiological functional indices are often evaluated by monitoring their improvement serially, during a nutrition intervention program (Solomons, 1985). Alternatively, the observed values may be compared with cutoff points, described below.

15.4.2 Cutoff points

Cutoff points are generally based on data from subjects with clinical and/or functional manifestations of a nutrient deficiency. In national nutrition surveys of industrialized countries, clinical signs of nutrient deficiencies (with the exception of iron) are rarely observed, and tests measuring physiological and/or behavioral functions have not been performed. Consequently, the cutoff points are generally based on ranges

Authority	Less than Acceptable (at Risk)		Acceptable
	Deficient (high risk)	Low (medium risk)	(low risk)
ICNND (1963)	< 0.1	0.1–0.2	> 0.2
Nutrition Canada	< 0.2	0.2–0.4	> 0.4

Table 15.4: Guidelines for the interpretation of serum vitamin C values (mg/dL), applicable to both sexes. The data for Nutrition Canada are from Health and Welfare Canada (1973) and are applicable to adults aged greater than twenty years. Reproduced with permission of the Minister of Supply and Services Canada. The ICNND (1963) guidelines are for all ages.

associated with clinical signs, or impairment in a biochemical or physiological function, reported in the literature (Pilch, 1985). Cutoff points may be age, race, and/or sex specific, depending on the laboratory index used.

In the Nutrition Canada National Survey (Health and Welfare Canada, 1973), and the U.S. Interdepartmental Committee on Nutrition for National Defence (ICNND, 1963) nutrition surveys, cutoff points were used to define several levels of nutritional status. The Nutrition Canada National Survey adopted a concept of likelihood of 'risk' of deficiency and designated three levels as: 'high risk', 'medium risk', and 'low risk'. High risk was defined as a high probability that a nutrient deficiency exists, moderate risk as an average probability that a nutrient deficiency is present or developing, and low risk as a low probability that a nutrient deficiency exists. The levels were based on the presence of clinical signs indicative of a nutritional disease, or on an abnormal level of a nutrient or metabolite in the blood or urine. The ICNND (1963) chose four levels, designated as 'deficient', 'low', 'acceptable', and 'high'. Table 15.4 compares the cutoff points for serum vitamin C values used by the Nutrition Canada National Survey (Health and Welfare Canada, 1973) and the ICNND (1963). As discussed earlier in Chapters 8 and 13, cutoff points can never separate the 'deficient' and the 'adequately nourished' without some misclassification occurring. There always exists some overlap between persons who actually have the deficiency and those falsely identified (i.e. false positives) (Figure 1.1). This arises because the physiological normal levels of laboratory indices vary among persons, depending on their individual nutrient requirements (Beaton, 1986).

The following nine chapters include details of the laboratory tests for those nutrients for which primary nutritional deficiency states in humans, have been described. Clinical assessment and the nutritional assessment of hospital patients is discussed in Chapters 25 and 26.

References

Assarian GS, Oberleas D. (1977). Effect of washing procedures on trace element content of hair. Clinical Chemistry 23: 1771–1772.

Bank HL, Robson J, Bigelow JB, Morrison J, Spell LH, Kantor R. (1981). Preparation of fingernails for trace element analysis. Clinica Chimica Acta 116: 179–190.

Bates SE, Suen JY, Tranum BL. (1979). Immunological skin testing and interpretation: A plea for uniformity. Cancer 43: 2306–2314.

Bayley N. (1969). Bayley Scales of Infant Development Manual. Psychological Corporation, New York.

Beaton GH. (1986). E.V. McCollum International Lectureship in nutrition. Toward harmonization of dietary, biochemical, and clinical assessments: the meanings of nutritional status and requirements. Nutrition Reviews 44: 349–358.

Binder HJ, Spiro HM. (1967). Tocopherol deficiency in man. American Journal of Clinical Nutrition 20: 594–603.

Bingham S, Cummings JH. (1983). The use of 4-aminobenzoic acid as a marker to validate the completeness of 24 hr urine collections in man. Clinical Science 64: 629–635.

Bingham S, Cummings JH. (1985). The use of creatinine output as a check on the completeness of 24-hour urine collections. Human Nutrition: Clinical Nutrition 39C: 343–353.

Brown RR. (1981). The tryptophan load test as an index of vitamin-B6 nutrition. In: Leklem JE, Reynolds RD (eds). Methods in Vitamin B-6 Nutrition. Analysis and Status Assessment. Plenum Press, New York–London, pp. 321–340.

Buzina R, Jusic M, Sapunar J, Milanovic N. (1980). Zinc nutrition and taste acuity in school children with impaired growth. American Journal of Clinical Nutrition 33: 2262–2267.

Caddell JL, Saier FL. Thomason CA. (1975). Parenteral magnesium load tests in *postpartum* American women. American Journal of Clinical Nutrition 28: 1099–1104.

Casey CE, Robinson MF. (1983). Some aspects of nutritional trace element research. In: Sigel H (ed). Metal Ions in Biological Systems. Volume 16. Methods Involving Metal Ions and Complexes in Clinical Chemistry. Marcel Dekker Inc., New York, pp. 1–26.

Chandra RK. (1974). Rosette-forming T lymphocytes and cell-mediated immunity in malnutrition. British Medical Journal 3: 608–609.

Chandra RK, Scrimshaw NS. (1980). Immunocompetence in nutritional assessment. American Journal of Clinical Nutrition 33: 2694–2697.

Chittleborough G. (1980). A chemist's view of the analysis of human hair for trace elements. Science of the Total Environment. 14: 53–75.

Creason JP, Hinners TA, Bumgarner JE, Pinkerton C. (1975). Trace elements in hair, as related to exposure in metropolitan New York. Clinical Chemistry 21: 603–612.

Davies TS. (1982). Hair analysis and selenium shampoos. Lancet 2: 935.

DeAntonio SM, Katz SA, Scheiner DM, Wood JD. (1982). Anatomically-related variations in trace-metal concentrations in hair. Clinical Chemistry 28: 2411–2413.

Desor JA, Mallor O. (1975). Taste corrrelates of disease states: cystic fibrosis. Journal of Pediatrics 87: 93–96.

Eads EA, Lambdin CE. (1973). A survey of trace metals in human hair. Environmental Research 6: 247–252.

Elin RJ. (1983). The status of cellular analysis. Journal of the American College of Nutrition 2: 329–330.

English JL, Hambidge KM, Jacobs Goodall M, Nelson D. (1987). Evaluation of some factors that may affect plasma or serum zinc concentrations. In: Hurley LS, Keen CL, Lönnerdal B, Rucker RB (eds). Trace Elements in Man and Animals 6, Plenum Press, New York–London, pp. 459-460.

Erten J, Arcasoy A, Caudar AO, Cin S. (1978). Hair zinc levels in healthy and malnourished children. American Journal of Clinical Nutrition 31: 1172–1174.

Fickel JF, Freeland-Graves JH, Roby MJ. (1986). Zinc tolerance tests in zinc deficient and zinc supplemented diets. American Journal of Clincial Nutrition 43: 47–58.

Gibson RS, Gibson IL. (1984). The interpretation of human hair trace element concentrations. Science of the Total Environment 39: 93–101.

Gibson RS, Smit-Vanderkooy PD, MacDonald AC, Goldman A, Ryan BA, Berry M. (1989). A growth limiting mild zinc deficiency syndrome in some Southern Ontario boys with low height percentiles. American Journal of Clinical Nutrition 49: 1266–1273.

Hambidge KM. (1982). Hair analysis: worthless for vitamins, limited for minerals. American Journal of Clinical Nutrition 36: 943–949.

Hambidge KM, Franklin ML, Jacobs MA. (1972a). Hair chromium concentration: effect of sample washing and external environment. American Journal of Clinical Nutrition 25: 384–389.

Hambidge KM, Hambidge C, Jacobs M, Baum JD. (1972b). Low levels of zinc in hair, anorexia, poor growth, and hypogeusia in children. Pediatric Research 6: 868–874.

Hambidge KM, Walravens PA, Neldner KH. (1977). The role of zinc in the pathogenesis and treatment of acrodermatitis enteropathica. In: Brewer GJ, Prasad AS (eds). Zinc Metabolism: Current Aspects in Health and Disease. Alan R. Liss Inc., New York, pp. 329–340.

Hammer DI, Finklea JF, Hendricks RH, Shy CM. (1971). Hair trace metal levels and environmental exposure. American Journal of Epidemiology 93: 84–92.

Harrison WW, Yurachek JP, Benson CA. (1969). The determination of trace elements in human hair by atomic absorption spectroscopy. Clinica Chimica Acta 23: 83–91.

Health and Welfare Canada (1973). Nutrition Canada National Survey. Health and Welfare, Ottawa.

Henkin RI. (1984). Review: zinc in taste function. A critical review. Biological Trace Element Research 6: 263–280.

Henkin RI, Patten BM, Peter K, Bronzert DA. (1975). A syndrome of acute zinc loss: cerebellar dysfunction, mental changes, anorexia, and taste and smell dysfunction. Archives of Neurology 32: 745–751.

Herbert V, Tisman G, Le-Teng-Go, Brenner L. (1973). The dU suppression test using ^{125}I-UdR to define biochemical megaloblastosis. British Journal of Haematology 24: 713–723.

Hess AF. (1913). The involvement of the blood and blood vessels in infantile scurvy. Proceedings of the Society for Experimental Biology and Medicine 11: 130–132.

Hilderbrand DC, White DH. (1974). Trace-element analysis in hair: An evaluation. Clinical Chemistry 20: 148–151.

Hodges RE. (1981). The fat-soluble vitamins. In: Nutritional Assessment — Present Status, Future Directions and Prospects. Report of the Second Ross Conference on Medical Research, Ross Laboratories, Columbus, Ohio, pp. 61–64.

Hopps HC. (1977). The biologic basis for using hair and nail for analyses of trace elements. Science of the Total Environment 7: 71–89.

ICNND (Interdepartmental Committee on Nutrition for National Defense) (1963). Manual for Nutrition Surveys, US Government Printing Office, Washington, D.C.

Jackson S. (1966). Creatinine in urine as an index of urinary excretion rate. Health Physics 12: 843–850.

Katz SA. (1979). The use of hair as a biopsy material for trace elements in the body. American Laboratory 11: 44–53.

Kumpulainen J, Salmela A, Vuori E, Lehto J. (1982). Effects of various washing procedures on the chromium content of human scalp hair. Analytica Chimica Acta 138: 361–364.

L'Abbé MR, Fischer PW. (1984). The effects of high dietary zinc and copper deficiency on the activity of copper-requiring metalloenzymes in the growing rat. Journal of Nutrition 114: 813–822.

Laker M. (1982). On determining trace element levels in man: the uses of blood and hair. Lancet 2: 260–262.

Lozoff B, Brittenham GM. (1986). Behavioral aspects of iron deficiency. In: Progress in Hematology. Volume XIV. Grune and Stratton, Duluth, Minnesota, pp. 23–51.

Maugh TH. (1978). Hair: A diagnostic tool to complement blood serum and urine. Science 202: 1271–1273.

McBean LD, Mahloudji M, Reinhold JG, Halsted JA. (1971). Correlations of zinc concentrations in human plasma and hair. American Journal of Clinical Nutrition 24: 506–509.

McKenzie JM. (1978). Alteration of the zinc and copper concentration of hair. American Journal of Clinical Nutrition 31: 470–476.

Mertz W. (1975). Trace-element nutrition in health and disease: contributions and problems of analysis. Clinical Chemistry 21: 468–475.

Miller CL. (1978). Immunological assays as measurements of nutritional status: a review. Journal of Parenteral and Enteral Nutrition 2: 554–566.

Mills CF. (1981). Some outstanding problems in the detection of trace element deficiency diseases. Philosophical Transactions of the Royal Society of London. Series B — Biological Sciences 294: 199–213.

Milne DB, Ralston NVC, Wallwork JC. (1985). Zinc content of cellular components of blood: methods for cell separation and analysis evaluated. Clinical Chemistry 31: 65–69.

Morris JS, Stampfer MJ, Willett W. (1983). Dietary selenium in humans: toenails as an indicator. Biological Trace Element Research 5: 529–537.

Noord PAH van, Collette HJA, Maas MJ, De Waard F. (1987). Selenium levels in nails of premenopausal breast cancer patients assessed prediagnostically in a cohort-nested case-referent study among women screened in the DOM project. International Journal of Epidemiology 16: 318–322.

Petering HG, Yeager DW, Witherup SO. (1971). Trace metal content of hair: I. Zinc and copper content of human hair in relation to age and sex. Archives of Environmental Health 23: 202–207.

Palti H, Pevsner B, Adler B. (1983). Does anemia in infancy affect achievement on developmental and intelligence tests? Human Biology 55: 189–194.

Pilch SM (ed). (1985). Assessment of the vitamin A nutritional status of the U.S. population based on data collected in the second National Health and Nutrition Examination Survey, 1976 — 1980. Life Sciences Research Office, Federation of the American Societies for Experimental Biology, Bethesda, Maryland.

Pilch SM, Senti FR (eds). (1984a). Assessment of the zinc nutritional status of the U.S. population based on data collected in the second National Health and Nutrition Examination Survey, 1976 — 1980. Life Sciences Research Office, Federation of the American Societies for Experimental Biology, Bethesda, Maryland.

Pilch SM, Senti FR (eds). (1984b). Assessment of the iron nutritional status of the U.S. population based on data collected in the second National Health and Nutrition Examination Survey, 1976 — 1980. Life Sciences Research Office, Federation of the American Societies for Experimental Biology, Bethesda, Maryland.

Pi-Sunyer FX, Woo R. (1984). Laboratory assessment of nutritional status. In: Simko MD, Cowell C, Gilbride JA (eds) Nutrition Assessment. A Comprehensive Guide for Planning Intervention. Aspen Systems Corporation, Rockville, Maryland, pp. 139–174.

Prasad AS, Cossack ZT. (1982). Neutrophil zinc: an indicator of zinc status in man. Transactions of the Association of American Physicians 95: 65–176.

Robberecht HJ, Deelstra HA. (1984). Review. Selenium in human urine: concentration levels and medical implications. Clinica Chimica Acta 136: 107–120.

Russell D McR, Jeejeebhoy KN. (1983). The assessment of the functional consequences of malnutrition. Nutrition Abstracts and Reviews 53: 863–877.

Salmela S, Vuori E, Kilpio JO. (1981). The effect of washing procedures on trace element content of human hair. Analytica Chimica Acta 125: 131–137.

Sauberlich HE, Dowdy RP, Skala JH. (1974). Laboratory Tests for the Assessment of Nutritional Status. CRC Press Inc., Cleveland, Ohio.

Schroeder HA, Nason PA. (1969). Trace metals in human hair. Journal of Investigative Dermatology 53: 71–78.

Seshadri S, Hirode K, Naik P, Malhotra S. (1982). Behavioural responses of young anaemic Indian children to iron-folic acid supplements. British Journal of Nutrition 48: 233–240.

Sky-Peck HH, Joseph BJ. (1983). The 'use' and 'misuse' of human hair in trace metal analysis. In: Brown SS, Savory J (eds) Chemical Toxicology and Clinical Chemistry of Metals. Academic Press, London, pp. 159–163.

Smith JC Jr, Holbrook JT, Danford DE. (1985). Analysis and evaluation of zinc and copper in human plasma and serum. Journal of the American College of Nutrition 4: 627–638.

Solomons NW. (1985). Assessment of nutritional status: functional indicators of pediatric nutriture. Pediatric Clinics of North America 32: 319–334.

Solomons NW, Allen LH. (1983). The functional assessment of nutritional status: principles, practice and potential. Nutrition Reviews 41: 33–50.

Sorenson JR, Melby EG, Nord PJ, Petering HC. (1973). Interferences in the determination of metallic elements in human hair. Archives of Environmental Health 27: 36–39.

Takagi Y, Matsuda S, Imai S, Ohmori Y, Masuda T, Vinson JA, Mehra MC, Puri BK, Kaniewski A. (1988). Survey of trace elements in human nails: an international comparison. Bulletin of Environmental Contamination and Toxicology 41: 690–695.

Taylor A. (1986). Usefulness of measurements of trace elements in hair. Annals of Clinical Biochemistry 23: 364–378.

Twomey P, Ziegler D, Rombeau J. (1982). Utility of skin testing in nutritional assessment: A critical review. Journal of Parenteral and Enteral Nutrition 6: 50–58.

Vance DE, Ehmann WD, Markesbery WR. (1988). Trace element imbalances in hair and nails of Alzheimer's disease patients. Neurotoxicology 9: 197–208.

Versieck J. (1984). Trace element analysis — a plea for accuracy. Trace Elements in Medicine 1: 2–12.

Versieck J, Vanballenberghe L, De Kesel A, Renterghem D van. (1987). Review. Accuracy of biological trace-element determinations. Biological Trace Element Research 12: 45–54.

Waterlow JC. (1985). Observations on the variability of creatinine excretion. Human Nutrition: Clinical Nutrition 40C: 125–129.

Watson AR, Stuart A, Wells FE, Houston IB, Addison GM. (1983). Zinc supplementation and its effects on taste acuity in children with chronic renal failure. Human Nutrition: Clinical Nutrition 37C: 219–225.

Webster J, Garrow JS. (1985). Creatinine excretion over 24 hours as a measure of body composition or of completeness of urine collection. Human Nutrition: Clinical Nutrition 39C: 101–106.

Wickramasinghe SM, Longland JE. (1974). Assessment of deoxyuridine suppression test in diagnosis of vitamin B-12 or folate deficiency. British Medical Journal 3: 148–150.

Wickramasinghe SN, Saunders JE. (1975). (Letter) Deoxyuridine suppression test. British Medical Journal 2: 87.

Wolf WR. (1982). Trace element analysis in food. In: Prasad AR (ed). Clinical, Biochemical and Nutritional Aspects of Trace Elements. Alan R. Liss Inc., New York, pp. 427–446.

Chapter 16

Assessment of protein status

The adult human body of a 70 kg reference man contains about 10 to 13 kg of protein, which is widely distributed throughout the different tissues of the body (Table 16.1). Proteins are essential for structural (e.g. collagen and elastin) and regulatory (e.g. hormones and enzyme) functions. They also act as specific carrier proteins and mediators of the immune response.

There are no dispensable protein stores in humans, and therefore loss of body protein results in loss of essential structural elements as well as impaired function. Most of the body protein is found in the skeletal muscle (approximately 30% to 50% of total body protein) and in the smaller visceral protein pool (Table 16.1). Visceral protein is made up of serum proteins, erythrocytes, granulocytes, and lymphocytes as well as the solid tissue organs such as liver, kidneys, pancreas, and heart. The skeletal muscle protein (termed somatic protein) and the visceral protein pool together compose the metabolically available protein known as the *body cell mass* (Section 14.4). The other major protein components of the body are found in the extracellular connective tissue and constitute the noncellular structural proteins of the cartilage, fibrous, and skeletal tissues. Such noncellular structural proteins are not readily exchangeable with other body pools of protein. Hence, although alterations may occur in the somatic and visceral protein components

	g/kg		g/kg
Muscle	22	Extracellular	17
Skeleton	20	Fat	6
Viscera & skin	18		

Table 16.1: The protein concentration of body tissues, calculated from Forbes et al. (1953) with permission. © The American Society for Biological Chemists, Inc.

during protein malnutrition and disease (Figure 14.1), much of the protein in the extracellular connective tissue cannot be mobilized to counteract these changes (Phinney, 1981).

Whole body protein can be estimated from the measurement of total body potassium or nitrogen described in Sections 14.2 and 14.5. Alternatively, *changes* in total body protein nutriture can be monitored indirectly, using anthropometric indices such as mid-upper-arm muscle area (Section 11.2.3). The latter provide an estimate of changes in skeletal muscle, a major component of body protein. Biochemical measurements such as urinary excretion of creatinine (Section 16.1.1) or 3-methylhistidine (Section 16.1.2) can also be used to estimate skeletal muscle protein.

Loss of muscle mass (and adipose tissue) characterizes the marasmic form of protein-energy malnutrition, the form most frequently encountered in developing countries. It generally results from a prolonged reduction of food intake. The latter may arise in hospital patients with chronic illnesses, or from the prolonged use of clear fluid diets and hypocaloric intravenous infusions of 5% dextrose.

Kwashiorkor, another form of protein-energy malnutrition, also occurs in children from certain regions of developing countries, as well as in hospital patients. In developing countries, kwashiorkor is often precipitated by a series of infections occurring successively or concurrently in the presence of a diet with a low protein content relative to energy. In hospital patients, kwashiorkor tends to arise from an inadequate intake of dietary protein concomitant with acute protein losses induced by stress associated with hypermetabolism (e.g. trauma and/or sepsis) (Jeejeebhoy, 1981). Unlike marasmus, kwashiorkor does not result in a depletion of skeletal muscle protein; instead, the visceral protein pool is depleted and edema occurs. Biochemical assessment of the visceral protein component (Section 16.2) usually involves measurement of serum proteins such as albumin and transferrin. Protein-energy malnutrition also results in metabolic changes, some of which can be used to distinguish between kwashiorkor and marasmus; others (e.g. nitrogen balance) can be used to monitor the effectiveness of nutritional support in hospital patients. These changes (and the related assessment procedures) are discussed in Section 16.3. Finally, selected physiological functional indices of nutritional status, such as tests of muscle and immune function, are given in Sections 16.4 and 16.5.

16.1 Assessment of somatic protein status

16.1.1 Urinary creatinine excretion

Creatinine, excreted in the urine, is derived from the catabolism of creatine phosphate, a metabolite present principally in muscle. Hence, the creatine pool of the body can be estimated from measurement of urinary creatinine excretion. If the creatine content of muscle is assumed to be constant, urinary creatinine can be used as an index of muscle mass. This assumption has been confirmed in animal studies involving chemical analysis of muscle mass and isotopic dilution of labeled creatine (Meador et al., 1968), and in humans by the existence of a highly significant linear relationship between muscle mass and creatinine excretion during growth (Cheek, 1968). Some investigators have suggested the use of a constant ratio of creatinine per unit of body composition. For example, in a twenty-four-hour urine sample, each gram of creatinine excreted is said to represent approximately 18 to 20 kg of fat-free muscle (Cheek et al., 1966; Cheek, 1968; Heymsfield et al., 1983). Other investigators, however, consider it is inappropriate to use a constant ratio of creatinine per kilogram of fat-free muscle in a population, unless factors such as age, gender, maturity, physical training, and metabolic state are controlled (Boileau et al., 1972; Forbes and Bruining, 1976).

When estimating muscle mass from urinary creatinine, it is assumed that: most creatine (i.e. 98%) is in the skeletal muscle; the diet is creatine-free; the total creatine pool and the average concentration of creatine per kg of muscle remain constant; creatine is converted to creatinine at a constant daily rate nonenzymatically and irreversibly; and creatinine undergoes a constant rate of renal excretion (Heymsfield et al., 1983). Unfortunately, these assumptions are not all true. Several factors are known to affect daily creatinine excretion (Table 16.2) and thus limit the validity of urinary creatinine as an index of muscle mass.

In general, the longer the collection period for the urinary creatinine determination, the more precise the prediction of muscle mass and hence lean body mass. In practice, three consecutive twenty-four-hour urine collections are generally used. Some investigators recommend placing subjects on a constant, low-creatine, meat-free diet containing 60 to 80 g protein per day to stabilize the creatinine excretion, prior to the collection of the urine samples. However, because the half-life of the creatine pool is long (approximately forty-three days), it takes many weeks to eliminate the creatine contribution, and consequently this approach is impractical in the clinical setting. Instead, meat should be eliminated from the diet only during the collection of the twenty-four-hour urine samples (Walser, 1987).

Several methods are used to express urinary creatinine excretion:

- Urinary creatinine excretion (mg) per twenty-four hours;
- Daily urinary creatinine excretion (mg) per cm body height;
- Creatinine height index (CHI) as percentage:

$$\text{CHI}(\%) = \frac{\text{Measured 24-hr urinary creatinine} \times 100\%}{\text{Ideal 24-hr urinary creatinine for height}}$$

- **Diurnal and day-to-day variations** within an individual occur, which are independent of diet and physical activity. These normally range from 4% to 8%, although larger variations ranging from 8.7% to 34.4% have been noted for obese subjects (Webster and Garrow, 1985). Use of several consecutive twenty-four-hour urine samples eliminates some of this variation (Waterlow, 1986).

- **Strenuous exercise** increases urinary creatinine excretion by 5% to 10% (Srivastava et al., 1957). The mechanism inducing such changes is unknown.

- **Emotional stress** affects the variability but not the absolute amount of creatinine excretion. The cause is unknown.

- **Dietary intakes of creatine and creatinine** from meat increase urinary creatinine excretion. Dietary protein also has a small effect on urinary creatinine excretion because it is the main source of the two dietary amino-acid precursors of creatine — arginine and glycine.

- **Menstruation** affects creatinine excretion. It increases by 5% to 10% late in the second half of the menstrual cycle, decreasing just before and during menstrual flow (Smith, 1942).

- **Age** influences creatinine excretion, a decline occurring with increasing age. This effect is attributed to a probable progressive decrease in lean body mass in absolute terms, a decrease in the proportion of muscle in lean body mass, especially in men, and a probable lower meat intake in older subjects (Walser, 1987).

- **Infection, fever, and trauma** result in an apparent increase in urinary creatinine excretion because noncreatinine chromogens interfere with the analysis (Walser, 1987).

- **Chronic renal failure** results in decreased excretion of creatinine. The decrease is not related to depletion in muscle mass, but to a recycling of creatinine to creatine, and intestinal degradation of creatinine to products other than creatine (Mitch et al., 1980). Hence, the use of urinary creatinine to estimate muscle mass or lean body mass in patients with chronic renal failure is invalid.

Table 16.2: Factors affecting daily creatinine excretion. Adapted from Heymsfield et al. (1983).

- CHI as a percentage deficit (mild deficit = 5% to 15%; moderate 15% to 30%; severe > 30%):

$$\text{Percentage deficit} = 100 - \text{CHI} (\%)$$

A creatinine height index of 60% to 80% of standard has been suggested to represent a moderate deficit in body muscle mass, whereas a value of less than 60% indicates a severe deficit of body muscle mass (Blackburn et al., 1977). These interpretive values for creatinine height index, however, should be used with caution because they have not been validated. Moreover, if the creatinine height index for a patient is at the upper end of the normal range before developing malnutrition, severe protein malnutrition will not be detected by measuring creatinine height index.

One of the biggest practical difficulties in estimating urinary creatinine excretion is ensuring that twenty-four-hour urine collections are complete. Forbes and Bruining (1976) stressed that an error as small as fifteen minutes in a collection period represents an error of 1% in the determination of twenty-four-hour urinary creatinine excretion. Creatinine excretion is generally expressed in relation to height in preference to body weight because height is not affected by adipose tissue and fluid imbalances (e.g. edema). For calculation of creatinine height index values, the ideal twenty-four-hour urinary creatinine excretion for height has been derived from a population of thirty healthy young adults receiving a creatine-free diet (Bistrian et al., 1975; Bistrian, 1977). These ideal values are not appropriate for the elderly, as a 20% decline in creatinine excretion (mg per cm body height) occurs from age sixty-five to seventy-four (Driver and McAlvey, 1980). Consequently, use of these reference data is likely to overestimate protein depletion in elderly patients.

To derive age-corrected creatinine excretion rates, Imbembo and Walser (1984) combined linear regression equations for predicting creatinine excretion (mg/kg/day) in relation to age, with 'ideal' weights for height derived from the 1983 Metropolitan Life Insurance Company Tables (Section 12.5.3). The resulting tables are shown in Appendix A16.1. These tables should be used to determine an age-corrected creatinine height index in subjects consuming self-selected diets, until observations of age-corrected creatinine excretion in a large series of healthy men and women of varying age are available.

The creatinine height index is most frequently used to assess the degree of depletion of muscle mass in creatinine height indexldren with the marasmic form of protein-energy malnutrition. In such subjects, there will be a decrease in creatinine height index as a result of loss of lean body mass to maintain serum protein levels. The creatinine height index can also be used to monitor the effects of long-term nutritional intervention on repletion of lean body mass in hospital patients. It is not sensitive to weekly changes in lean body mass and should be used over longer periods. The creatinine height index is also useful for patients for whom measurements of weight and/or skinfolds are unobtainable or inaccurate (e.g. in patients with severe edema, marked obesity, and/or pendulous skinfolds).

Urinary creatinine is commonly assayed by the Jaffé reaction (Cook, 1975) using precise automated methods (Boileau et al., 1972). Urinary acetoacetate interferes with this method, making the creatinine height index an unsuitable index for insulinopenic (type I) diabetic patients who excrete large amounts of this metabolite in their urine (Bleiler and Schedl, 1962). So far, studies have revealed no predictive value of creatinine height index for morbidity and mortality (Mullen et al., 1979a).

16.1.2   3-Methylhistidine excretion

3-Methylhistidine (3-MH) is an amino acid present almost exclusively in
the actin of all skeletal muscle fibers and the myosin of white fibers. It is
formed by the methylation of histidine residues after the synthesis of actin
and myosin. When the proteins actin and myosin are catabolized, 3-MH
is released, but not recycled and reincorporated into protein. Instead,
it is excreted quantitatively into the urine without further metabolism.
Therefore, if muscle protein synthesis and catabolism in adults are
in balance, 3-MH excretion should reflect muscle mass, provided that
exogenous sources of 3-MH have been eliminated. The latter can be
achieved by placing the subjects on a meat-free diet for at least three
days prior to the urine collection. After such a period, mean daily 3-MH
excretion is relatively constant with a coefficient of variation of 4.5%
(Lukaski et al., 1981). Complete twenty-four-hour urine collections are
also essential for the measurement of 3-MH and should preferably be
collected over three consecutive twenty-four-hour periods. When the diet
contains meat, 3-MH excretion is significantly greater, the magnitude of
the increase depending on the 3-MH content of the meat consumed.

Several investigators have attempted to validate the relationship between 3-MH excretion and muscle mass in adults fed meat-free diets
(Lukaski et al., 1981). Results confirm that skeletal muscle mass, estimated from a mathematical model based on the measured ratio of total
body potassium to total body nitrogen, is related to endogenous urinary
3-MH excretion. Nevertheless, the use of 3-MH excretion as a routine index of muscle mass is not recommended at the present time. The precise
effects of factors such as sex, age, maturity, nutrition, hormonal status,
fitness, recent intense exercise, injury, and disease on excretion of 3-MH
have not been quantified (Buskirk and Mendez, 1985). For example, the
level of 3-MH excretion increases for up to forty-eight hours after periods of exercise. The effect appears to be greater after weight lifting than
running and is independent of meat consumption (Dohm et al., 1982).
Moreover, any catabolic state, such as fever, starvation, trauma, infection, etc., will increase muscle turnover and alter the relationship between
muscle mass and excretion of 3-MH, thus invalidating the index. Urinary
3-MH excretion may be useful for monitoring the effectiveness of nutritional support; the latter should result in a reduction in muscle protein
breakdown, indicated by a decrease in urinary 3-MH excretion. So far,
the predictive value of 3-MH as an index of morbidity and mortality has
not been extensively investigated.

Several precise methods are available for the analysis of 3-MH in urine.
Some involve the use of ion-exchange chromatography with ninhydrin or
ninhydrin-orthophthalaldehyde (Young et al., 1973; Ward, 1978; Vielma
et al., 1981), whereas others use high-performance liquid chromatography
(Wassner et al., 1980).

Protein	Half-Life	Body Pool Size g/kg body weight
Serum albumin	14–20 days	3–5
Serum transferrin	8–10 days	< 0.1 g
Serum thyroxine-binding pre-albumin (TBPA)	2–3 days	0.01
Serum retinol-binding protein (RBP)	12 hours	0.002

Table 16.3: Serum proteins of hepatic origin.

16.2 Assessment of visceral protein status

Visceral protein status is frequently assessed by the measurement of one or more of the serum proteins shown in Table 16.3. The main site of synthesis for most of these is the liver, one of the first organs to be affected by protein malnutrition. In such circumstances, the limited supply of protein substrate impairs the synthesis of serum proteins, resulting in a decline in serum protein concentrations.

Many non-nutritional factors influence the concentration of serum proteins (Table 16.4) and reduce their specificity and sensitivity (Golden, 1982). For example, reductions in many serum protein levels arising from stress occur so frequently in critically ill hospital patients that many investigators recommend using serum proteins *only* during convalescence. During this latter period, serum protein concentrations probably correlate with total body protein, although their rate of change may not be related to the relative change in body protein (Grant, 1986). During convalescence, serum proteins with short half-lives may provide an index of the effectiveness of nutritional therapy (Carpentier et al., 1982).

Serum proteins useful for measuring short-term changes in protein status have: a small body pool, a rapid rate of synthesis, a major proportion present within the vascular space, a fairly constant catabolic rate that responds specifically to protein-energy deprivation but is not affected by extraneous factors, and a very short biological half-life (Fischer, 1981).

16.2.1 Total serum protein

Total serum protein has been used as an index of visceral protein status in several national nutrition surveys (Health and Welfare Canada, 1973). It is easily measured, but is a rather insensitive index of protein status. For example, the total serum protein concentration is maintained initially within normal limits despite restricted protein intake and is only significantly depleted when clinical signs of protein malnutrition are apparent. The observed decline results largely from a marked decrease in the serum albumin concentrations which represent 50% to 60% of the total serum protein.

In severely ill hospital patients, blood products such as albumin are sometimes administered which may significantly affect the concentration of total serum protein. Furthermore, many other factors influence the concentration of total serum protein and hence compromise the specificity and sensitivity of this index (Table 16.4).

Table 16.5 presents the interpretive guidelines for total serum protein used by the ICNND (Sauberlich et al., 1974) and those used by the Nutrition Canada National Survey (Health and Welfare Canada, 1973).

16.2.2 Serum albumin

There is a relatively large body pool (3 to 5 g/kg body weight) of albumin, more than 50% of which is present outside the vascular space. Serum albumin reflects changes occurring within the intravascular space and not the total visceral protein pool. Serum albumin is not very sensitive to short-term changes in protein status; it has a long half-life, of fourteen to twenty days (Table 16.3). In addition, any reduction in hepatic synthesis of serum albumin is largely compensated by reduced catabolism. Redistribution of albumin from the extravascular to the intravascular space also occurs, and hence the net change in serum albumin level may be very small. Shetty et al. (1979), for example, observed no significant changes in serum albumin over a five-week period, after unstressed, obese subjects received a daily protein intake of only 20 g with and without energy restriction.

Serum albumin levels are also influenced by a variety of other conditioning factors, some of which are noted in Table 16.4. Low serum

---

- **Inadequate protein intake** resulting from:low dietary intakes, anorexia, unbalanced diets, hypocaloric intravenous infusions.

- **Altered metabolism** generated by: trauma, stress, sepsis, and hypoxia.

- **Specific deficiency of plasma proteins** caused by: protein-losing enteropathy, and liver disease.

- **Reduced protein synthesis** resulting from inadequate energy intake, electrolyte deficiency, trace element deficiencies (e.g. iron and zinc), vitamin deficiency (e.g. vitamin A).

- **Pregnancy** induces changes in the amount and distribution of body fluids.

- **Capillary permeability** changes.

- **Drugs** (e.g. oral contraceptive agents).

- **Strenuous exercise.**

Table 16.4: Factors affecting serum protein concentrations. Adapted from Jeejeebhoy (1981).

Subjects	Less than Acceptable		Acceptable (low risk)
	Deficient (high risk)	Low (medium risk)	
Sauberlich et al. (1974)			
Infants 0 to 11 months	—	< 5.0	≥ 5.0
Children 1 to 5 years	—	< 5.5	≥ 5.5
Children 6 to 17 years	—	< 6.0	≥ 6.0
Adults	< 6.0	6.0 to 6.4	≥ 6.5
Pregnant, 2nd and 3rd trimester	< 5.5	5.5 to 5.9	≥ 6.0
Health and Welfare Canada (1973)			
Infants 0 to 5 months	—	—	—
6 months to 71 months	< 5.0	5.0 to 6.0	> 6.0
≥ 6 years	< 6.0	6.0 to 6.4	> 6.4
Pregnant Women	< 5.5	5.5 to 6.0	> 6.0

Table 16.5: Guidelines for the interpretation of total serum protein concentrations (g/dL). Conversion factor to SI units (g/L) = × 10.0. Reproduced with permission from Sauberlich HE, Dowdy RP, Skala JH. (1974). Laboratory Tests for the Assessment of Nutritional Status. CRC Press, Inc., Boca Raton, FL., and the Minister of Supply and Services Canada.

albumin levels (hypo-albuminemia) may be generated in certain gastrointestinal and renal diseases by loss of protein, in liver disease and hypothyroidism by reduced protein synthesis, in congestive heart failure by increases in plasma volume, and in pregnancy by hemodilution. Infection and zinc depletion also reduce serum albumin levels (Taylor et al., 1949; Wahlqvist et al., 1981). In the presence of traumatic injury or ongoing stress, a shift of albumin from the intravascular to the extravascular space also results in a transient fall in serum albumin, whereas in semistarvation the opposite effect occurs. As a result, serum albumin concentrations are artificially elevated in semistarvation (James and Hay, 1968). In patients with dehydration, hyperalbuminemia may also occur as a result of diminished plasma volume. Age also influences serum albumin, concentrations declining in the elderly. This trend is probably associated with a decreased rate of albumin synthesis which responds slowly to increases in protein intake (Misra et al., 1975).

In developing countries, serum albumin concentrations may be used to identify malnourished children susceptible to edema, because hypoalbuminemia is a major contributory factor in the development of this condition (Whitehead et al., 1971). In such cases, a deficit in weight for age is not apparent (Table 16.6), and therefore an alternative index for identifying marginal kwashiorkor is essential. In contrast, in marasmus, there is no change in serum albumin concentration but deficits in weight for age are severe.

Group	Serum Albumin (g/dL) Mean ± SEM	Weight for Age Mean ± SEM
Children with early signs of edema (n = 33)	2.59 ± 0.09	76 ± 2
Children with no signs of edema (n = 65)	3.26 ± 0.5	79 ± 3
Significance of difference	$p < 0.001$	NS

Table 16.6: Comparison of serum albumin levels (g/dL) and weights for age (as percentage of Tanner and Whitehouse reference median) in two groups of Ugandan children. Conversion to SI units (g/L) = × 10. From Whitehead et al. (1971) with permission.

The use of serum albumin levels as a prognostic index for the development of postoperative complications has been extensively studied. Results have been inconsistent. Mullen et al. (1979b) reported that serum albumin levels less than 3.0 g/dL were associated with a complication rate two and half times greater than that of patients with levels above 3.0 g/dL. In contrast, Ryan and Taft (1980) found no relationship between plasma albumin levels and complication rate after major abdominal surgery.

Serum albumin is assayed in most clinical laboratories via an automated dye-binding method using bromocresol green (McPherson and Everard, 1972). Other methods include standard electrophoresis and salt fractionation. Values for serum albumin depend on the separation method used; salting out procedures give consistently higher values than those using electrophoresis. These differences should be taken into account when interpreting serum albumin levels. The interpretive guidelines for serum albumin compiled by Sauberlich et al. (1974) are shown in Table 16.7.

16.2.3   Serum transferrin

Transferrin is a serum β-globulin protein synthesized primarily in the liver but, unlike albumin, it is located almost totally intravascularly. Transferrin serves as the iron transport protein, each molecule of transferrin binding with two molecules of iron. Normally, in well nourished persons, 30% to 40% of transferrin is used for iron transport. Transferrin is also bacteriostatic: it binds with free iron and prevents the growth of gram-negative bacteria which require iron for growth.

Transferrin has a shorter half-life of eight to ten days (Table 16.3) and a smaller body pool (< 100 mg/kg body weight) than albumin and therefore responds more rapidly to changes in protein status. Nevertheless, there is a wide range of serum transferrin concentrations among malnourished subjects, both before and during refeeding (Ingenbleek et al., 1975). Unfortunately, serum transferrin concentrations, like serum albumin concentrations, are affected by a variety of factors, including gastrointestinal,

Subjects	Less than Acceptable		Acceptable (low risk)
	Deficient (high risk)	Low (medium risk)	
Infants 0 to 11 months	—	< 2.5	≥ 2.5
Children 1 to 5 years	< 2.8	< 3.0	≥ 3.0
Children 6 to 17 years	< 2.8	< 3.5	≥ 3.5
Adults	< 2.8	2.8 to 3.4	≥ 3.5
Pregnant, 1st trimester	< 3.0	3.0 to 3.9	≥ 4.0
Pregnant, 2nd and 3rd trimester	< 3.0	3.0 to 3.4	≥ 3.5

Table 16.7: Interpretive guidelines for serum albumin concentrations (g/dL). Conversion to SI units (g/L) = × 10.0. Reproduced with permission from Sauberlich HE, Dowdy RP, Skala JH. (1974). Laboratory Tests for the Assessment of Nutritional Status. CRC Press, Inc., Boca Raton, FL.

	Group I Mean ± SE	Group II Mean ± SE	p
Age (months)	32.8 ± 2.3	27.6 ± 2.5	NS
Weight for height (%)	90.6 ± 1.6	91.4 ± 1.9	NS
Height for age (%)	93.8 ± 0.6	91.0 ± 0.9	< 0.05
Fe (μmol/L)	11.7 ± 1.1	7.8 ± 1.0	< 0.01
Transferrin (mg/L)	3513 ± 86	3907 ± 175	< 0.05
% Transferrin sat.	15.8 ± 1.5	9.8 ± 1.3	< 0.01
Prealbumin (mg/L)	125 ± 6	97 ± 7	< 0.01

Table 16.8: Biochemical and other comparative data for two groups children from northern Cameroon, grouped according to their blood hemoglobin concentrations (Group I: > 100 g/L; Group II: < 80 g/L). From Delpeuch F, Cornu A, Chevalier P. (1980). The effect of iron-deficiency anaemia on two indices of nutritional status, prealbumin and transferrin. British Journal of Nutrition 43: 375–379. With permission of Cambridge University Press.

renal, and liver diseases, congestive heart failure, and inflammation. Concentrations also fall when the requirements for iron transport are reduced because of decreased iron absorption (e.g. in conditions of chronic infection, iron overload, and pernicious anemia). Conversely, iron deficiency leads to an increased transferrin synthesis in response to increased iron absorption, producing elevated serum transferrin levels. The latter also occur in pregnancy, during estrogen therapy, and during acute hepatitis. In concomitant protein-energy malnutrition and iron deficiency, therefore, a decrease in transferrin concentrations may be masked by an increase caused by iron deficiency (Table 16.8).

In cases of severe kwashiorkor, when liver function is impaired, there may be no concomitant increase in transferrin synthesis in the liver despite the presence of iron deficiency. In general, serum transferrin is not an appropriate index of protein status where both iron deficiency anemia and chronic protein-energy malnutrition are widespread. Instead, alternative serum proteins should be selected.

Despite these confounding effects, some associations between serum transferrin concentrations and poor prognosis in children with kwashiorkor (McFarlane et al., 1969; McFarlane et al., 1970; Gabr et al., 1971) and marasmus (Reeds and Laditan, 1976) have been reported. Reeds and Laditan demonstrated a linear relationship between serum transferrin concentrations and deficits in weight and length for age in undernourished children. The response of serum transferrin levels to dietary treatment has been less predictable (Ingenbleek et al., 1975; Shetty et al., 1979). Studies of the value of serum transferrin to predict morbidity and mortality in hospital patients have produced conflicting results. Some studies suggest that the concentration of serum transferrin, either individually or as part of a multi-parameter index (Section 26.2), is one of the strongest predictors of patient morbidity and mortality (Kaminski et al., 1977; Mullen et al., 1979a) whereas others have not confirmed these findings (Ryan and Taft, 1980).

Serum transferrin concentrations are assayed by a radial-immuno-diffusion technique. This method is expensive, time consuming, and not routinely performed in most clinical laboratories. Instead, serum transferrin is estimated indirectly, using a prediction equation based on total iron-binding capacity. If this practice is adopted, a prediction equation specific for the analytical methods used for serum transferrin and total iron-binding capacity (TIBC) should be established (Stromberg et al., 1982) and the confounding effect of concurrent disorders such as iron deficiency, iron overload, pregnancy, and chronic infections on the TIBC transferrin relationship recognized. Leonberg et al. (1987) have developed an accurate and precise assay for plasma transferrin based on an antigen-antibody reaction using commercially available transferrin antibody. The method requires only 15 µL of plasma and is rapid (sixty to ninety minutes) and easily performed. Interpretive guidelines for serum transferrin values are shown in Table 16.9.

16.2.4 Serum retinol-binding protein

Retinol-binding protein (RBP) is the carrier protein for retinol, with a single binding site for one molecule of retinol. The resultant complex of retinol-binding protein + retinol is the smallest of the circulatory serum proteins. The complex travels together with one molecule of plasma thyroxine-binding pre-albumin (TBPA) to form a trimolecular complex of retinol, retinol-binding protein, and TBPA. In this way, loss of retinol during filtration at the kidney glomerulus is prevented.

Parameter	Protein Deficit			
	None	Mild	Moderate	Severe
Transferrin (mg/dL)	> 200	150–200	100–150	< 100
Retinol-binding Protein (mg/dL)	2.6–7.6	—	—	—
Thyroxine-binding Prealbumin (mg/dL)	15.7–29.6	10–15	5–10	< 5

Table 16.9: Interpretive guidelines for serum transferrin, retinol-binding protein, and thyroxine-binding pre-albumin. Conversion factors to SI units (g/L) = × 0.01. Modified from Grant et al. (1981).

As the half-life of RBP is about twelve hours (Table 16.3), and the body pool is small (2 mg/kg body weight), serum RBP concentrations tend to fall rapidly in response to protein and, to a lesser extent, energy deprivation, and respond quickly to dietary treatment (Shetty et al., 1979). For example, low levels were observed in obese subjects following a low-protein diet with and without energy restriction (Table 16.10) (Shetty et al., 1979), and in children with marasmus, kwashiorkor, and marasmic kwashiorkor (Smith et al., 1975). Later more detailed studies of children with both vitamin A deficiency and protein-energy malnutrition indicated that retinol-binding protein synthesis is, in fact, less affected in marasmus than kwashiorkor (Large et al., 1980).

Unfortunately, like other serum transport proteins, the specificity of RBP as an index of protein status is low. Some of the factors affecting concentrations of RBP are similar to those described earlier for serum albumin and serum transferrin. For example, concentrations generally fall in liver diseases such as cirrhosis and hepatitis, presumably as a result of interference with the storage and synthesis of retinol-binding protein in the liver. Likewise, serum RBP concentrations are reduced in vitamin A deficiency, acute catabolic states, postsurgery, and hyperthyroidism. In chronic renal disease, serum RBP may actually increase, because RBP is catabolized in the renal proximal tubular cell. As a result, the half-life of RBP in increased.

A fall in serum RBP levels is also observed during deficiencies of vitamin A or zinc, in response to a reduced demand for the vitamin A transport protein. The latter occurs because deficiencies of both vitamin A and zinc inhibit the mobilization of RBP from the liver (Muhilal and Glover, 1974; Jacob et al., 1978). Following vitamin A or zinc supplementation, serum RBP levels rise. Decreased levels of serum RBP have been noted in cases of cystic fibrosis, possibly associated with a defect at the molecular level and/or release of retinol-binding complex from the liver (Smith et al., 1972; Jacob et al., 1978). Retinol-binding protein, unlike serum transferrin, is not affected by iron-deficiency anemia.

Energy Intake	80 g Protein/Day	60 g Protein/Day	40 g Protein/Day	20 g Protein/Day
	Plasma-RBP (Mean ± SEM mg/dL)			
High-energy diet				
Day 10	5.7 ± 0.5	6.9 ± 0.2 *	5.4 ± 0.5	3.7 ± 0.4
Low-energy diet				
Day 6	5.1 ± 0.3	5.3 ± 0.3	3.5 ± 0.6	—
Day 12	5.4 ± 0.3	4.4 ± 0.5	3.3 ± 0.9	2.9 ± 1.1
Day 24	3.6 ± 0.5	3.6 ± 0.1	3.4 ± 0.9	3.3 ± 0.5
Refeeding (Day 4)	—	7.2 ± 0.9	—	—
	Plasma-TBPA (Mean ± SEM mg/dL)			
High-energy diet				
Day 10	29.8 ± 1.4	29.8 ± 0.5 *	29.0 ± 4.0	24.0 ± 3.2
Low-energy diet				
Day 6	28.0 ± 1.8	16.6 ± 1.4	20.8 ± 3.2	15.3 ± 1.2
Day 12	20.8 ± 4.3	19.9 ± 1.4	16.7 ± 2.0	14.7 ± 3.4
Day 24	19.3 ± 1.9	16.9 ± 2.7	15.0 ± 1.0	12.7 ± 2.9
Refeeding (Day 4)	—	24.0 ± 5.3	—	—

Table 16.10: Changes in plasma-RBP and -TBPA on energy and/or protein restriction with four obese adults in each treatment group. * observation from day 7. Conversion to SI units (g/L) = × 0.01. Modified from Shetty et al. (1979) with permission.

Serum retinol-binding protein, like transferrin, is also measured by radial-immunodiffusion techniques. As the normal levels are low (2.6 to 7.6 mg/dL; mean 5.1 ± 2.5 mg/dL), it is difficult to measure precisely. Interpretive guidelines for serum RBP concentrations are not clearly established (Table 16.9).

16.2.5   Serum thyroxine-binding pre-albumin

Thyroxine-binding pre-albumin (TBPA) serves as a transport protein for thyroxine, and as a carrier protein for RBP (Section 16.2.4). Although TBPA has a half-life of two days (Table 16.3) and a slightly larger body pool (10 mg/kg body weight) than that of RBP, the sensitivities of these two serum proteins to protein deprivation and treatment are similar. Serum levels of TBPA are four to five times higher than those of RBP and are easier to assay. Concentrations are determined by overall energy and nitrogen balance (Golden, 1982). Serum TBPA is a more sensitive index of protein status and responds more rapidly to dietary treatment than serum albumin or transferrin (Shetty et al., 1979). Indeed, TBPA concentrations have been normalized after giving total parenteral nutrition to severely depleted patients for only four days (Carpentier et al., 1982).

The presence of other diseases, such as gastrointestinal diseases, renal and kidney diseases, surgical trauma, stress, inflammation, and infection, all lead to modifications in the metabolism of TBPA and reduce its specificity as an index of protein status (Farthing, 1982). Furthermore, because TBPA, like RBP, is extremely sensitive to even minor stress and inflammation, decreasing markedly in such conditions, it is not a very useful index for critically ill patients. Patients with acute renal failure may have increased serum TBPA values because of the role of the kidneys in thyroxine pre-albumin catabolism (Young et al., 1975). Deficiencies of vitamin A, zinc, and iron do not affect the levels of TBPA, but may modify the concentrations of RBP and/or transferrin, as noted previously.

Smith et al. (1975) found that serum TBPA concentrations were equally low in kwashiorkor, marasmic kwashiorkor, and marasmus. Shetty et al. (1979), however, reported that serum TBPA concentrations did not respond to a short-term protein restriction (e.g. ten days) when energy intake was maintained, but levels fell markedly when both energy, and to a lesser extent protein intakes, were restricted (Table 16.10). Ogunshina and Hussain (1980) noted an inverse relationship between plasma TBPA values and the severity of malnutrition, assessed by the anthropometric classification of Waterlow (1972) (Figure 16.1) (Section 13.2.5).

Radial-immunodiffusion techniques are also used to determine TBPA. Thyroxine-binding pre-albumin values appear to vary according to age, and sex (Carpentier and Ingenbleek, 1983), and possibly ethnic group and geographical area (Ingenbleek et al., 1975), although the reasons for these differences are unclear at present. Genetic, nutritional factors, and/or the presence of infections have all been implicated. Therefore, it is preferable to compare values for TBPA with those for a control group matched by age, geographical area, and ethnic group. Serum TBPA values for preschool children are lower than for adults, rising markedly at the onset of puberty. Healthy adult females have lower values than males. Reported mean concentrations for healthy adult males and females vary widely (Buckell et al., 1979; Ingenbleek and De Visscher, 1979); the normal lower limit ranges from 100 mg/L (Buckell et al., 1979) to 240 mg/L (Carpentier and Ingenbleek 1983). Age- and sex-specific interpretive values are not yet available. Tentative interpretive values are given in the summary Table 16.9.

16.2.6 Serum somatomedin-C

Somatomedins are growth-hormone dependent serum growth factors produced by the liver. They have a proinsulin-like structure and broad anabolic properties. Somatomedins circulate bound to carrier proteins and have a half-life of several hours (Phillips and Vassilopoulou-Sellin, 1980). In studies of children with chronic undernutrition, decreased concentrations of circulating somatomedin in the serum occur, which respond rapidly to dietary treatment (Smith et al., 1981). When acutely malnourished patients receive nutritional support for three to sixteen days, somatomedin-C levels increase from initial levels, although no significant changes in serum albumin, transferrin, RBP, or TBPA concentrations

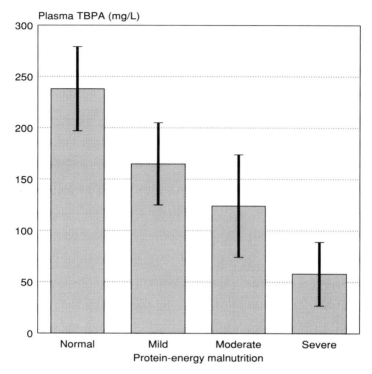

Figure 16.1: Plasma TBPA (mean ± SE) levels in children classified as normal, or with mild, moderate, and severe protein-energy
malnutrition according to the Waterlow classification of protein-energy malnutrition. From Ogunshina and Hussain (1980).
© Am. J. Clin. Nutr. American Society for Clinical Nutrition.

occur (Unterman et al., 1985). These results suggest that serum
somatomedin-C may be more sensitive to acute changes in protein status
than the other serum proteins. Nevertheless, more studies are necessary
to establish the sensitivity and specificity of somatomedin-C measurements as an index of malnutrition and as a marker for the response
to nutritional therapy. Reductions in serum somatomedin-C values occur in patients with hypothyroidism, and with estrogen administration.
Somatomedin-C can be assayed using a radio-immunoassay method
(Furlanetto et al., 1977).

16.3   Metabolic changes as indices of protein status

Several striking changes in metabolism develop in protein-energy malnutrition, some of which can be used to distinguish between marasmus and
kwashiorkor. For example, in marasmus, fasting serum insulin levels are
low, whereas in kwashiorkor they are elevated (Coward and Lunn, 1981).

This latter hyperinsulinemia results in characteristic alterations in serum amino-acid concentrations via its effect on muscle protein synthesis. Other metabolic changes, such as reduced urinary hydroxyproline excretion and increased urinary nitrogen excretion, occur in both the kwashiorkor and marasmic forms of protein-energy malnutrition, and are used as less specific indices of protein-energy malnutrition.

16.3.1 Serum amino-acid ratio

Measurement of the serum ratio of nonessential (NEAA) to essential amino acids (EAA) as an index of kwashiorkor was developed by Whitehead and Dean (1964). The EAA, particularly the branched-chain amino acids leucine, isoleucine, and valine, as well as methionine, fall to low concentrations in the serum of children with kwashiorkor, whereas the NEAA, especially glycine, tend to remain normal, or even rise. Hence, the ratio of NEAA to EAA rises in these children. In addition, phenylalanine hydroxylase activity declines, and conversion of phenylalanine to tyrosine is impaired. Consequently, the serum ratio of phenylalanine to tyrosine also rises. Such changes in serum amino-acid levels are not found in normal children, or those with marasmus, and are attributed to changes in hormonal profiles of children with kwashiorkor (Coward and Lunn, 1981). Children with kwashiorkor generally have serum NEAA : EAA ratios above three, whereas for normal children and those with marasmus, ratios are usually less than two (Simmons, 1970).

$$\text{Amino-acid ratio (NEAA : EAA)} = \frac{\text{Glycine + serine + glutamine + taurine}}{\text{Isoleucine + leucine + valine + methionine}}$$

The absence of an elevated serum NEAA : EAA ratio in children with marasmus may result from the metabolic adaptation to an inadequate energy intake. Children with marasmus have low serum insulin concentrations in response to their reduced food intake (Coward and Lunn, 1981). Low serum insulin concentrations may induce the release of energy metabolites from endogenous sources (Cahill, 1970). As a result, EAA are released from skeletal muscle for gluconeogenesis and probably for serum protein synthesis in the liver, maintaining the serum amino acid ratio within normal levels.

The serum NEAA : EAA ratios are not always consistent with the type or severity of protein-energy malnutrition. Such inconsistencies have been attributed to the confounding effects of infections, diarrhea, energy deficits, etc. (Simmons, 1970). Marked changes in the ratios are evident only in children with frank kwashiorkor.

A simplified technique to determine serum amino-acid ratios using one-dimensional paper chromatography and a finger prick blood sample was developed for field survey use (Whitehead and Dean, 1964). Three of the separated amino acids are then detected by spraying the dried chromatogram with a solution of ninhydrin in acetone. The amino acids

	Less than Acceptable		Acceptable (low risk)
	Deficient (high risk)	Low (medium risk)	
Nonessential : essential amino acid ratio (NEAA : EAA) (all ages)	> 3.0	2.0–3.0	< 2.0
Hydroxyproline index (3 months to 10 years of age)	< 1.0	1.0–2.0	> 2.0
Creatinine height index (3 months to 17 years of age)	< 0.5	0.5–0.9	> 0.9
Urea nitrogen : creatinine ratio	< 6.0	6.0–12.0	> 12.0

Table 16.11: Guidelines for the interpretation of serum nonessential : essential amino-acid ratios, urinary hydroxyproline index, creatinine height index, and urinary urea nitrogen : creatinine ratios. Reproduced with permission from Sauberlich HE, Dowdy RP, Skala JH. (1974). Laboratory Tests for the Assessment of Nutritional Status. CRC Press, Inc., Boca Raton, FL.

combine with the ninhydrin to give a blue-violet-colored compound and hence appear as blue-violet spots on the paper. The spots corresponding to the NEAA glycine, and the EAA leucine + valine are cut out, eluted, and the absorption of the eluate measured spectrophotometrically. The following ratio can then be calculated:

$$\text{Simplified amino-acid ratio} = \frac{\text{Glycine}}{\text{Leucine} + \text{valine}}$$

Fasting blood samples are recommended because serum amino-acid patterns can be influenced by recent dietary intake. Alternatively, blood samples can be taken four hours after the most recent meal. Interpretive guidelines suggested by Whitehead and Dean (1964) for serum NEAA : EAA ratios are shown in Table 16.11.

In general, serum amino-acid concentrations are not sensitive indices of protein-energy malnutrition because the regulatory systems for the maintenance of serum amino-acid concentrations are very effective. Future laboratory tests may include a test which measures the rate of clearance of a standard amino-acid load from blood (Harper, 1981).

16.3.2   Urinary 3-hydroxyproline excretion

Urinary 3-hydroxyproline, principally in the peptide form, is an excretory product derived from the soluble and insoluble collagens of both soft and calcified tissues. In malnourished children with impaired growth, resulting from kwashiorkor, marasmus, or marasmic kwashiorkor, urinary hydroxyproline excretion levels are significantly lower compared to age-matched well-nourished controls. In adults, levels of 3-hydroxyproline in the urine are often used to diagnose certain bone and connective tissue or endocrine disorders.

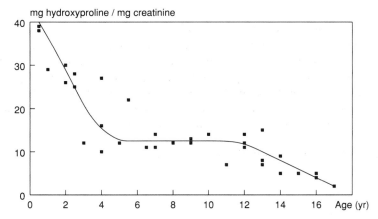

Figure 16.2: The hydroxyproline : creatinine ratio of normal individuals from six months to seventeen years. From Allison DJ, Walker A, Smith QT. (1966). Urinary hydroxyproline : creatinine ratio of normal humans at various ages. Clinica Chimica Acta 14: 729–734. With permission of authors and Elsevier Science Publishers BV (Biomedical Division).

Several extraneous factors influence urinary hydroxyproline excretion. These include the ingestion of collagen or gelatin, sex, age, the presence of certain disease states, and hookworm and/or malarial infestations (Whitehead, 1967). Males, for example, have greater amounts of soft and calcified tissue and excrete larger amounts of hydroxyproline. Differences in growth velocity account for the age-related changes, excretion rising rapidly during periods of fast growth. Increases in the excretion of hydroxyproline also occur in diseases associated with disturbances in collagen metabolism, such as rheumatoid arthritis, and in sprue and rheumatic fever (LeRoy, 1967).

The marked changes in hydroxyproline excretion with age and sex necessitate the use of age- and sex-specific interpretive reference data. Consequently, investigators have developed alternative methods for evaluating urinary hydroxyproline excretion levels which are independent of age. Methods for expressing hydroxyproline excretion include:

The hydroxyproline : creatinine ratio

This ratio corrects at least partially for differences in adult body size.

$$\frac{\text{Hydroxyproline (mg) per 24 hr}}{\text{Creatinine (mg) per 24 hr}}$$

As a result, ratios in adults are independent of age and are the same for males and females. For children, however, the ratio changes rapidly with age (Figure 16.2); hydroxyproline decreases with age while creatinine excretion increases.

% Standard Weight for Age	n	Hydroxyproline Index
< 70%	6	1.1 ± 0.4
71–80%	9	1.4 ± 0.5
81–90%	15	1.7 ± 0.6
> 90%	26	2.7 ± 1.0
Kwashiorkor	10	0.9 ± 0.3
Marasmus	8	1.1 ± 0.4
Upper-middle-class children < 4 yr	42	2.9 ± 0.9

Table 16.12: Hydroxyproline index (mean ± SD) in relation to weight deficit (n = number of subjects). Modified from Whitehead (1965) with permission.

The hydroxyproline index

In an attempt to take body weight into account, Whitehead (1965) developed the hydroxyproline index as an age-independent interpretive standard for children.

$$\text{Hydroxyproline index} = \frac{\text{mg hydroxyproline per mL urine}}{\text{mg creatinine per mL urine}} \times \text{kg body weight}$$

In normal children, between one and six years of age, the hydroxyproline index is relatively constant and is approximately 3.0. In malnourished children, however, the hydroxyproline index is low, irrespective of the type of malnutrition, but is statistically related to the extent of the growth deficit (Whitehead, 1965) (Table 16.12).

Interpretive guidelines for the hydroxyproline index, applicable to infants and children from three months to ten years of age, are: deficient (high risk) < 1.0; low (medium risk) 1.0 to 2.0; and acceptable (low risk) > 2.0 (Sauberlich et al., 1974).

Several methods have been used to analyze hydroxyproline in urine (Prockop and Udenfriend, 1960; LeRoy, 1967; Dabev and Struck, 1971). For the method of Prockop and Udenfriend (1960), the urine samples are first hydrolyzed, then decolorized and neutralized prior to oxidation to pyrrole. The pyrrole is estimated colorimetrically after coupling with 4-dimethylaminobenzaldehyde.

16.3.3 Nitrogen balance

Nitrogen balance is a measure of net changes in total body protein mass. The method is based on the assumption that nearly all of total body nitrogen is incorporated into protein. As protein contains 16% nitrogen:

$$\text{Nitrogen (g)} = \frac{\text{Protein (g)}}{6.25}$$

In healthy adults with adequate energy and nutrient intakes, nitrogen losses are dependent primarily on the amounts and proportions of essential amino acids in the diet, and the total nitrogen intake. When such intakes are adequate to replace the endogenous nitrogen losses and for the growth of hair and nails, the subject is said to be in nitrogen balance. A numerical expression for nitrogen balance is:

$$\text{Nitrogen balance} = I - (U - U_e) + (F - F_e) + S$$

where I = nitrogen intake (grams protein / 6.25); U = total urinary nitrogen; U_e = endogenous urinary nitrogen; F = nitrogen voided in feces (as unabsorbed protein); F_e = endogenous fecal nitrogen losses; S = dermal nitrogen losses.

When nitrogen intake exceeds nitrogen output, subjects are in positive balance. This occurs during growth, late pregnancy, athletic training, and recovery from illness. In contrast, when nitrogen output exceeds nitrogen intake, subjects are in negative nitrogen balance. A negative nitrogen balance of 1 g/day is equivalent to a reduction in total body protein of 6.25 g/day. If the negative balance persists, the resultant protein depletion may have adverse effects on all organ systems. Factors which may precipitate a negative nitrogen balance include: inadequate protein and/or energy intakes; an imbalance in EAA : NEAA; conditions of accelerated protein catabolism (e.g. trauma, infection, sepsis, and burns) and excessive loss of nitrogen arising from fistulas or excessive diarrhea. The range of nitrogen balance values observed in hospital patients can vary from +4 to -20 grams of nitrogen per day. An estimate of the *change* in nitrogen balance, rather than a single measurement, is preferred to monitor the effectiveness of nutritional therapy.

Approximately 90% to 95% of daily nitrogen losses is excreted in the urine, the remainder being lost through the skin, stools, hair, and nails. Consequently, measurements of urinary nitrogen excretion and nitrogen intake over a defined period of time can be used to estimate the state of nitrogen balance. Total urinary nitrogen levels are seldom measured in routine hospital clinical laboratories because the conventional Kjeldahl technique is very time consuming and laborious. Instead, urinary urea nitrogen is more frequently determined. The method is simple and can be modified for an auto-analyzer. In addition, more than 80% to 90% of the total nitrogen in the urine is normally excreted as urea; excretion of the nonurea nitrogen components (e.g. creatinine nitrogen 6.4%, ammonia nitrogen 7.4%, uric acid nitrogen 2% to 3%, and other minor nitrogenous compounds 1% to 2%) remains fairly stable on a general diet (Allison and Bird, 1977). Figure 16.3 depicts the relationship between measured total urinary nitrogen and measured urinary urea nitrogen observed in 81 patients for 564 study days and with a variety of clinical and nutritional conditions. The difference between the total nitrogen and the urea nitrogen in the urine averaged 1.8 g/day (range 0 to 5.8 g/day) with

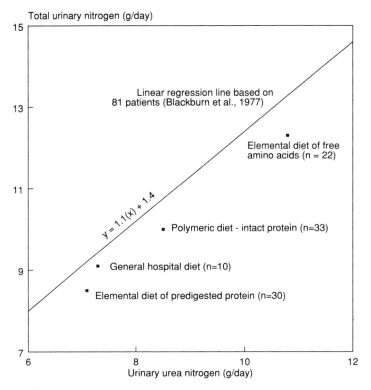

Figure 16.3: The relationship of total urinary nitrogen to urinary urea nitrogen for eighty-one subjects and four groups of hospital patients. From Blackburn GL, Bistrain BR, Maini BS, Schlamm HT, Smith MF. (1977). Nutritional and metabolic assessment of the hospitalized patient. Journal of Parenteral and Enteral Nutrition 1: 11–22. © Am. Soc. for Parenteral and Enteral Nutrition, 1977, and from Allison JB, Bird JWC (1977). Elimination of nitrogen from the body. In: Munro HN, Allison JB (eds). Mammalian Protein Metabolism. Volume 1. American Medical Association, pages 141–146. © Academic Press.

a standard deviation of 0.9 g/day (Blackburn et al., 1977; MacKenzie et al., 1985). On the basis of these results, an estimate of 2 g of nitrogen per day is commonly used for the nonurea nitrogen components of the urine.

When protein intakes are low, urinary nitrogen excretion falls and the urea nitrogen accounts for a decreasing percentage of total urinary nitrogen (e.g. 61% to 70%) (Allison and Bird, 1977) (Figure 16.4). In such circumstances, urinary urea nitrogen excretion is no longer a valid index of total urinary nitrogen excretion, and total urinary nitrogen must be determined. In contrast, increased excretion of urea (ureagenesis) occurs when diets are based on proteins of low biological

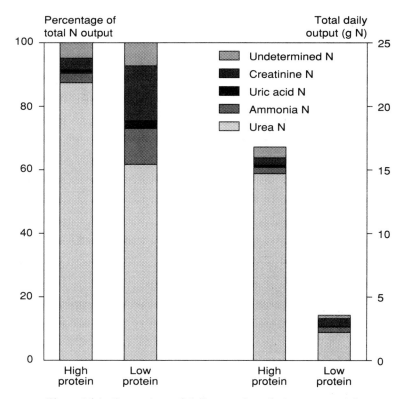

Figure 16.4: Comparison of daily excretion of nitrogen-containing compounds for subjects on high- and low-protein diets. Modified from Allison JB, Bird JWC (1977). Elimination of nitrogen from the body. In: Munro HN, Allison JB (eds). Mammalian Protein Metabolism. Volume 1. American Medical Association, pages 141–146. With permission © Academic Press.

value, or parenteral or enteral solutions containing certain amino acids (e.g. arginine and glutamine) are administered.

Nitrogen intake is generally estimated from the protein intake. For mixed diets, approximately 16% of the protein intake can be assumed to be nitrogen. For parenteral solutions containing free amino acids, specific conversion factors can be used to calculate the nitrogen content exactly. Alternatively, nitrogen intakes can be determined accurately by analyzing the nitrogen content of the diets or parenteral/enteral formulas using the micro-Kjeldahl technique.

When urinary urea nitrogen is used to estimate nitrogen balance, two correction factors are necessary: (a) 2 g for the dermal and fecal losses of nitrogen which also occur but are not measured; and (b) 2 g for the nonurea nitrogen components of the urine (e.g. ammonia, uric acid, and creatinine (MacKenzie et al., 1985). The equation most commonly employed is therefore:

$$\text{Estimated nitrogen balance} = \frac{\text{Protein intake (g)}}{6.25} - (\text{urinary urea nitrogen (g)} + 4)$$

This equation is not appropriate in certain circumstances. For example, the unmeasured nitrogen losses from the integument, sweat, exfoliated skin, and growing hair and nails vary, and may be greater or less than normal in patients with certain disease states and burns, or increase with sweating and nitrogen intake (Kopple, 1987). Calloway et al. (1971) estimated skin nitrogen loss as 5 mg/kg body weight per day on a normal mixed diet, and 3 mg/kg body weight per day on a protein-free formula. Likewise, fecal losses of nitrogen can also vary. In patients with malabsorption, fecal losses may be as high as 3.5 g/day (41%), whereas for patients on free-amino-acid formula feedings, fecal losses are much lower (i.e. 0.2 g/day). Therefore, for patients with malabsorption, fecal nitrogen should be measured on a timed stool specimen. Furthermore, the equation is not appropriate for calculating nitrogen balance during severe energy restriction or starvation. In such circumstances, the production of renal ammonia is increased to such an extent that the nonurea nitrogen correction factor of 2 g is inadequate (Winterer et al., 1980). Increases in urinary ammonia also occur in metabolic acidosis; in metabolic alkalosis, decreases are noted. The equation also has limited use in nitrogen-retention diseases such as renal or hepatic failure. In such cases, the nitrogen balance must be adjusted for changes in body urea nitrogen (BUN) by using the following equations:

$$\text{Adjusted N balance} = \text{Measured N balance} - \text{change in body urea nitrogen (BUN)}$$

$$\text{Change in BUN (g)} = ((\text{SUN}_f - \text{SUN}_i) \times \text{BW}_i \times 0.6) + ((\text{BW}_f - \text{BW}_i) \times \text{SUN}_f \times 1.0)$$

where BW = body weight (kg), SUN = serum urea nitrogen (g/L), and the suffixes i and f indicate the initial and final values of the measurement (Harvey et al., 1980). In this equation, the fraction of the body weight that is water is assumed to be 0.6. Unfortunately, although this fraction varies depending on the age and condition of the patient, no simple corrections are available. For example, in lean patients or those with edema, the fraction (i.e. 0.6) is too low whereas in obese or very young persons, the fraction is too high (Kopple, 1987).

To assess nitrogen balance in hospital patients, it is preferable to use at least three consecutive, complete twenty-four-hour urine collections, because intra-subject variation for urinary nitrogen excretion can be large. The urine collections should be made after an equilibrium period, to allow for readjustment to a new, steady-state level of nitrogen balance. The length of the readjustment period required depends on the relative change in protein intake. Care must be taken to avoid spills, discards, or inadvertent omissions of urine during collection, because these lead to a positive error in the nitrogen balance. A simplified system has

- Balance studies are expensive to perform.

- Balance procedures require substantial time of the patient and staff.

- Losses of foods that adhere to dishware, cooking, and eating utensils lead to an overestimate of intake.

- Losses of feces or urine on toilet paper and in stool and urine containers lead to an underestimate of output.

- Unmeasured losses from skin (including exfoliated cells, sweat, hair and nail growth), flatus respiration, toothbrushing, menstrual fluid, semen, and blood sampling lead to an underestimate of output. Some of these unmeasured outputs are not constant and can vary with intake (e.g. nitrogen), the degree of sweating, and disease state.

- Difficulty in precise collections of fistula or wound drainage, or, in incontinent individuals, of urine or stool, leads to errors in measurement of output.

- The intake and excretion of nitrogenous compounds are not measured by standard techniques (e.g. nitrate) and may introduce errors.

- The balance value is usually a relatively small number calculated as the difference between two much larger numbers (intake and output). Hence, small percentage errors in these latter measurements can lead to large errors in the calculated balance.

- Cumulative balance measurements (e.g. calculation of the total positive or negative balance over the entire period of study) are particularly likely to be erroneous.

- Balance studies are a type of 'black box' procedure: the fate of the compounds ingested, their intermediary metabolism, and the tissue or cellular sources of the nitrogen outputs are not defined by the balance technique.

Table 16.13: Limitations and sources of error in balance studies. From Kopple JD. (1987). Uses and limitations of the balance technique. Journal of Parenteral and Enteral Nutrition 11: 79S–85S. © Am. Soc. for Parenteral and Enteral Nutrition, 1987.

been devised for collecting twenty-four-hour urine samples in the field, which is easily transported, and readily cleaned (Mann, 1988). Using this system, subjects can collect an accurate aliquot of each urine sample voided during a twenty-four-hour period, in a container which can later be mailed to the laboratory. Urea nitrogen in the urine can be assessed by an enzymatic method of Searcy et al. (1965). Table 16.13 lists some of the sources of error and limitations of the nitrogen balance studies, which must be kept in mind when interpreting nitrogen balance results.

Once nitrogen intake and urinary urea nitrogen excretion have been determined, an estimate of the apparent net protein utilization can be derived using the following relationship:

$$\text{Apparent net protein utilization} = \frac{P}{6.25} - \frac{(UUN + 2 - N_L) \times 6.25}{P}$$

where P = protein intake (g), UUN = urinary urea nitrogen (g), and N_L = obligatory nitrogen loss (approximately 0.1 g for each kilogram of ideal body weight) (Blackburn et al., 1977).

16.3.4   Urinary urea nitrogen : creatinine ratios

Estimations of nitrogen balance are seldom made in field surveys because twenty-four-hour urine collections are impractical. Instead, first-voided, fasting urine specimens are sometimes collected and urinary urea nitrogen : creatinine ratios determined. Urea, as discussed above, is the largest source of urinary nitrogen and is synthesized in the liver by the Krebs-Henseleit cycle. Urinary urea nitrogen : creatinine ratios have been used as an index of dietary protein intake because several studies have reported a relationship between the level of protein intake and the ratio (Simmons, 1972; Allison and Bird, 1977). The ratios do not, however, provide an index of long-term protein status.

Creatinine excretion is measured in an attempt to take into account variations in urine volume, on the assumption that excretion of creatinine is relatively constant over a twenty-four-hour period. Nevertheless, many factors affect urinary creatinine excretion (Section 16.1.1) and thus severely limit the use of this ratio as an index of protein intake of individuals. If this ratio is used to compare the adequacy of dietary protein intakes of groups, the time of day for urine collection should be standardized — preferably by using the next urine sample after the first-voided, morning, fasting sample. Such samples will minimize the effect of diuresis on urea output. If possible, dietary intake data should also be collected to provide confirmatory information on dietary protein intakes.

Several extraneous factors can affect urinary urea nitrogen : creatinine ratios. Those specific for urinary creatinine have been discussed in Section 16.1.1. Conditions such as trauma, sepsis, infections, burns, fistulas, and diarrhea all increase the level of urinary nitrogen excretion and hence, in turn, excretion of urea. The latter is also influenced by the presence of urinary tract infections which reduce the glomerular filtration rate. Interpretive guidelines used for urinary urea nitrogen : creatinine ratios are shown in Table 16.11 (Sauberlich et al., 1974). Guidelines are very tentative because of the uncertain effects of age.

16.4   Muscle function tests

Muscle wasting characterizes the marasmic form of protein-energy malnutrition. Changes in muscle function, such as muscle contractility, relaxation rate, and endurance, may precede body composition changes and, as a result, detect functional impairment at the subclinical level (Lopes et al., 1982). Impairment in hand grip strength has also been observed. In critically ill patients, changes in muscle function may alter respiratory function and precipitate respiratory failure.

16.4.1 Skeletal muscle function after electrical stimulation

Skeletal muscle function tests generally measure the function of the adductor pollicis muscle after electrical stimulation of the ulnar nerve. Changes in the adductor pollicis muscle appear to be representative of muscle function as a whole.

For the test, the right arm and hand are placed in an arm support with a fixation device for the arm and hand. The ulnar nerve at the wrist is then electrically stimulated with a square wave impulse of 50 to 100 microsecond duration, and between 80 and 120 volts at frequencies increasing from 10 to 100 Hz. The force produced by the adductor pollicis muscle is measured using a force transducer and a strip chart pen recorder. Electromyograms (EMG) of the adductor pollicis muscle are recorded. Supramaximal nerve stimulation during the study is ensured by placing surface electrodes over the adductor pollicis muscle and on the tip of the index finger (Edwards et al., 1977). The force generated depends on the frequency of stimulation and on whether the muscle is fresh or fatigued. In malnourished patients, tetany occurs at a lower stimulation frequency. There is also a loss of force at high-frequency stimulation so that the force at 10 Hz (expressed as a percentage of the force at 100 Hz) is increased. This procedure can also be used to measure muscle relaxation rate and muscle endurance (Lopes et al., 1982).

The method has been investigated using both animal models and human studies of nutritional deprivation and refeeding. In patients with clinical and biochemical features of severe nutritional depletion, three abnormalities of muscle function have been noted, all of which can be

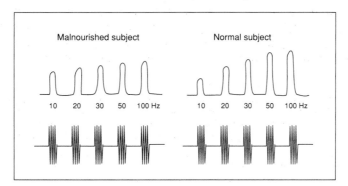

Figure 16.5: Comparison of the force of contraction with electrical stimulation at 10, 20, 30, 50, and 100 Hz in a malnourished and a normal subject. The typical malnourished patient shows an increased force at 10 Hz (expressed as the percentage of the force at 100 Hz) compared with a normal subject. The lower tracing shows diagrammatically the surface EMG, demonstrating constant nerve stimulation. Modified after Russell and Jeejeebhoy (1983) with permission of Nutrition Abstracts and Reviews, A (Human and Experimental).

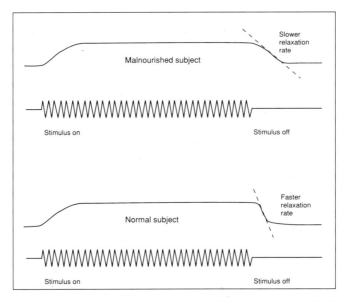

Figure 16.6: Comparison of the force of contraction (and EMG recording) at 30 Hz in typical malnourished and normal subjects. The maximal relaxation rate is calculated from the gradient of the initial phase of relaxation (dotted line), and is slower in the malnourished subject. Modified from Russell and Jeejeebhoy (1983) with permission of Nutrition Abstracts and Reviews, A (Human and Experimental).

reversed by refeeding. These include: (1) an altered force-frequency pattern with an increased force at 10 Hz stimulation expressed as a percentage of the maximal force (Figure 16.5); (2) a lower maximal relaxation rate, expressed as percentage force loss/10 ms (Figure 16.6); and (3) an increased susceptibility to muscle fatigue (Figure 16.7). These abnormalities have also been reported in obese patients during a period of fasting and were restored to normal within two weeks of refeeding.

In contrast, no significant changes in anthropometric measurements of body composition and selected biochemical indices (e.g. serum albumin and transferrin, creatinine height index, and total body nitrogen and potassium) were observed in these obese patients during fasting and refeeding (Russell et al., 1983a). Similar results were also reported in patients with primary anorexia nervosa (Russell et al., 1983b). These results suggest that changes in skeletal muscle function may be more sensitive to nutritional deprivation and repletion than other nutritional assessment indices. Nevertheless, the changes which occur after five days of total starvation are still too small to detect short-term nutritional depletion (Lennmarken et al., 1986). Moreover, when both body composition (assessed by multiple-isotope dilution, Section 14.4) and skeletal

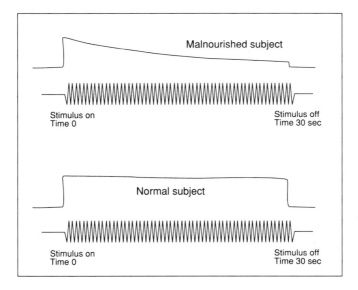

Figure 16.7: Comparison of the force of contraction (and EMG recording) at 20 Hz stimulation for thirty seconds, in typical malnourished and normal subjects. The malnourished subject shows noticeable muscle fatigue. Modified from Russell and Jeejeebhoy (1983) with permission of Nutrition Abstracts and Reviews, A (Human and Experimental).

muscle function were simultaneously evaluated in a group of malnourished and normally nourished patients, no significant correlations were noted between the two measurements (Shizgal et al., 1986). More work is therefore required before the validity of skeletal muscle function tests as indices of nutritional status is firmly established.

16.4.2 Hand grip strength

Hand grip strength has also been used as a test of skeletal muscle function. This can be measured with a strain gauge with a graded scale (0 to 90 units). Subjects are asked to perform a maximal contraction, generally with the nondominant hand. This is repeated three to four times and the highest value achieved is recorded. Age- and sex-specific lower limits of acceptable grip strength have been compiled by Webb et al. (1989). Psychological factors, such as motivation and anxiety, may also influence hand grip strength and confound the interpretation of the results (Lennmarken et al., 1986).

16.5 Immunological tests

During protein-energy malnutrition and deficiencies of specific nutrients such as iron and zinc, consistent changes in immunological responses have been observed, which have been reversed with nutritional repletion

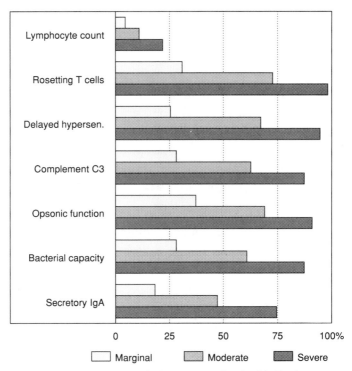

Figure 16.8: Immunological changes associated with the immune response in marginal, moderate, and severe malnutrition. Modified from Chandra RK (1981). Immunodeficiency in undernutrition and overnutrition. Nutrition Reviews 39: 225–231, with permission.

(Meakins et al., 1977). As a result, immunocompetence has been used as a functional index of nutritional status. Immunological tests, however, are not specific enough to detect individual nutrient deficiencies; many other factors affect the immunocompetence. These include emotional and physical stress, such as surgery, anesthesia, major burns, neoplasia, and viral infections. Hence, to correctly interpret the results, information on nutritional intake, concurrent illness, exposure to infectious agents, duration of the deficit, and genetic factors is also required. Furthermore, the immunological tests must be used in conjunction with other nutritional assessment indices for specific nutrient deficiencies. Figure 16.8 shows the immunological changes associated with the immune response which occur in marginal, moderate, and severe malnutrition (Chandra, 1981).

The immune system consists of two central lymphoid organs, the thymus and the bone marrow, as well as peripheral lymphoid organs such as lymph nodes, the spleen, tonsils, mucous membrane-associated lymphoid tissue, and other diffuse lymphoid tissues of the body. Lymphocytes of thymus origin are called T-cells; they are responsible for mediating cell-mediated immunity reactions. B-lymphocytes (bursal-equivalent derived)

	Average (Cells/mm^3)	Normal Range (Cells/mm^3)	Percentage of Total White Cells
Total WBC	9000	4000–11,000	
Granulocytes			
Neutrophils	5400	3000–6000	50–70
Eosinophils	275	150–300	1–4
Basophils	35	0–100	0.4
Lymphocytes	2750	1500–4000	20–40
Monocytes	540	300–600	2–8

Table 16.14: Classes of leukocytes in the peripheral blood of the average adult. Conversion factor to SI units $(10^9/L) = \times 0.001$.

are derived from the bone marrow and, in general, are responsible for humoral immunity, producing antibodies (IgM, -A, -D, -E, -G) in response to specific antigens. In general, humoral immunity is said to be less affected by nutritional status than cell-mediated immunity (Stiehm, 1980). B-lymphocytes make up 20% to 30% of peripheral blood lymphocytes.

Nearly all aspects of the immune system can be impaired by nutritional deficiencies. No single test can measure the adequacy of the immune response. Only those tests more frequently used in nutritional assessment will be discussed below.

16.5.1 Lymphocyte count

Lymphocytes comprise 20% to 40% of the total white blood cells (WBC) (leukocytes) (Table 16.14). Measurement of the total lymphocytes in the peripheral circulation is usually performed routinely on almost all hospital patients in industrialized countries. In healthy subjects, the average lymphocyte count in peripheral blood is generally above 2750 cells per mm^3. In malnutrition, the blood lymphocyte count is reduced (Figure 16.8). A level between 900 and 1500 cells per mm^3 is said to indicate moderate depletion, whereas below 900 per mm^3 represents severe depletion (Blackburn et al. 1977). Figure 16.8 shows the change in lymphocyte counts (as %) in marginal, moderate, and severe malnutrition (Chandra, 1981). The total lymphocyte count is derived from the percentage of lymphocytes multiplied by the white blood cell count and divided by 100:

$$\text{Total lymphocyte count} = \frac{\% \text{ lymphocytes} \times \text{WBC}}{100}$$

Many other factors can affect the absolute lymphocyte count, notably stress, sepsis, infection, neoplasia, and steroids. Therefore the specificity and sensitivity of this test is low. The relationship of total lymphocyte count to patient prognosis has not been extensively investigated, although Riesco (1970) observed a relationship between depressed total lymphocyte count in cancer patients and prognosis. This test does not provide any information on which specific lymphocyte subpopulation is responsible for the lowered total lymphocyte count.

16.5.2 Measurement of thymus-dependent lymphocytes

Approximately 75% to 80% of the circulating lymphocytes are thymus-dependent lymphocytes (T-cells). During protein-energy malnutrition, both the proportion and absolute number of T-cells in the peripheral blood may be reduced (Chandra, 1974). In most cases, these changes can be rapidly reversed with nutritional therapy. Hence, sequential measurements of T-cell numbers provide an index of the effectiveness of nutrition intervention, and nutritional recovery in malnourished patients.

For the test, the lymphocytes are first isolated from a venous blood sample (approximately 5 mL) using density gradient centrifugation on Ficoll-Hypaque. After washing, the lymphocytes are mixed with sheep red blood cells and incubated briefly (five to ten minutes) at 37°C. This is followed by incubation at 4°C for three to fifteen hours, during which time the T-cells bind to the sheep red blood cells forming rosettes. Prior treatment of sheep red blood cells with neuraminidase increases the number of rosettes. The cell pellet is then gently resuspended, mounted on a counting chamber, and the proportion of lymphocytes forming rosettes with three or more sheep red blood cells are counted as T-cells; alternatively, T-cell numbers can be measured using the CD3 surface marker. Results should be expressed as the number of T-cells per microliter of whole blood, and compared with standard values derived from normal healthy individuals for each laboratory (Chandra and Scrimshaw, 1980). Thymus-dependent lymphocytes can be segregated into suppressor, helper, and killer cells. The test described above measures total T-cells. Hence, immune dysfunctions that result from increased numbers of suppressor T-cells cannot be detected by this test (Miller, 1978). In such cases, total T-cell numbers may rise, as has been noted in some marasmic children (Schlesinger et al., 1977).

16.5.3 Lymphocyte mitogen assays

To assess human lymphocyte function, lymphocytes are incubated in the presence of mitogens, which stimulate carbohydrate receptors on lympho-cyte surfaces causing them to divide. In cases of immune dysfunction, decreases in the mitogen-induced proliferation occur. Mitogens com-monly used include concanavalin A (Con A) and phytohemagglutinin (PHA) which primarily stimulate division of T-cells, and the thymus-dependent B-lymphocyte mitogen, pokeweed mitogen (PWM). For the test, lymphocytes are first purified from heparinized peripheral whole blood by density gradient centrifugation on Ficoll-Hypaque, as noted above. Cultures are then set up in triplicate in microtiter plates containing a lymphocyte concentration of 2×10^5 per mL viable lymphocytes in $200\,\mu L$ volume. The culture medium is supplemented with 10% to 20% serum — either autologous, heterologous, or pooled human sera. Mitogens are added at levels including 1, 2.5, 5, and $10\,\mu g/mL$, for Con A and PHA, and 0.5, 2.5, 10, and $15\,\mu g/mL$ for PWM. Control cultures contain no mitogen. Cultures are incubated at $37°C$ in a 5% CO_2 atmosphere for seventy-two hours, a time period during which most mitogens produce their maximal effect on DNA synthesis. The cultures are then labeled with tritiated thymidine, and incubated for a further sixteen- to twenty-four-hour period. The rate of DNA synthesis can then be determined by counting the amount of tritiated thymidine incorporated per culture, using a liquid scintillation spectrophotometer. Results should be expressed as both disintegrations per minute and as stimulation indices, to facilitate interpretation of the results.

The results must be interpreted with caution because technical variations and difficulties in the assays can influence the results (Miller, 1978). Confounding technical factors include the concentration of the cells, the geometry of the culture vessel, contamination of the cultures, differences in the mitogen preparations and dose, incubation time used, and the technique used to harvest the cells (Miller, 1978). Furthermore, the proportion of suppressor or helper T-, B-, and mononuclear cells present in the culture will affect the degree of multiplication of the lymphocytes. A normal mitogen response does not necessarily indicate normal immunocompetence. Patients with certain immuno-defects may have normal or elevated mitogen responses. The mitogen assays should always be performed with normal healthy controls as well as the patients, and the responses of the cells of the controls should not vary by more than 15% between tests.

16.5.4 Delayed cutaneous hypersensitivity

When healthy persons are re-exposed to recall antigens intradermally, T-cells respond by proliferation, and release of soluble mediators of inflammation. This produces an induration (hardening) and erythema (redness). These skin reactions are often decreased in malnourished persons with marasmus and/or kwashiorkor and/or nutrient deficiencies such as vitamin A, zinc, iron, and pyridoxine, but are reversed after nutritional rehabilitation. For this test, a battery of specific antigens are injected intradermally in the forearm and the acquired immunity response noted at selected time intervals. The recall skin test antigens commonly used are: purified protein derivative (PPD), mumps, trichophyton, *Candida albicans*, and dinitrochlorobenzene (DNCB).

Many non-nutritional factors affect skin test reactivity and hence reduce the specificity and sensitivity of the test; a summary of these appears in

- Infections — sepsis as a result of viral, bacterial, and granulomatous infections can suppress normal DCH

- Metabolic disorders — uremia, cirrhosis, hepatitis, inflammatory bowel diseases, and sarcoidosis suppress normal DCH

- Malignant diseases — most solid tumors, leukemias, lymphomas, chemotherapy, and radiotherapy impair DCH

- Drugs — steroids, immunosuppressants, cimetidine, coumadin, and possibly aspirin

- Surgery and anaesthesia — can alter DCH

- Patient factors — age, race, geographic location, prior exposure to antigen, circadian rhythm, psychological state.

Table 16.15: Non-nutritional factors affecting the delayed cutaneous hypersensitivity response. Adapted from Twomey P, Ziegler D, Rombeau J. (1982). Utility of skin testing in nutritional assessment: A critical review. Journal of Parenteral and Enteral Nutrition 6: 50–58. © Am. Soc. Parenteral and Enteral Nutrition, 1982.

Table 16.15. Some of the effects of the technical factors can be minimized if standard procedures are adopted for delayed cutaneous hypersensitivity (DCH) testing. Technical factors include reader variability, dilution of the antigens used, time course of interpretation, and the 'booster effect' of repeated antigen administration. The latter effect is particularly significant when DCH is tested serially, and applied at the same site each time. In such cases, the responses will be enhanced. Table 16.16 presents recommendation by Bates et al. (1979) for standardization of DCH testing procedures.

The time course used for interpreting the DCH test is also an important consideration. Usually, skin tests are measured twenty-four and forty-eight hours after the antigen injection. However, some individuals being tested for the first time may develop reactions more slowly, so that seventy-two hours may be needed (Sokal, 1975), whereas in others who have undergone repeated testing, accelerated reactions may occur. Consequently, multiple readings should be taken, and the largest reading used. If only one reading can be taken, the peak reaction is most likely to occur at forty-eight hours. An example of a form used for classifying and recording skin test responses is given in Appendix A16.2.

Several investigators have studied the usefulness of DCH testing for assessing risk of morbidity and mortality in hospital patients. In general, anergic hospitalized patients have an increased risk for complications after surgery (Mullen et al., 1979b), such as sepsis and death (Meakins et al., 1977), compared to patients with normal responses to skin test antigens. Indeed, DCH was selected as one of the four indices in the prognostic nutritional index developed by Mullen and associates (Mullen et al., 1979a) (Section 26.2). The DCH response does not appear to be

> • Use uniform dilutions for the antigens.
>
> • Use uniform measurement techniques: the ball-point pen technique of Sokal (1975) is recommended. In this method, a ball-point pen is placed on the skin 1 to 2 cm away from the margin of the skin reaction and is moved slowly toward the center. When resistance at the edge of induration is reached, the pen is lifted, and the procedure is repeated from the opposite side. The distance between the opposite lines is the diameter of induration.
>
> • Record measurements of erythema (redness) and induration (hardening).
>
> • Use a uniform interpretation method. A modification of the gradual scale of Sokal (1975) is recommended in which the size of both the erythema and induration is noted:- 1+ erythema 10 mm or more, without induration or induration 1 to 5 mm; 2+ induration 6 to 10 mm; 3+ induration 11 to 20 mm; 4+ induration greater than 20 mm.

Table 16.16: Recommendations for standardization of delayed cutaneous hypersensitivity testing. From Bates SE, Suen JY, Tranum BL. (1979). Immunological skin testing and interpretation. A plea for uniformity. Cancer 43: 2306–2314. With permission of Lippincott/Harper & Row.

useful, however, for assessing the effectiveness of nutrition intervention involving total parenteral nutrition (Law et al., 1973).

A new technique — the Multi-test Cell Mediated Immunity (CMI) Delayed Hypersensitivity Skin test kit — has been developed by the Institut Merieux (Lyons, France) (Kniker et al., 1979). This kit eliminates some of the methodological problems associated with the traditional skin testing method. It consists of a sterile, disposable plastic multipuncture applicator consisting of eight test heads preloaded with standardized doses of seven antigens (tuberculin, tetanus toxoid, diphtheria toxoid, *Streptococcus*, *Candida*, trichophyton, and proteus) in glycerin solution and a glycerin control. Use of seven antigens reduces the number of false-negatives and increases the sensitivity of the test.

16.5.5 Other methods

Mixed leukocyte culture is another method used to assess immune function, which involves measuring the ability of cells to divide in response to a specific antigen challenge, again using tritiated thymidine incorporation. The method reflects immunocompetence more accurately than simple mitogen assays (Section 16.5.3) (Miller, 1978).

The level of specific antibodies such as IgA in body fluid samples such as saliva can also be measured; levels are reduced in malnutrition. Samples can be stored for prolonged periods at $-20°C$ prior to assay for IgA by radial-immunodiffusion in agar.

Complement levels, particularly C3 which acts as an acute phase reactant, can be quantified by radial-immunodiffusion or by rocket immuno-electrophoresis. In well-nourished persons, serum C3 levels rise in response to infection. In malnourished individuals serum C3 is generally low, and decreases further with infection. For this test, serum must be separated immediately after the blood has clotted at room temperature. Serum samples can then be stored at $-20°C$ prior to testing.

16.6 Summary

Laboratory indices of protein status measure (1) somatic protein status; (2) visceral protein status; (3) metabolic changes; (4) muscle function; and (5) immune function.

Indices of somatic protein status include urinary excretion of creatinine (frequently expressed as a creatinine height index) and 3-methylhistidine. The former is used to assess the degree of depletion of muscle mass in marasmic patients, and degree of repletion, after long-term nutrition intervention, provided that accurately timed seventy-two-hour urine collections are made. Urinary excretion of 3-methylhistidine appears promising as a marker of muscle protein except in conditions of severe sepsis or major physical trauma, although it has not been widely used.

To assess visceral protein status, concentrations of one or more serum proteins are measured. Of the four serum proteins — albumin, transferrin, retinol-binding protein, and thyroxine-binding pre-albumin — albumin and transferrin are most frequently used in hospital assessment protocols. They are not necessarily the most appropriate, particularly for monitoring short-term changes in protein status. They show a relatively slow response which, like most serum proteins, may be complicated by the effects of such confounding factors as stress, sepsis, and hydration, severely limiting their use in critically ill patients. As a result, serum albumin and transferrin are more usefully applied for monitoring long-term changes during convalescence. To monitor short-term changes in visceral protein status during convalescence, serum retinol-binding protein and thyroxine-binding pre-albumin should be used. These serum proteins have a smaller total body pool, a shorter half-life, and a relatively high specificity, compared to serum albumin and transferrin. Future studies may include measurement of serum somatomedin-C; it is said to be more sensitive to acute changes in protein status than the other serum proteins.

Some metabolic changes which occur in protein-energy malnutrition are also used as indices of protein status. For example, in field settings where both kwashiorkor and marasmus may occur, tests which differentiate between subclinical cases of these two forms of protein-energy malnutrition are desirable. The hydroxyproline index, in combination with the serum nonessential (NEAA) : essential amino-acid (EAA) ratio, has been used in such circumstances, although the rather low sensitivity and specificity of the NEAA : EAA ratio has limited its use. For hospital patients, urinary urea nitrogen excretion on at least three twenty-four-hour urine samples, in association with nitrogen intake data, can provide an estimate of nitrogen balance. Such estimates are used most effectively to monitor changes in the nutritional status of hospital patients during the course of nutritional therapy. In field surveys, twenty-four-hour urine collections are impractical. Instead, the urinary urea nitrogen : creatinine ratio on casual urine samples can be calculated to assess the adequacy of protein intake.

Functional indices of protein status include muscle function and immunological tests. The former measure changes in muscle contractility, relaxation rate, and endurance, as well as hand grip strength, in malnourished patients. Such tests may be more sensitive to nutritional deprivation than some other indices of protein nutriture, provided that the period of depletion is not too acute. Tests of immunocompetence are sometimes used as functional indices of protein status, although their specificity and sensitivity are low. Nearly all aspects of the immune system can be impaired by nutritional deficiencies, and no single test can measure the adequacy of the immune response. The immunological tests may include lymphocyte count, delayed cutaneous hypersensitivity, measurement of thymus-dependent lymphocytes, and lymphocyte mitogen assays.

References

Allison JB, Bird JWC. (1977). Elimination of nitrogen from the body. In: Munro HN, Allison JB (eds). Mammalian Protein Metabolism. Volume 1. American Medical Association, Chicago, pp. 141–146.

Allison DJ, Walker A, Smith QT. (1966). Urinary hydroxyproline : creatinine ratio of normal humans at various ages. Clinica Chimica Acta 14: 729–734.

Bates SE, Suen JY, Tranum BL. (1979). Immunological skin testing and interpretation. A plea for uniformity. Cancer 43: 2306–2314.

Bistrian BR. (1977). Nutritional assessment and therapy of protein-calorie malnutrition in the hospital. Journal of the American Dietetic Association 71: 393–397.

Bistrian BR, Blackburn GL, Sherman M, Scrimshaw NS. (1975). Therapeutic index of nutritional depletion in hospitalized patients. Surgery, Gynecology and Obstetrics 141: 512–516.

Blackburn GL, Bistrian BR, Maini BS, Schlamm HT, Smith MF. (1977). Nutritional and metabolic assessment of the hospitalized patient. Journal of Parenteral and Enteral Nutrition 1: 11–22.

Bleiler RE, Schedl HP. (1962). Creatinine excretion: variability and relationship to diet and body size. Journal of Laboratory and Clinical Medicine 59: 945–955.

Boileau RB, Horstman DH, Buskirk ER, Mendez J. (1972). The usefulness of urinary creatinine excretion in estimating body composition. Medicine and Science in Sports and Exercise 4: 85–90.

Buckell NA, Lennard-Jones JE, Hernandez MA, Kohn J, Riches PG, Wadsworth J. (1979). Measurement of serum proteins during attacks of ulcerative colitis as a guide to patient management. Gut 20: 22–27.

Buskirk ER, Mendez J. (1985). Lean body tissue assessment, with emphasis on skeletal muscle mass. In: Roche AF (ed) Body Composition Assessment in Youth and Adults. Report of the Sixth Ross Conference on Medical Research. Ross Laboratories, Columbus, Ohio, pp. 59–65.

Cahill GF, Jr. (1970). Starvation in man. In: Sherwood, L.M. (ed). Seminars in Medicine of the Beth Israel Hospital, Boston. New England Journal of Medicine 282: 668–675.

Calloway DH, Odell ACF, Margen S. (1971). Sweat and miscellaneous nitrogen losses in human balance studies. Journal of Nutrition 101: 775–786.

Carpentier YA, Ingenbleek Y. (1983). Serum thyroxine-binding prealbumin: an unreliable index of nutritional status? Nutrition Research 3: 617–620.

Carpentier YA, Barthel J, Bruyns J. (1982). Plasma protein concentration in nutritional assessment. Proceedings of the Nutrition Society 41: 405–417.

Chandra RK. (1974). Rosette-forming T-lymphocytes and cell-mediated immunity in malnutrition. British Medical Journal 3: 608–609.

Chandra RK. (1981). Immunodeficiency in undernutrition and overnutrition. Nutrition Reviews 39: 225–231.

Chandra RK, Scrimshaw NS. (1980). Immunocompetence in nutritional assessment. American Journal of Clinical Nutrition 33: 2694–2697.

Cheek DB. (1968). Human Growth: Body Composition, Cell Growth, Energy, and Intelligence. Lea and Febiger, Philadelphia, pp. 31–47.

Cheek DB, Brasel JA, Elliot D, Scott R. (1966). Muscle cell size and number in normal children and in dwarfs (pituitary, cretins, and primordial) before and after treatment. Bulletin of Johns Hopkins Hospital 119: 46–62.

Cook JGH. (1975). Factors influencing the assay of creatinine. Annals of Clinical Biochemistry 12: 219–232.

Coward WA, Lunn PG. (1981). The biochemistry and physiology of kwashiorkor and marasmus. British Medical Bulletin 37: 19–24.

Dabev D, Struck H. (1971). Microliter determination of free hydroxyproline in blood serum. Biochemical Medicine 5: 17-21.

Delpeuch F, Cornu A, Chevalier P. (1980). The effect of iron-deficiency anaemia on two indices of nutritional status, prealbumin and transferrin. British Journal of Nutrition 43: 375–379.

Dohm GL, Williams RT, Kasperek GJ, Rij AM van. (1982). Increased excretion of urea and N tan-methylhistidine by rats and humans after a bout of exercise. Journal of Applied Physiology 52: 27–33.

Driver AG, McAlvey MT. (1980). Creatinine height index as a function of age. American Journal of Clinical Nutrition 33: 2057.

Edwards RH, Young A, Hosking GP, Jones DA. (1977). Human skeletal muscle function: description of tests and normal values. Clinical Science and Molecular Medicine 52: 283–290.

Farthing MJG. (1982). Serum thyroxine-binding prealbumin: an unreliable index of nutritional status in chronic intestinal disease. Nutrition Research 2: 561–568.

Fischer JE. (1981). Plasma proteins as indicators of nutritional status. In: Levenson SM (ed). Nutritional Assessment — Present Status, Future Directions and Prospects. Ross Laboratories, Columbus, Ohio, pp. 25–26.

Forbes GB, Bruining GJ. (1976). Urinary creatinine excretion and lean body mass. American Journal of Clinical Nutrition 29: 1359–1366.

Forbes RM, Cooper AR, Mitchell HH. (1953). Composition of adult human body as determined by chemical analysis. Journal of Biological Chemistry 203: 359–366.

Furlanetto RW, Underwood LE, VanWyk JJ, D'Ercole A. (1977). Estimation of somatomedin-C levels in normals and patients with pituitary disease by radio-immunoassay. Journal of Clinical Investigation 60: 648–657.

Gabr M, El-Hawary MF S, El-Dali M. (1971). Serum transferrin in kwashiorkor. Journal of Tropical Medicine and Hygiene 74: 216–221.

Golden MNH. (1982). Transport proteins as indices of protein status. American Journal of Clinical Nutrition 35: 1159–1165.

Grant JP. (1986). Nutritional assessment in clinical practice. Nutrition in Clinical Practice 1: 3–11.

Grant JP, Custer PB, Thurlow J. (1981). Current techniques of nutritional assessment. Surgical Clinics of North America 61: 437–463.

Harper AE. (1981). Plasma amino acid concentrations in relation to evaluation of nutritional status. In: Nutritional Assessment — Present Status, Future Directions and Prospects. Ross Laboratories, Columbus, Ohio, pp. 29–33.

Harvey KB, Blumenkrantz MJ, Levine SE, Blackburn GL. (1980). Nutritional assessment and treatment of chronic renal failure. American Journal of Clinical Nutrition 33: 1586–1597.

Health and Welfare Canada (1973). Nutrition Canada National Survey. Health and Welfare, Ottawa.

Heymsfield SB, Arteaga C, McManus CB, Smith J, Moffitt S. (1983). Measurement of muscle mass in humans: validity of the twenty-four-hour urinary creatinine method. American Journal of Clinical Nutrition 37: 478–494.

Imbembo AL, Walser M. (1984). Nutritional assessment. In: Walser M, Imbembo AL, Margolis S, Elfert GA (eds). Nutritional Management. The John Hopkins Handbook. W.B. Saunders Co., Philadelphia pp. 9–30.

Ingenbleek Y, De Visscher M. (1979). Hormonal and nutritional status: Critical conditions for endemic goiter epidemiology? Metabolism 28: 9–19.

Ingenbleek Y, Schrieck HG van den, De Nayer PL, De Visscher M. (1975). Albumin, transferrin and the thyroxine-binding prealbumin/retinol-binding protein (TBPA-RBP) complex in assessment of malnutrition. Clinica Chimica Acta 63: 61–67.

Jacob RA, Sandstead HH, Solomons NW, Rieger C, Rothberg R. (1978). Zinc status and vitamin A transport in cystic fibrosis. American Journal of Clinical Nutrition 31: 638–644.

James WP, Hay AM. (1968). Albumin metabolism: effect of the nutritional state and the dietary protein intake. Journal of Clinical Investigation 47: 1958–1972.

Jeejeebhoy KN. (1981). Protein nutrition in clinical practice. British Medical Bulletin 37: 11–17.

Kaminski MV, Jr., Fitzgerald MJ, Murphy RJ, Pagast P, Hoppe M, Winborn AL. (1977). Correlation of mortality with serum transferrin and anergy. Journal of Parenteral and Enteral Nutrition 1: 27–29.

Kopple JD. (1987). Uses and limitations of the balance technique. Journal of Parenteral and Enteral Nutrition 11: 79S–85S.

Kniker WT, Anderson CT, Roumiantzeff M. (1979). The multi-test system: A standardized approach to evaluation of delayed hypersensitivity and cell-mediated immunity. Annals of Allergy 43: 73–79.

Large S, Neal G, Glover J, Thanangkul O, Olson RE. (1980). The early changes in retinol-binding protein and prealbumin concentrations in plasma of protein-energy malnourished children after treatment with retinol and an improved diet. British Journal of Nutrition, 43: 393–402.

Law DK, Dudrick SJ, Abdou NI. (1973). Immunocompetence of patients with protein-calorie malnutrition: The effects of nutritional repletion. Annals of Internal Medicine 79: 545–550.

Lennmarken C, Sandstedt S, Schenck HV, Larsson J. (1986). The effect of starvation on skeletal muscle function in man. Clinical Nutrition 5: 99–103.

Leonberg BL, Crosby LO, Buzby GP. (1987). A rapid, accurate, precise assay for determination of plasma transferrin. Journal of Parenteral and Enteral Nutrition 11: 74–76.

LeRoy EC. (1967). The technique and significance of hydroxyproline measurement in man. Advances in Clinical Chemistry 10: 213–253.

Lopes J, Russell D McR, Whitwell J, Jeejeebhoy KN. (1982). Skeletal muscle function in malnutrition. Americal Journal of Clinical Nutrition 36: 602–610.

Lukaski HC, Mendez J, Buskirk ER, Cohn SR. (1981). Relationship between endogenous 3-methylhistidine excretion and body composition. American Journal of Physiology 240: E302–E307.

Mann GV. (1988). A simplified system for collecting twenty-four-hour urine samples. Journal of the American College of Nutrition 7: 141–145.

MacKenzie TA, Clark NG, Bistrian BR, Flatt JP, Hallowell EM, Blackburn GL. (1985). A simple method for estimating nitrogen balance in hospitalized patients: a review and supporting data for a previously proposed technique. Journal of the American College of Nutrition 4: 575–581.

McFarlane H, Ogbeide MI, Reddy S, Adcock KJ, Adestina H, Gurney JM, Cooke A, Taylor GO, Mordie JA. (1969). Biochemical assessment of protein-calorie malnutrition. Lancet 1: 392–395.

McFarlane H, Reddy S, Adcock KJ, Adestina H, Cooke AR, Akene J. (1970). Immunity, transferrin and survival in kwashiorkor. British Medical Journal 4: 268–270.

McPherson IG, Everard DW. (1972). Serum albumin estimation: modification of the bromocresol green method. Clinica Chimica Acta 37: 117–121.

Meador CK, Kreisberg RA, Friday JP, Bowdoin B, Coan P, Armstrong J, Hazelrig JB. (1968). Muscle mass determination by isotopic dilution of creatine-^{14}C. Metabolism 17: 1104–1108.

Meakins JL, Pietsch JB, Bubernick O, Kelly R, Rode H, Gordon J, MacLean LD. (1977). Delayed hypersensitivity: Indicator of acquired failure of host defenses in sepsis and trauma. Annals of Surgery 186: 241–250.

Miller CL. (1978). Immunological assays as measurements of nutritional status: a review. Journal of Parenteral and Enteral Nutrition 2: 554–566.

Misra DP, Loudon JM, Staddon GE. (1975). Albumin metabolism in elderly patients. Journal of Gerontology 30: 304-306.

Mitch WE, Collier VU, Walser M. (1980). Creatinine metabolism in chronic renal failure. Clinical Science 58: 327–335.

Muhilal H, Glover J. (1974). Effects of dietary deficiencies of protein and retinol on the plasma level of retinol-binding protein in the rat. British Journal of Nutrition 32: 549–558.

Mullen JL, Buzby GP, Waldman MT, Gertner MH, Hobbs CL, Rosato EF. (1979a). Prediction of operative morbidity and mortality by preoperative nutritional assessment. Surgical Forum 30: 80–82.

Mullen JL, Gertner MH, Buzby GP, Goodhart GL, Rosato EF. (1979b). Implications of malnutrition in the surgical patient. Archives of Surgery 114: 121–125.

Ogunshina SO, Hussain MA. (1980). Plasma thyroxine-binding prealbumin as an index of mild protein-energy malnutrition in Nigerian children. American Journal of Clinical Nutrition 33: 794–800.

Phillips LS, Vassilopoulou-Sellin R. (1980). Somatomedins (first of two parts). New England Journal of Medicine 302: 371–380.

Phinney SD. (1981). The assessment of protein nutrition in the hospitalized patient. Clinics in Laboratory Medicine 1: 767–774.

Prockop DJ, Udenfriend S. (1960). A specific method for the analysis of hydroxyproline in tissues and urine. Analytical Biochemistry 1: 228–239.

Reeds PJ, Laditan AAO. (1976). Serum albumin and transferrin in protein-energy malnutrition. British Journal of Nutrition, 36: 255–263.

Riesco A. (1970). Five-year cancer cure: relation to total amount of peripheral lymphocytes and neutrophils. Cancer 25: 135-140.

Russell D McR, Jeejeebhoy KN. (1983). The assessment of the functional consequences of malnutrition. Nutrition Abstracts and Reviews 53: 863–877.

Russell DM, Leiter LA, Whitwell J, Marliss EB, Jeejeebhoy KN. (1983a). Skeletal muscle function during hypocaloric diets and fasting: a comparison with standard nutritional assessment parameters. American Journal of Clinical Nutrition 37: 133–138.

Russell DM, Prendergast PJ, Darby PL, Garfinkel PE, Whitwell J, Jeejeebhoy KH. (1983b). A comparison between muscle function and body composition in anorexia nervosa: the effect of refeeding. American Journal of Clinical Nutrition 38: 229–237.

Ryan JA, Taft DA. (1980). Preoperative nutritional assessment does not predict morbidity and mortality in abdominal operations. Surgical Forum 31: 96–98.

Sauberlich HE, Dowdy RP, Skala, JH. (1974). Laboratory Tests for the Assessment of Nutritional Status. CRC Press Inc., Cleveland, Ohio.

Schlesinger L, Ohlbaum A, Grez T, Stekel A. (1977). Cell-mediated immune studies in marasmic children from Chile: delayed hypersensitivity, lymphocyte transformation, and interferon production. Malnutrition and the Immune Response 7: 91–98.

Searcy RL, Simms NM, Foreman JA, Bergquist LM. (1965). A study of the specificity of the Berthelot color reaction. Clinica Chimica Acta 12: 170–175.

Shetty PS, Jung RT, Watrasiewicz KE, James WPT. (1979). Rapid-turnover transport proteins: an index of subclinical protein-energy malnutrition. Lancet 2: 230–232.

Shizgal HM, Vasilevsky CA, Gardiner PF, Wang W, Quellette Tuitt DA, Brabant GV. (1986). Nutritional assessment and skeletal muscle function. American Journal of Clinical Nutrition 44: 761–771.

Simmons WK. (1970). The plasma amino acid ratio as an indicator of the protein nutrition status: A review of recent work. Bulletin of the World Health Organization 42: 480–484.

Simmons WK. (1972). Urinary urea nitrogen-creatinine ratio as an indicator of recent protein intake in field studies. American Journal of Clinical Nutrition 25: 539–542.

Smith IF, Latham MC, Azubuike JA, Butler WR, Phillips LS, Pond WG, Enwonwu CO. (1981). Blood plasma levels of cortisol, insulin, growth hormone and somatomedin in children with marasmus, kwashiorkor, and intermediate forms of protein-energy malnutrition. Proceedings of the Society for Experimental Biology and Medicine 167: 607–611.

Smith OW. (1942). Creatinine excretion in women: Data collected in the course of urinalysis for female sex hormones. Journal of Clinical Endocrinology 2: 1–12.

Smith FR, Suskind R, Thanangkul O, Leitzmann C, Goodman DS, Olson RE. (1975). Plasma vitamin A, retinol-binding protein and prealbumin concentrations in protein-calorie malnutrition. III. Response to varying dietary treatments. American Journal of Clinical Nutrition 28: 732–738.

Smith FR, Underwood BA, Denning CR, Varma A, Goodman DS. (1972). Depressed plasma retinol-binding protein levels in cystic fibrosis. Journal of Laboratory and Clinical Medicine 80: 423–433.

Sokal JE. (1975). Measurement of delayed skin-test responses. New England Journal of Medicine 293: 501–502.

Srivastava SS, Mani KV, Soni CM, Bhati J. (1957). Effect of muscular exercises on urinary excretion of creatine and creatinine. Indian Journal of Medical Research 55: 953–960.

Stiehm ER. (1980). Humoral immunity in malnutrition. Federation Proceedings 39: 3093–3097.

Stromberg BV, Davis RJ, Danziger LH. (1982). Relationship of serum transferrin to total iron binding capacity for nutritional assessment. Journal of Parenteral and Enteral Nutrition 6: 392–394.

Taylor HL, Mickelsen O, Keys A. (1949). Effects of induced malaria, acute starvation and semistarvation on the electrophoretic diagram of the serum proteins of normal young men. Journal of Clinical Investigation 28: 273–281.

Twomey P, Ziegler D, Rombeau J. (1982). Utility of skin testing in nutritional assessment: A critical review. Journal of Parenteral and Enteral Nutrition 6: 50–58.

Unterman TG, Varquez RM, Slas AJ, Martyn PA, Phillips LS. (1985). Nutrition and somatomedin. XIII. Usefulness of somatomedin-C in nutritional assessment. American Journal of Medicine 78: 228–234.

Vielma H, Mendez J, Durckenmiller M, Lukaski H. (1981). A practical and reliable method for determination of urinary 3-methylhistidine. Journal of Biochemistry and Biophysics Methods 5: 75–82.

Wahlqvist ML, Flint DM, Prinsley DM, Dryden PA. (1981). Effect of zinc supplementation on serum albumin and folic acid concentrations in a group of hypo- albuminaemic and hypozincaemic aged persons. In: Howard AN, Baird I M (eds). Recent Advances in Clinical Nutrition. Volume 1. John Libbey, London, pp. 83–84.

Walser M. (1987). Creatinine excretion as a measure of protein nutrition in adults of varying age. Journal of Parenteral and Enteral Nutrition 11: 73S–78S.

Ward LC. (1978). A ninhydrin-orthophthalaldehyde reagent for the determination of N-methylhistidine. Analytical Biochemistry 88: 598–604.

Wassner SJ, Schlitzer JL, Li JB. (1980). A rapid, sensitive method for the determination of 3-methylhistidine levels in urine and plasma using high pressure liquid chromatography. Analytical Biochemistry 104: 284–289.

Waterlow JC. (1972). Classification and definition of protein-calorie malnutrition. British Medical Journal 3: 566–569.

Waterlow JC. (1986). Observations on the variability of creatinine excretion. Human Nutrition: Clinical Nutrition 40C: 125–129.

Webb AR, Newman LA, Taylor M, Keogh JB. (1989). Handgrip dynamometry as a predictor of post operative complications: reappraisal using age standardized grip strengths. Journal of Parenteral and Enteral Nutrition 13: 30–33.

Webster J, Garrow JS. (1985). Creatinine excretion over 24 hours as a measure of body composition or of completeness of urine collection. Human Nutrition: Clinical Nutrition 39C: 101–106.

Whitehead JDL, Frood JDL, Poskitt EME. (1971). Value of serum-albumin measurements in nutritional surveys. A reappraisal. Lancet 2: 287–289.

Whitehead RG. (1965). Hydroxyproline creatinine ratio as an index of nutritional status and rate of growth. Lancet 2: 567–570.

Whitehead RG. (1967). Biochemical tests in differential diagnosis of protein and calorie deficiencies. Archives of Disease in Childhood. 42: 479–484.

Whitehead RG, Dean RFA. (1964). Serum amino acids in kwashiorkor. I. Relationship to clinical conditions. American Journal of Clinical Nutrition 14: 313–319.

Winterer J, Bistrian BR, Bilmazes C, Blackburn GL, Young VR. (1980). Whole body protein turnover studied with 15N-glycine, and muscle protein breakdown in mildly obese subjects during a protein-sparing diet and a brief total fast. Metabolism 29: 575–581.

Young VR, Haverberg LN, Bilmazes C, Munro HN. (1973). Potential use of 3-methylhistidine excretion as an index of progressive reduction in muscle protein catabolism during starvation. Metabolism 22: 1429–1436.

Young GA, Keogh GB, Parsons FM. (1975). Plasma amino acids and protein levels in chronic renal failure and changes caused by oral supplements of essential amino acids. Clinica Chimica Acta 61: 205–213.

Chapter 17

Assessment of iron status

The assessment of the iron status of population groups is particularly important, as iron deficiency is the commonest micronutrient deficiency in both developing and industrialized countries. It is particularly prevalent among infants, young children, and pregnant women. The deficiency may arise from inadequate intakes of dietary iron, poor absorption, excessive loss, or a combination of these factors. The quantity of iron in the body is controlled by absorption from the gut, which is in turn determined by the nutritional needs of the individual and by factors influencing the bioavailability of iron (Narasinga Rao, 1981). Such factors may include high intakes of phytate, dietary fiber, and tannins — components known to inhibit the absorption of nonheme iron — as well as intakes of enhancing factors such as vitamin C and flesh foods (Morck and Cook, 1981). In North American omniverous diets, grain products are a major source of nonheme iron, because many of these products are fortified with iron; flesh foods provide almost all of the heme iron.

Clinical manifestations of iron deficiency include anemia, angular stomatitis, glossitis, dysphagia, hypochlorhydria, koilonychia (spoon nails), and pagophagia (ice eating). Other less specific signs and symptoms frequently associated with iron deficiency include loss of energy, tiredness, anorexia, increased susceptibility to infection, certain behavioral abnormalities, and reduction in intellectual performance and work capacity (Oppenheimer and Hendrickse, 1983).

Iron overload occurs most frequently with the disorder idiopathic hemo-chromatosis. This is a hereditary disease characterized by the progressive accumulation of iron in the parenchymal tissue. In some circumstances, iron overload may also result from excessive intakes of medicinal or dietary iron, injections of therapeutic iron, or blood transfusions. The excessive iron accumulates in the tissues as hemosiderin, resulting in hemosiderosis or siderosis (Crosby, 1978).

The four to five grams of elemental iron present in a normal adult can be divided into three components: essential iron, transport iron, and storage iron. The essential component includes iron in the hemoglobin

349

of the red blood cells (70% of total iron), iron in the oxygen-binding protein found in muscle (myoglobin, 4%), and the iron in enzymes such as cytochromes, catalases, and peroxidases (less than 1%). Transport iron occurs in small amounts in the blood, bound to the iron transport protein transferrin.

Twenty-five percent of body iron is in the form of storage iron, which is found predominantly in the liver. Smaller amounts occur in the reticulo-endothelial cells of the bone marrow, liver, and spleen (Oski, 1979). Storage iron averages 1 g in an adult male and 300 mg in an adult menstruating female (Brittenham et al., 1981). Of this, approximately two-thirds consists of ferritin, the soluble fraction of the nonheme iron stores. Small quantities of ferritin can be synthesized in all cells of the body, even those with no special iron storage function (Cook and Finch, 1979). Ferritin also occurs in small concentrations in the serum, but does not contribute to iron transport. The remainder of storage iron is insoluble hemosiderin, a heterogeneous material composed principally of the breakdown products of denatured ferritin.

Three stages characterize the development of iron-deficiency anemia (Cook and Finch, 1979); these stages are discussed in detail in the sections describing the indices of iron status. The three stages are:

Iron depletion

The first stage is characterized by a progressive reduction in the amount of storage iron in the liver. At this stage, levels of transport iron and hemoglobin are normal, but the depletion of iron stores will be reflected by a fall in serum ferritin concentrations.

Iron-deficient erythropoiesis

Complete exhaustion of iron stores characterizes the second stage. As a result, the plasma iron supply to the erythropoietic cells is progressively reduced, and decreases in transferrin saturation occur (Section 17.4). In contrast, erythrocyte protoporphyrin concentrations increase. Erythrocyte protoporphyrin is a precursor of heme which accumulates in the red blood cells when the supply of iron is not adequate for heme synthesis (Section 17.6). Hemoglobin levels may decline slightly, but usually remain within the normal range during iron-deficient erythropoiesis. Exercise performance also appears to be reduced at this stage (Schoene et al., 1983).

Iron-deficiency anemia

The third and final stage of iron deficiency, caused by exhaustion of iron stores and declining levels of circulating iron, is characterized by frank microcytic, hypochromic anemia. The main feature of this stage is a reduction in the concentration of hemoglobin in the red blood cells,

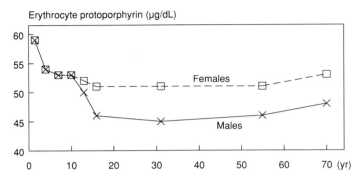

Figure 17.1: Median values for hemoglobin by age and sex. Conversion factor to SI units (g/L) = × 10. Modified from Yip et al. (1984). © Am. J. Clin. Nutr. American Society for Clinical Nutrition.

arising from the restriction of iron supply to the bone marrow. Decreases in the hematocrit and red cell indices also occur (Sections 17.2 and 17.3). Study of a stained blood film allows confirmation of the presence of hypochromic microcytosis.

17.1   Hemoglobin

Iron is an essential component of the hemoglobin molecule, the oxygen-carrying pigment of the red blood cells. Each hemoglobin molecule is a conjugate of a protein (globin) and four molecules of heme. Measurement of the concentration of hemoglobin in whole blood is probably the most widely used screening test for iron-deficiency anemia. A low hemoglobin concentration is associated with hypochromia, a characteristic feature of iron-deficiency anemia. The use of hemoglobin as an index of iron status has several limitations. These are outlined below:

Age, sex, and race dependence

Median hemoglobin values rise during the first ten years of childhood, with a further increase at puberty (Figure 17.1). Sex differences are apparent by the second decade of life, and are most marked in young adults when the hemoglobin concentration for men is on average about 2.0 g/dL (20 g/L) higher than in women. These sex-related differences diminish gradually with increasing age (Yip et al., 1984). Individuals of African descent have hemoglobin values which are 0.3 to 1.0 g/dL (3 to 10 g/L) lower than Caucasians, irrespective of age and income (Garn et al., 1981a).

Insensitivity

Hemoglobin is relatively insensitive, concentrations falling only during the third stage of iron deficiency. Considerable overlap exists in the hemoglobin values of normal nonanemic and iron-deficient individuals (Garby et al., 1969).

Low specificity

Low hemoglobin values also arise in chronic infections and inflammations, hemorrhage, protein-energy malnutrition, thalassemia minor, vitamin B-12 or folate deficiency, hemoglobinopathies, pregnancy, and other states in which there is overhydration or acute plasma volume expansion. In contrast, elevated hemoglobin values occur in polycythemia and hemoconcentration caused by dehydration.

Other factors

Hemoglobin concentrations are also modified by a variety of other factors, including diurnal variation and cigarette smoking. Hemoglobin values tend to be lower in the evening than in the morning, by amounts of up to 1.0 g/dL (10 g/L). Cigarette smoking is associated with higher concentrations of hemoglobin (0.3 to 0.5 g/dL) (3 to 5 g/L) in adults (Pilch and Senti, 1984).

Age- and sex-specific interpretive reference data for hemoglobin must be used. Several data sets are available (Table 17.1 and Table 17.3) (Garn et al., 1981b). The most recent U.S. cutoff values for hemoglobin are based on the distribution of hemoglobin values in venous blood obtained from a white, ostensibly healthy, nonpregnant population (Table 17.1) (Pilch and Senti, 1984). All subjects with evidence of iron deficiency and chronic disease were excluded. Hemoglobin values below the lower limit of the 95% confidence interval for each age/sex group for white subjects (i.e. below the 2.5th percentile) were considered low. Some misclassification will always arise because of the overlap of values in normal nonanemic, and iron-deficient persons. As the sample size was small for young children, the value obtained for three- and four-year-old children was also used for subjects aged one to years.

This approach was not used for American Negro subjects because too few were included in the survey for reliable determinations of the 95% confidence interval. Moreover, it is not clear whether separate hemoglobin criteria should be used for black and white subjects (Garn et al., 1981a).

Tables of means, standard deviations, standard errors of the mean, and selected percentiles are also available from the NHANES II survey for hemoglobin levels of persons one to seventy-four years old, by race, sex, and age (Pilch and Senti, 1984). Data tables are for all persons in the

Age (yr)	Males and Females	Hemoglobin (g/dL) Males	Females
NHANES II. From Pilch and Senti (1984)[a]			
1–2	10.9	—	—
3–4	10.9	—	—
5–10	11.2	—	—
11–14	—	12.0	11.8
15–19	—	13.1	11.7
20–44	—	13.4	11.9
45–64	—	13.2	11.8
65–74	—	12.6	11.9
WHO. From World Health Organization (1972)[b]			
0.5–6	11.0	—	—
6–14	12.0	—	—
> 14	—	13.0	12.0
Nutrition Canada. From Health and Welfare Canada (1973)[c]			
0–1	10.0	—	—
2–5	11.0	—	—
6–12	11.5	—	—
13–16	—	13.0	11.5
> 17	—	14.0	12.0

Table 17.1: Three different sets of criteria used for analysis of hemoglobin data. [a] Hemoglobin cutoff points derived from the NHANES II population (white subjects only). [b] Concentrations of hemoglobin below which anemia is likely to be present. [c] Criteria given as the upper limit of 'moderate' risk of deficiency. Conversion factor to SI units (g/L) = × 10. Reproduced with permission of the World Health Organization and the Minister of Supply and Services Canada.

NHANES II population, as well as for a reference sample formed by excluding persons with evidence of iron deficiency and chronic disease. Selected percentiles for the reference sample for children (all races) are given in Table 17.2 and for both children and adults in Appendix A17.1.

Percentile curves for hemoglobin concentrations in white infants and children, living at sea level, have also been compiled by Dallman and Siimes (1979). For these curves, children with laboratory evidence of iron deficiency, thalassemia minor, and/or hemoglobinopathy were excluded. Again, the applicability of these percentile curves to an American Negro population is not clearly established.

Hemoglobin can be determined using venous blood, anticoagulated with EDTA. Alternatively, capillary blood from heel, ear, or finger pricks, collected in heparized capillary tubes, can be used. Hemoglobin concentrations determined using capillary blood are less precise than corresponding measurements on venous blood. The cyanmethemoglobin method is the most reliable (Drabkin and Austin, 1932), provided that the blood specimen has been accurately diluted. Incorrect dilution of

Age	Hemoglobin Percentiles (g/dL)						
(yr)	5	10	25	50	75	90	95
Males							
1–2	—	11.2	11.5	11.9	12.4	12.9	—
3–4	11.3	11.6	12.0	12.6	13.0	13.4	13.6
5–10	11.5	11.8	12.3	12.9	13.5	13.9	14.3
11–14	12.1	12.4	13.1	13.8	14.5	15.1	15.4
15–19	13.3	13.6	14.2	15.0	15.6	16.3	16.6
Females							
1–2	—	—	11.9	12.4	12.8	—	—
3–4	10.9	11.2	11.7	12.3	12.9	13.4	13.9
5–10	11.5	11.8	12.3	12.9	13.5	14.0	14.3
11–14	11.8	12.1	12.7	13.3	13.9	14.3	14.7
15–19	12.0	12.3	12.8	13.4	14.0	14.7	15.0

Table 17.2: Selected percentiles for hemoglobin (g/dL) for male and female children of all races. Percentiles are for the NHANES II 'reference population'. A more complete data set, including information for adults, is given in the appendix. Abstracted from comprehensive tabulations of Pilch and Senti (1984), which includes additional information on the standard deviation, standard error of the mean, and the number of subjects studied in each age range. Conversion factor to SI units (g/L) = × 10.

the sample is one of the main sources of error in this method (Pilch and Senti, 1984). The method involves converting all of the usually encountered forms of hemoglobin in blood (oxyhemoglobin, methemoglobin, carboxyhemoglobin) to cyanmethemoglobin. The analysis can be performed with a spectrophotometer, or by an electronic counter. The coefficients of variation for hemoglobin by the cyanomethemoglobin method using venous blood, for both analytical and biological variation, are less than 4% (Dallman, 1984).

17.2 Hematocrit

The hematocrit is defined in SI units as the volume fraction of packed red cells. During iron deficiency, the hematocrit falls only after hemoglobin formation has become impaired. Consequently, in early cases of moderate iron deficiency, a marginally low hemoglobin value may be associated with a near-normal hematocrit (Graitcer et al., 1981). Only in more severe iron-deficiency anemia are both hemoglobin and hematocrit reduced. Limitations associated with the hematocrit determination include:

- The relative insensitivity of the method; hematocrit falls only in the third stage in the development of iron deficiency.
- The method lacks specificity. Hematocrit is affected by all the factors influencing the hemoglobin concentration.

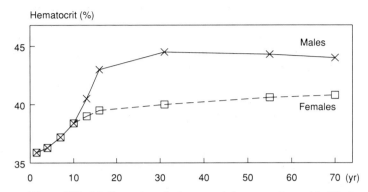

Figure 17.2: Median values for hematocrit by age and sex. Modified from Yip et al. (1984). Conversion factor to SI units = × 0.01. © Am. J. Clin. Nutr. American Society for Clinical Nutrition.

- The values are dependent on age and sex. Age- and sex-related trends in the hematocrit values are similar to those described for hemoglobin (Figure 17.2) (Yip et al., 1984).
- The method is not very precise, particularly when capillary blood samples are used.

Hematocrit, like hemoglobin, can be readily determined on capillary blood or EDTA-anticoagulated blood from veni-puncture blood samples. It is a relatively easy and rapid test, and is therefore often used in screening for iron-deficiency anemia. Surprisingly, hematocrit measurements generally detect lower rates of anemia than hemoglobin determinations, possibly because of the greater technical errors which occur when hematocrit is measured. Such errors may include: poorly packed iron-deficient cells resulting in spuriously elevated values; improper mixing of blood caused by intermittent blood flow from the puncture site; excessive anticoagulant in the collection tube; and elevated white blood cell counts leading to a poorly defined boundary between the red blood cells and the plasma in the hematocrit tube (Graitcer et al., 1981).

Hematocrit is measured by centrifuging a minute amount of blood in a heparinized capillary tube until the red cells have been reduced to a constant packed cell volume. The hematocrit is calculated by comparing the height of the column of packed red cells with the height of the entire column of red cells and plasma. Cutoff values for hematocrit, compiled by Dallman (1977), are shown in Table 17.3.

17.3 Red cell indices

Red cell indices derived from measurements of hemoglobin, hematocrit, and red blood cell count provide additional information for the diagnosis

Age (yr)	Hemoglobin (g/dL)		Hematocrit (%)		MCV (fL)	
	Mean	Lower limit	Mean	Lower limit	Mean	Lower limit
0.5–2	12.0	11.0	36	33	77	70
2–6	12.5	11.0	37	34	81	74
6–12	13.5	11.5	40	35	86	76
12–18						
Female	14.0	12.0	41	36	88	78
Male	14.5	13.0	43	38	88	78
18–49						
Female	14.0	12.0	41	36	90	80
Male	15.5	13.5	47	41	90	80

Table 17.3: Normal mean and lower limit (mean − 2 SD) of normal for hemoglobin, hematocrit, and MCV. Conversion factors to SI units are: hemoglobin (g/L) = × 10; hematocrit = × 0.01; MCV (fL). From Dallman PR. (1977). New approaches to screening for iron deficiency. Journal of Pediatrics 90: 678–681 with permission.

Red Cell Index	Iron Deficiency Anemia (microcytic hypochromic)	Macrocytic Anemia (normochromic)	Anemia of Chronic Disease (normocytic normochromic)
MCV	Low	High	Normal
MCHC	Low	Normal	Normal
MCH	Low	High	Normal

Table 17.4: Expected changes in red cell indices during iron-deficiency anemia, macrocytic anemia, and anemia of chronic disease. From Wintrobe MM, Lee GR, Boggs DR, Bithell TC, Foerster J, Athens JW, Lukens JN (eds). (1981). Clinical Hematology. Eight edition, Lea and Febiger, with permission.

of different types of anemia. Their accuracy, precision, and use have increased with the advent of automated equipment. A comparison of the expected changes in red cell indices during iron-deficiency anemia, macrocytic anemia resulting from vitamin B-12 and/or folic acid deficiency, and the anemia of chronic disease is summarized in Table 17.4. The anemia of chronic disease is caused by a defect in the transfer of iron from the reticulo-endothelial cells to serum transferrin. The anemia is generally mild and the peripheral blood appears normocytic and normochromic, or slightly hypochromic. Changes in red cell indices during vitamin B-12 and folic acid deficiency are described in more detail in Section 22.1.1.

Age (yr)	Serum Ferritin (ng/mL)	Transferrin Saturation (%)	Erythrocyte Protoporphyrin µg/dL RBC	MCV (fL)
1–2	—	< 12	> 80	< 73
3–4	< 10	< 14	> 75	< 75
5–10	< 10	< 15	> 70	< 76
11–14	< 10	< 16	> 70	< 78
15–74	< 12	< 16	> 70	< 80

Table 17.5: Cutoff points used for identifying abnormal values of iron status indices in the analysis of the NHANES II data. Conversion factors to SI units are: serum ferritin (µg/L) = × 1.00; erythrocyte protoporphyrin (µmol/L) = × 0.0177. From Pilch and Senti (1984).

17.3.1 Mean cell volume

Mean cell volume (MCV) is a measure of the average size of the red blood cell. It is best determined directly with electronic counters as results obtained are highly reproducible. Furthermore, MCV is less affected by sampling errors in skin puncture capillary blood samples than hemoglobin, because red cell size is unaffected if the sample is diluted by the tissue fluid. Low values of MCV only occur when iron deficiency becomes severe. If an electronic counter is not available, mean cell volume can be calculated from the hematocrit and red blood cell count:

$$\text{MCV (fL)} = \frac{\text{Hematocrit (volume fraction)}}{\text{Red blood cell count per liter}}$$

A low MCV is a relatively specific index for iron deficiency anemia, provided that the anemias of infection, chronic inflammatory disease, thalassemia minor, and lead poisoning have been excluded. In macrocytic anemias associated with vitamin B-12 or folate deficiency, MCV values are high (Table 17.4). The mean cell volume changes progressively during infancy, childhood and early adult life (Dallman and Siimes, 1979; Yip et al., 1984) (Figure 17.3). Red blood cells are generally larger at birth than during adulthood; they decrease in size rapidly during the first six months of life, gradually increasing in size during childhood. Differences according to sex are small; MCV is slightly higher in young adult females than males. For the NHANES II survey, a cutoff value of 80 fL was accepted as the lower limit of normal for adults, a value within the range 80 to 84 fL recommended by other investigators (Wintrobe et al., 1981). For children in the NHANES II survey, cutoff values for four age groups were set, and are shown in Table 17.5. The MCV values in the NHANES II survey were not determined by direct measurements, but were derived from the hematocrit and red blood cell count.

Reference data for MCV levels by race, sex, and age, for all persons aged one to seventy-four years in the NHANES II population, and

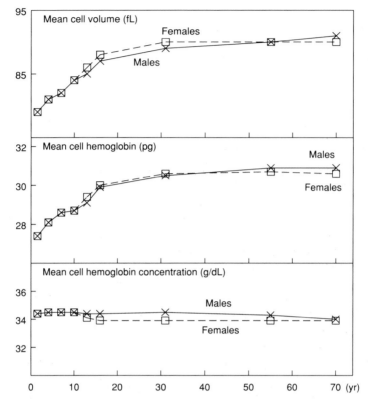

Figure 17.3: Median values for red blood cell indices by age and sex
Conversion factors to SI units are: MCHC (g/L) = × 10; MCH (pg);
MCV (fL) Modified from Yip et al. (1984). © Am. J. Clin. Nutr.
American Society for Clinical Nutrition.

for a reference sample, are available, as described for hemoglobin (Section 17.1) (Pilch and Senti, 1984). Selected percentiles for the reference sample for children and adults (all races) are given in Appendix A17.2.

17.3.2 Mean cell hemoglobin concentration

If the hemoglobin concentration and the hematocrit are known, the concentration of hemoglobin in the red blood cells can be determined. This is known as the mean cell hemoglobin concentration (MCHC). Mean cell hemoglobin concentration is less affected by age, after the first few months of life, than any other red cell index (Matoth et al., 1971) (Figure 17.3). This index is, however, the least useful of the red cell indices; it is the last to fall during iron deficiency.

$$\text{MCHC (g/L)} = \frac{\text{Hemoglobin (g/L)}}{\text{Hematocrit (vol. fraction)}}$$

Mean cell hemoglobin concentrations are low in iron-deficiency anemia, but normal in the macrocytic anemia of vitamin B-12 and folic acid deficiency and the anemia of chronic disease (Table 17.4).

17.3.3 Mean cell hemoglobin

Mean cell hemoglobin (MCH) refers to the hemoglobin content of the individual red blood cells. It can be measured using an electronic counter, and is derived from the ratio of hemoglobin to red blood cell count. The MCH changes progressively throughout life (Figure 17.3) and undergoes similar changes in iron-deficiency anemia to the MCV; it is low in iron-deficiency anemia but high in the macrocytic anemias of vitamin B-12 and folate deficiency (Table 17.4). In the latter, the red blood cells are laden with hemoglobin but are reduced in number. In severe iron deficiency, the relative fall in MCH is greater than the corresponding fall in MCV (Dallman, 1977).

$$\text{MCH (pg)} = \frac{\text{Hemoglobin (g/L)}}{\text{Red blood cell count } (10^{12}/\text{L})}$$

If subnormal values for the red cell indices are noted in the absence of thalassemia trait and the anemia of chronic disease, additional tests of iron status are generally performed to confirm the diagnosis of iron deficiency. The confirmatory tests commonly used are serum iron and total iron-binding capacity, serum ferritin, and erythrocyte protoporphyrin. These tests are discussed in detail below.

17.4 Serum iron, TIBC, and transferrin saturation

Serum iron, total iron-binding capacity (TIBC), and transferrin saturation are particularly useful for differentiating between nutritional deficiencies of iron and iron deficits arising from chronic infections, inflammation, or chronic neoplastic diseases. The concentrations of serum iron and the total iron-binding capacity reflect the iron in transit from the reticulo-endothelial system to the bone marrow. The serum iron content is a measure of the number of atoms of iron bound to the iron transport protein transferrin. Each molecule of transferrin (MW = 80,000) can be bound to one or two atoms of iron, although rarely are both the binding sites occupied. The total iron-binding capacity is related to the total number of *free* iron-binding sites on the transport protein transferrin. Determination of serum iron and total iron-binding capacity is usually performed simultaneously, and transferrin saturation calculated as shown below. The latter measures the iron supply to the erythroid bone marrow.

$$\text{Transferrin saturation (\%)} = \frac{\text{Serum iron (µmol/L)}}{\text{TIBC (µmol/L)}} \times 100\%$$

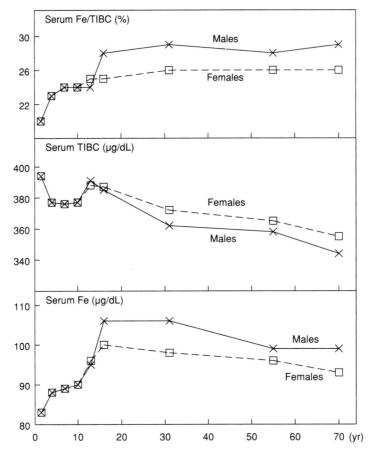

Figure 17.4: Median values for serum Fe/total iron-binding capacity (TIBC) (%), serum TIBC (μg/dL), and serum iron (μg/dL), by age and sex. Conversion factors to SI units are: TIBC (μmol/L) = × 0.179; serum Fe (μmol/L) = × 0.179. Modified from Yip et al. (1984). © Am. J. Clin. Nutr. American Society for Clinical Nutrition.

Several factors influence concentrations of serum iron, total iron-binding capacity, and hence transferrin saturation. Their effects are discussed below.

Age

Serum iron and, to a lesser extent, total iron-binding capacity are age-dependent. Serum iron levels rise during childhood, whereas total iron-binding capacity falls (Figure 17.4). Values for both indices are highest in young adults, and decline steadily with advancing age (Yip et al., 1984).

Sex

The sex of the subject does not have an important effect on serum iron or total iron-binding capacity levels. Nevertheless, in the NHANES II survey, there was a tendency for serum iron levels to be higher in males than females after the middle of the second decade of life (Figure 17.4) (Pilch and Senti, 1984).

Oral contraceptive agents

In the NHANES II survey, women taking oral contraceptives had elevated levels of total iron-binding capacity characteristic of iron deficiency (Pilch and Senti, 1984).

Iron deficiency

Iron deficiency results in a fall in serum iron levels, and an associated rise in total iron-binding capacity arising from the increase in the number of free iron-binding sites. Consequently, transferrin saturation is low. These changes appear during the second stage of iron deficiency, when iron stores are depleted. Hence, transferrin saturation is a more sensitive index of iron status than the red cell indices discussed in Section 17.3. It is also more consistently useful for diagnosing iron deficiency than the values for either serum iron or total iron-binding capacity alone, because a low transferrin saturation in association with an elevated total iron-binding capacity is more specific for iron deficiency.

Iron overload

In conditions such as hemochromatosis, hemolytic anemia, acute liver damage, excessive absorption of iron from the gut, transfusions, and iron therapy, iron overload may occur. It results in elevated body iron stores and thus high serum iron levels. Hence, there are fewer free iron-binding sites on the transferrin molecules, and total iron-binding capacity falls. Such changes produce an elevated transferrin saturation level. In the NHANES II survey, a transferrin saturation $> 70\%$ was used as a criterion for detecting iron overload in adults (Pilch and Senti, 1984).

Chronic disease states

Infection, inflammation, and malignancy typically produce low serum iron *and* low total iron-binding levels, and hence a transferrin saturation which tends towards the low end of the normal range. Such trends arise from defects in the release of iron from the reticulo-endothelial cells and the subsequent transport of iron from these stores to transferrin. Together, these defects — termed the 'mucosal block' — result in a shortage of iron in the bone marrow, despite adequate or even slightly increased iron stores. As the iron stores are adequate, the body does not respond to the fall in serum iron by increasing absorption of iron from the diet.

Consequently, transferrin synthesis is not increased, and levels of total iron-binding capacity remain low. Hence, the determination of total iron-binding capacity allows one to distinguish between the low transferrin saturation of chronic disease and that of true iron deficiency.

Decreased erythropoiesis

Vitamin B-12 or folic acid deficiency, and the action of certain drugs and toxins, may be associated with decreased erythropoiesis. In these circumstances, serum iron levels are normal or slightly above normal because of decreased utilization of iron for hemoglobin synthesis; levels of total iron-binding capacity are often normal or low. Consequently, transferrin saturation may be high.

Increased erythropoiesis

Increased erythropoiesis often occurs after recovery from bone marrow depression, in response to vitamin B-12 and folate therapy, in hemolysis, and in some cases of polycythemia. In such cases, the serum iron concentration may fall below normal limits whereas the total iron-binding capacity is often high-normal or even high, a trend comparable to that observed in iron deficiency. Consequently, alternative indices of iron status (e.g. serum ferritin) should also be used to distinguish between iron deficiency and increased erythropoiesis.

Biological variation of serum iron values can be very high and sometimes coefficients of variation approach 30% — perhaps as a result of large diurnal effects which may be inconsistent among individuals (Dallman, 1984). In general, serum iron values tend to be elevated in the morning, decreasing in the afternoon and evening (Bothwell and Mallett, 1955; Wiltink et al., 1973). As a result, measurements of serum iron should preferably be determined on fasting morning blood samples. In this way, the effects of both recent dietary intake and diurnal variation are minimized. Day-to-day variation in serum iron also occurs (Statland and Winkel, 1977). Total iron-binding capacity is less subject to biological variation — especially diurnal effects — than serum iron, but is more susceptible to analytical errors.

In adults, a transferrin saturation below 16% indicates iron-deficient erythropoiesis (Bainton and Finch, 1964; Dallman, 1977), provided that infection and inflammation are excluded (Cook, 1982). Age-related differences in normal serum iron (but not TIBC) occur in infants and children, resulting in corresponding changes in the normal levels of transferrin saturation (Dallman et al., 1980). Uncertainties still exist in the extent of these changes. Consequently, cutoff points are not as clearly defined for infants and children as for adults. Pilch and Senti (1984) used cutoff values ranging from < 12% to < 16% for transferrin saturation in children from one to fourteen years of age when assessing the prevalence of iron deficiency in the NHANES II survey (Table 17.5). Transferrin saturation values > 70% were used as a criterion for detecting iron overload in adults, in conjunction with elevated serum ferritin levels (Section 17.5).

Tables of selected percentiles, means, standard deviations, and standard errors of the mean by race, age, and sex, for percentage transferrin saturation, derived from all the persons in the NHANES II survey, and for a reference sample, are also given in Pilch and Senti (1984). Selected percentiles for children and adults (all races) for the reference population are given in Appendix A17.3. Serum iron and total iron-binding capacity measurements are technically more difficult than the determination of hemoglobin and hematocrit. Precision can be low, particularly for manual methods. The analytical coefficient of variation for serum iron determined manually can be up to 9.6% compared 3.2% to 4.6% for the automated method. Comparable analytical coefficients of variation have been documented for total iron-binding capacity (Dallman, 1984).

Colorimetric procedures for determining serum iron frequently use ferrozine as the chromogen to react with Fe(II) to form a violet complex (Giovanniello et al., 1968). In this method, total iron-binding capacity is determined by saturating the serum with excess iron, followed by the addition of magnesium carbonate. The latter removes the iron not bound to serum transferrin. Other commonly used chromogens for the colorimetric assay of serum iron include bathophenanthroline sulfonate and tripyridyltriazine (Zak et al., 1980). Alternatively, serum iron can be assayed by atomic absorption spectrophotometry.

Potential sources of error in the measurement of serum iron and total iron-binding capacity by all methods include contamination by exogenous iron, and a copper interference with the colorimetric determination. Variations in the type and amount of magnesium carbonate used to remove unbound iron when the ferrozine method is used, and uncertainties in the concentration of the saturating iron solution, may also be a problem (Pilch and Senti, 1984). Quality control sera, with certified values for serum iron and total iron-binding capacity covering a wide range, should be included with each assay, and iron-free water used. In the future, an electrochemical method may be used which is not sensitive to copper interference, and which requires only a small blood sample.

17.5 Serum ferritin

Ferritin was first identified in human serum by Addison et al. (1972); its function in serum is unknown. Ferritin appears to enter the plasma by secretions from the reticulo-endothelial system (Cook and Skikne, 1982). In most individuals the concentration of serum ferritin parallels the total amount of storage iron (Cook et al., 1974), and serum ferritin is the only iron status index that can reflect a deficient, excess, and normal iron status.

Evidence for the quantitative relationship between serum ferritin and storage iron includes:

- a positive correlation between serum ferritin levels and stainable bone marrow stores;
- a fall in serum ferritin in response to iron removal by phlebotomy, the decline parallelling changes in liver iron stores as measured by liver biopsy (Jacobs et al., 1972; Walters et al., 1973);
- a positive response of serum ferritin levels to iron therapy and repeated transfusions (Kimber et al., 1983).

Quantification of iron stores based on serum ferritin levels is difficult, because there is considerable inter-subject variation in the relationship between serum ferritin and tissue iron. In normal adults with serum ferritin concentrations within the range of 20 to 300 µg/L, a serum ferritin concentration of 1 µg/L is equivalent to approximately 10 mg of storage iron (Cook and Skikne, 1982). Once iron stores have become depleted, however, serum ferritin no longer reflects the *severity* of the iron deficiency.

Several factors affect serum ferritin levels, some of which may coexist with iron deficiency. These are discussed below.

Iron deficiency

Serum ferritin values fall during iron deficiency before the characteristic changes in serum iron and total iron-binding capacity. In conditions of frank iron-deficiency anemia, when classical microcytic hypochromic anemia occurs, serum ferritin levels are very low or zero, reflecting the exhaustion of storage iron. It is important to note that a low concentration of serum ferritin is characteristic *only* of iron deficiency (Dallman et al., 1980).

Iron overload

This results in a rise in body iron stores and an associated increase in ferritin synthesis and hence a rise in serum ferritin. Serum ferritin provides similar information to that of serum iron and total iron-binding capacity in conditions of iron overload.

Chronic disease states

Infection, inflammation, and certain neoplastic diseases produce the defect known as the 'mucosal block' (Section 17.4). One of the results of this defect is an increased rate of ferritin synthesis in the reticulo-endothelial system, which is reflected by an elevated concentration of ferritin in the serum. Hence, serum ferritin should not be used as an index of iron status in countries where iron deficiency coexists with infection or inflammation; values may be in the normal range despite the presence of iron deficiency (Wickramasinghe et al., 1985). In such cases, alternative indices of iron status, such as red blood cell protoporphyrin, and/or serum iron and total iron-binding capacity, should be used.

Decreased erythropoiesis

A deficiency of specific nutrients such as vitamin B-12 and folic acid and certain drugs and toxins may be associated with decreased erythropoiesis. In such cases, serum ferritin levels may be normal or slightly above normal limits, as the utilization of iron for hemoglobin synthesis is decreased.

Increased erythropoiesis

This is associated with *normal* serum ferritin levels, which decline slowly as storage iron is used for hemoglobin synthesis. In contrast, increased erythropoiesis induces rapid changes in serum iron and total iron-binding capacity comparable to those observed during iron deficiency. Hence it is advisable to measure serum ferritin as well as serum iron and total iron-binding capacity in conditions of increased erythropoiesis.

Acute and chronic liver disease

Abnormally high serum ferritin concentrations are often observed in patients with acute and chronic liver disease, probably the result of the release of ferritin from the damaged degenerating liver cells, which contain appreciable amounts of ferritin. Such damage is one of the factors contributing to the elevated serum ferritin concentrations observed in children with protein-energy malnutrition (Wickramasinghe et al., 1985). These elevated serum ferritin levels do not reflect a high intracellular concentration of ferritin (Worwood, 1979).

Leukemia and Hodgkin's disease

Raised serum ferritin concentrations are also observed in patients with leukemia or Hodgkin's disease. In leukemia, these may be associated with: (a) increased deposition of iron in cells of the reticulo-endothelial system; (b) circulating leukemic cells containing high levels of ferritin; and/or (c) increased release of ferritin from damaged cells, as in liver disease. In Hodgkin's disease, the increased ferritin in the serum possibly comes from the lymphocytes (Worwood, 1979).

Age

At birth, serum ferritin concentrations are relatively high, as iron stores in the liver are abundant. During the first two months, serum ferritin levels rise further, as iron is released from the fetal red cells and the

	Age (yr)	Serum Ferritin (µg/L)		
		Sexes combined	Males	Females
NHANES II				
Normal children	3–4	15	14	17
	5–10	19	18	19
	11–14	18	18	18
	15–19	25	35	18
Normal adults	20–44	50	89	28
	45–64	81	110	63
	65–74	83	98	74
From Worwood (1979)				
Iron deficiency anemia	3–14	< 10	—	—
	15–74	< 12	—	—
Idiopathic hemochromatosis	adults	1000–10,000	—	—
Liver disease	adults	400–3000+	—	—
Inflammation	adults	10–1650	—	—
Acute infections	children	100–510	—	—

Table 17.6: Changes in serum ferritin concentrations with age and disease states. The NHANES II data are from Pilch and Senti (1984), and are the median values and representative of all races.

rate of erythropoiesis is slow. Serum ferritin concentrations then fall throughout later infancy and childhood. Adult men and the elderly have higher levels than children and premenopausal women (Table 17.6).

Sex

In women, levels are relatively constant until the menopause, and then increase gradually, whereas in men concentrations rise progressively after adolescence (Cook et al., 1976).

Diurnal and day-to-day variation

This is less important for serum ferritin levels than for serum iron. Pilon et al. (1981) reported the average intra-subject day-to-day coefficient of variation for serum ferritin to be 14.5% compared to 28.5% for serum iron, although analytical variation for the serum ferritin assay was greater than for the serum iron assay. Diurnal variation appears to be minimal.

In the NHANES II survey, a cutoff value for serum ferritin of $< 10\,\mu g/L$ was used for children up to fourteen years of age and a value of $< 12\,\mu g/L$ for all older subjects (Pilch and Senti, 1984). Serum ferritin concentrations $< 12\,\mu g/L$ are almost always indicative of depletion of iron stores (Jacobs et al., 1972). Elevated values are useful in diagnosing iron overload disorders. Table 17.7 shows the cutoff values for serum ferritin indicative of iron overload in adults used in the NHANES II survey, in conjunction with transferrin saturation $> 70\%$ (Pilch and Senti, 1984).

Age Group	Males	Females
20–44 yr	> 200	> 150
45–64 yr	> 300	> 200
65–74 yr	> 400	> 300

Table 17.7: Cutoff values for serum ferritin (ng/mL) indicative of iron overload in adults. Conversion factor to SI units (µg/L) = × 1.0. From Pilch and Senti (1984).

Nevertheless, these high levels are not specific to iron overload disorders, as they also occur in liver disease, neoplasms, and inflammatory disease (Dallman, 1977).

Reference data, by race, age, and sex, are also available for serum ferritin for all persons aged three to seventy-four years in the NHANES II survey, and for the reference sample, discussed earlier (Section 17.1) (Pilch and Senti, 1984). Selected percentiles for children and adults (all races) for the reference sample are given in Appendix A17.4.

Serum ferritin is commonly assayed using a two-site immunoradiometric method (Miles et al., 1974). Capillary blood samples can be used (Segall et al., 1979). The method requires a gamma counter and a trained technician, and is therefore a relatively expensive procedure. The within- and between-assay analytical coefficients of variation for serum ferritin are approximately 3% and 7% respectively (Dallman, 1984). Use of an international standard preparation of ferritin should improve the precision of assays in the future. Sensitive, enzyme-linked immunosorbent (ELISA), which eliminate the need for radioisotopes, have been developed (Anaokar et al., 1979). These methods allow the assay of ferritin concentrations in the serum/plasma obtained from a single microhematocrit tube (Lu et al., 1987).

17.6 Erythrocyte protoporphyrin

Protoporphyrin, a precursor of heme, normally occurs in erythrocytes in very low concentrations. In the second stage of iron deficiency, when iron stores are completely exhausted, protoporphyrin IX accumulates in the developing erythrocytes because the supply of iron is not adequate for the synthesis of heme. Consequently, a rise in erythrocyte protoporphyrin concentration is a sensitive indicator of an inadequate iron supply. Erythrocyte protoporphyrin provides the same information as percentage transferrin saturation but is a more stable measurement and responds more gradually to changes in the iron supply to the marrow (Langer et al., 1972). In adults, a transferrin saturation indicative of iron deficiency (i.e. of less than 16%), corresponds to an erythrocyte protoporphyrin concentration of greater than 70 µg/dL (1.24 µmol/L) red blood

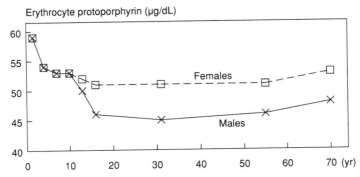

Figure 17.5: Median values for erythrocyte protoporphyrin by age and sex. Conversion factor to SI units (μmol/L) = × 0.0177. Modified from Yip et al. (1984). © Am. J. Clin. Nutr. American Society for Clinical Nutrition.

cells (RBC) (Langer et al., 1972). This value was used as a cutoff point by Pilch and Senti (1984) for assessing the prevalence of iron deficiency in adults in the NHANES II survey. Factors affecting erythrocyte protoporphyrin values are discussed below. Iron deficiency of increasing severity produces progressively elevated protoporphyrin concentrations. In classical iron deficiency, when microcytic hypochromic anemia occurs, erythrocyte protoporphyrin levels may rise to values ranging from 83 to 457 μg/dL (1.47 to 8.09 μmol/L) RBC. A week after transferrin saturation values have fallen to less than 15%, erythrocyte protoporphyrin concentrations are markedly elevated.

Chronic disease states, such as infection, inflammation, and certain neoplastic diseases, are associated with elevated protoporphyrin levels resulting from the mucosal block defect (Section 17.4). Therefore, erythrocyte protoporphyrin values, unlike serum ferritin, cannot be used to differentiate between iron deficiency caused by total body depletion of iron, and that arising from the mucosal block defect. In both situations, erythrocyte protoporphyrin levels are elevated. Hence additional measurements of iron status, such as serum ferritin and total iron-binding capacity, must be used to distinguish between these two conditions.

Lead toxicity produces elevated erythrocyte protoporphyrin levels via interference with heme synthesis. In the NHANES II survey, erythrocyte protoporphyrin values were elevated in children aged one to four years with high blood lead values.

Age- and sex-related changes in erythrocyte protoporphyrin values were documented in the NHANES II survey. Values were highest in the case of infants and young children, declining rapidly, and remaining relatively stable during adulthood (Figure 17.5). The reason for such elevation of levels during infancy is unclear at the present time. The range in erythrocyte protoporphyrin values was greatest in children and among the elderly. Differences according to sex were small (Yip et al., 1984).

Protoporphyrin concentrations in the whole blood samples are expressed as µmol/L RBC using the following formula, where hematocrit is expressed as the volume fraction of packed red cell:

$$\text{Protoporphyrin in red blood cells (µmol/L)} = \frac{\text{Protoporphyrin in whole blood (µmol/L)}}{\text{Hematocrit (vol. fraction)}}$$

Erythrocyte protoporphyrin is useful for distinguishing iron deficiency from thalassemia minor, being elevated in the former but not in the latter (Stockman et al., 1975). Measurements of erythrocyte protoporphyrin do not, however, distinguish between the anemia of iron deficiency and that occurring in chronic inflammatory disorders. Concentrations may also be increased in response to other conditions that interfere with heme synthesis, such as lead poisoning, erythropoietic protoporphyria, and acute myelogenous leukemia (Piomelli et al., 1982). In adults, a protoporphyrin level greater than 70 µg/dL (1.24 µmol/L) RBC has been associated with depleted iron stores, and was used as the cutoff point for abnormal values in the NHANES II survey. The cutoff points selected for children aged one to fourteen years are shown in Table 17.5 and represent < 90th percentile of the NHANES II reference population data. Tables of selected percentiles, means, standard deviations, and standard errors of the mean, by race, sex, and age are available for erythrocyte protoporphyrin values from all persons in the NHANES II survey, and for the reference sample only (Pilch and Senti, 1984). Appendix A17.5 gives selected percentiles for children and adults (all races) for the reference sample. Hershko et al. (1981) recommend the use of erythrocyte protoporphyrin, in combination with MCH, to screen for iron-deficiency anemia in children with a high incidence of minor inter-current infections. Their recommendation was based on the high sensitivity and specificity of these indices, their low cost, and the ease of use of fingertip blood samples. Any abnormal results found should be confirmed by direct measurement of transferrin saturation

Erythrocyte protoporphyrin can be measured rapidly by a technically simple and inexpensive fluorometric procedure. A hematofluorometer has been designed for field use, in which erythrocyte protoporphyrin is determined by the reflected fluorescence of a thin film of capillary whole blood (Poh Fitzpatrick and Lamola, 1976). The blood film must be mixed vigorously to ensure oxygenation and complete dissolution of red cell aggregates. Several readings should be made until successive values are stable (within 10%). Artificial calibration slides are provided by the manufacturer to check instrument stability. This field method should be standardized against quality control samples in which erythrocyte protoporphyrin has been measured by an alternative extraction method (Sassa et al., 1973). The latter also measures the fluorescence and is more readily standardized. Values by the extraction procedure tend to be lower than those measured by the hematofluorometer (Lu et al., 1987). The

Frequency

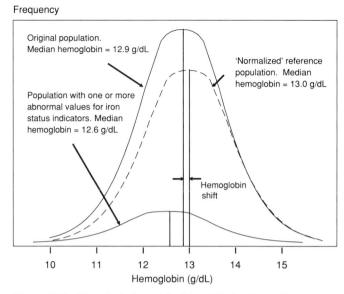

Figure 17.6: Hypothetical model of the shift in the median hemoglobin after exclusion of persons with abnormal values for iron status
indices. From Pilch and Senti (1984).

inter-assay coefficients of variation are lower for the hematofluorometer
(1.4% to 2.5%) than for the extraction method (5.0%) (Dallman, 1984).

17.7   Multi-parameter indices

The use of several indices of iron status simultaneously provides a more
accurate measure of iron status than any single index (Cook et al., 1976).
Several combinations of indices have been used. Generally, the presence
of two or more abnormal values for iron status   indices is considered
indicative of impaired iron status.   In the NHANES II survey (Pilch
and Senti, 1984), three different models were used to assess the relative
prevalence of impaired iron status and anemia in selected groups of the
U.S. population: (a) the ferritin model; (b) the MCV model, and (c) the
hemoglobin percentile shift model (Figure 17.6).

In the ferritin model (a), serum ferritin, transferrin saturation, and erythrocyte protoporphyrin were included.   The MCV model (b) included
MCV, transferrin saturation, and erythrocyte protoporphyrin, indices independently representing the three stages characterizing the development
of iron-deficiency anemia. For example, serum ferritin detects the first
stage of iron deficiency — depletion of storage iron — whereas the decrease in transport iron which accompanies the second stage is reflected

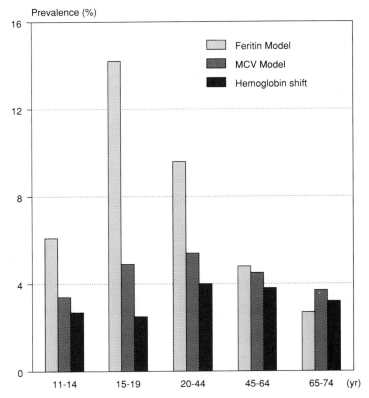

Figure 17.7: Prevalence of impaired iron status in subjects of varying ages estimated using the ferritin model, the MCV model, and the hemoglobin percentile shift model: NHANES II, 1976–1980. From Pilch and Senti (1984).

by a fall in transferrin saturation. The third and final stage of iron deficiency, characterized by frank microcytic, hypochromic anemia, is detected by the MCV index. If model (a) is used, the prevalence of impaired iron status, indicated by two or more abnormal values, will be higher than that based on the MCV model (b), as serum ferritin is the most sensitive index of the *early* depletion of body iron stores (see Figure 17.7). Neither model, however, can provide a definitive diagnosis of iron deficiency because none of the indices (with the exception of serum ferritin) distinguishes between changes resulting from iron deficiency and those arising from infection or inflammation. The cutoff values for these indices indicative of abnormal values of iron status and used in the NHANES II survey are shown in Table 17.1 and Table 17.5 (Pilch and Senti, 1984).

For population studies, the hemoglobin percentile shift model (c) is used (Figure 17.6). It is based on the premise that the presence of anemia arising from iron deficiency or inflammatory disease causes a lowering of the hemoglobin concentration (Meyers et al., 1983; Dallman et al., 1984).

Hence, the relative prevalence of anemia can be estimated by determining the change, or shift, in the median hemoglobin concentrations after excluding subjects who have one or more biochemical indices indicative of iron deficiency (Figure 17.6) (Pilch and Senti, 1984). In the NHANES II survey, two criteria were used for excluding subjects from the reference sample: those with transferrin saturation $< 16\%$ and those with erythrocyte protoporphyrin $> 70\,\mu g/dL$ ($> 1.24\,\mu mol/L$) RBC. The hemoglobin percentile shift was then estimated by plotting the cumulative percentage distribution curves for the total sample of the NHANES II survey and for the reference sample. A straight line is then drawn at the median. The hemoglobin percentile shift, indicative of the prevalence of anemia, is the distance between the reference sample line and the total sample line at the median (Expert Scientific Working Group, 1985).

Figure 17.7 compares the estimates of the prevalence of impaired iron status (arising from iron deficiency and/or inflammatory disease) for females from eleven to seventy-four years of age in the NHANES II survey. As expected, the estimates obtained using the MCV model and the hemoglobin percentile shift model are in general similar, whereas the prevalence estimates based on the ferritin model are higher in almost all age groups. Nevertheless, the prevalence estimates obtained by all three models were relatively low.

17.8 Summary

Table 17.8 summarizes the changes in the biochemical indices of iron status that occur during each of the three phases in the development of iron-deficiency anemia. The first phase is a decrease in iron stores, reflected by a decline in serum/plasma ferritin concentrations. The second phase, iron-deficient erythropoiesis, is characterized by a decrease in serum/plasma iron ($< 60\,\mu g/dL$) and an elevation in total iron-binding capacity, resulting in a fall in percentage transferrin saturation ($< 15\%$). At the same time, erythrocyte protoporphyrin concentrations will be increased ($> 100\,\mu g/dL$), because the supply of iron is no longer adequate for heme synthesis; the hemoglobin remains within the normal range for age and sex. In the third and final stage of iron deficiency, frank microcytic, hypochromic anemia occurs, when decreases in both the hemoglobin concentration and the hematocrit occur, resulting in a low MCHC. At this stage, further decreases in plasma iron ($< 40\,\mu g/dL$) and ferritin ($< 10\,\mu g/L$) will be apparent, and increases in erythrocyte protoporphyrin ($> 200\,\mu g/dL$) and total iron-binding capacity ($> 410\,\mu g/dL$). The presence of hypochromic microcytosis can be confirmed at this stage by using a stained blood film. Table 17.8 also presents the changes in the iron status indices which occur during iron overload. As elevated serum ferritin

	Iron Overload	Normal	Iron Depletion	Iron-Deficient Erythro-poiesis	Iron-Deficiency Anemia
RE marrow Fe	4 +	2–3 +	0–1 +	0	0
TIBC (μg/dL)	< 300	330 ± 30	360	390	410
Plasma ferritin (μg/L)	> 300	100 ± 60	20	10	< 10
Iron absorption (%)	> 15	5–10	10–15	10–20	10–20
Plasma iron (μg/dL)	> 175	115 ± 50	115	< 60	< 40
Transferrin saturation (%)	> 60	35 ± 15	30	< 15	< 15
Sideroblasts (%)	40–60	40–60	40–60	< 10	< 10
RBC protoporphyrin (μg/dL)	30	30	30	100	200
Erythrocytes	Normal	Normal	Normal	Normal	Microcytic/ Hypochromic

Table 17.8: Sequential stages in the development of iron deficiency and iron overload. RE = reticuloendothelial; TIBC = total iron-binding capacity; RBC = red blood cell. To convert μg iron to SI units (nmol) multiply by 17.9. Modified from Herbert (1987). © Am. J. Clin. Nutr. American Society for Clinical Nutrition.

concentrations also occur during chronic inflammatory conditions, measurements of serum iron and total iron-binding capacity are the preferred screening tests for iron overload.

To provide the best measure of iron status, several indices should be used simultaneously. The presence of two or more abnormal values generally indicates impaired iron status. The selection of the most appropriate combination depends on the health of the individual(s), and the study objectives. Diagnosis of iron deficiency is particularly difficult in the presence of other conditions which confound the interpretation of the laboratory results. For example, the diagnosis of iron deficiency may be obscured by the simultaneous effects of chronic inflammation, unless tests such as total iron-binding capacity and serum ferritin are performed. Erythrocyte protoporphyrin can be used to distinguish iron deficiency from thalassemia minor, but not to differentiate between the anemia of iron deficiency and that associated with chronic inflammatory disorders. Prevalence values for impaired iron status will vary according to the combination of indices selected. When serum ferritin is included, prevalence values will always be higher, because serum ferritin is the most sensitive index of early depletion of body iron stores.

References

Addison GM, Beamish MR, Hayles CN, Hodgkins M, Jacobs A, Llewellyn P. (1972). An immunoradiometric assay for ferritin in the serum of normal subjects and patients with iron deficiency and iron overload. Journal of Clinical Pathology 25: 326–329.

Anaokar S, Garry PJ, Standefer JC. (1979). Solid-phase enzyme immunoassay for serum ferritin. Clinical Chemistry 25: 1426–1431.

Bainton DF, Finch CA. (1964). The diagnosis of iron deficiency anemia. American Journal of Medicine 37: 62–70.

Bothwell TH, Mallet B. (1955). Diurnal variation in turnover of iron through plasma. Clinical Science 14: 235–239.

Brittenham GM, Danish EH, Harris JW. (1981). Assessment of bone marrow and body iron stores: old techniques and new technologies. Seminars in Hematology 18: 194–221.

Cook JD. (1982). Clinical evaluation of iron deficiency. Seminars in Hematology 19: 6–18.

Cook JD, Finch CA. (1979). Assessing iron status of a population. American Journal of Clinical Nutrition 32: 2115–2119.

Cook JD, Finch CA, Smith NJ. (1976). Evaluation of the iron status of a population. Blood 48: 449–455.

Cook JD, Lipschitz DA, Miles LEM, Finch CA. (1974). Serum ferritin as a measure of iron stores in normal subjects. American Journal of Clinical Nutrition 27: 681–687.

Cook JD, Skikne BS. (1982). Serum ferritin: a possible model for the assessment of nutrient stores. American Journal of Clinical Nutrition 35: 1180–1185.

Crosby WH. (1978). The effect of nutrient toxicities in animals and man: Iron. In: Recheigl M Jr (ed). CRC Handbook Series in Nutrition and Food. Section E: Nutritional Disorders Volume 1. Effect of Nutrient Excesses and Toxicities in Animals and Man. CRC Press Inc., West Palm Beach, Florida, pp. 177–192.

Dallman PR. (1977). New approaches to screening for iron deficiency. Journal of Pediatrics 90: 678–681.

Dallman PR. (1984). Diagnosis of anemia and iron deficiency: analytic and biological variations of laboratory tests. American Journal of Clinical Nutrition 39: 937–941.

Dallman PR, Siimes MA. (1979). Percentile curves for hemoglobin and red cell volume in infancy and childhood. Journal of Pediatrics 94: 26–31.

Dallman PR, Siimes MA, Stekel A. (1980). Iron deficiency in infancy and childhood. American Journal of Clinical Nutrition 33: 86–118.

Dallman PR, Yip R, Johnson C. (1984). Prevalence and causes of anemia in the United States, 1976 to 1980. American Journal of Clinical Nutrition 39: 437–445.

Drabkin DL, Austin JH. (1932). Spectrophotometric studies: spectrophotometric constants for common hemoglobin derivatives in human, dog and rabbit blood. Journal of Biological Chemistry 98: 719–733.

Expert Scientific Working Group (1985). Summary of a report on assessment of the iron nutritional status of the United States population. American Journal of Clinical Nutrition 42: 1318–1330.

Garby L, Irnell L, Werner I. (1969). Iron deficiency in women of fertile age in a Swedish community. III. Estimation of prevalence based on response to iron supplementation. Acta Medica Scandinavica 185: 113–117.

Garn SM, Ryan AS, Owen GM, Abraham S. (1981a). Income matched black-white hemoglobin differences after correction for low transferrin saturations. American Journal of Clinical Nutrition 34: 1645–1647.

Garn SM, Ryan AS, Abraham S, Owen G. (1981b). Suggested sex and age appropriate values for 'low' and 'deficient' hemoglobin levels. American Journal of Clinical Nutrition 34: 1648–1651.

Giovanniello TJ, DiBenedetto G, Palmer DW, Peters T Jr. (1968). Fully- and semi-automated methods for the determination of serum iron and total iron-binding capacity. Journal of Laboratory and Clinical Medicine 71: 874–883.

Graitcer PL, Goldsby JB, Nichaman MZ. (1981). Hemoglobins and hematocrits: are they equally sensitive in detecting anemias? American Journal of Clinical Nutrition 34: 61–64.

Health and Welfare Canada (1973). Nutrition Canada National Survey. Health and Welfare, Ottawa.

Herbert V. (1987). The 1986 Herman Award Lecture. Nutrition Science as a continually unfolding story: the folate and vitamin B-12 paradigm. American Journal of Clinical Nutrition 46: 387–402.

Hershko C, Bar-Or D, Gaziel Y, Naparstek E, Konijn AM, Grossowicz N, Kaufman N, Izak G. (1981). Diagnosis of iron deficiency anemia in a rural population of children. Relative usefulness of serum ferritin, red cell protoporphyrin, red cell indices, and transferrin saturation determinations. American Journal of Clinical Nutrition. 34: 1600–1610.

Jacobs A, Miller F, Worwood M, Beamish MR, Wardrop CA. (1972). Ferritin in the serum of normal subjects and patients with iron deficiency and iron overload. British Medical Journal 4: 206–208.

Kimber RJ, Rudzki Z, Blunden RW. (1983). Clinching the diagnosis: 1. Iron deficiency and iron overload: serum ferritin and serum iron in clinical medicine. Pathology 15: 497–503.

Langer EE, Haining RG, Labbe RF, Jacobs P, Crosby EF, Finch CA. (1972). Erythrocyte protoporphyrin. Blood 40: 112–128.

Lu Y, Lynch SR, Cook JD, Madan N, Bayer WL. (1987). Use of capillary blood for the evaluation of iron status. American Journal of Hematology 24: 365–374.

Matoth Y, Zaizov R, Varsoni I. (1971). Postnatal changes in some red cell parameters. Acta Paediatrica Scandinavica 60: 317–323.

Meyers LD, Habricht JP, Johnson CL, Brownie C. (1983). Prevalences of anemia and iron deficiency anemia in black and white women in the United States estimated by two methods. American Journal of Public Health 73: 1042–1049.

Miles LEM, Lipschitz DA, Bieber CP, Cook JD. (1974). Measurement of serum ferritin by a 2-site immunoradiometric assay. Annals of Biochemistry 61: 209–224.

Morck TA, Cook JD. (1981). Factors affecting the bioavailability of dietary iron. Cereal Foods World 26: 667–672.

Narasinga Rao BS. (1981). Physiology of iron absorption and supplementation. British Medical Bulletin 37: 25–30.

Oppenheimer S, Hendrickse R. (1983). The clinical effects of iron deficiency and iron supplementation. Nutrition Abstracts and Reviews 53: 585–598.

Oski, FA. (1979). The nonhematologic manifestations of iron deficiency. American Journal of Diseases of Children 133: 315–322.

Pilon VA, Howanitz PJ, Domres N. (1981). Day-to-day variation in serum ferritin concentrations in healthy subjects. Clinical Chemistry 27: 78–82.

Pilch SM, Senti FR (eds). (1984). Assessment of the iron nutritional status of the US population based on data collected in the second National Health and Nutrition Examination Survey, 1976–1980. Life Sciences Research Office, Federation of the American Societies for Experimental Biology, Bethesda, Maryland.

Piomelli S, Seaman C, Zullow D, Curran A, Davidow B. (1982). Threshold for lead damage to heme synthesis in urban children. Proceedings of the National Academy of Sciences of the United States of America — Biological Sciences 79: 3335–3339.

Poh Fitzpatrick M, Lamola AA. (1976). Direct spectrofluorometry of diluted erythrocytes and plasma: A rapid diagnostic method in primary and secondary porphyrinemias. Journal of Laboratory and Clinical Medicine 87: 362–370.

Sassa S, Granick JL, Granick S, Kappas A, Levere RD. (1973). Studies in lead poisoning. I. Microanalysis of erythrocyte protoporphyrin levels by spectrophotometry in the detection of chronic lead intoxication in the subclinical range. Biochemical Medicine 8: 135–148.

Schoene RB, Escourrou P, Robertson HT, Nilson KL, Parsons JR, Smith NJ. (1983). Iron repletion decreases maximal exercise lactate concentrations in female athletes with minimal iron-deficiency anemia. Journal of Laboratory and Clinical Medicine 102: 306–312.

Segall ML, Heese H B, Dempster WS. (1979). Estimation of serum ferritin in blood obtained by heelstick. Journal of Pediatrics 95: 65–67.

Statland BE, Winkel P. (1977). Relationship of day-to-day variation of serum iron concentrations to iron-binding capacity in healthy young women. American Journal of Clinical Pathology 67: 84–90.

Stockman JA, Weiner LB, Simon Ge, Stuart MJ, Oski FA. (1975). The measurement of free erythrocyte porphyrin (FEP) as a simple means of distinguishing iron deficiency from beta thalassemia trait in subjects with microcytosis. Journal of Laboratory and Clinical Medicine 85: 113–119.

Walters GO, Miller FM, Worwood M. (1973). Serum ferritin concentration and iron stores in normal subjects. Journal of Clinical Pathology 26: 770–772.

Wickramasinghe SN, Gill DS, Broom GN, Akinyanju OO, Grange A. (1985). Limited value of serum ferritin in evaluating iron status in children with protein-energy malnutrition. Scandinavian Journal of Haematology 35: 292–298.

Wiltink WF, Kruithof J, Mol C, Bas MG, Eijk HG van. (1973). Diurnal and nocturnal variations of the serum iron in normal subjects. Clinica Chimica Acta 49: 99-104.

Wintrobe MM, Lee GR, Boggs DR, Bithell TC, Foerster J, Athens JW, Lukens JN (eds). (1981). Clinical Hematology. Eighth edition, Lea and Febiger, Philadelphia.

WHO (World Health Organization) (1972). Nutritional Anemia. WHO Technical Report Series No. 3. World Health Organization, Geneva.

Worwood M. (1979). Serum ferritin. CRC Critical Reviews in Clinical Laboratory Sciences 10: 171–204.

Yip R, Johnson C, Dallman PR. (1984). Age-related changes in laboratory values used in the diagnosis of anemia and iron deficiency. American Journal Clinical Nutrition 39: 427–436.

Zak B, Baginski ES, Epstein E. (1980). Modern iron ligands useful for the measurement of serum iron. Annals of Clinical and Laboratory Science 10: 276–289.

Chapter 18

Assessment of the status of vitamins A, D, and E

The fat-soluble vitamins A, D, and E have a structure based on the isoprene unit: $[-CH_2-C(CH_3)=CH-CH_2)-]$. The major body storage sites for vitamin A and E are the liver and adipose tissue, respectively. Very little vitamin D is stored in the body. Vitamin D can, however, be synthesized by the action of ultraviolet light on a precursor of vitamin D present in the skin. Generally, deficiencies of vitamin A, D, and E develop more slowly than those for the water-soluble vitamins; secondary deficiencies may occur in patients with malabsorption syndromes and other disease states, and in association with certain drug therapies.

Although vitamin A has other physiological functions, only its role in vision is clearly understood. Vitamin D, after hydroxylation to a biologically active form, is involved in calcium metabolism, whereas vitamin E acts as a lipid anti-oxidant. Major food sources of both vitamins A and D include liver and fish liver oils; precursors of vitamin A also occur in plants as carotenoids. Vegetable and seed oils are important sources of vitamin E.

Vitamin A, D, and E status is generally assessed by measurements of the vitamins and/or their metabolites in serum. High-performance liquid chromatography is the preferred method of analysis. Urinary excretion of metabolites is not used because it does not reflect the nutritional status of these fat-soluble vitamins. Some functional physiological tests are also available for assessing vitamin A and E status, but they are complex and not suitable for routine use.

Vitamin K is not considered in this chapter because a primary deficiency is very rare in healthy persons. Vitamin K is widely distributed in plant and animal tissues, and is synthesized by the microbiological flora of the normal gut. Deficiency of vitamin K may be secondary to certain disease states (e.g. biliary obstruction, malabsorption syndromes, and liver disease). Use of drugs such as broad-spectrum antibiotics which destroy

377

the intestinal flora, or anticoagulant drugs such as salicylates, hydantoins, and 4-hydroxycoumarins, may also produce secondary vitamin K deficiency. No static biochemical tests exist for assessing vitamin K status. Instead, functional tests which depend on the measurement of blood clotting time and prothrombin time are used.

18.1   Vitamin A

Vitamin A is a generic term for all retinoids that qualitatively exhibit the biological activity of all-trans retinol. The various biologically active forms of vitamin A are shown in Figure 18.1. Certain carotenoids have provitamin A activity. Of these β-carotene is the most biologically active, and the most widely distributed in plant products; α-carotene and γ-carotene have about half the biological activity of β-carotene. Preformed vitamin A is found only in foods of animal origin: fish-liver oils, liver, butter fat, fortified margarine, and egg yolk are major sources. Muscle meats, nuts, grains, and vegetable oils are poor sources of preformed vitamin A. Provitamin A carotenoids are found in both plant and animal products, the most important sources being yellow, yellowish-red, and dark green leafy vegetables and fruits.

The most clearly defined role of vitamin A is in vision: when retinal tissue is deprived of vitamin A, both rod and cone function are impaired. Vitamin A also has a role in growth, reproduction, cellular differentiation, glycoprotein synthesis, membrane stabilization, and the immune response. The precise mechanism of vitamin A in these latter processes, however, remains unclear.

Early signs of vitamin A deficiency in humans include growth failure, loss of appetite, and impaired immune response with lowered resistance to infection. Night blindness develops when liver reserves of vitamin A are nearly exhausted. Later, ocular lesions such as conjunctival xerosis, Bitot's spots, keratomalacia, and xerophthalmia may occur. Xerophthalmia and vitamin A deficiency blindness are endemic in southern and eastern Asia, parts of Latin America, and in many countries in Africa and the Middle East. Vitamin A deficiency may occur secondary to certain disease states such as cystic fibrosis, severe intestinal and liver diseases, and with severe defects in lipid absorption (e.g. cholestasis) (Sauberlich et al., 1974). In developed countries, the prevalence of frank nutritional deficiency of vitamin A is low. For example, characteristic ocular lesions were seen in less than 0.1% of the subjects in the NHANES surveys. Nevertheless, more than 20% of the children in these surveys had serum vitamin A levels indicative of suboptimal vitamin A status (Pilch, 1985). In the Nutrition Canada National Survey, 25% of infants and toddlers and 15% of school-aged children had serum vitamin A concentrations classified as 'moderate risk' (10 to 30 µg/dL) (Health and Welfare Canada, 1973). These findings may be particularly important

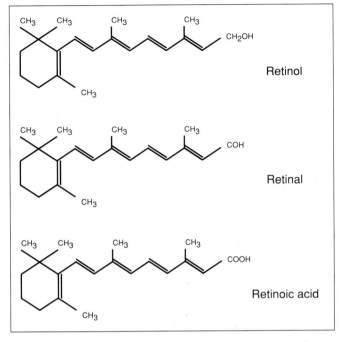

Figure 18.1: The various forms of vitamin A: retinol, retinal, and retinoic acid.

if serum vitamin A is related to cancer risk (Wald et al., 1980; Kark et al., 1981; Willet et al., 1984).

Suggestions that vitamin A and its carotenoid precursors are possible cancer-preventive agents have led to increased consumption of large doses of vitamin A. This is a serious health hazard: vitamin A toxicity can occur when daily doses are greater than ten times the recommended dietary intakes. Clinical manifestations of vitamin A toxicity include a pseudobrain tumor, skeletal pain, desquamating dermatitis, and hepatic inflammation (Frame et al., 1974; Russell et al., 1974).

Most of the vitamin A in the body is stored in the form of retinyl ester in the liver. Therefore, a measure of liver stores of vitamin A is the best index of vitamin A nutriture. Unfortunately, liver biopsies are impractical in population studies. Instead, total plasma/serum vitamin A or retinol concentrations are frequently determined. The plasma contains only about 1% of the total body reserve of vitamin A, and does not reflect body stores until they are severely depleted. Consequently, other biochemical and functional tests of vitamin A status should be used in combination with serum vitamin A levels; some of these tests are discussed in the following sections.

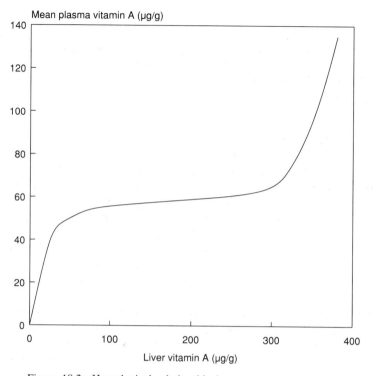

Figure 18.2: Hypothetical relationship between mean plasma vitamin A levels and liver vitamin A concentrations. From Olson (1984).

18.1.1 Serum retinol concentrations

Vitamin A in the serum circulates largely in the form of a 1:1 complex of retinol and retinol-binding protein (RBP); the remainder is in the form of retinyl ester (approximately 8%) and very small amounts of retinoic acid and other metabolites (Olson, 1984). Until recently, total serum vitamin A, rather than retinol, was assayed. Results for the two assays are in general comparable for levels below 35 µg/dL (1.22 µmol/L) (Driskell et al., 1982). At higher concentrations, the discrepancy between the two assays is greater; approximately 4 µg/dL (0.14 µmol/L) higher for total serum vitamin A compared to that for serum retinol.

Serum retinol levels reflect vitamin A status only when liver vitamin A stores are severely depleted (below 20 µg/g liver) or excessively high (above 300 µg/g liver) (Figure 18.2). When liver vitamin A concentrations are between these limits, serum retinol concentrations are homeostatically controlled; levels remain relatively constant and do not reflect total body reserves of vitamin A (Olson, 1984).

Functional impairment has been seen in malnourished Indian and Indonesian children with extremely low serum vitamin A values. For example, results of studies in India (Pirie and Anbunathan, 1981), and

	n	Percent with Serum Vitamin A:		
		< 10 µg/dL	10–19 µg/dL	≥ 20 µg/dL
Normal children	252	8	37	55
Children with night-blindness or Bitot's spots	325	30	55	15
Children with corneal xeropthalmia	98	75	24	1

Table 18.1: Serum vitamin A levels in a sample of Indonesian children with and without ocular lesions. Conversion factor to SI units (µmol/L) = × 0.035. From Sommer et al. (1980). © Am. J. Clin. Nutr. American Society for Clinical Nutrition.

Indonesia (Sommer, 1982), showed that at least 75% of the children with corneal xerophthalmia had serum vitamin A levels below 10 µg/dL (< 0.35 µmol/L). In contrast, in a sample of 252 clinically normal Indonesian children, only 8% had serum vitamin A levels within this low range (Table 18.1).

Marginally low (i.e. < 20 µg/dL; < 0.70 µmol/L) serum vitamin A values are a less specific index of vitamin A deficiency; their ability to predict vitamin A deficiency varies widely by region, probably depending on the presence and severity of other risk factors. For example, serum vitamin A levels less than 20 µg/dL were found in only 28% of 29 children from Sri Lanka with clinical signs of vitamin A deficiency (Bitot's spots, corneal scars, or blindness) and in 5% of the children without positive eye findings (Brink et al., 1979), whereas in Indonesia, 85% of 325 children under six years of age with either night-blindness and/or Bitot's spots had serum vitamin A levels less than 20 µg/dL (< 0.70 µmol/L) (Sommer et al., 1980). In contrast, 28% of the children with eye findings and 48% of the children without eye findings had serum vitamin A values greater than 30 µg/dL (> 1.05 µmol/L). Additional indices may therefore be required to confirm marginal vitamin A depletion.

A variety of extraneous factors may affect plasma vitamin A or retinol concentrations, which are independent of the size of vitamin A stores in the liver. These are summarized in Table 18.2.

The ingestion of meals containing relatively large amounts of dietary vitamin A, or supplemental vitamin A during the previous four hours, does not alter serum retinol concentrations in children or adults (Mejia and Arroyave, 1983; Mejia et al., 1984). Consequently, the collection of fasting blood samples is not necessary for serum retinol determinations.

Interpretive guidelines for low serum vitamin A concentrations for three age groups have been developed (Table 18.3) (Pilch, 1985). Such age-specific criteria should always be used to interpret serum vitamin A values; age-related changes in serum vitamin A concentrations were noted

- **Liver disease** decreases plasma retinol levels, probably as a result of a combination of decreased synthesis and secretion of RBP.

- **Stress** decreases plasma retinol levels.

- **Protein-energy malnutrition** decreases RBP production because of a limited supply of protein substrate. Consequently hepatic release of vitamin A is impaired resulting in decreased serum retinol levels.

- **Zinc deficiency** decreases plasma retinol levels via its role in the synthesis of RBP.

- **Chronic renal disease** increases plasma retinol levels with the reduced catabolism of vitamin A and its carriers.

- **Infections and parasitic infections** lower plasma retinol levels.

- **Cystic fibrosis** is associated with a defect in the transport of vitamin A from the hepatic stores to the periphery resulting in decreased levels of circulating retinol and RBP.

- **Low fat diets** impair absorption of vitamin A, lowering plasma retinol concentrations.

- **Estrogens**, either endogenous or those used in contraceptive agents, increase plasma retinol and RBP apparently as a result of increased mobilization of vitamin A from the liver.

- **Age, sex, and race** influence serum retinol levels, as indicated by the NHANES II survey results (Pilch, 1985). Only age-specific interpretive criteria are used at the present time for serum vitamin A values.

Table 18.2: Extraneous factors that may affect plasma vitamin A or retinol levels.

in the NHANES II survey (Pilch, 1985) and by Garry et al. (1987) in their study of healthy elderly U.S. adults. No comparable criteria are available for marginally low serum vitamin A levels. The guidelines are based on their relationship with clinical signs of vitamin A deficiency such as impaired dark adaptation, night blindness, and ocular lesions, and on the serum vitamin A distributions from the data of the NHANES surveys (Pilch, 1985). Whether these guidelines are appropriate for other countries is unknown. Serum vitamin A concentrations $\geq 30\,\mu g/dL$ are considered indicative of adequate vitamin A status in U.S. persons (Pilch, 1985). Age-, sex-, and race-specific means and percentile distribution data for serum vitamin A of U.S. persons aged three to seventy-four years, together with a reference sample for the same age group, have also been compiled from the NHANES I and II surveys for comparisons of populations (Pilch, 1985). The reference sample excluded all individuals taking vitamin-mineral supplements, pregnant women, and women using oral contraceptive agents. These serum vitamin A reference data can be used for U.S. white children, children of Negro descent, and Mexican-American children. Looker et al. (1988) reported no ethnic differences in serum vitamin A concentrations in their study of children from four to eleven years old.

Vit. A Levels	3–11 yr	12–17 yr	18–74 yr
< 10 µg/dL	Vitamin A status is very likely to improve with increased consumption of vitamin A. Impairment of function is likely.		
< 20 µg/dL	Vitamin A status is likely to improve with increased consumption of vitamin A.	Vitamin A status is likely to improve with increased consumption of vitamin A; some individuals may exhibit impairment of function.	Vitamin A status is likely to improve with increased consumption of vitamin A; impairment of function likely.
20–29 µg/dL	Vitamin A status of some subjects may improve with increased consumption of vitamin A. Improvement is most likely in those with values 20–24 µg/dL	Vitamin A status may improve with increased consumption of vitamin A. Improvement is more likely in those with values 20–24 µg/dL	Vitamin A status may improve with increased consumption of vitamin A. Some individuals may exhibit impairment of function

Table 18.3: Guidelines recommended by the NHANES II committee for interpreting low serum total vitamin A concentrations in three age categories. Vitamin A status refers to serum and tissue levels of the nutrient. Impairment of function may include impaired dark adaptation, night blindness, ocular lesions, and possibly impaired immune function. Conversion factor to SI units (µmol/L) = × 0.035. From Pilch (1985).

18.1.2 Serum retinyl ester concentrations

In normal healthy persons, retinyl esters constitute less than 5% of the total vitamin A content of fasting serum samples. However, when the capacity of the liver to store vitamin A is exceeded, as may occur after the chronic ingestion of high levels of vitamin A (i.e. hypervitaminosis A) and in liver disease, elevated concentrations of serum retinyl esters are observed. For example, in three patients with hypervitaminosis A, retinyl esters made up 67%, 65%, and 33% of the total vitamin A present in the plasma (Smith and Goodman, 1976). Fasting blood samples are essential for serum retinyl ester measurements; concentrations rise transiently after ingestion of a vitamin A-rich meal or vitamin A supplement.

18.1.3 Serum carotenoid concentrations

About fifty carotenoids show provitamin A activity, and provide about 50% of the total vitamin A intake in the United States, and larger percentages in Asia, Africa, and parts of South America. Levels of carotenoids in the serum reflect the current dietary intake of carotenoids (Olson, 1984). Major components of serum carotenoids are β-carotene, lycopene, and various hydroxylated carotenoids. Serum carotenoids are of increasing interest because of their possible relationship to cancer risk.

In countries where dietary carotenoids provide the only source of vitamin A and where dietary patterns are relatively constant, serum carotenoids may serve as a useful secondary index of vitamin A deficiency

Liver vitamin A (μg/g wet weight)

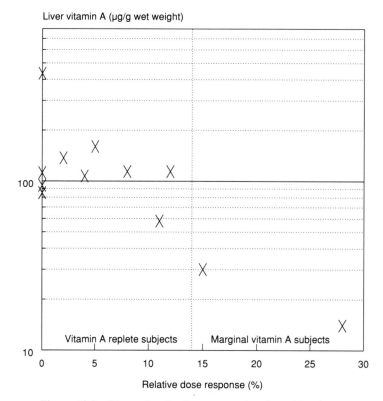

Relative dose response (%)

Figure 18.3: Liver vitamin A concentration from biopsies compared with corresponding RDR test results in a group of adult American surgical patients. From Amédée-Manesme et al. (1984). © Am. J. Clin. Nutr. American Society for Clinical Nutrition.

(Le Francois et al., 1981). For populations receiving most of their vitamin A from animal sources, however, serum carotenoid concentrations provide no information on vitamin A status (Olson, 1984). Carotenoids can be separated and measured by high-performance liquid chromatography combined with ultraviolet/visual detection.

18.1.4   Relative dose response

The relative dose response (RDR) is a test used in the estimation of liver stores of vitamin A, and can be used to identify those individuals with marginal vitamin A deficiency. The test is based on the observation that in vitamin A deficiency, retinol-binding protein (RBP) accumulates in the liver as apo-RBP (i.e. RBP that is not bound to retinol). Following a test dose of vitamin A, the latter binds to this relative excess of apo-RBP in the liver, and holo-RBP (i.e. RBP bound to retinol) is subsequently

Serum Retinol (µg/dL)	%	Number Tested
≤ 20	100	12
21–29	86	21
30–40	26	19
> 40	3	39
Total tested		91

Table 18.4: Percentage of children with a positive RDR test classified by serum retinol levels. From Flores et al. (1984). © Am. J. Clin. Nutr. American Society for Clinical Nutrition.

released from the liver (Loerch et al., 1979). Consequently, in vitamin A-depleted individuals, a rapid sustained increase in serum retinol occurs after the ingestion of a small dose of vitamin A.

For the test, a baseline blood sample is taken immediately before the administration of a small oral dose (450 µg) of vitamin A (as retinyl acetate or retinol palmitate), followed by a second blood sample, five hours later. The RDR (%) is calculated as:

$$RDR(\%) = \frac{\text{Plasma retinol at 5 hr} - \text{Plasma retinol at 0 hr}}{\text{Plasma retinol at 5 hr}} \times 100$$

Vitamin-A-replete subjects have RDR values ranging from 0% to 14%. Relative dose response values greater than 14% to 20% are indicative of marginal vitamin A status in humans, the cutoff value depending on the coefficient of variation for the analytical method used to measure serum retinol (Flores et al., 1984).

The validity of the RDR test as an index of body stores of vitamin A has been studied by comparing vitamin A concentrations in liver biopsy samples with corresponding RDR test results in otherwise healthy surgical patients (Figure 18.3). The two subjects with the lowest liver vitamin A concentrations had the highest RDR values (i.e. 14 µg/g and RDR 28%; 30 µg/g and RDR 15%). Following supplementation with vitamin A, RDR values fell to < 5%. Subjects with liver vitamin A concentrations ranging from 58 to 434 µg/g had corresponding RDR values ranging from 0% to 12% (Amédée-Manesme et al., 1984).

In a study of Brazilian children from low-income families, all children with serum retinol concentrations < 20 µg/dL (<0.70 µmol/L) had elevated RDR values. Moreover, 86% of the children with serum retinol concentrations 21 to 29 µg/dL (0.74 to 1.02 µmol/L), and 26% with serum retinol concentrations 30 to 40 µg/dL (1.05 to 1.40 µmol/L) had elevated RDR values (Flores et al., 1984) (Table 18.4). Following supplementation with vitamin A, all the elevated RDR values reverted to normal. These results indicate that RDR is a more sensitive index of marginal vitamin A status than using serum vitamin A levels < 20 µg/dL.

Other factors associated with low RDR values include malabsorption, liver disease, and severe protein-energy malnutrition. Such factors reduce the sensitivity and the specificity of the RDR test (Russell et al., 1983; Mobarhan et al., 1984). For example, when an oral dose of vitamin A was given to patients with varying degrees of liver dysfunction and protein-energy malnutrition, no correlation was observed between the vitamin A content of liver biopsies and the RDR test result (Russell et al., 1983; Mobarhan et al., 1984). These results were attributed to vitamin A malabsorption because when an *intravenous* injection of retinyl palmitate was given to children with liver disease, the RDR test proved to be a reliable and sensitive index of vitamin A status (Amédée-Manesme et al., 1987).

18.1.5 Rapid dark adaptation test

An early sign of vitamin A deficiency is night blindness, which can be assessed using dark adaptation tests. The conventional test, formal dark adaptometry, is a tedious and time-consuming procedure (Russell et al., 1973). A rapid dark adaptation test (RDAT), suitable for field conditions, has been developed which is based on the measurements of the time of occurrence of the Purkinje shift (Thornton, 1977). In the latter, the peak wavelength sensitivity of the retina shifts from the red toward the blue end of the visual spectrum during the transition from phototopic or cone-mediated day vision to scotopic or rod-mediated night vision. This shift causes the intensity of blue light to appear brighter than that of red light under scotopic lighting conditions. The test requires a light-proof room, a light source, a dark, nonreflective work surface, a standard X-ray view box, and sets of red, blue, and white discs. The discs can be distinguished only by their relative brightness rather than color once the lights are dimmed. For the test, subjects are light-adapted for a fixed time (one minute), and then asked to separate out the white and the blue discs as fast as possible. The time taken to achieve 100% accuracy of sorting is recorded (in seconds). The test is usually repeated three times to allow for learning and standardization. Results of the RDAT correlate with those obtained by the classical dark adaptation method (Vinton and Russell, 1981). The RDAT was also found to be precise over a two-week period, and had a specificity of 91% and sensitivity of 95%. Nevertheless, false positives can occur with all tests of visual function for vitamin A deficiency because of congenital night blindness, and because of deficiencies of other nutrients such as zinc and protein. Inter-examiner variability may also produce inconsistencies in the results. The RDAT is not appropriate for preschool children, who are too young to perform the test accurately, and is not sensitive enough to detect early signs of vitamin A deficiency (Duarte Favaro et al., 1986). Age influences dark-adaptation and hence must be taken into account when determining the normal range of the rapid test adaptation times for healthy reference populations (Vinton and Russell, 1981).

18.1.6 Conjunctival impression cytology

Conjunctival impression cytology detects early physiological changes occurring in vitamin A deficiency. Such changes include the progressive loss of goblet cells in the conjunctiva and elsewhere, and the appearance of enlarged, partially keratinized, epithelial cells (Wittepen et al., 1986). For the test, an impression of the conjunctival surface of the eye is taken. The procedure involves carefully placing a 25×5 mm strip of cellulose acetate filter paper on the temporal conjunctiva and gently pressing the paper for three to five seconds with a blunt, smooth-ended forcep, or with the fingers. The filter paper is then peeled off gently and placed in a fixative solution for ten minutes. After fixing, the specimens can be stored indefinitely until they are stained, preferably with Gill's modified Papanicolaou stain, prior to microscopic examination (Tseng, 1985; Amédée-Manesme et al., 1988). The staining and examination takes only ten to fifteen minutes, once the biopsy tissue has been obtained. The procedure can be undertaken without topical anesthesia. It is usually painless, although if a layer of cells is pulled off with the filter paper, a pricking sensation may be felt. Subjects with confirmed xeropthalmia show complete loss of goblet cells. These changes are reversed after treatment with vitamin A (Wittepenn et al., 1986).

The validity of this test to distinguish between subjects with physiologically significant but preclinical vitamin A deficiency, and those with normal vitamin A status, has been demonstrated (Amédée-Manesme et al., 1988). Patients with chronic cholestasis and biochemical evidence of vitamin A deficiency had no goblet cells and enlarged epithelial cells despite apparently normal clinical ocular examination. After receiving retinyl palmitate for two months, goblet cells reappeared and epithelial cells reverted to normal (Amédée-Manesme et al., 1988). Nevertheless, more work is required to establish the specificity and sensitivity of conjunctival impression cytology for assessing vitamin A status and its feasibility for field use (Gadomski et al., 1989; Kjolhede et al., 1989).

18.1.7 Future developments

Stable isotope dilution procedures for assessing total body stores of vitamin A may be used in the future, after the recent synthesis of deuterium-labeled vitamin A suitable for human use. The method is based on the principle that when deuterium-labeled vitamin A is administered, it equilibrates with the total body vitamin A. After equilibration, a sample of blood is taken from which the deuterium : hydrogen ratio is measured. The ratio is a measure of total body stores of vitamin A (Olson, 1982).

Serum retinoic acid concentrations may also be a useful index of body stores of vitamin A.

18.1.8   Analysis of vitamin A, retinol, and retinyl esters in serum

Several methods are available for the analysis of total serum vitamin A, retinol, or retinyl esters in serum. These include colorimetry, UV spectrophotometry, fluorometry, and high-performance liquid chromatography (HPLC) linked to a UV detector. Only HPLC can distinguish retinol from retinyl esters in the serum. All the other methods measure total serum vitamin A, and generally give comparable results provided that conditions of collection, storage and analysis are clearly defined and controlled.

Colorimetric methods

Colorimetric methods were originally based on the Carr-Price reaction, in which the blue color formed by complexing vitamin A with antimony trichloride as the oxidizing agent is measured at 620 nm (Carr and Price, 1926). Corrections must be made for any carotenes in the sample. Traces of moisture produce turbidity in the antimony trichloride reagent, but this problem can be overcome by using trifluoroacetic acid in place of antimony trichloride (Neeld and Pearson, 1963). A modification of the Neeld-Pearson method was used in the NHANES I and II surveys (Pilch, 1985).

UV Spectrophotometric technique

The spectrophometric method generally used to measure total serum vitamin A is that of Bessey et al. (1946a). In this method, the absorbance of serum vitamin A after extraction with an organic solvent is measured at 328 nm before and after destruction of vitamin A by irradiation with a mercury discharge lamp. Some extractable impurities, such as phytofluene (widely found in vegetables), interfere with the method as they absorb at 328 nm and are also destroyed by the irradiation.

Fluorometry

Methods based on the direct measurement of fluorescence in serum extracts are popular for measuring total serum vitamin A. The methods are highly sensitive, simple, and critical timing is not necessary (Thompson et al., 1971). Nevertheless, other highly fluorescent substances, notably phytofluene, interfere but can be removed by column chromatography or by the use of a correction factor (Thompson et al., 1971).

High-performance liquid chromatography

High-performance liquid chromatography (HPLC) is the preferred method for the separation and analysis of serum retinol because of the ease and specificity of the method. Either reverse-phase (Bieri et al., 1979; Furr et al., 1984) or normal-phase (Bankson et al., 1986) HPLC is used. The former technique is preferred for serum and was used in the US 1982–1984 Hispanic Health and Nutrition Examination Survey (HHANES). All interfering compounds, such as phytofluene and retinyl esters, can be separated from retinol using HPLC methods. If normal-phase HPLC is used, the low levels of serum retinyl ester usually found in fasting serum can be measured concurrently with serum retinol concentrations.

Special precautions must be taken in the preparation and storage of serum samples for vitamin A, retinol, and/or carotenoid analysis. For instance, the serum should be centrifuged soon after the blood is drawn, and hemolysis and exposure to bright light avoided. If serum is to be stored for prolonged periods of time prior to analysis, it should be quickly frozen in temperature resistant tubes, flushed with argon or oxygen-free nitrogen, and the tubes closed tightly with a screw top. Only a small gas space should be left within the tube. Tubes should be stored, together with a reference serum sample, in the dark at temperatures below $-40°C$ (Olson, 1984). Thawing and refreezing should be kept to a minimum, although under controlled conditions such procedures do not appear to significantly affect serum retinol values (Kark et al., 1981).

18.2   Vitamin D

Vitamin D is required primarily by humans to ensure adequate intestinal absorption of calcium and phosphorus, and to regulate bone mineralization. The vitamin D requirement can be met by dietary intake and/or by skin synthesis (Holmes and Kummerow, 1983).

Vitamin D is a generic term for all steroids that exhibit the biological activity of vitamin D_3 (calciol). They occur only in animal tissues. The principal dietary form of vitamin D is vitamin D_2 (ercalciol), unless large amounts of oily fish products are consumed which contain vitamin D_3 (calciol) (Figure 18.4). Ingested vitamin D_2 and vitamin D_3 are absorbed in the small intestine and enter the circulation bound to a vitamin D-binding protein. Vitamin D_3 is also synthesized in the skin, where it is formed in two stages: the photochemical transformation of 7-dehydrocholesterol to previtamin D_3, followed by thermal isomerization of the previtamin to vitamin D_3. Variables influencing the formation of previtamin D_3 in the skin include the intensity of the ultraviolet radiation and skin pigmentation (Holick et al., 1981; Lo et al., 1986).

To function biochemically in the tissues, vitamin D_3 from the diet or skin must be hydroxylated in the liver to 25-hydroxyvitamin D_3 (25-OH-D_3 or calcidiol) and in the kidney to either 1,25-dihydroxyvitamin D_3 (1,25-$(OH)_2D_3$ or calcitriol), the biologically active form, or 24,25-dihy-droxyvitamin D_3 (24,25-$(OH)_2$-D_3; 24-hydroxycalcidiol), a less

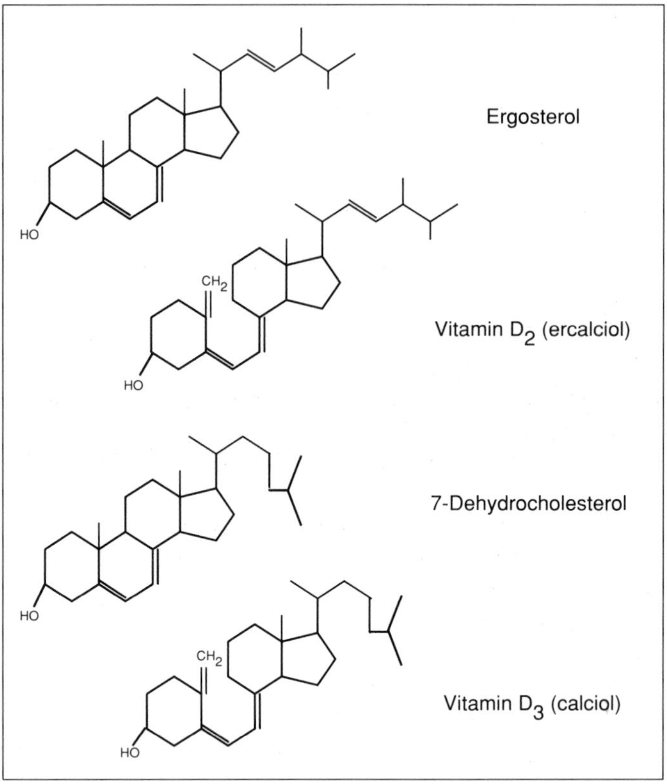

Figure 18.4: Various forms of vitamin D and major chemical structure of vitamin D metabolites.

active metabolite, depending on physiological circumstances. Ingested vitamin D_2 is metabolized to the analogous metabolites 25-OH-D_2 (ercalcidiol) in the liver and 1,25-(OH)$_2$-D_2 (ercalcitriol) in the kidney. Vitamin D and its metabolites are transported in the plasma bound to the vitamin D-binding protein.

Persons who are housebound or living in institutions may be primarily dependent on dietary sources of vitamin D (Lawson et al., 1979; Lester et al., 1980; McKenna et al., 1985; Gibson et al., 1986), whereas free-living individuals obtain their requirement largely from the synthesis of vitamin D_3 by the action of ultraviolet light on 7-dehydrocholesterol in the skin (Fraser, 1983). Thus population groups vulnerable to vitamin D deficiency include those with inadequate skin exposure to sunlight (e.g. the housebound elderly) (Dattani et al., 1984; McKenna et al., 1985) or persons living in northern geographical latitudes (Lester et al.,1980).

Severe vitamin D deficiency in normal adults produces osteomalacia, a condition characterized by a failure in the mineralization of the organic matrix of bone, resulting in weak bones, diffuse skeletal bone tenderness, proximal muscle weakness, and increased frequency of fractures. Suboptimal vitamin D status in the elderly may also be responsible for decreased absorption of calcium, a factor associated with a lowering of the bone mineral content during postmenopausal aging (Heaney et al., 1978). Adult patients with chronic renal failure, gastrectomy, intestinal malabsorption and steatorrhea arising from celiac sprue, inflammatory bowel disease, pancreatic insufficiency, or massive bowel resection may also develop osteomalacia.

In infants and children, deficiency in vitamin D may result in rickets, in which abnormal softness of the skull (craniotabes) occurs, accompanied by enlargement of the epiphyses of the long bones and of the costochondral junction (rachitic rosary). Bow legs and knock knees may arise from these bone deformities. Rickets, arising from primary vitamin D deficiency, is rarely seen today in children from industrialized countries because of widespread vitamin D supplementation of some dairy products. Cases have been described in Asian immigrant children living in the United Kingdom. Rickets can arise in association with certain metabolic defects such as vitamin D-resistant rickets (familial hypophosphatemia) and vitamin D-dependency rickets, as well as in children with malabsorption syndromes.

Indiscriminate self-dosing with excessive amounts of vitamin D supplements has been described, but considerable individual variation exists in the amount required to induce vitamin D toxicity (Parfitt et al., 1982). Clinical manifestations of vitamin D toxicity include hypertension, hypercalcemia, and extra-osseous calcification (Blum et al., 1977; Parfitt and Kleerekoper, 1980).

Until recently, vitamin D status was assessed indirectly by measurement of alkaline phosphatase activity, and calcium and phosphorus concentrations in serum, all very unspecific indices. Now methods are available for the direct measurement of vitamin D metabolites in serum, and these are described below.

18.2.1   Serum 25-hydroxyvitamin D concentrations

Measurement of serum total 25-hydroxyvitamin D (25-OH-D) is the most useful index of vitamin D status in humans because in general it reflects the amount of vitamin D in the liver, the major tissue store of vitamin D (Parfitt et al., 1982; Fraser, 1983). Serum 25-OH-D concentrations reflect the total supply of vitamin D from both endogenous and exogenous sources (Parfitt et al., 1982). It is the most abundant circulating metabolite of vitamin D, and has the longest half-life of all vitamin D derivatives.

Subjects	n	Summer	n	Winter	p
Men	258	16.2 ± 8.66	250	11.1 ± 5.72	< 0.005
Women	199	13.1 ± 7.04	209	9.9 ± 4.15	< 0.005
All	457	14.9 ± 8.0	459	10.5 ± 5.06	< 0.005

Table 18.5: Serum 25-OH-D concentrations (ng/mL) in summer and winter (Mean ± SD) in United Kingdom elderly men and women. Conversion factor to SI units (nmol/L) = × 2.5. From Dattani et al. (1984) with permission.

Several factors influence serum total 25-OH-D concentrations and confirm the validity of this index as a measure of vitamin D status. These include:

Seasonal effects

The highest serum 25-OH-D levels occur in the summer and the lowest in the winter. This trend parallels the seasonal change in solar ultraviolet light in temperate regions. For example, Dattani et al. (1984) reported that plasma 25-OH-D levels of men and women aged sixty-five years and over (Table 18.5) were significantly higher in the summer than in the winter and correlated with exposure to sunlight as measured by a 'sunshine' score. The latter was based on the estimated number of hours spent in the open air, as well as the type of exposure and holidays. Similar findings have been reported by others for the elderly (Lester et al., 1973; Stamp and Round, 1974; Delvin et al., 1988) and for persons living in several different countries (Sedrani et al., 1983; Lamberg-Allardt, 1984; McKenna et al., 1985).

Place of work

Outdoor workers from Dundee, Scotland, exposed to increased levels of solar radiation, had significantly higher levels of serum 25-OH-D at all seasons compared to the indoor workers consuming similar diets (Devgun et al., 1981).

Vitamin D supplement usage

In a study of an American elderly population, higher 25-OH-D concentrations were observed in both male and female subjects taking vitamin D supplements compared to levels for unsupplemented subjects (Table 18.6), irrespective of the season (Omdahl et al., 1982).

Clinical signs

Overt rickets in children and osteomalacia in adults, clinical signs of vitamin D deficiency, have been associated with serum 25-OH-D concentrations below 3.0 ng/mL (7.5 nmol/L) (Haddad and Stamp, 1974; Preece

	Males		Females	
	without Vit. D supplements	with Vit. D supplements	without Vit. D supplements	with Vit. D supplements
25-OH-D (ng/mL)	13.2 ± 6.5 (37)	15.4 ± 4.8 (22)	10.5 ± 5.3 (45)	12.1 ± 4.7 (29)
Alk. phosphatase (u/mL)	94.4 ± 23.1 (37)	76.9 ± 23.7 (23)	95.7 ± 23.6 (49)	90.5 ± 19.6 (29)
Calcium (mg/dL)	9.7 ± 0.3 (37)	9.7 ± 0.4 (24)	9.8 ± 0.4 (49)	9.8 ± 0.4 (29)
Phosphorus (mg/dL)	2.8 ± 0.4 (37)	2.9 ± 0.4 (24)	3.2 ± 0.4 (48)	3.3 ± 0.4 (29)

Table 18.6: Plasma 25-OH-D, alkaline phosphatase, calcium, and phosphorus levels of male and female healthy American elderly subjects in relation to vitamin D supplementation. Both sex and supplementation effects on the plasma 25-OH-D and alkaline phosphatase levels are significant ($p < 0.05$). Conversion factors to SI units: 25-OH-D (nmol/L) = × 2.5; calcium (mmol/L) = × 0.25; phosphorus (mmol/L) = × 0.32. Adapted from Omdahl et al. (1982). © Am. J. Clin. Nutr. American Society for Clinical Nutrition.

et al., 1975). Following treatment of osteomalacia patients with vitamin D supplements, serum 25-OH-D values rose and radiological lesions healed (Preece et al., 1975).

Age and sex

Serum 25-OH-D levels decline with age, but the change has been attributed, in part, to a more limited exposure to solar radiation. Low dietary intakes of vitamin D, lesions in dermal synthesis of vitamin D, and/or impaired intestinal absorption of ingested vitamin D may also be involved. Serum 25-OH-D levels are generally, but not consistently, lower in women than men (Omdahl et al., 1982; Dattani et al., 1984; McKenna et al., 1985) irrespective of season or vitamin D supplement usage (Tables 18.5 and 18.6). Reasons for these sex differences are unclear. Absorption of dietary vitamin D may be less in elderly women or, alternatively, their activity pattern may result in less sunlight exposure than men (Omdahl et al., 1982).

Latitude

Subjects from lower latitudes, again exposed to increased levels of solar radiation, have higher values when the effects of variation in dietary intake and season have been taken into account (Figure 18.5).

Low serum 25-OH-D concentrations in association with rickets and osteomalacia may occur in patients with intestinal malabsorption and

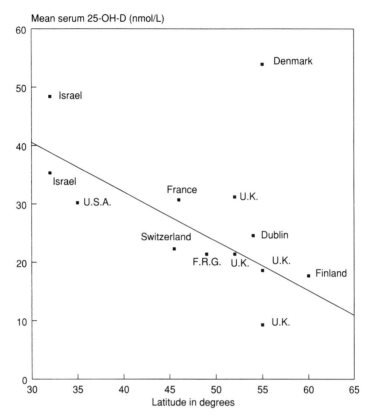

Figure 18.5: Relationship between latitude of country and serum 25-OH-D levels in groups of healthy elderly subjects studied in winter-spring. The regression equation, excluding the Danish results, is: $y = 67 - 0.88x$, $r = -0.85$, $p < 0.001$. From McKenna et al. (1985). © Am. J. Clin. Nutr. American Society for Clinical Nutrition.

steatorrhea caused by celiac sprue, inflammatory bowel disease, pancreatic insufficiency, or massive bowel resection. In these cases, vitamin D depletion arises from malabsorption of dietary vitamin D. Gastrectomy patients sometimes have low serum 25-OH-D concentrations associated with osteomalacia. The latter appears to result from poor dietary intake of vitamin D rather than from impaired absorption (Gertner et al., 1977).

Prolonged use of certain anticonvulsant drugs, such as diphenylhydantoin and phenobarbital, is also associated with low serum 25-OH-D concentrations and the development of rickets or osteomalacia (Hahn et al., 1975). The latter can be prevented or reversed by vitamin D therapy. The origin of these conditions is unclear; they may result from calcium malabsorption caused by suppression of both absorption and metabolism of vitamin D by the drug. Low serum 25-OH-D levels may also occur in diseases affecting organs involved in vitamin D metabolism (e.g. hepatic disorders and chronic renal failure).

Serum 1,25-dihydroxyvitamin D concentrations are not useful indices of vitamin D status because they are under stringent homeostatic regulation at the site of $1,25\text{-}(OH)_2D$ synthesis in the kidney. Synthesis is stimulated by low serum concentrations of calcium or phosphorus, and is inhibited by excess $1,25\text{-}(OH)_2D$. Serum levels are increased by parathyroid hormone (which responds to a decrease in serum calcium) and decreased by renal disease (which affects the hydroxylase enzyme). Levels are very low in anephric patients (DeLuca and Schnoes, 1983).

18.2.2 Analysis of 25-hydroxyvitamin D in serum

Two methods have been developed to measure 25-OH-D levels in serum: competitive protein binding assays and HPLC (Edelstein et al., 1974; Eisman et al., 1977; Shepard and DeLuca, 1980). Only the HPLC method is capable of separating the vitamin D-2 and vitamin D-3 forms of vitamin D and their metabolites. High-performance liquid chromatography is used for separation of serum 25-OH-D from other metabolites. Serum 25-OH-D can then be estimated from its ultraviolet absorption at 254 nm. Alternatively, after separating serum 25-OH-D by HPLC, it can be assayed by a competitive binding assay. The latter method is more specific. The competitive protein binding assay uses either mammalian serum or tissue-binding protein for 25-OH-D (Haddad and Chyu, 1971; Preece et al., 1974). In both methods, the sterols must first be extracted from the serum with an organic solvent. Recovery of the sterol is monitored by adding tracer amounts of tritiated 25-OH-D_3 to the serum prior to extraction and chromatography (Duncan and Haddad, 1981).

At present, the cutoff point for serum 25-OH-D values indicative of vitamin D deficiency is poorly defined; few studies have correlated clinical signs of vitamin D deficiency with serum 25-OH-D concentrations. Moreover, in adults, vitamin D deficiency may exist for several years before clinical signs of the vitamin D deficiency appear. Generally, concentrations below 3.0 ng/mL (7.5 nmol/L) have been associated with clinical signs of vitamin D deficiency in children and adults (Haddad and Stamp, 1974; Preece et al., 1974; Preece et al., 1975). Concentrations in the marginal range (3 to 10 ng/mL) (7.5 to 25 nmol/L) should be interpreted cautiously.

Interpretive guidelines for identifying vitamin D toxicity are also not clearly defined. Serum 25-OH-D values above 200 ng/mL (500 nmol/L), with concomitant hypercalcemia, suggest excessive accumulation of vitamin D (Haddad and Stamp, 1974). The distribution of serum 25-OH-D values is often skewed in population studies, and log transformations

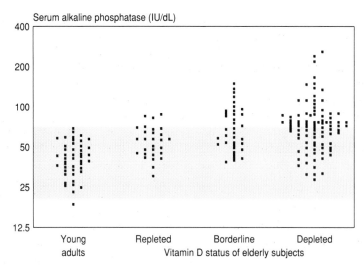

Figure 18.6: Serum alkaline phosphatase values in elderly subjects with serum 25-OH-D concentrations classified as replete, borderline, or depleted. From McKenna et al. (1985). © Am. J. Clin. Nutr. American Society for Clinical Nutrition.

are often performed in the statistical analysis to counteract the skewness.

18.2.3 Serum alkaline phosphatase activity

Alkaline phosphatase activity in serum can be used as an indirect measure of vitamin D status (Guzman et al., 1961). Activity increases in osteomalacia in adults and childhood rickets. Increases in the enzyme activity are generally proportional to the severity of vitamin D depletion. McKenna et al. (1985) showed that elderly Irish individuals with serum 25-OH-D levels indicative of severe and marginal vitamin D depletion had significantly higher serum alkaline phosphatase activity than those with 25-OH-D levels classified as replete (Figure 18.6). Seasonal changes in serum alkaline phosphatase activity have been observed in cross-sectional studies of Irish and American elderly persons, levels decreasing with seasonal rises in serum 25-OH-D levels (Omdahl et al., 1982; McKenna et al., 1985).

   Serum alkaline phosphatase activity is also affected by sex and age, again in the opposite direction to changes in serum 25-OH-D levels. For instance, significantly higher serum alkaline phosphatase activity occurs in females than males and in older versus younger persons. The activity of serum alkaline phosphatase is also altered by a variety of other disease states such as Paget's disease and hyperparathyroidism (Table 18.7). The

Condition	Serum Alk. Phos. (U/L)	Serum Calcium (mg/dL)	Serum Phosphorous (mg/dL)
Normal infants	99–298	10	5–8
Normal adults	57–99	10	3–4.5
Rickets (children)	> 390	8–9	3
Osteomalacia	298	9	2–3
Hyperparathyroidism	78–390	12–16	2–8
Osteoporosis	36	10–12	4–5
Paget's disease	994	10	4
Neoplasm: osteoblastic	604	10	4

Table 18.7: Approximate levels of serum alkaline phosphatase, calcium, and phosphorus in normal, healthy subjects and in various disease states. Conversion factors to SI units: calcium (mmol/L) = × 0.25; phosphorus (mmol/L) = × 0.32. Reproduced with permission from Sauberlich HE, Dowdy RP, Skala JH. (1974). Laboratory Tests for the Assessment of Nutritional Status. © CRC Press, Inc., Boca Raton, FL.

method of Bessey et al. (1946b) is often used for the assay of alkaline phosphatase.

18.2.4   Calcium and phosphorus concentrations in serum and urine

Many studies of vitamin D status have included measurement of calcium and phosphorus concentrations in serum and/or urine as additional biochemical parameters. In vitamin D deficiency in children, serum calcium and phosphorus levels are usually reduced. Nevertheless, measurement of total serum calcium is not the best index of vitamin D depletion, but is useful for identifying possible cases of vitamin D intoxication. In such cases, concentrations of serum 25-OH-D and serum calcium are elevated and provide additional evidence for hypervitaminosis D.

The response of urinary calcium and phosphorus concentrations to changes in vitamin D status varies, as excretion of these minerals is also affected by dietary calcium and phosphorus intakes. Hence changes in urinary calcium and phosphorus concentrations are not specific for vitamin D status and their use is not recommended.

18.3   Vitamin E

Vitamin E is the generic term for a group of lipid-soluble tocol and tocotrienol derivatives possessing vitamin E activity. The tocotrienols have similar structures to their corresponding tocol, but their side chains are unsaturated, as shown in Figure 18.7. Four tocols and four tocotrienols occur naturally, of which five have significant vitamin E activity. Of

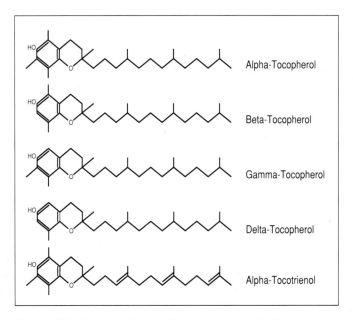

Figure 18.7: Structure of naturally occurring vitamin E compounds.

these, α-tocopherol is the most abundant and active isomer. Major food sources of vitamin E in North American diets are vegetable and seed oils (e.g. corn, soyabean, and safflower oils), and margarine. Animal products are poor sources of vitamin E. Details of the method used to calculate the vitamin E activity of mixed diets is given in Section 4.3.5.

Vitamin E functions as a lipid anti-oxidant. It prevents cellular damage by inhibiting the peroxidation of polyunsaturated fatty acids in cell membranes. It performs this function by scavenging free radicals formed by the reaction of these acids with oxygen. This function is related to that of selenium and sulphur amino acids (Bieri, 1984).

In animals, various syndromes of vitamin E deficiency have been identified. These syndromes include sterility in male rats, fetal resorption in female rats, muscular dystrophy in rabbits and guinea pigs, encephalomalacia in chicks, and hematological disorders in monkeys. Vitamin E deficiency in animals has also been associated with increased prostaglandin synthesis, platelet aggregation, impaired membrane function, and red cell defects. In humans, a clear-cut deficiency syndrome has not been recognized. However, signs of vitamin E deficiency, such as muscle weakness, ceroid deposition, and decreased erythrocyte survival time *in vivo*, have been reported in malabsorption syndromes (Farrell et al., 1977; Sokol et al., 1985). In premature infants with vitamin E deficiency, hemolytic anemia is observed (Hassan et al., 1966; Oski and Barness, 1967; Johnson et al., 1974). Some evidence of neurological dysfunction in children

Plasma Lipid Component	Plasma		Platelet	
Used for Correlations	α-tocopherol	γ-tocopherol	α-tocopherol	γ-tocopherol
Total lipid	0.79*	0.60*	0.22	0.15
Cholesterol	0.58*	0.46*	0.27	0.17
Triglyceride	0.78*	0.61*	0.08	0.09

Table 18.8: Correlation coefficients showing the relation of α- and γ-tocopherol in plasma and platelets to total lipid, cholesterol, and triglyceride concentrations in 49 healthy male subjects. * indicates that correlations are statistically significant with $p < 0.001$. From Vatassery et al. (1983a). © Am. J. Clin. Nutr. American Society for Clinical Nutrition.

with chronic cholestasis, which improves with vitamin E treatment, has been documented (Sokol et al., 1984).

Recently, self-supplementation with vitamin E has become increasingly common in many industrialized countries because of an assumed beneficial effect on sexuality, aging, and the prevention of cancer. Fortunately, excessive doses of vitamin E, unlike vitamins A and D, do not appear to produce deleterious effects (Farrell and Bieri, 1975). Nevertheless, further research is needed before it can be concluded that long-term self-supplementation with vitamin E is without risk.

At present, there is no suitable index which accurately reflects dietary intakes or body stores of vitamin E. Several indices have been investigated and these are described below.

18.3.1 Serum tocopherol concentrations

The concentration of total tocopherols in serum is the most frequently used biochemical index of vitamin E nutritional status. Nevertheless, its use as an index of vitamin E intake or tissue stores is questionable. Vitamin E is transported in human plasma mainly in the LDL-lipoprotein fractions (Behrens et al., 1982). In adults, both α- and γ-tocopherol levels in serum are highly correlated with serum cholesterol and total lipid concentrations (Horwitt et al., 1972; Vatassery et al., 1983a) (Table 18.8). As a result, tocopherol/lipid ratios are sometimes used (Horwitt et al., 1972). A ratio of 0.6 mg total tocopherols per gram of total serum lipids is said to indicate adequate vitamin E nutritional status (Farrell et al., 1978). Horwitt et al. (1972) recommended the use of this ratio to prevent persons with low serum lipid levels from being misclassified as vitamin E deficient. Conversely, some subjects with elevated serum lipid concentrations may have normal serum total tocopherol concentrations despite clinical evidence of vitamin E deficiency (Sokol et al., 1984). For example, Sokol et al. reported that in patients with chronic cholestasis, tocopherol/lipid ratios correlated more strongly with the vitamin E deficiency neurological syndrome than serum tocopherol concentrations. Moreover, tocopherol/lipid ratios less than 0.6 mg/g have been associated

Age Group	Concentration	Reference
Normal subjects		
Infants, full term	0.22 ± 0.10*	Gordon et al. (1958)
Children ≤ 12 yr	0.38 − 1.55	Farrell et al. (1978)
Adults (20–39 yr)	1.096 ± 0.057	Vandewoude and Vandewoude (1987)
Adults (40–59 yr)	1.462 ± 0.164	Vandewoude and Vandewoude (1987)
Adults (60–79 yr)	1.342 ± 0.100	Vandewoude and Vandewoude (1987)
Adults (80–94 yr)	0.937 ± 0.061	Vandewoude and Vandewoude (1987)
Disease states		
Cystic fibrosis 1–19 yr	0.15 ± 0.15*	Gordon et al. (1958)
Primary biliary cirrhosis	1.21 ± 0.09	Sokol et al. (1985)
Chronic liver disease	1.39 ± 0.15	Sokol et al. (1985)
Chronic cholestasis in children, 6–12 yr	> 0.1	Sokol et al. (1984)

Table 18.9: Serum tocopherol concentrations (mg/dL ± SEM or * SD) for subjects of various ages and with disease states. Conversion factor to SI units (μmol/L) = × 23.22.

with reductions in erythrocyte malondialdehyde formation in children with cholestasis who are less than six months of age. Erythrocyte malondialdehyde release *in vitro* is a functional measure of vitamin E status (Section 18.3.8) (Cynamon et al., 1985). Not all investigators, however, advocate the use of tocopherol/lipid ratios (Gutcher et al., 1984; Cynamon and Isenberg, 1987).

Total serum tocopherol concentrations are often lower in persons in less industrialized countries, where they are associated with lower tocopherol intakes. Rahman et al. (1964) reported that 21% of persons living in rural East Pakistan had serum tocopherol levels less than 0.5 mg/dL (< 11.6 μmol/L) compared to 1.1% of adults (of a total of 379 apparently healthy adults) living in Canada (Desai, 1968). Agricultural migrant workers in Southern Brazil, however, had a mean plasma vitamin E concentration (1.14 ± 0.33 mg/dL; 26.5 ± 7.7 μmol/L) comparable to that for adults from North America, and no workers had levels below 0.5 mg/dL (< 11.6 μmol/L) (Desai et al., 1980). Their average dietary intake of α-tocopherol was similar to that for well-nourished populations.

Serum total tocopherol values vary according to age, physiological state, and the method of analysis. Hence, a wide range of values has been reported for apparently healthy subjects (Table 18.9).

Some (Lewis et al., 1973; Vandewonde and Vandewonde, 1987), but not all (Vatassery et al., 1983b), investigators have noted increases in serum total tocopherol concentrations with age in adults up to the sixth decade of life, which have been associated with an increase in blood lipids. Children up to twelve years of age have lower serum tocopherol levels than adults, whether expressed as total tocopherol in the plasma or as tocopherol per unit of total serum lipids (Goldbloom, 1960; Farrell et al., 1978). Concentrations of serum tocopherol in premature infants are also low (Dju et al., 1958; Hågå and Lunde, 1978; DeVito et al., 1986), arising from low reserves and transient malabsorption. Pregnant and *postpartum* women with adequate intakes of vitamin E have elevated serum total tocopherol values.

In general, serum total tocopherol concentrations of less than 0.5 mg/dL ($< 11.6\,\mu$mol/L) have been associated with greater than 5% hemolysis of erythrocytes in the peroxide hemolysis test in adults (Section 18.3.6), and with low vitamin E status (Sauberlich et al., 1974). This cutoff value is not appropriate for pediatric populations. Many infants and children have serum tocopherol concentrations less than 0.5 mg/dL ($< 11.6\,\mu$mol/L) because of lower lipid concentrations, but no evidence of vitamin E deficiency (Farrell et al., 1978).

18.3.2 Erythrocyte tocopherol concentrations

Studies of erythrocyte tocopherol concentrations as an index of vitamin E status are limited, perhaps because it is technically more difficult to determine tocopherol in the erythrocytes than in the serum. Initial studies in rats suggested that tocopherol levels in erythrocytes and plasma were closely correlated (Poukka and Bieri, 1970). In later studies, marked variations in erythrocyte tocopherol levels were noted in rats fed the same dietary levels of vitamin E, especially at low dosage levels (Lehmann, 1981). Such discrepancies may be associated with differences in the analytical methods used. At present there appears to be no justification for using erythrocyte tocopherol as an index of vitamin E status.

18.3.3 Platelet tocopherol concentrations

Platelets contain mostly α-tocopherol (80%); the rest is γ-tocopherol. Platelet tocopherol content appears to be a promising index of vitamin E nutritional status in rats (Lehmann, 1981), and probably in humans. A linear relationship between platelet tocopherol content and dosage of DL-α-tocopherol was noted in five human subjects, up to the daily dose of 1800 IU (Vatassery et al., 1983a). These findings were confirmed by Lehmann et al. (1988), who concluded that platelets were more sensitive for measuring dose response when compared to plasma, red blood cells, or lymphocytes. Platelet tocopherol concentrations are independent of serum lipid levels, an important advantage relative to serum tocopherol concentrations (Vatassery et al., 1983a) (Table 18.8). Platelet α-, γ-, and total tocopherol concentrations decline significantly with age, but it is not known whether such decreases affect platelet function in the aged (Vatassery et al., 1983b).

18.3.4   Tissue tocopherol concentrations

Analysis of liver biopsy or adipose tissue samples for tocopherol may be a useful index of body stores of vitamin E and thus long-term vitamin E status. For example, adipose tissue with a low vitamin E content was observed in vitamin-E-deficient children with chronic cholestasis (Sokol et al., 1983) and adults with α-β-lipoproteinemia (Kayden et al., 1983). The methods, however, are not suitable for large population studies because they are too invasive.   More work is required to develop both standardized techniques for sampling subcutaneous tissues and interpretive guidelines for evaluating adipose tocopherol concentrations in biopsy samples.

18.3.5   Analysis of tocopherol in blood components and tissues

Gas liquid chromatography (GLC) and, more recently, HPLC are the methods most commonly used to measure the tocopherols in blood, blood components, and tissues. In the GLC method, the individual tocopherols can be estimated as trimethylsilyl ethers using methyl silicon rubber SE-30 or Apiezon L as a liquid phase in concentrations from 1% to 10% and at a temperature of 235°C. It is possible to separate α-tocopherol from β- and γ-tocopherols; δ-tocopherol constitutes a third fraction (Bieri and Andrews, 1963).

The HPLC techniques are relatively simple, rapid, noninvasive, and suitable for studies of pediatric populations because only small volumes of serum are required (Vatassery et al., 1978; Bieri et al., 1979). Some HPLC techniques (e.g. normal phase HPLC) are capable of analyzing α-, β-, and γ-tocopherols separately (Tangney et al., 1979). In others (e.g. reverse-phase HPLC), very small concentrations of β-tocopherol remain as contaminants in the γ-tocopherol fraction (Vatassery et al., 1983a; Handelman et al., 1985).   Nevertheless, reverse-phase HPLC, with a high sensitivity fluorescence detector, is very sensitive for analyzing γ-tocopherol provided that characterization of the minor component β-tocopherol is not required.

Earlier chemical methods involved saponification, solvent extraction of tocopherols, molecular distillation, and separation of the tocopherols by two-dimensional reverse-phase paper chromatography or column chromatography.   Following elution, the various tocopherol fractions were assayed by the Emmerie-Engel method (Emmerie and Engel, 1938).

18.3.6   Erythrocyte hemolysis test

The erythrocyte hemolysis test has been used as a functional index of vitamin E status.   The rate of hemolysis correlates inversely with serum total tocopherol levels, increasing in vitamin E deficiency (Binder and Spiro, 1967) (Figure 18.8).   The technique must be rigorously standardized (Farrell et al., 1977; Mino et al., 1978). The test, however,

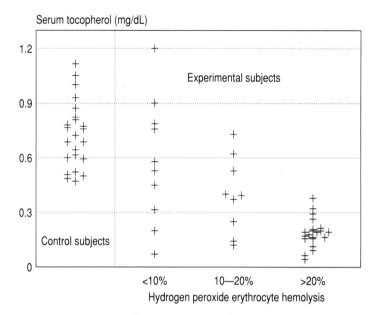

Figure 18.8: Relationship between serum tocopherol levels and hydrogen peroxide hemolysis of red blood cells in human subjects. From Binder and Spiro (1967). © Am. J. Clin. Nutr. American Society for Clinical Nutrition.

lacks specificity; changes in the status of other nutrients can also influence the rate of erythrocyte hemolysis (Melhorn et al., 1971). In children with cholestasis, the hemolysis test is said to underestimate the degree of vitamin E deficiency, as indicated by plasma vitamin E, vitamin E lipid ratio, and malondialdehyde formation (Section 18.3.8) (Cynamon and Isenberg, 1987).

Freshly prepared samples of erythrocytes must be used for the erythrocyte hemolysis test, making it an impractical method for field studies. Isotonic dialuric acid, oxygen-containing isotonic saline, or hydrogen peroxide has been used as the hemolyzing agent; hydrogen peroxide is most commonly used in human studies (Sauberlich et al., 1974). The test involves incubating washed erythrocytes in a 2% to 2.4% hydrogen peroxide solution for a period of three hours, followed by determining the amount of hemoglobin produced by hemolysis. Comparison is then made with the amount of hemoglobin produced by incubation with distilled water, and the result expressed as a percentage. A normal result (i.e. less than 5% hemolysis during the three-hour incubation in 2% H_2O_2) generally indicates the absence of vitamin E deficiency. Serum vitamin E concentrations in such patients will generally be > 0.5 mg/dL, whereas for subjects in whom the test results are greater than 5% hemolysis, serum vitamin E concentrations will be < 0.5 mg/dL (< 11.6 µmol/L).

Hemolysis *in vivo* only occurs when serum vitamin E concentrations are $\leq 0.2\,\text{mg/dL}$ ($\leq 4.6\,\mu\text{mol/L}$).

18.3.7   Breath pentane measurements

Measurements of the exhalation of ethane and pentane, peroxidation products of linoleic and linolenic acids respectively, have been used to evaluate oxidative changes in animals and may be potential methods for assessing vitamin E deficiency states in humans. Lemoyne et al. (1987) standardized a technique for collecting and measuring breath pentane in humans. They compared their results with plasma vitamin E concentrations in vitamin-E-deficient and normal subjects and found a significant negative correlation between plasma vitamin E levels and breath pentane. Moreover, after supplementing five normal subjects with vitamin E for ten days, breath pentane levels were significantly decreased. Hence, measurement of breath pentane appears promising as a functional test of vitamin E status in humans. Further studies, however, utilizing alternative indices of vitamin E status for comparison with breath pentane measurements are necessary, before the validity of this test can be firmly established. The effects of other anti-oxidants and pro-oxidant toxins also need further study.

18.3.8   Erythrocyte malondialdehyde release *in vitro*

This functional test is based on quantifying the formation of malondialdehyde generated from the lipid peroxidation of polyunsaturated fatty acids of erythrocytes exposed to hydrogen peroxide *in vitro* (Cyanamon et al., 1985). Cyanamon and Isenberg (1987) evaluated this test in twenty-four children with cholestatic liver disease at risk to vitamin E deficiency and eleven healthy controls. The test was said to reflect vitamin E deficiency accurately, as indicated by low plasma vitamin E concentrations, and a low ratio of plasma vitamin E to plasma total lipids. The test is easy to perform and results appear reproducible. More studies are needed, however, to confirm the validity of this test for assessing vitamin E status, particularly in marginal vitamin E deficiency states.

18.4   Summary

Vitamin A

Ocular lesions, characteristic of vitamin A deficiency, are endemic in some developing countries. Total serum vitamin A/serum retinol concentrations are the most frequently determined biochemical index of vitamin A status. They reflect total body reserves of vitamin A when liver vitamin A stores are either severely depleted or excessively high, but not when liver vitamin A concentrations are between these limits. Several confounding factors affect serum vitamin A or retinol concentrations, and hence limit their specificity and sensitivity as an index of vitamin A status. Age-specific interpretive guidelines are available for low serum vitamin A concentrations for U.S. persons. Whether these guidelines are appropriate for other population groups is unknown. Generally, serum total vitamin A values of $\geq 30\,\mu g/dL$ ($\geq 1.05\,\mu mol/L$) are indicative of adequate vitamin A status. Vitamin A toxicity can be assessed by the presence of elevated serum retinyl ester concentrations in fasting blood samples. Physiological functional tests for vitamin A status include the relative dose response, the rapid dark adaptation test, and conjunctival impression cytology. The last test may also detect subclinical vitamin A deficiency. Newer methods for measuring vitamin A body stores include stable isotope dilution procedures and the determination of serum retinoic acid. Analytical methods for total vitamin A, retinol, and retinyl esters in serum include colorimetry, spectrophotometry, fluorometry, and HPLC. The methods give comparable results provided that conditions of collection, storage, and analysis of serum samples are clearly defined and controlled. High-performance liquid chromatography is capable of distinguishing retinol from retinyl esters in the serum.

Vitamin D

In industrialized countries, suboptimal vitamin D status may occur in persons with inadequate skin exposure to sunlight, and in those living in northern geographical latitudes. Additionally, conditions such as malabsorption, or the prolonged use of certain anti-convulsant drugs, may precipitate secondary vitamin D deficiency. Severe vitamin D deficiency may result in rickets in infants and children and osteomalacia in adults. Indiscriminate self-dosing with excessive intakes of vitamin D may produce vitamin D toxicity.

Serum 25-hydroxyvitamin D concentrations are the most useful index of vitamin D status; they reflect the amount of vitamin D in the liver, the major tissue store of vitamin D. Positive relationships between serum 25-OH-D concentrations and season, place of work, use of vitamin D supplements, latitude, and clinical signs of vitamin D deficiency provide further evidence for the validity of serum 25-OH-D as a measure of vitamin D status. The preferred method for assaying serum 25-OH-D is by a competitive binding assay, after separating it from other metabolites by HPLC. Interpretive guidelines for serum 25-OH-D concentrations indicative of vitamin D deficiency or toxicity are poorly defined; very few studies have correlated clinical signs of deficiency or excess of vitamin D with serum 25-OH-D concentrations.

Although serum alkaline phosphatase activity has been used as an indirect index of vitamin D status, it is also affected by a variety of other disease states. Hence its specificity and sensitivity as an index of vitamin D status is poor. Serum calcium can be used to identify vitamin D intoxication; in such cases, both serum calcium and serum 25-OH-D are elevated. Urinary excretion levels of calcium and phosphorus are not specific for vitamin D status, and their use as an index of vitamin D status is not recommended.

Vitamin E

Various syndromes of vitamin E deficiency have been identified in animals, but no clearly defined deficiency syndrome has been recognized in humans. Nevertheless, signs of vitamin E deficiency have been reported in premature infants and persons with chronic cholestasis and certain intestinal malabsorption conditions. Serum total tocopherol is most frequently used to assess vitamin E status, although its use as an index of vitamin E tissue stores or dietary intake is questionable, except in a deficiency state. Concentrations of total serum tocopherol vary according to age, physiological state, method of analysis, and total serum lipid levels. Some investigators prefer to use the ratio of total serum tocopherol to total serum lipids as an index of vitamin E status, ratios of ≥ 0.6 mg tocopherol per gram of total serum lipids indicating adequate nutritional status. Red blood cell tocopherol concentrations are not useful as an index of vitamin E status. Platelet tocopherol concentrations are independent of serum lipid concentrations, but isolation of platelets is impractical for surveys. New functional tests which appear promising include measurement of breath pentane and erythrocyte malondialdehyde release *in vitro*. More studies are needed, however, before the validity of these functional tests for assessing marginal vitamin E deficiency states is established. Interpretive guidelines for serum tocopherol concentrations are based on their relationship with erythrocyte hemolysis, which increases in vitamin E deficiency. Hemolysis *in vivo* occurs when serum tocopherol concentrations fall to ≤ 0.2 mg/dL (≤ 4.6 µmol/L). Serum tocopherol concentrations of < 0.5 mg/dL (< 11.6 µmol/L) and > 0.5 mg/dL (> 11.6 µmol/L) are associated with greater and less than 5% hemolysis *in vitro*, respectively, during a three hour incubation in 2% H_2O_2. Although vitamin E levels of liver or adipose tissue samples provide a measure of tissue stores of vitamin E, such techniques are too invasive for population studies and are difficult to standardize. Analysis of tocopherol in tissues, blood, and/or its components is best performed by HPLC.

References

Amédée-Manesme O, Anderson D, Olson JA. (1984). Relation of the relative dose response to liver concentrations of vitamin A in generally well nourished surgical patients. American Journal of Clinical Nutrition 39: 898–902.

Amédée-Manesme O, Luzeau R, Wittepen JR, Hanck A, Sommer A. (1988). Impression cytology detects subclinical vitamin A deficiency. American Journal of Clinical Nutrition 47: 875–878.

Amédée-Manesme O, Mourey MS, Hanck A, Therasse J. (1987). Vitamin A relative dose response test: validation by intravenous injection in children with liver disease. American Journal of Clinical Nutrition 46: 286–289.

Bankson DD, Russell RM, Sadowski JA. (1986). Determination of retinyl esters and retinol in serum or plasma by normal-phase high-performance liquid chromatography: method and applications. Clinical Chemistry 32: 35–40.

Behrens WA, Thompson JN, Madère R. (1982). Distribution of α-tocopherol in human plasma lipoproteins. American Journal of Clinical Nutrition 35: 691–696.

Bessey OA, Lowry OH, Brock MJ, Lopez JA. (1946a). Determination of vitamin A and carotene in small quantities of blood serum. Journal of Biological Chemistry 166: 177–188.

Bessey OA, Lowry OH, Brock MJ. (1946b). Method for rapid determination of alkaline phosphatase with 5 cubic millimeters of serum. Journal of Biological Chemistry 164: 321–329.

Bieri JG. (1984). Vitamin E. In: Present Knowledge in Nutrition. Fifth edition. The Nutrition Foundation Inc., Washington, D.C., pp. 226–240.

Bieri JG, Andrews EL. (1963). The determination of α-tocopherol in animal tissues by gas liquid chromatography. Iowa State Journal of Science 38: 3–12.

Bieri JG, Tolliver TJ, Catignani GL. (1979). Simultaneous determination of alpha-tocopheral and retinol in plasma or red cells by high pressure liquid chromatography. American Journal of Clinical Nutrition 32: 2143–2149.

Binder HJ, Spiro HM. (1967). Tocopherol deficiency in man. American Journal of Clinical Nutrition 20: 594–603.

Blum M, Kirsten M, Worth MH Jr. (1977). Reversible hypertension: caused by the hypercalcemia of hyperparathyroidism, vitamin D toxicity, and calcium infusion. Journal of American Medical Association 237: 262–263.

Brink EW, Perera WD, Broske SP, Cash RA, Smith JL, Sauberlich HE, Bashor MM. (1979). Vitamin A status of children in Sri Lanka. American Journal of Clinical Nutrition 32: 84–91.

Carr FH, Price EA. (1926). Color reactions attributed to vitamin A. Biochemical Journal 20: 497–501.

Cynamon HA, Isenberg JN. (1987). Characterization of vitamin E status in cholestatic children by conventional laboratory standards and a new functional assay. Journal of Pediatric Gastroenterology and Nutrition 6: 46–50.

Cynamon HA, Isenberg JN, Nguyen CH. (1985). Erythrocyte malondialdehyde release *in vitro*: a functional measure of vitamin E status. Clinica Chimica Acta 151: 169–176.

Dattani JT, Exton-Smith AN, Stephen JM. (1984). Vitamin D status of the elderly in relation to age and exposure to sunlight. Human Nutrition: Clinical Nutrition 38C: 131–137.

DeLuca HF, Schnoes HK. (1983). Vitamin D: Recent advances. Annual Review of Biochemistry 52: 411–439.

Desai ID. (1968). Plasma tocopherol levels in normal adults. Canadian Journal of Physiology and Pharmacology 46: 819–822.

Devgun MS, Patterson CR, Johnson BE, Cohen C. (1981). Vitamin D nutrition in relation to season and occupation. American Journal of Clinical Nutrition 34: 1501-1504.

Delvin EE, Imback A, Copti M. (1988). Vitamin D nutritional status and related biochemical indices in an autonomous elderly population. American Journal of Clinical Nutrition 48: 373–378.

Desai ID. (1968). Plasma tocopherol levels in normal adults. Canadian Journal of Physiology and Pharmacology 46: 819–822.

Desai ID, Swann MA, Garcia Tavares ML, Dutra de Oliveira BS, Duarte FAM, Dutra de Oliveira JE. (1980). Vitamin E status of agricultural migrant workers in Southern Brazil. American Journal of Clinical Nutrition 33: 2669–2673.

DeVito V, Reynolds JW, Benda GI, Carlson C. (1986). Serum vitamin E levels in very low-birth weight infants receiving vitamin E in parenteral nutrition solutions. Journal of Parenteral and Enteral Nutrition 10: 63–65.

Dju MY, Mason KE, Filer LJ Jr. (1958). Vitamin E (tocopherol) in human tissues from birth to old age. American Journal of Clinical Nutrition 6: 50–60.

Driskell WJ, Neese JW, Bryant CC, Bashor MM. (1982). Measurement of vitamin A and vitamin E in human serum by high performance liquid chromatography. Journal of Chromatography. 231:439–444.

Duarte Favaro RM, de Souza NV, Vannucchi H, Desai ID, Dutra de Oliveira JE. (1986). Evaluation of rose bengal staining test and rapid dark-adaptation test for the field assessment of vitamin A status of preschool children in Southern Brazil. American Journal of Clinical Nutrition 43: 940–945.

Duncan WE, Haddad JG. (1981). Vitamin D assessment. The assays and their applications. In: Labbé RE (ed). Laboratory Assessment of Nutritional Status. Clinics in Laboratory Medicine 1: 713–727.

Edelstein S, Charman M, Lawson DEM, Kodicek E. (1974). Competitive protein-binding assay for 25-hydroxycholecalciferol. Clinical Science and Molecular Medicine 46: 231–240.

Eisman JA, Shepard RM, DeLua HF. (1977). Determination of 25-hydroxyvitamin D_2 and 25-hydroxyvitamin D_3 in human plasma using high-pressure liquid chromatography. Analytical Biochemistry 80: 298–305.

Emmerie A, Engel C. (1938). Colorimetric determination of dl-α-tocopherol (vitamin E). Nature 142:873.

Farrell PM, Bieri JG. (1975). Megavitamin E supplementation in man. American Journal of Clinical Nutrition 28: 1381–1386.

Farrell PM, Bieri JG, Fraantoni JF, Wood RE, Di Sant Agnese PA. (1977). The occurrence and effects of human vitamin E deficiency: a study in patients with cystic fibrosis. Journal of Clinical Investigation 60: 233–241.

Farrell PM, Levine SL, Murphy MD, Adams AJ. (1978). Plasma tocopherol levels and tocopherol-lipid relationships in a normal population of children as compared to healthy adults. American Journal of Clinical Nutrition 31: 1720–1726.

Flores H, Compos F, Araujo CRC, Underwood BA. (1984). Assessment of marginal vitamin A deficiency in Brazilian children using the relative dose response procedure. American Journal of Clinical Nutrition 40: 1281–1289.

Frame B, Jackson CE, Reynolds WA, Umphrey JE. (1974). Hypercalcemia and skeletal effects in chronic hypervitaminosis A. Annals of Internal Medicine 80: 44–48.

Fraser DR. (1983). The physiological economy of vitamin D. Lancet 1: 969–972.

Furr HC, Amédée-Manesme O, Olson JA. (1984). Gradient reversed-phase high-performance liquid chromatographic separation of naturally occurring retinoids. Journal of Chromatography 309: 229–307.

Gadomski AM, Kjolhede CL, Wittpen J, Bulux J, Rosas AR, Forman MR. (1989). Conjunctival impression cytology (CIC) to detect subclinical vitamin A deficiency: comparison of CIC with biochemical assesments. American Journal of Clinical Nutrition 49: 495–500.

Garry PJ, Hunt WC, Brandrofchak JL, VanderJagt D, Goodwin JS. (1987). Vitamin A intake and plasma retinol levels in healthy elderly men and women. American Journal of Clinical Nutrition 46: 989–994.

Gertner JM, Lilburn M, Domeneck M. (1977). 25-hydroxycalciol absorption in steatorrhoea and postgastrectomy osteomalacia. British Medical Journal 1:1310–1312.

Gibson RS, Draper HH, McGirr LG, Nizan P, Martinez OB. (1986). The vitamin D status of a cohort of postmenopausal noninstitutionalized Canadian women. Nutrition Research 6: 1179–1187.

Goldbloom RB. (1960). Investigations of tocopherol deficiency in infancy and childhood: Studies of serum tocopherol levels and of erythrocyte survival. Canadian Medical Association Journal 82: 1114–1117.

Gordon HH, Nitowsky HM, Tildon JT, Levin S. (1958). Studies of tocopherol deficiency in infants and children. V. An interim summary. Pediatrics 21: 673–681.

Gutcher GR, Raynor WR, Farrell PM. (1984). An evaluation of vitamin E status in premature infants. American Journal of Clinical Nutrition 40: 1078–1089.

Guzman MA, Arroyave G, Scrimshaw NS. (1961). Serum ascorbic acid, riboflavin, carotene, vitamin A, vitamin E and alkaline phosphatase values in Central American school children. American Journal of Clinical Nutrition 9: 164–169.

Haddad JG, Chyu KJ. (1971). Competitive protein-binding radioassay for 25-hydroxy-cholecalciferol. Journal of Clinical Endocrinology and Metabolism 33: 992–995.

Haddad JG, Stamp TCB. (1974). Circulating 25-hydroxyvitamin D in man. American Journal of Medicine 57: 57–62.

Hågå P, Lunde G. (1978). Selenium and vitamin E in cord blood from preterm and full term infants. Acta Paediatrica Scandinavia 67: 735–739.

Hahn TJ, Hendin BA, Scharp CR, Boisseau VC, Haddad JG. (1975). Serum 25-hydroxy-calciferol levels and bone mass in children on chronic anticonvulsant therapy. New England Journal of Medicine 292: 550–554.

Handelman GJ, Machlin LJ, Fitch K, Weiter JJ, Dratz EA. (1985). Oral α-tocopherol supplements decrease plasma γ-tocopherol levels in humans. American Journal of Clinical Nutrition 115: 807–813.

Hassan H, Hashim SA, Itallie TB van, Sebrell WH. (1966). Syndrome in premature infants associated with low plasma vitamin E levels and high polyunsaturated fatty acid diet. American Journal of Clinical Nutrition 19: 147–157.

Health and Welfare Canada. (1973). Nutrition Canada National Survey. Health and Welfare, Ottawa.

Heaney RP, Recker RR, Saville PD. (1978). Menopausal changes in calcium balance performance. Journal of Laboratory and Clinical Medicine 92: 953–963.

Holick MF, MacLaughlin JA, Doppelt SH. (1981). Regulation of cutaneous previta-min D_3 photosynthesis in man: skin pigment is not an essential regulator. Science 211: 590–593.

Holmes RP, Kummerow FA. (1983). The relationship of adequate and excessive intake of vitamin D to health and disease. Journal of the American College of Nutrition 2: 173–199.

Horwitt MK, Harvey CC, Dahm CH Jr, Searcy MT. (1972). Relationship between toco-pherol and serum lipid levels for determination of nutritional adequacy. Annals of New York Academy of Sciences 203: 223–236.

Johnson L. Schaffer D, Boggs TR Jr. (1974). The premature infant, vitamin E deficiency and retrolental fibroplasia. American Journal of Clinical Nutrition 27: 1158–1173.

Kark JD, Smith AH, Switzer BR, Hames CG. (1981). Low serum vitamin A (retinol) and cancer incidence in Evans County, Georgia. Journal of the National Cancer Institute 66: 7–16.

Kayden HJ, Hatam LJ, Traber MG. (1983). The measurement of nanograms of tocopherol from needle aspiration biopsies of adipose tissue: normal and abetalipoproteinemic subjects. Journal of Lipid Research 24: 652–656.

Kjolhede CL, Gadomski AM, Wittepenn J, Bulux J, Rosas A, Solomons NW, Brown KH, Forman MR. (1989). Conjunctival impression cytology: feasibility of a field trial to detect subclinical vitamin A deficiency. American Journal of Clinical Nutrition 49: 490–494.

Lamberg-Allardt C. (1984). Vitamin D intake, sunlight exposure and 25-hydroxyvit-amin D levels in the elderly during one year. Annals of Nutrition and Metabolism 28: 144–150.

Lawson DE, Paul AA, Black AE, Cole JJ, Mandal AR, Davie M. (1979). Relative contributions of diet and sunlight to vitamin D state in the elderly. British Medical Journal 2: 303–305.

Le Francois P, Chevassus-Agnes S, Ndiaye AM. (1981). Plasma carotenoids as a useful indicator of vitamin A status. American Journal of Clinical Nutrition 34: 434.

Lehmann J. (1981). Comparative sensitivities of tocopherol levels of platelets, red blood cells and plasma for estimating vitamin E nutritional status in the rat. American Journal of Clinical Nutrition 34: 2104–2110.

Lehmann J, Rao DD, Canary JJ, Judd JT. (1988). Vitamin E and relationships among tocopherols in human plasma, platelets, lymphocytes, and red blood cells. American Journal of Clinical Nutrition 47: 470–474.

Lemoyne M, Gossum A van, Kurian R, Ostro M, Axler J, Jeejeebhoy KN. (1987). Breath pentane analysis as an index of lipid peroxidation: a functional test of vitamin E status. American Journal of Clinical Nutrition 46: 267–272.

Lester E, Skinner RK, Willis MR. (1973). Seasonal variation in serum 25-hydroxy-vitamin D in the elderly in Britain. Lancet 1: 979–980.

Lester E, Skinner RK, Foo AY, Lund B, Sørenson OH. (1980). Serum 25-hydroxy-vitamin D levels and vitamin D intake in healthy young adults in Britain and Denmark. Scandinavian Journal of Clinical and Laboratory Investigation 40: 145–150.

Lewis JS, Pian AK, Baer MT, Acosta PB, Emerson GA. (1973). Effect of long-term ingestion of polyunsaturated fat, age, plasma cholesterol, diabetes mellitus and supplemental tocopherol upon plasma tocopherol. American Journal of Clinical Nutrition 26: 136–143.

Lo CW, Paris PW, Holick MF. (1986). Indian and Pakistani immigrants have the same capacity as Caucasians to produce vitamin D in response to ultraviolet irradiation. American Journal of Clinical Nutrition 44: 683-685.

Loerch JD, Underwood BA, Lewis KC. (1979). Response of plasma levels of vitamin A to a dose of vitamin A as an indicator of hepatic vitamin A reserves in rats. Journal of Nutrition 109: 778–786.

Looker AC, Johnson CL, Wotek CE, Yetley EA, Underwood BA. (1988). Ethnic and racial differences in serum vitamin A levels of children aged 4–11 years. American Journal of Clinical Nutrition 47: 247–252.

McKenna MJ, Freaney R, Meade A, Muldowney FP. (1985). Hypovitaminosis D and elevated serum alkaline phosphatase in elderly Irish people. American Journal of Clinical Nutrition 41: 101-109.

Mejia LA, Arroyave G. (1983). Determination of vitamin A in blood. Some practical considerations on the time of collection of the specimens and the stability of the vitamin. American Journal of Clinical Nutrition 37: 147–151.

Mejia LA, Pineda O, Noriega JF, Benitez J, Fall G. (1984). Significance of postprandial blood concentrations of retinol, retinol-binding protein, and carotenoids when assessing the vitamin A status of children. American Journal of Clinical Nutrition 39: 62–65.

Melhorn DK, Gross S, Lake GA, Leu JA. (1971). The hydrogen peroxide fragility test and serum tocopherol level in anemias of various etiologies. Blood 37: 438–446.

Mino M, Nishida Y, Morata K, Takegawa M, Katsui G, Yuguchi Y. (1978). Studies on the factors influencing the hydrogen peroxide hemolysis test. Journal of Nutritional Science and Vitaminology 24: 383–395.

Mobarhan S, Russell RM, Underwood BA, Wallingford J, Mathieson RD, Al-Midani H. (1984). Evaluation of the relative dose response test for vitamin A nutriture in cirrhotics. American Journal of Clinical Nutrition 34: 2264–2270.

Neeld JB, Pearson WN. (1963). Macro- and micro-methods for the determination of serum vitamin A using trifluoroacetic acid. Journal of Nutrition 79: 454–462.

Olson JA. (1982). New approaches to methods for the assessment of nutritional status of the individual. American Journal of Clinical Nutrition 35:1166–1168.

Olson JA. (1984). Serum levels of vitamin A and carotenoids as reflectors of nutritional status. Journal of the National Cancer Institute 73: 1439–1444.

Omdahl JL, Garry PJ, Hunsaker LA, Hunt WC, Goodwin JS. (1982). Nutritional status in a healthy elderly population: vitamin D. American Journal of Clinical Nutrition 36: 1225–1233.

Oski FA, Barness IA. (1967). Vitamin E deficiency: a previously unrecognized cause of hemolytic anemia in the premature infant. Journal of Pediatrics 70: 211–220.

Parfitt AM, Gallagher JC, Heaney RP, Johnston CC, Neer R, Whedon GD. (1982). Vitamin D and bone health in the elderly. American Journal of Clinical Nutrition 36: 1014–1031.

Parfitt AM, Kleerekoper M. (1980). Clinical disorders of calcium, phosphorus and magnesium metabolism. In: Maxwell MH, Kleman CR (eds). Clinical Disorders of Fluid and Electrolyte Metabolism. Third edition. McGraw Hill Inc., New York, pp. 947–1152.

Pilch SM. (ed). (1985). Assessment of the vitamin A nutritional status of the U.S. population based on data collected in the Health and Nutrition Examination Surveys. Life Sciences Research Office, Federation of American Biological Societies, Bethesda, Maryland.

Pirie A, Anbunathan P. (1981). Early serum changes in severely malnourished children with corneal xerophthalmia after injection of water-miscible vitamin A. American Journal of Clinical Nutrition 34: 34–40.

Poukka RKH, Bieri, JG. (1970). Blood alpha-tocopherol: erythrocyte and plasma relationships in vitro and in vivo. Lipids 5: 757–761.

Preece MA, O'Riordan JL, Lawson DE, Kodicek E. (1974). A competitive protein-binding assay for 25-hydroxycalciol and 25-hydroxyercalciol in serum. Clinical Chemistry Acta 54: 235–242.

Preece MA, Tomlinson S, Ribot CA, Pietrek J, Korn HT, Davies DM, Ford JA, Dunnigan MG, O'Riordan JLH. (1975). Studies of vitamin D deficiency in man. Quarterly Journal of Medicine 44: 575–589.

Rahman MM, Hossain S, Talukdar SA, Ahmad K, Bieri JE. (1964). Serum vitamin E levels in the rural population of East Pakistan. Proceedings of the Society of Experimental Biology and Medicine 117: 133–135.

Russell RM, Boyer JL, Bagheri SA, Hruban Z. (1974). Hepatic injury from chronic hypervitaminoisis A resulting in portal hypertension and ascites. New England Journal of Medicine 291: 435–440.

Russell RM, Iber FL, Krasinski SD, Miller P. (1983). Protein-energy malnutrition and liver dysfunction limit the usefulness of the relative dose response (RDR) test for producing vitamin A deficiency. Human Nutrition: Clinical Nutrition 37C: 361–371.

Russell RM, Smith VC, Multack R, Krill AE, Rosenburg IH. (1973). Dark adaptation testing for diagnosis of subclinical vitamin A deficiency and evaluation of therapy. Lancet 2: 1161–1164.

Sauberlich HE, Dowdy RP, Skala JH. (1974). Laboratory Tests for the Assessment of Nutritional Status. CRC Press Inc., Cleveland, Ohio.

Sedrani SH, Elidrissy AW, El Arabi KM. (1983). Sunlight and vitamin D status in normal Saudi subjects. American Journal of Clinical Nutrition 38: 129–132.

Shepard RM, DeLuca HF. (1980). Determination of vitamin D and its metabolites in plasma. Methods in Enzymology 67: 393–413.

Smith FR, Goodman DS. (1976). Vitamin A transport in human vitamin A toxicity. New England Journal of Medicine 294: 805–808.

Sokol RJ, Balistreri WF, Hoofnagle JH, Jones EA. (1985). Vitamin E deficiency in adults with chronic liver disease. American Journal of Clinical Nutrition 41: 66–72.

Sokol RJ, Heubi JE, Iannaccone ST, Bove KE, Balistreri WF. (1983). Mechanism causing vitamin E deficiency during chronic childhood cholestasis. Gastroenterology 85: 1172–1182.

Sokol RJ, Heubi JE, Iannaccone ST, Bove KE, Balistreri WF. (1984). Vitamin E deficiency with normal serum vitamin E concentrations in children with chronic cholestasis. New England Journal of Medicine 310: 1209–1212.

Sommer A. (1982). Nutritional Blindness: Xerophthalmia and Keratomalacia. Oxford University Press, New York.

Sommer A, Hussaini G, Muhilal G, Tarwotjo I, Susanto D, Saroso JS. (1980). History of nightblindness: a simple tool for xerophthalmia screening. American Journal of Clinical Nutrition 33: 887–891.

Stamp TC, Round JM. (1974). Seasonal changes in human plasma levels of 25-hydroxyvitamin D. Nature 247: 563–565.

Tangney CC, Driskell JA, McNair HM. (1979). Separation of vitamin E isomers by high-performance liquid chromatography. Journal of Chromatography 172: 513–515.

Thompson JN, Erdody P, Brien R, Murray TK. (1971). Fluorometric determination of vitamin A in human blood and liver. Biochemical Medicine 5: 67–89.

Thornton SP. (1977). A rapid test for dark adaption. Annals of Ophthalmology 9: 731–734.

Tseng SCG. (1985). Staging of conjunctival squamous metaplasia by impression cytology. Opthalmology 92: 728–733.

Vandewonde MFJ, Vandewonde MG. (1987). Vitamin E status in a normal population: the influence of age. Journal of the American College of Nutrition 6: 307–311.

Vatassery GT, Maynard VR, Hagen DF. (1978). High performance liquid chromatography of various tocopherols. Journal of Chromatography 161: 299–302.

Vatassery GT, Kezowski AM, Eckfeldt JH. (1983a). Vitamin E concentrations in human blood plasma and platelets. American Journal of Clinical Nutrition 37: 1020–1024.

Vatassery GT, Johnson GJ, Krezowski AM. (1983b). Changes in vitamin E concentrations in human plasma and platelets with age. Journal of the American College of Nutrition 2: 369–375.

Vinton NE, Russell RM. (1981). Evaluation of a rapid test of dark adaptation. American Journal of Clinical Nutrition 34: 1961–1966.

Wald N, Idle M, Boreham J, Bailey A. (1980). Low serum-vitamin-A and subsequent risk of cancer. Preliminary results of a prospective study. Lancet 2: 813–815.

Willet WC, Polk BF, Underwood BA, Stampfer MJ, Pressel S, Rosner B, Taylor JO, Schneider K, Hames CG. (1984). Relation of serum vitamins A and E and carotenoids to the risk of cancer. New England Journal of Medicine 310: 430–434.

Wittepenn JR, Tseng SCG, Sommer A. (1986). Detection of early xerophthalmia by impression cytology. Archives of Opthalmology 104:237–239.

Chapter 19

Assessment of vitamin C status

For centuries, the consumption of citrus fruit has been associated with the prevention of the vitamin C deficiency disease scurvy, but it was not until 1932 that the active compound was isolated (King and Waugh, 1932; Svirbely and Szent-Györgyi, 1932). A year later, ascorbic acid was characterized and synthesized. Both L-ascorbic acid and dehydroascorbic acid, the partially oxidized form, have vitamin C activity; their structures are shown in Figure 19.1. Major food sources of ascorbic acid in North America are fresh fruits and fruit juices, and some fresh vegetables. Meat, fish, eggs, and dairy products are poor sources of ascorbic acid.

Ascorbic acid acts predominantly as a cosubstrate in oxygen-requiring hydroxylation reactions, notably in the hydroxylation of proline and lysine in procollagen, of dopamine to norepinephrine, and of tryptophan to 5-hydroxytryptophan. As well, it acts as an electron donor in the metabolism of tyrosine, folic acid, histamine, and certain drugs, and has a role in the synthesis of carnitine and steroids, the degradation of cholesterol, and in iron absorption and wound healing (Bates, 1981). More recently, ascorbic acid has also been implicated in the immune response, allergic reactions, and in leukocyte function. The mechanism of ascorbic acid in most of these processes has not been clearly defined (Sauberlich, 1981).

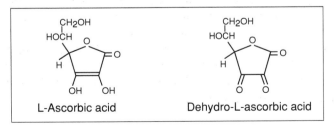

Figure 19.1: Structure of L-ascorbic and dehydroascorbic acid.

413

Clinical manifestations of scurvy, such as weakness, petechial hemorrhages in the skin, ecchymoses, gingival and subperiosteal hemorrhage, and defects in bone development in children, are rare in industrialized countries today (Hodges et al., 1971). Nevertheless, suboptimal vitamin C status has been observed in some elderly subjects living in institutions in the United Kingdom, United States, and Canada, and arises from a low dietary intake of vitamin C (Andrews and Brook, 1966; Taylor, 1966; Burr et al., 1974; Newton et al., 1985). Alcoholic patients (Lemoine et al., 1980) and some Canadian Eskimos (Health and Welfare Canada, 1973) are also vulnerable to vitamin C deficiency. Subclinical vitamin C deficiency frequently occurs secondary to certain disease states such as gastrointestinal disorders, liver disease, cancer, and rheumatoid disease. Rheumatoid patients may utilize ascorbic acid at a faster rate, perhaps as a result of an interaction between aspirin and ascorbic acid (Basu, 1981).

Some cases of rebound scurvy have been reported in persons who abruptly stopped taking large doses of vitamin C (Rhead and Schrauzer, 1971; Siegel et al., 1982). An ascubutic condition has also been reported in some infants of mothers apparently ingesting daily mega-doses of ascorbic acid during pregnancy (Cochrane, 1965). Such occasional observations must be confirmed by well controlled studies before the existence of rebound scurvy can be firmly established (Rivers, 1987).

Therapeutic benefits from the consumption of high doses of ascorbic acid on the common cold (Pauling, 1971) and cancer (Cameron and Pauling, 1976) have been reported but not confirmed by objective, well-controlled studies (Chalmers, 1975; Moertel et al., 1985). Nevertheless such reports have stimulated the increased consumption of large doses of vitamin C, which may in some cases produce adverse effects such as diarrhea, uricosuria, oxaluria, hypoglycemia, allergic skin reactions, and increased absorption of dietary iron (Stein et al., 1976; Sauberlich, 1981). In some instances, kidney stones have been attributed to the increased excretion of oxalic or uric acid (McMichael, 1978). Evidence to date is insufficient, however, to implicate high intakes of ascorbic acid as a risk factor in oxalate stone formation.

As precise information on the metabolic functions of vitamin C is limited, static biochemical tests, such as the measurement of serum and leukocyte ascorbic acid concentrations, are most frequently used to assess vitamin C status. These are discussed below.

19.1 Serum ascorbic acid concentrations

Serum ascorbic acid concentrations are the most frequently used and practical index of vitamin C status in humans. Levels are influenced by any recent intake of the vitamin, especially when intakes are high, making fasting blood samples essential (Omaye et al., 1979).

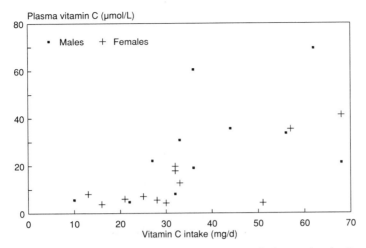

Figure 19.2: The between-subject correlation of plasma vitamin C and vitamin C intake (mg/day) in healthy elderly men and women. From Bates CJ, Rutishauser HE, Block AE, Paul AA. (1977). Long-term vitamin status and dietary intake of healthy elderly subjects. 2. Vitamin C. British Journal of Nutrition 42: 43–56. With permission of Cambridge University Press.

Serum ascorbic acid concentrations increase with dietary intakes until a serum concentration of approximately 1.4 mg/dL (79.5 μmol/L) is reached. This trend was noted by Dodds and MacLeod (1947) in a series of studies conducted from 1942 to 1947 on young women receiving controlled intakes of ascorbic acid. Nevertheless, a wide range of plasma ascorbic acid concentrations at each of the three levels of intake was observed in this study. Such findings emphasize that estimates of ascorbic acid intake, based on plasma ascorbic acid values, cannot be well defined. A similar trend was demonstrated by Bates et al. (1977) in their 18-month study of the vitamin C status of twenty-three relatively healthy U.K. elderly persons living at home (Figure 19.2). Serum concentrations rarely exceed this threshold concentration of 1.4 mg/dL despite very large doses, because the renal clearance of the vitamin rises sharply with daily intakes greater than 100 mg (Friedman et al., 1940). Consequently, serum ascorbic acid levels cannot be used to identify persons regularly consuming excessive amounts of vitamin C. In persons consuming chronically low ascorbic acid intakes, however, serum ascorbic acid concentrations probably reflect body ascorbic acid content and are probably as accurate an index as leukocyte ascorbic acid concentrations (Section 19.2) (Jacob et al., 1987).

Serum ascorbic acid levels are lowered by several non-nutritional factors, some of which do not relate to changes in body stores of ascorbic acid. These factors include acute stress, imposed by cold or elevated temperatures, surgery, and trauma, oral contraceptive agents, chronic inflammatory diseases, acute and chronic infections (e.g. tuberculosis and rheumatic fever), and probably cigarette smoking (Sauberlich et al., 1974). Kallner et al. (1981) showed that heavy smokers required a greater daily intake of ascorbic acid to ensure plasma ascorbic acid levels comparable to those of nonsmokers. Other investigators have found smaller or no effects of heavy smoking on plasma levels of vitamin C (Irwin and Hutchins, 1976). Nevertheless, human studies using isotopically labeled ascorbic acid have demonstrated increased metabolic turnover of ascorbic acid in smokers (70.0 ± 20.2 mg/day versus 35.7 ± 9.3 for nonsmokers), resulting in a 40% greater requirement for vitamin C. Women appear to have higher plasma ascorbic acid levels than men on similar intakes of vitamin C, suggesting physiological differences in the metabolism or retention of vitamin C (Dodds, 1969; Garry et al., 1982; VanderJagt et al., 1987). Such sex differences are not apparent before adolescence. In contrast, women using oral contraceptive agents have lower serum vitamin C levels than nonusers (Rivers, 1975). Reasons for these differences are unclear.

Protracted low intakes of vitamin C (i.e. less than 20 mg/day) cause serum ascorbic acid levels to decrease rapidly to levels of 0.20 mg/dL (11.4 μmol/L) or less (Hodges et al., 1971; Jacob et al., 1987). Clinical signs of scurvy such as follicular hyperkeratosis, swollen or bleeding gums, petechial hemorrhages, and joint pain are usually associated with levels less than 0.20 mg/dL (11.4 μmol/L) (Hodges et al., 1969). The cutoff values for serum ascorbic acid concentrations used to define *marginal* vitamin C status vary. In the United States, serum ascorbic acid values commonly considered as low (i.e. medium risk) range from 0.20 to 0.29 mg/dL (11 to 17 μmol/L) (Table 19.1), whereas in the Nutrition Canada National Survey serum ascorbic acid values of 0.20 to 0.39 mg/dL (11 to 22 μmol/L) were used to indicate moderate risk. Interpretive criteria commonly used for serum ascorbic acid levels in the United States are shown in Table 19.1

19.2   Leukocyte ascorbic acid concentrations

Leukocyte ascorbic acid concentrations are a more reliable index of tissue stores of ascorbic acid than corresponding levels in the serum, erythrocytes, or whole blood (Loh, 1972; Omaye et al., 1979; Turnbull et al., 1981). They are less responsive to short-term fluctuations in recent vitamin C intakes than serum, slowly reflecting changing tissue ascorbic acid concentrations (Jacob et al., 1987). Nevertheless, the preparation and assay of the leukocytes for ascorbic acid is technically difficult and requires relatively large blood samples (2 to 4 mL), making it unsuitable for infants. Furthermore, the contribution of platelets to the leukocyte ascorbic acid content has generally been ignored.

	Serum Ascorbic Acid (mg/dL)	Leukocyte Ascorbic Acid (mg/dL)	Leukocyte Ascorbic Acid (μg per 10^8 cells)
Acceptable (low risk)	> 0.3	> 15 mg	> 20
Low (medium risk)	0.2–0.3	8–15	10–20
Deficient (high risk)	< 0.2	< 8	< 10

Table 19.1: Interpretive criteria for serum and leukocyte ascorbic acid concentrations, modified after Sauberlich et al. (1981) with permission. Conversion factors to SI units: (μmol/L) = $\times$ 56.78; (nmol/10^8 cells) = $\times$ 5.678.

The ratio of platelets:leukocytes, however, can vary widely among individuals (Bates et al., 1977). Vallance (1986) noted that the apparent fall in buffy layer (leukocytes and platelets) vitamin C concentrations after surgical operations was associated with changes in the ratio of leukocytes and platelets in the buffy layer. Hence, platelets should be completely separated from leukocytes prior to leukocyte ascorbic acid assays to enable subclinical vitamin C deficiency states to be identified reliably. At present, the precision and accuracy of leukocyte ascorbic acid measurements is low (Jacob et al., 1987). In patients with scurvy, leukocyte ascorbic acid levels of 7 mg/dL (400 μmol/L) or less occur; normal levels are above 15 mg/dL (850 μmol/L) (Table 19.1). Alternatively, leukocyte ascorbic acid can be expressed in terms of μg per 10^8 cells. Clinical signs of scurvy, such as swollen or bleeding gums, petechial hemorrhages, and joint pain, have been associated with leukocyte concentrations of < 2 μg/10^8 cells (11.4 nmol/10^8 cells).

Erythrocyte ascorbic acid concentrations are not widely used as an index of ascorbic acid status. Levels respond to changes in vitamin C intake over a narrow range, and hence are not as sensitive as plasma ascorbic acid concentrations (Hodges et al., 1971). Moreover, intra- and inter-subject and analytical variance are greater (Jacob et al., 1987).

19.3 Urinary excretion of ascorbic acid and metabolites

Urine is the major excretory route for absorbed ascorbic acid and its metabolites. The main urinary metabolites of ascorbic acid are dehydro-ascorbate, 2,3-diketo-L-gulonate, ascorbate-2-sulfate, and oxalate. Oxalate is the major urinary metabolite when ascorbic acid intakes are less than 100 mg/day (568 μmol/day), but at higher intakes (i.e. > 1 g/day), ascorbic acid is excreted largely in its unmetabolized form (Olson and Hodges, 1987).

Urinary excretion of ascorbic acid reflects recent dietary intake. Levels in the urine decline progressively with increasing depletion of vitamin C until, in persons with scurvy, levels are undetectable. Urinary excretion is not a very sensitive index of ascorbic acid status; differences between persons with adequate or deficient intakes of ascorbic acid are small (Jacob et al., 1987). Specificity is also low. Drugs such as amino-pyrine, aspirin, barbiturates, hydantoins, and paraldehyde increase urinary ascorbic acid excretion (Sauberlich, 1981). An additional disadvantage of this test as an index of vitamin C status in humans is the requirement for twenty-four-hour urine specimens. The latter are impractical in field studies; they can only be collected in clinical or research settings.

The ascorbic acid saturation test is sometimes used as an alternative index of vitamin C status in research studies. In this test, ascorbic acid is administered orally (usually 0.50 to 2.0 g of ascorbic acid per day) in divided doses for four consecutive days, and the amount of the dose excreted in the urine is determined. Recovery of the test dose in the urine should be between 60% and 80% for subjects with normal tissue saturation of ascorbic acid (Lowry et al., 1946).

Excretion of urinary ascorbitol may be a useful index of vitamin C status; the urinary excretion of this metabolite appears to be proportional to body pool size of vitamin C (Klasing and Pilch, 1985). Ascorbitol is also more stable than ascorbic acid. So far, no reference data for comparison of urinary ascorbitol concentrations exists.

19.4   Salivary ascorbic acid concentrations

The use of saliva as a biopsy material for assessing vitamin C status has been investigated because the collection of saliva is noninvasive and simple to perform in population surveys. Results have not been promising. Ascorbic acid concentrations in whole mixed saliva are relatively low, ranging from 0.02 to 0.4 mg/dL (1.1 to 22.7 μmol/L) (Hess and Smith, 1949), and change very little; they are apparently not correlated with vitamin C intake (Jacob et al., 1987).

A lingual vitamin C test has also been used to assess vitamin C status (Cheraskin and Ringsdorf, 1968a,b,c; Loh, 1973). For this test, the time taken to decolorize an aqueous solution of 2,6-dichloroindophenol by the tongue is measured with a stop watch. Theoretically, the higher the vitamin C concentration, the shorter the decoloration time. The method is not a valid index of vitamin C status and has low precision (MacLennan and Hamilton, 1976; Saracci et al., 1976).

19.5   Body pool size

Isotope dilution techniques are the most reliable methods of assessing vitamin C status (Baker et al., 1971; Kallner et al., 1977). They determine body pool size by administering an oral dose of ^{14}C-labeled ascorbic acid, followed by measurement of the specific activity of blood or urine ascorbate within twenty-four to forty-eight hours. ^{14}C-labeled ascorbic acid, however, is a long-lived radioactive isotope, so that use of ^{13}C, a shorter-lived isotope, is recommended. In studies of adult men, total-body pool of vitamin C ranged from < 20 mg to approximately 3000 mg, depending on daily intake of L-ascorbate. At levels below 600 mg (3.4 mmol) of vitamin C, psychological abnormalities have been observed (Kinsman and Hood, 1971), whereas below 300 to 400 mg (1.7 to 2.3 mmol), signs of scurvy have been noted (Hodges et al., 1971). In young healthy male adults, the pool size is approximately 1500 mg (i.e. 20 mg/kg body weight) (Baker et al., 1971). No comparable data exist for women or the elderly.

19.6 Capillary fragility

Capillary fragility has been used as a functional test of vitamin C deficiency. For the test, pressure is applied to the veins of the upper arm, and the venous pressure at which petechial hemorrhages appear is measured with a blood pressure cuff (Hess, 1913; Göthlin, 1933). This test produces inconsistent results in individuals with vitamin C deficiency, and is not specific to vitamin C deficiency states. Other diseases increase capillary fragility (Vilter, 1967), and consequently alternative functional tests of ascorbic acid status need to be developed.

19.7 Analysis of ascorbic acid in biological tissues and fluids

Several methods are available for measuring vitamin C in the reduced form or as total ascorbic acid (Sabry and Dodds, 1958; Pelletier, 1985). For all methods, metaphosphoric acid or trichloroacetic acid is used to precipitate the protein in the samples and to stabilize the ascorbic acid.

The 2,6-dichloroindophenol method

This method measures only the reduced form, L-ascorbic acid, which reduces the blue dye 2,6-dichloroindophenol at a specific pH (3.0 to 4.5), causing a lowering of the absorption at 520 nm (Omaye et al., 1979). The color of the dye fades so that the measurements with the spectrophotometer must be timed exactly. The method is easy to perform, rapid, and can be adapted for small samples, but is not suitable for urine samples as it cannot measure their dehydroascorbic acid content.

The α, α'-dipyridyl method

In this method, the reduction of ferric iron to ferrous iron by ascorbic acid is followed by the determination of the ferrous iron as the red-orange α, α'-dipyridyl complex. The method is specific and sensitive and can be used for finger prick blood samples. The effect of interfering substances can be inhibited by the addition of orthophosphoric acid (Omaye et al., 1979).

The 2,4-dinitrophenylhydrazine method

Dehydroascorbic acid and total ascorbic acid can be measured separately by this method, so that the reduced ascorbic acid (L-ascorbic acid) can be determined by difference. The ascorbic acid is oxidized by copper to form dehydroascorbic and diketogluconic acids, which, when dissolved in sulphuric acid and treated with 2,4-dinitrophenylhydrazine, form hydrazone. Hydrazone forms an orange-red product that absorbs at 520 nm (Roe and Kuether, 1943). The method can be adapted for small samples, but is more time consuming than the 2,6-dichloroindophenol method. Ascorbate sulfate in the samples interferes with 2,4-dinitrophenylhydrazine if the reaction is carried out at temperatures above 37°C.

Fluorometric methods

Ascorbic acid is oxidized to dehydroascorbic acid in the presence of iodine, and the excess iodine destroyed by sodium thiosulfate. A fluorescent quinoxaline is then formed from the dehydroascorbic acid by condensation with *o*-phenylenediamine. The method is specific, rapid, and straightforward, although some investigators suggest that the sensitivity is lower than for some other methods (Omaye et al., 1979).

High-performance liquid chromatography

High-performance liquid chromatography may prove to be a sensitive, specific, and nondestructive alternative for measuring all forms of vitamin C in the future. It was used by Omaye et al. (1986) for ascorbic acid analysis of isolated leukocytes, after deproteinization with 6% metaphosphoric acid, and by VanderJagt et al. (1987) for plasma ascorbic acid analysis. For plasma ascorbic acid concentrations below 1.3 mg/dL (74 µmol/L), the HPLC method apparently gives lower values compared to an automated dichloroindophenol method, with an average difference of 0.07 mg/dL (4 µmol/L) (VanderJagt et al., 1986).

19.8   Summary

Ascorbic acid is involved in a variety of biological processes, although in many cases, its precise mechanism is still unclear. Clinical deficiency of vitamin C produces scurvy, a rare disease in industrialized countries today. Nevertheless, marginal vitamin C deficiency has been described in selected vulnerable groups. Excess intakes of vitamin C may produce adverse effects including kidney stones. Static biochemical indices such as serum and leukocyte ascorbic acid concentrations are most frequently used to assess vitamin C status. The former reflect recent dietary intake rather than tissue stores, except when individuals are consuming chronically low ascorbic acid intakes. Therefore, fasting blood samples are preferred for serum ascorbic acid assays. Serum ascorbic acid levels increase linearly with dietary intake but only up to about 1.4 mg/dL (79.5 µmol/L), making them unsuitable for detecting excessive intakes of vitamin C. Several non-nutritional factors affect serum ascorbic acid concentrations and hence reduce their specificity and sensitivity. Cutoff points for serum ascorbic acid concentrations indicative of moderate risk of vitamin C deficiency are disputed and values from 0.20 to 0.39 mg/dL (11 to 22 µmol/L) have been used. Leukocyte ascorbic acid concentrations (expressed as mg/dL or µg per 10^8 cells) are a more reliable index of tissue ascorbic acid stores; they are less responsive to short-term fluctuations in vitamin C intakes than serum but their assay is difficult and requires a relatively large blood sample.

Urinary excretion of ascorbic acid is also influenced by recent dietary intake. Moreover, sensitivity and specificity of this index are low and twenty-four-hour urine samples are required. In research studies, the ascorbic acid saturation test is sometimes used. Excretion of urinary ascorbitol appears promising as an index which reflects the body pool size of vitamin C, although interpretive standards are not yet available. The most reliable method of assessing body pool size of ascorbic acid involves isotope dilution techniques. Capillary fragility is the only functional physiological test for assessing vitamin C status, but is rarely used because of its low specificity. Methods for assaying ascorbic acid measure either the reduced form using the 2,6-dichloroindophenol and α, α'-dipyridyl method, or total ascorbic acid. The latter is measured by the 2,4-dinitrophenylhydrazine method or the fluorometric method. In the future, HPLC may be used because it is sensitive, specific, and capable of measuring all forms of vitamin C.

References

Andrews J, Brook M. (1966). Leucocyte-vitamin-C content and clinical signs in the elderly. Lancet 1: 1350–1351.

Baker EM, Hodges RE, Hood J, Sauberlich HE, March SC, Canham JE. (1971). Metabolism of ^{14}C- and ^{3}H-labeled L-ascorbic acid in human scurvy. American Journal of Clinical Nutrition 24: 444–454.

Basu TK. (1981). The influence of drugs with particular reference to aspirin on the bioavailability of vitamin C. In: Counsell JN, Hornig DH (eds). Vitamin C (Ascorbic Acid). Applied Science Publishers, London, pp. 273–281.

Bates CJ. (1981). The function of vitamin C in man. In: Counsell JN, Hornig DH (eds). Vitamin C (Ascorbic Acid). Applied Science Publishers, London, pp. 1–22.

Bates CJ, Rutishauser HE, Block AE, Paul AA. (1977). Long-term vitamin status and dietary intake of healthy elderly subjects. 2. Vitamin C. British Journal of Nutrition 42: 43–56.

Burr ML, Elwood PC, Hole DJ, Hughes RE, Hurley RJ. (1974). Plasma and leukocyte ascorbic acid levels in the elderly. American Journal of Clinical Nutrition 27: 144–151.

Cameron E, Pauling L. (1976). Supplemental ascorbate in the supportive treatment of cancer: Prolongation of survival times in terminal human cancer. Proceedings of the National Academy of Sciences USA 73: 3685–3689.

Chalmers TC. (1975). Effects of ascorbic acid on the common cold. An evaluation of the evidence. American Journal of Medicine 58: 532–536.

Cheraskin E, Ringsdorf WM Jr. (1968a). A lingual vitamin C test. I. Reproducibility. Internationale Zeitschrift für Vitaminforschung 38: 114–117.

Cheraskin E, Ringsdorf WM Jr. (1968b). A lingual vitamin C test. II. Daily constancy. Internationale Zeitschrift für Vitaminforschung 38: 118–119.

Cheraskin E, Ringsdorf WM Jr. (1968c). A lingual vitamin C test. III. Relation to plasma ascorbic acid levels. Internationale Zeitschrift für Vitaminforschung 38: 120–122.

Cochrane WA. (1965). Overnutrition in prenatal and neonatal life: a problem? Canadian Medical Association Journal 93: 893–899.

Dodds ML. (1969). Sex as a factor in blood levels of ascorbic acid. Journal of the American Dietetic Association 54: 32–33.

Dodds ML, MacLeod FL. (1947). Blood plasma ascorbic acid levels on controlled intakes of ascorbic acid. Science 106: 67.

Friedman GJ, Sherry S, Ralli EP. (1940). Mechanism of excretion of vitamin C by the human kidney at low and normal plasma levels of ascorbic acid. Journal of Clinical Investigation 19: 685–689.

Garry PJ, Goodwin JS, Hunt WC, Gilbert BA. (1982). Nutritional status in a healthy elderly population: vitamin C. American Journal of Clinical Nutrition 36: 332–339.

Göthlin GF. (1933). Outline of a method for the determination of the strength of the skin capillaries and the indirect estimation of the individual vitamin C standard. Journal of Laboratory and Clinical Medicine. 18: 484–490.

Health and Welfare Canada. (1973). Nutrition Canada National Survey. Health and Welfare, Ottawa.

Hess AF. (1913). Involvement of the blood and blood vessels in infantile scurvy. Proceedings of the Society for Experimental Biology and Medicine 11: 130–132.

Hess WC, Smith BT. (1949). Ascorbic acid content of saliva of carious and noncarious individuals. Journal of Dental Research 28: 507–511.

Hodges RE, Baker EM, Hood J, Sauberlich HE, March SC. (1969). Experimental scurvy in man. American Journal of Clinical Nutrition 22: 535–548.

Hodges RE, Hood J, Canham JE, Sauberlich HE, Baker EM. (1971). Clinical manifestations of ascorbic acid deficiency in man. American Journal of Clinical Nutrition 24: 432–443.

Irwin MI, Hutchins BK. (1976). A conspectus of research on vitamin C requirements of man. Journal of Nutrition 106: 823–879.

Jacob RA, Skala JH, Omaye ST. (1987). Biochemical indices of human vitamin C status. American Journal of Clinical Nutrition 46: 818–826.

Kallner AB, Harman D, Hornig DH. (1981). On the requirements of ascorbic acid in man. Steady-state turnover and body pool in smokers. American Journal of Clinical Nutrition 34: 1347–1355.

Kallner A, Hartmann D, Hornig DH. (1977). Determination of body pool size and turnover rate of ascorbic acid in man. Nutrition and Metabolism 21 (Supplement 1): 31–35.

King CG, Waugh WA. (1932). Chemical nature of vitamin C. Science 75: 357–358.

Kinsman RA, Hood J. (1971). Some behavioral effects of ascorbic acid deficiency. American Journal of Clinical Nutrition 24: 455–464.

Klasing SA, Pilch SM (eds). (1985). Suggested Measures of Nutritional Status and Health Conditions for the Third National Health and Nutrition Examination Survey. Life Sciences Research Office, Federation of American Societies for Experimental Biology, Bethesda, Maryland, pp. 35–45.

Lemoine A, Le Devehat C, Codaccioni JL, Monges A, Bermond P, Salkeld RM. (1980). Vitamin B_1, B_2, B_6, and C status in hospital inpatients. American Journal of Clinical Nutrition 33: 2595–2600.

Loh HS. (1972). The relationship between dietary ascorbic acid intake and buffy coat and plasma ascorbic acid concentrations at different ages. International Journal for Vitamin and Nutrition Research 42: 80–85.

Loh HS. (1973). Screening for vitamin-C status (letter). Lancet 1: 944–945.

Lowry OH, Bessey OA, Brock MJ, Lopez JA. (1946). The interrelationship of dietary, serum, white blood cell and total ascorbic acid. Journal of Biological Chemistry 166: 111–119.

MacLennan WJ, Hamilton J. (1976). Quick assessment of vitamin C status. Lancet 1: 585.

McMichael AJ. (1978). Kidney stone hospitalization in relation to change in vitamin C consumption in Australia 1966–1976. Community Health Studies 2: 9–13.

Moertel CG, Fleming TR, Creagan ET, Rubin J, O'Connell MJ, Ames MM. (1985). High-dose vitamin C versus placebo in the treatment of patients with advanced cancer who have had no prior chemotherapy. A randomized double-blind comparison. New England Journal of Medicine 312: 137–141.

Newton HMV, Schorah CJ, Habibzadeh N, Morgan DB, Hullin RP. (1985). The cause and correction of low blood vitamin C concentrations in the elderly. American Journal of Clinical Nutrition 42: 656–659.

Olson JA, Hodges RE. (1987). Recommended dietary intakes (RDI) of vitamin C in humans. American Journal of Clinical Nutrition 45: 693–703.

Omaye ST, Turnbull JD, Sauberlich HE. (1979). Selected methods for the determination of ascorbic acid in animal cells, tissues, and fluids. Methods in Enzymology 62: 3–11.

Omaye ST, Skala JH, Jacob RA. (1986). Plasma ascorbic acid in adult males: effects of depletion and supplementation. American Journal of Clinical Nutrition 44: 257–264.

Pauling L. (1971). The significance of the evidence about ascorbic acid and the common cold. Proceedings of the National Academy of Sciences USA 68: 2678–2681.

Pelletier O. (1985). Vitamin C (L-ascorbic acid and dehydro-L-ascorbic acids). In: Augustin J, Klein BP, Becker D, Venugopal PB (eds). Methods of Vitamin Assay. Fourth edition. John Wiley and Sons Inc., New York, pp. 303–347.

Roe JH, Kuether CA. (1943). Determination of ascorbic acid in whole blood and urine through the 2,4-dinitrophenylhydrazine derivative of dehydroascorbic acid. Journal of Biological Chemistry 147: 399–407.

Rhead WJ, Schrauzer GN. (1971). Risk of long-term ascorbic acid overdosage. Nutrition Reviews 29: 262–263.

Rivers JM. (1975). Oral contraceptives and ascorbic acid. American Journal of Clinical Nutrition 28: 550–554.

Rivers JM. (1987). Safety of high-level vitamin C ingestion. In: Burns JL, Rivers JM, Machlin LJ (eds). Third Conference on Vitamin C. The New York Academy of Sciences, New York. pp. 445–454.

Roderuck C, Burrill L, Campbell LJ Brakke BE, Childs MT, Leverton R, Chaloupa M, Jebe EH, Swanson PP. (1958). Estimated dietary intake, urinary excretion and blood vitamin C in women of different ages. Journal of Nutrition 66: 15–27.

Sabry JH, Dodds ML. (1958). Comparative measurements of ascorbic acid and total ascorbic acid of blood plasma. Journal of Nutrition 64: 467–473.

Saracci R, Bardelli D, Mariani F. (1976). Quick assessment of vitamin C status. Lancet 1: 490-491.

Sauberlich HE. (1981). Ascorbic acid (vitamin C). In: Labbé RF (ed). Symposium on Laboratory Assessment of Nutritional Status. Clinics in Laboratory Medicine 1: 673–684.

Sauberlich HE, Dowdy RP, Skala JH. (1974). Laboratory Tests for the Assessment of Nutritional Status. CRC Press Inc., Cleveland, Ohio, pp. 13–22.

Siegel C, Baker B, Kunstadter M. (1982). Conditional oral scurvy due to megavitamin C withdrawal. Journal of Peridontology 53: 453–455.

Stein HB, Hasan A, Fox IH. (1976). Ascorbic acid-induced uricosuria. A consequence of megavitamin therapy. Annals of Internal Medicine 84: 385–388.

Svirbely JL, Szent–Györgyi A. (1932). Chemical nature of vitamin C. Biochemistry Journal 26: 865–870.

Taylor G. (1966). Diet of elderly women. Lancet 1: 926.

Turnbull JD, Sudduth JH, Sauberlich HE, Omaye ST. (1981). Depletion and repletion of ascorbic acid in the Rhesus monkey: relationship between ascorbic acid concentration in blood components with total body pool and liver concentration of ascorbic acid. International Journal for Vitamin and Nutrition Research 51: 47–53.

Vallance S. (1986). Platelets, leucocytes and buffy layer vitamin C after surgery. Human Nutrition: Clinical Nutrition 40C: 35–41.

VanderJagt DJ, Garry PJ, Bhagavan HN. (1987). Ascorbic acid intake and plasma levels in healthy elderly people. American Journal of Clinical Nutrition 46: 290–294.

VanderJagt DJ, Garry PJ, Hunt WC. (1986). Ascorbate in plasma measured by liquid chromatography and by dichloroindophenol colorimetry. Clinical Chemistry 32: 1004–1006.

Vilter RW. (1967). Effects of ascorbic acid deficiency in man. In: Sebrell WH Jr, Harris RS (eds). The Vitamins: Chemistry, Physiology, Pathology, Methods. Volume I. Academic Press, New York, pp. 457–485.

Chapter 20

Assessment of the status of thiamin, riboflavin, and niacin

The water-soluble B vitamins, thiamin, riboflavin, and niacin, participate as coenzymes or prosthetic groups in a variety of reactions involved in the catabolism of carbohydrates, fats, and proteins. All three vitamins are stored for a relatively short time, are rapidly excreted in the urine, and have a fast rate of catabolism. Consequently, deficiencies develop within a shorter period than that for the fat-soluble vitamins or vitamin B-12.

Clinical deficiency signs for these B vitamins are not very specific, and hence static and functional biochemical tests are frequently used to confirm the clinical diagnosis, and to detect subclinical deficiency states. In the latter, nonspecific, subjective effects such as insomnia, irritability, loss of appetite, and weight loss may occur (Brin, 1980), and the metabolism of certain drugs may be altered. Static biochemical tests for thiamin, riboflavin, and niacin measure the vitamin or its metabolites in blood and/or urine. Functional biochemical tests exist for thiamin and riboflavin, but not for niacin; they measure the activity of an enzyme that requires the vitamin as a coenzyme, with and without the addition of saturating amounts of the coenzyme *in vitro* (Bamji, 1981). The choice of the biochemical test depends on the objectives of the study; generally, more than one is used.

20.1 Assessment of thiamin status

The isolation and synthesis of thiamin was carried out in 1932 by Williams and Cline (1936). The structure of thiamin is shown in Figure 20.1; it consists of a pyrimidine and a thiazole moiety. Whole grain cereals, pork, and legumes are the richest food sources of thiamin, followed by other meats, fish, green vegetables, fruits, and milk. Polished rice, sugar, alcohol, fat, and other refined foods are poor sources of thiamin. Thiamin is destroyed at elevated temperatures unless the pH is below 5. In alkaline solution, thiamin may be oxidized to the fluorescent

425

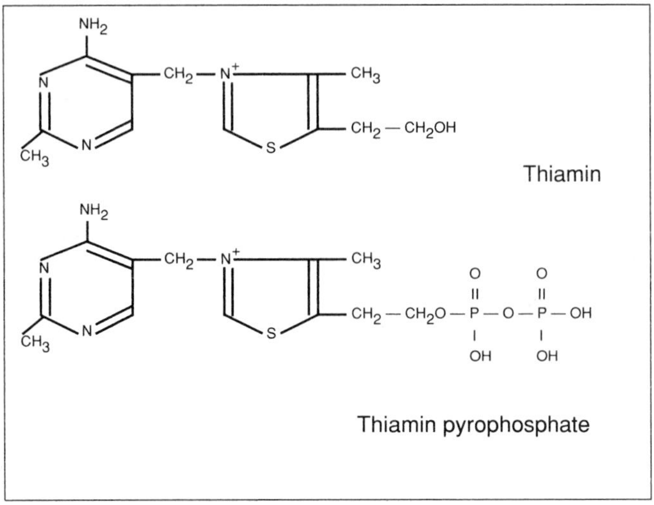

Figure 20.1: Structure of thiamin and the coenzyme thiamin pyrophosphate.

compound thiochrome. This reaction is widely used for measuring thiamin in biological tissues and fluids.

The classical syndrome of thiamin deficiency is beriberi, which occurs in countries where polished rice is the staple food. The deficiency affects the cardiovascular, muscular, nervous, and gastrointestinal systems and is characterized by polyneuritis, bradycardia, peripheral edema, muscle tenderness, and neurological signs. In areas where fermented raw fish is consumed (e.g. parts of Thailand and Southeast Asia), thiamin deficiency may occur because thiaminases, present in certain fish and shellfish, catalyze the cleavage of thiamin (Sauberlich, 1985). Thiamin deficiency has almost completely disappeared in Western countries, except in selected population groups such as chronic alcoholics, some elderly persons, and individuals with disease states involving chronic emesis, diarrhea, and marked anorexia. Subclinical and clinical thiamin deficiency has also been described in Japan among university students (Kawai et al., 1980; Hatanaka and Ueda, 1981). Severe deficiency among alcoholics is often associated with Wernicke's encephalopathy, a neurological disorder arising from prolonged thiamin deficiency. No adverse effects of excessive intakes of thiamin have been described other than occasional anaphylactoid responses (Viteri, 1983).

Thiamin, as a component of the coenzyme thiamin pyrophosphate (TPP), has an important role in carbohydrate metabolism. Thiamin pyrophosphate (Figure 20.1) is required for the oxidative decarboxylation of α-keto acids and for the action of transketolase in the pentose phosphate pathway. Thiamin pyrophosphate also functions as a cofactor in the condensation of glyoxylate and α-ketoglutarate to form 2-hydroxy-3-ketoadipate. The activity of the transketolase enzyme in erythrocytes is currently the most reliable index of thiamin nutritional status; it reflects the adequacy of body stores. Measurements of thiamin in urine, whole blood, serum, and erythrocytes, described below, are also used, but do not adequately assess the status of body stores.

20.1.1 Erythrocyte transketolase activity

Transketolase is a thiamin pyrophosphate-dependent enzyme. Measurement of the activity of this enzyme in the erythrocytes is most frequently used as an index of thiamin nutritional status as the erythrocytes are among the first tissues to be affected by thiamin depletion (Brin, 1967). The principle of this test and that of similar procedures used for riboflavin and pyridoxine is outlined below:

1. The basal activity of enzyme in erythrocytes is measured. This represents the endogenous enzyme activity and is dependent on the amount of the coenzyme in the erythrocytes;

2. The enzyme activity with excess coenzyme added *in vitro* is determined. This represents the maximum potential enzyme activity and is referred to as total or 'stimulated' activity;

3. (1) and (2) are compared to indicate the degree of unsaturation of the enzyme with the coenzyme;

4. The data are expressed in terms of an activity coefficient (AC) or 'percentage stimulation'. The relationship between the two is as follows:

$$AC = \frac{\text{Enzyme activity (with added coenzyme)}}{\text{Basal enzyme activity (without added coenzyme)}}$$

Percentage stimulation = (Activity coefficient × 100) − 100

The basal and stimulated enzyme activities can be expressed per gram of hemoglobin, per number of erythrocytes, or in terms of the volume of erythrocytes (in mL). In general, the higher the value of the AC or 'percentage stimulation', the greater the degree of vitamin deficiency. The ratio of stimulated to basal enzyme activity is used because: (a) the inter-subject variation in basal erythrocyte enzyme activity measurements is large, and (b) it is assumed that apoenzyme levels are not affected by vitamin deficiencies. This latter assumption, however, may be incorrect. Vitamin deficiency or excess, and other factors such as the presence of certain diseases, and the administration of hormones and drugs, may affect apoenzyme levels and confound the interpretation. Hence, it is advisable to take into account the basal enzyme activity as well as its activation with coenzyme when interpreting the results (Bamji, 1981).

Transketolase, a TPP-requiring enzyme, catalyzes the following two reactions in the pentose phosphate pathway:

(1)   Xylulose-5-phosphate + ribose-5-phosphate ⇌

Sedoheptulose-7-phosphate + glyceraldehyde-3-phosphate

(2)   Xylulose-5-phosphate + erythrose-4-phosphate ⇌

Fructose-6-phosphate + glyceraldehyde-3-phosphate

In thiamin deficiency, the basal level of erythrocyte transketolase activity is low, and an enhancement in enzyme activity after the addition of TPP is generally observed. This is known as the 'TPP effect'. Prolonged experimentally induced thiamin deficiency, however, induces a reduction in the apoenzyme level. Consequently, both basal and stimulated erythrocyte transketolase activities tend to fall, with no change in TPP effect. In such cases, therefore, the basal enzyme activity should also be considered.

Several factors, independent of thiamin nutriture, affect erythrocyte transketolase activity. For example, the erythrocyte enzyme activity declines as the cells age, so that the basal enzyme activity depends on the mean age of the erythrocytes (Powers and Thurnham, 1981). Hence, in patients undergoing treatment for iron deficiency, the basal level of erythrocyte transketolase activity will be increased as a result of the reticulocytosis. A similar effect is observed in patients responding positively to treatment for pernicious anemia (Kjøsen and Sein, 1977). Conversely, patients with polyneuritis, uremic neuropathy, cancer, disorders of the gastrointestinal tract, and early-onset diabetes have low erythrocyte transketolase activity values (Kjøsen and Sein, 1977), in some cases as a result of a reduced apoenzyme level associated with the disease. In cancer patients, the TPP effect is enhanced despite adequate intakes of thiamin because the conversion of thiamin to thiamin pyrophosphate is apparently impaired (Basu and Dickerson, 1976). Certain drugs, such as 5-fluorouracil and acytotoxin, used in the treatment of cancer, and furosemide, a diuretic used in the treatment of congestive heart failure, may also influence the activity of erythrocyte transketolase (Thurnham, 1981). Their precise mechanism is unclear.

The criteria usually used for interpreting transketolase activity, which are based on percentage stimulation and activity coefficients, are shown in Table 20.1. Measurement of erythrocyte transketolase activity is difficult. Numerous methods have been developed (Basu et al., 1974; Bayoumi and Rosalki, 1976), some including features to increase sensitivity, precision, and quality control (Buttery et al., 1982). Spectrophotometric procedures measure either the products formed (i.e. synthesis of sedoheptulose-7-phosphate per unit time) or the amount of substrate used in the reaction

Reference	Classification	TPP Percentage Stimulation	Activity Coefficient
ICNND (1963)	Acceptable (low risk) Low (medium risk) Deficient (high risk)	0–15% 16–20% > 20%	1.0–1.15 1.16–1.20 > 1.20
Brin (1967)	Normal (adequate) Marginally deficient (marginal) Severely deficient (deficient)	0–14% 14–24% ≥ 25%	1.0–1.14 1.14–1.24 ≥ 1.25

Table 20.1: The criteria commonly used for interpreting transketolase activity. The guidelines may require adjustment depending on the specific method used to measure transketolase activity. From Sauberlich HE, Dowdy RP, Skala JH. (1974). Laboratory Tests for the Assessment of Nutritional Status. © CRC Press, Inc., Boca Raton, FL.

(i.e. ribose-5-phosphate), before and after the addition of TPP. Preferred methods are semi-automated, eliminate hemoglobin interference by incorporating dialyzers in the system, and use glyceraldehyde-3-phosphate as an internal standard (Waring et al., 1982). Erythrocyte hemolysates are used for the assay rather than intact erythrocytes because they can be stored in the frozen state for up to two months without loss of transketolase activity (Pearson, 1962).

The activity of transketolase in leukocytes appears to be a sensitive and specific index of thiamin status in the rat, responding to dietary intakes of thiamin (Cheng et al., 1976). The use of this index in humans has not been extensively investigated.

20.1.2 Urinary thiamin excretion

Earlier population studies (e.g. Nutrition Canada, NHANES I) measured urinary excretion of thiamin per gram of creatinine as an index of thiamin status. Thiamin levels in the urine do not adequately reflect body stores but instead provide an index of the dietary intake, levels responding particularly to excessive intakes of thiamin. For example, positive correlations have been observed between thiamin intakes and excretion in twenty-four-hour urine specimens in young adults receiving controlled diets ranging from 0.6 to 2.0 mg thiamin per day (Oldham et al., 1946; Plough and Bridgeforth 1960; Oldham, 1962). A relationship between dietary intakes and urinary excretion of thiamin has also been reported in population studies in which casual urine samples have been collected and thiamin excretion expressed in terms of thiamin per gram of creatinine. Figure 20.2 shows the relationship between mean thiamin intake (mg/1000 kcal per day) and mean urinary thiamin excretion (per gram of creatinine) in casual urine samples in adults. At lower intakes, only small changes in urinary thiamin excretion occur, and most of the excretion is in the form of metabolites.

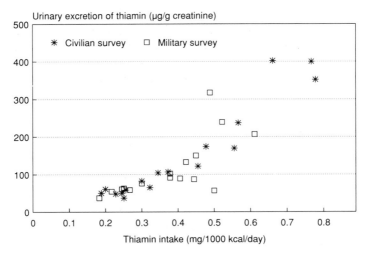

Figure 20.2: Relationship between thiamin intake and thiamin urinary excretion in adults as observed in nutrition surveys conducted in eighteen countries by ICNND. From a Report of a Joint Food and Agriculture Organization/World Health Organization Expert Group (1967). Figure 6, page 33 with permission.

In general, the interpretation of urinary thiamin excretion in individual casual urine samples is difficult, particularly in children. The latter have higher levels of thiamin excretion than adults when expressed on a creatinine basis, so age-specific interpretive criteria are necessary (Sauberlich et al., 1974). Consequently, thiamin concentrations measured in twenty-four-hour urine samples are preferred, and have been used to confirm suspected clinical deficiency states (Viteri, 1983). Table 20.2 presents age-specific guidelines for the interpretation of urinary excretion of thiamin expressed per gram of creatinine and over a twenty-four-hour period (Sauberlich et al., 1974).

A thiamin load test has also been used as an index of thiamin status. Excretion of thiamin in a four-hour period after the parenteral administration of 5 mg of thiamin is measured. If subjects are deficient in thiamin, usually less than 20 μg of the 5 mg thiamin load during the four-hour period is excreted (Table 20.2).

The classical method for measuring thiamin in urine is the fluorometric thiochrome procedure. In the direct method, thiamin is measured before and after destruction of the thiochrome fluorescence by the addition of benzylsulfonyl chloride (Leveille, 1972). Alternatively, the interfering compounds in the urine can be removed using a cation-exchange resin, before the conversion of the eluted thiamin to the fluorescent thiochrome derivative, which is measured with a spectrofluorometer (ICNND, 1963). Other methods utilize HPLC techniques (Roser et al., 1978).

Subjects	Less than Acceptable (at Risk)		Acceptable (low risk)
	Deficient (high risk)	Low (medium risk)	
	(μg/g creatinine)		
1–3 years	< 120	120–175	≥ 176
4–6 years	< 85	85–120	≥ 121
7–9 years	< 70	70–180	≥ 181
10–12 years	< 60	60–180	≥ 181
13–15 years	< 50	50–150	≥ 151
Adults	< 27	27–65	≥ 66
Pregnant, 2nd trimester	< 23	23–54	≥ 55
Pregnant, 3rd trimester	< 21	21–49	≥ 50
	Other interpretive guidelines		
Adults μg/24 hr	< 40	40–99	≥ 100
Adults μg/6 hr	< 10	10–24	≥ 25
Adults μg in 4 hr following 5 mg thiamin load	< 20	20–79	≥ 80

Table 20.2: Interpretive guidelines for the urinary excretion of thiamin. From Sauberlich HE, Dowdy RP, Skala JH. (1974). Laboratory Tests for the Assessment of Nutritional Status. © CRC Press, Inc., Boca Raton, FL.

20.1.3 Thiamin in serum, erythrocytes, and whole blood

Concentrations of thiamin in serum, erythrocytes, and whole blood have been investigated as potential indices of thiamin status. In general, these are insensitive indices of thiamin status, as relatively modest declines are observed even in cases of frank beriberi (Kawai et al., 1980). Thiamin in whole blood or its components can be separated using HPLC procedures, and then analyzed as thiochrome (Sauberlich, 1984).

Future methods of assessing thiamin nutriture may include measurement of erythrocyte thiamin pyrophosphate levels. Studies with thiamin-deficient rats showed that erythrocyte thiamin pyrophosphate levels fell before any changes in erythrocyte transketolase activity were apparent (Warnock et al., 1979).

20.2 Assessment of riboflavin status

Riboflavin was first synthesized in 1935. Its structure consists of an isalloxine ring attached to a ribityl side chain (Figure 20.3). Riboflavin is a component of two coenzymes, flavin mononucleotide (FMN) and flavin adenine dinucleotide (FAD), both of which are essential for a number of oxidative enzyme systems involved in electron transport. These coenzymes occur naturally in food. Small amounts of flavin bound covalently to protein are also found in foods, but are largely unavailable as nutritional sources of riboflavin; only limited amounts apparently undergo

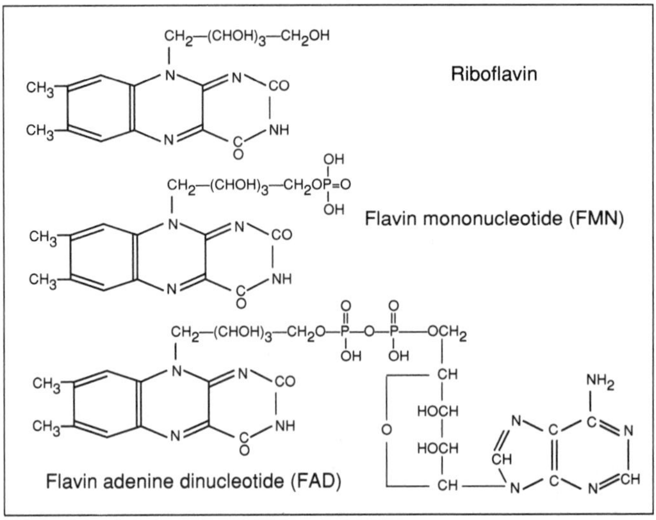

Figure 20.3: Structure of riboflavin and the two coenzymes derived from flavin, FMN and FAD.

digestion and absorption (Chia et al., 1978). The physiological roles of these covalently bound flavins are unclear.

Classical signs of riboflavin deficiency, termed ariboflavinosis, are angular stomatitis, cheilosis, and glossitis. Certain ocular symptoms, dermatological changes, neurological alterations, and hematological defects may also occur, but are not specific for ariboflavinosis (Thurnham, 1981). Ariboflavinosis usually occurs in association with other vitamin deficiency states, and has been most frequently documented during pregnancy in undernourished populations (Bates et al., 1981). In industrialized countries such as North America and the United Kingdom, suboptimal riboflavin status has been reported in vulnerable population groups such as the elderly (Rutishauser et al., 1979) and pregnant and nonpregnant adolescents of low socio-economic status (Lopez et al., 1980; Nicholalds, 1981). Several conditions, including alcoholism, diabetes mellitus, liver disease, and gastrointestinal and biliary obstruction, may also precipitate and/or exacerbate riboflavin deficiency (Nicholalds, 1981). Drugs, such as tetracycline, theophylline, and caffeine, and metals, such as zinc, copper, and iron, may chelate or form complexes with riboflavin and hence affect its bioavailability (Sauberlich, 1985).

Major dietary sources of riboflavin are meat, milk, and dairy products. In humans, there is no evidence for riboflavin toxicity produced by excessive intakes. Absorption of orally administered riboflavin in both vitamin supplements and natural foodstuffs is poor, and high intakes are rapidly excreted in the urine.

As the signs and symptoms of riboflavin deficiency are not very specific, diagnosis of a deficiency state is difficult when based exclusively on clinical assessment. Consequently, biochemical methods are essential for confirming clinical cases of riboflavin deficiency, and for establishing subclinical deficiencies. Several methods are available and these are discussed in the following sections.

20.2.1   Erythrocyte glutathione reductase activity

Measurement of the activity coefficient (AC) of erythrocyte glutathione reductase (EGR) has been increasingly used in recent years as an index of subclinical riboflavin deficiency. Glutathione reductase is a nicotinamide adenine dinucleotide phosphate (NADPH) and FAD-dependent enzyme, and is the major flavoprotein in erythrocytes. It catalyzes the oxidative cleavage of the disulfide bond of oxidized glutathione (GSSG) to form reduced glutathione (GSH) as shown below:

$$GSSG + NADPH + H^+ \rightarrow 2\ GSH + NADP^+$$

The activity of erythrocyte glutathione reductase is measured spectrophotometrically by monitoring the oxidation of NADPH to NADP$^+$ at 340 nm, with and without the presence of added FAD coenzyme. Alternatively, the production of reduced glutathione (GSH) can be determined colorimetrically. The activity coefficient, or percentage stimulation, is then derived following the principle described for erythrocyte transketolase activity (Section 20.1.1):

$$EGR\ AC = \frac{\text{Enzyme activity (with added FAD)}}{\text{Basal enzyme activity (without added FAD)}}$$

The degree of *in vitro* stimulation of EGR activity depends on the FAD saturation of the apoenzyme, which in turn depends on the availability of riboflavin. In persons with riboflavin deficiency, erythrocyte glutathione reductase activity falls and the *in vitro* stimulation by FAD rises.

Both animal and human depletion/repletion studies have confirmed that the EGR AC is a useful and sensitive measure of impaired riboflavin status. For instance, significant correlations between the EGR AC and overall riboflavin status were reported in a number of tissues taken from both acutely and chronically riboflavin-deficient rats (Tillotson and Sauberlich, 1971). In experimentally controlled human studies, concomitant increases in EGR AC in response to graded decreases in intakes of riboflavin have also been reported (Tillotson and Baker, 1972). Nevertheless, the increase does not continue indefinitely; riboflavin intakes below 0.5 mg/1000 kilocalories do not produce any further increases in EGR AC (Sterner and Price, 1973). Consequently, the extent to which the EGR AC is elevated does not necessarily indicate the degree of riboflavin deficiency. Hence, it is not surprising that consistent correlations

Subject #	July–Aug. 1975	Sept.–Nov. 1975	Dec.–Feb. 1975/6	Mar.–May 1976	June–July 1976	Aug.–Oct. 1976	Mean for All Six Clinics
1 (M)	1.27	1.17	1.24	1.23	1.19	1.11	1.20
2 (M)	1.36	1.35	1.31	1.37	1.30	1.23	1.33
3 (M)	1.28	1.26	1.30	1.07	1.21	1.19	1.22
13 (F)	1.20	1.21	1.22	1.25	1.19	1.15	1.20
14 (F)	1.25	1.21	1.22	1.11	1.07	1.17	1.17
15 (F)	1.17	1.32	1.29	1.36	1.16	1.30	1.27
Mean (n = 23)		1.21	1.20	1.18	1.14	1.17	1.19

Table 20.3: Individual and mean values for the activity coefficient (AC) of erythrocyte glutathione reductase (EGR). Abstracted from data from an eighteen-month longitudinal study of healthy U.K. elderly men (n = 12) and women (n = 11). From Rutishauser IH, Bates CJ, Paul AA, Black AE, Mandel AR, Patnaik BK. (1979). Long term vitamin status and dietary intake of healthy elderly subjects. I. Riboflavin. British Journal of Nutrition 42: 33–42. With permission of Cambridge University Press.

between EGR AC values and clinical signs of riboflavin deficiency have not been observed (Bates et al., 1981). Environmental factors may also influence the clinical manifestations of riboflavin deficiency.

Measurement of EGR AC has been used to monitor the riboflavin status of apparently healthy elderly persons from the United Kingdom (Rutishauser et al., 1979). The EGR AC remained fairly constant for each individual over the eighteen-month period (see data for six typical subjects in Table 20.3), suggesting that a single measurement of EGR AC may be a reliable index of long-term biochemical riboflavin status of individuals.

The EGR AC appears to be relatively independent of gender, and a single interpretive criterion for acceptable (< 1.2), low (1.2–1.4), or deficient (> 1.4) states has been used (McCormick, 1985). These guidelines are tentative, as several factors are known to affect EGR AC values. For example, the concentration of FAD used in the assay to stimulate EGR affects the EGR AC values obtained. Concentrations of FAD greater than $5\,\mu\text{mol}$ result in lower normal ranges of EGR ACs compared to FAD concentrations ranging from 1 to $3\,\mu\text{mol}$ (Garry and Owen, 1976; Rutishauser et al., 1979). Results of studies with fractionated erythrocytes suggest that the age of erythrocytes may also influence the ERG activity (Powers and Thurnham, 1981). In addition, some (Garry et al., 1982), but not all (Glatzle et al., 1970), investigators have noted a trend toward lower EGR ACs with increasing age. If this trend is more firmly established, specific guidelines for EGR AC values for the elderly may be required.

The appropriateness of the EGR AC test to assess the riboflavin status of subjects with glucose-6-phosphate dehydrogenase deficiency, a condition affecting approximately 10% of Americans of African descent, has been questioned (Prentice et al., 1981). Increased avidity of the EGR for FAD occurs in this condition, resulting in ACs within the normal range, even in the presence of clinical signs of riboflavin deficiency (Thurnham, 1972). Pyridoxine deficiency also interferes with the EGR AC test, resulting in a decreased erythrocyte glutathione reductase activity but no change in the activity coefficient, probably as a result of a decrease in apoenzyme. No comparable effects have been observed for other vitamin deficiencies such as thiamin, vitamin C, and folic acid (Sharda and Bamji, 1972). Increased erythrocyte glutathione reductase activity has been documented in persons with iron deficiency anemia (Ramachandran and Iyer, 1974), and in patients with severe uremia and cirrhosis of the liver.

Only small samples of blood are required for the EGR assay and fasting samples are not necessary (Komindr and Nichoalds, 1980). Either EDTA or heparin can be used as an anticoagulant. Erythrocytes must be prepared immediately after the blood samples are drawn. Hemolyzed samples can be kept frozen for up to three months at $-25°C$ without loss of EGR activity. Generally, glutathione reductase activity is measured using enzyme-coupled kinetic assays, although some colorimetric methods have been developed (Sauberlich, 1984). Very small volumes of whole blood can also be used for the measurement of GR activity, but the method, although simpler, is less sensitive than using erythrocytes for the assay.

20.2.2 Urinary riboflavin excretion

Riboflavin concentrations (per gram of creatinine) in casual urine samples were used to assess riboflavin status in the population studies of the Nutrition Canada National Survey, the US Ten State Nutrition Survey and in the NHANES I survey. Urinary riboflavin values tend to reflect recent dietary intake rather than body stores, and vary widely. Factors unrelated to riboflavin status, such as physical activity and sleep, decrease riboflavin excretion, whereas increased excretion is generated by elevated environmental temperatures, a negative nitrogen balance, and enforced bed rest (Tucker et al., 1960). Thus increased urinary riboflavin may not reflect improved riboflavin status. The administration of antibiotics and certain psychotropic (phenothiazine) drugs also increases urinary riboflavin excretion. Use of oral contraceptive agents decreases riboflavin excretion, as tissue retention of the vitamin is increased.

For survey use, nonfasting casual or six-hour urine collections can be used, although twenty-four-hour urine specimens are preferred. For adults, when dietary intakes are adequate, more than 120 µg riboflavin per day, or more than 30 µg per six hours, should be excreted (Table 20.4). For children, the rate of riboflavin excretion, when expressed as µg per gram of creatinine, is greater than for adults. Interpretive guidelines for

Subjects	Less than Acceptable (at Risk)		Acceptable (low risk)
	Deficient (high risk)	Low (medium risk)	
		(μg/g creatinine)	
1–3 years	< 150	150–499	≥ 500
4–6 years	< 100	100–299	≥ 300
7–9 years	< 85	85–269	≥ 270
10–15 years	< 70	70–199	≥ 200
Adults	< 27	27–79	≥ 80
Pregnant, 2nd trimester	< 39	39–119	≥ 120
Pregnant, 3rd trimester	< 30	30–89	≥ 90
		Other interpretive guidelines	
Adults μg/24 hr	< 40	40–119	≥ 120
Adults μg/6 hr	< 10	10–29	≥ 30
Adults μg in 4 hr following 5 mg riboflavin load	< 1000	1000–1399	≥ 1400

Table 20.4: Interpretive guidelines for the urinary excretion of riboflavin. From Sauberlich HE, Dowdy RP, Skala JH. (1974). Laboratory Tests for the Assessment of Nutritional Status. © CRC Press, Inc., Boca Raton, FL.

urinary riboflavin per gram of creatinine for both children and adults are shown in Table 20.4. Occasionally, a riboflavin load test has been performed. An oral dose of 5 mg riboflavin is given and the excretion of riboflavin in the urine collected during the following four hours is measured (Lossy et al., 1951; ICNND, 1963); it should also be compared with the level in the urine before the test load. Under conditions of adequate riboflavin intake, more than 1400 μg of riboflavin should be excreted in a four-hour period, whereas in a deficiency state, less than 1000 μg of riboflavin will be excreted during the same time period.

Fluorometric or microbiological assays have generally been used to determine riboflavin concentrations in urine. The former measure either the fluorescence of the flavins directly or convert the flavins to lumi-flavin and determine its fluorescence. The microbiological methods use *Ochromonas danica*. More recent developments include HPLC procedures capable of detecting urinary riboflavin levels as low as 0.01 μg/mL (Gatautis and Naito, 1981) and the competitive binding protein methods (Tillotson and Bashor, 1980). The latter are rapid, sensitive, and require no treatment of the urine sample prior to analysis. Discrepancies between the competitive protein binding and the microbiological methods have been documented and warrant further investigation (Sauberlich, 1984). In general, urinary riboflavin excretion, preferably measured on twenty-four-hour urine samples, should be used to confirm the results of EGR AC.

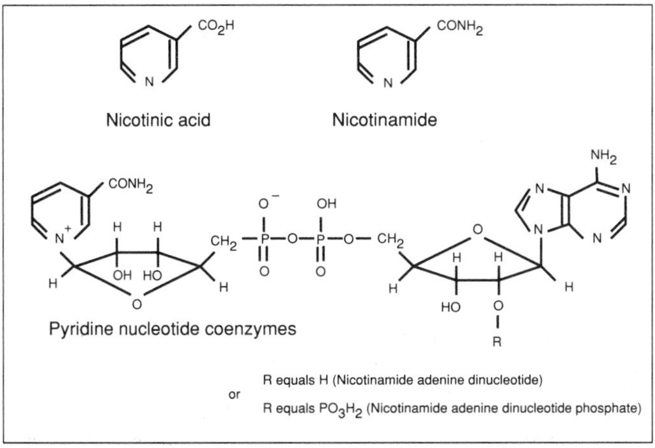

Figure 20.4: Structure of nicotinic acid and nicotinamide, and the two coenzyme forms containing the nicotinamide moiety.

20.2.3 Riboflavin concentrations in blood or its components

Generally, analysis of riboflavin in blood or its components is of limited value. Serum riboflavin concentrations are influenced by recent dietary intake and are too variable to serve as a useful index, whereas levels in whole blood and erythrocytes are relatively insensitive to small changes in riboflavin status (Bessey et al., 1956; Sauberlich et al., 1974).

20.3 Assessment of niacin status

Niacin is the term used to describe two compounds with the biological activity of the vitamin, nicotinic acid and nicotinamide. Their structures are shown in Figure 20.4. Nicotinic acid and nicotinamide have similar but not identical properties and they are both found in plant and animal foodstuffs, largely in the form of nicotinamide nucleotides. Niacin can also be derived from the amino acid tryptophan. Approximately 60 mg of tryptophan yields 1 mg of niacin after digestion and absorption. Oil seeds, cereals, legumes, and lean meats are rich sources of niacin. Niacin in cereals is present in the bran, bound as niacytin; most of the niacytin is biologically unavailable, although a small fraction may be biologically available when hydrolyzed by gastric acid (Bender and Bender, 1986). Treatment of cereals with alkali, baking with alkaline baking powders, and roasting whole grain maize all result in the release of niacin from the bound form (Kodicek et al., 1974).

Niacin is a component of two coenzymes, nicotinamide adenine dinucleotide (NAD) and nicotinamide adenine dinucleotide phosphate (NADP) (Figure 20.4). Both serve as proton and electron carriers in a variety of oxidation and reduction reactions.

Pellagra is the characteristic syndrome of niacin deficiency. Early symptoms include lassitude, anorexia, weakness, digestive disturbances, anxiety, irritability, and depression. Later, photosensitive dermatitis and a depressive psychosis develop. No known metabolic lesion has been associated with the photosensitive dermatitis. The mental symptoms are probably associated with a relative deficit of the essential amino acid tryptophan, which reduces synthesis of the neuro-transmitter amine 5-hydroxy-tryptamine (Bender and Bender, 1986).

The absence of pellagra in most industrialized countries today is attributed, in part, to the practice of fortifying certain foods (e.g. flour), with niacin. Some cases of pellagra do occur in association with chronic alcoholism, when the absorption of niacin is impaired. Pellagra can also develop as a result of prolonged use of isoniazid and 3-mercapto-purine, drugs used in the treatment of tuberculosis and leukemia respectively. Pellagra continues to be a major problem in South Africa, Egypt, and India, where maize and millet jowar (*Sorghum vulgare*) are the dietary staples (Sauberlich, 1984). Both these cereals have a relatively high concentration of leucine; excess leucine in the diet inhibits the conversion of tryptophan to niacin (Gopalan and Krishnaswamy, 1976; Bender, 1983). Additional factors possibly involved in the development of pellagra include lipid-soluble toxins, mycotoxins resulting from fungal spoilage of maize and other grains, other carcinogenic alkylating agents, and concurrent pyridoxine deficiency (Gopalan and Krishnaswamy, 1976; Bender and Bender, 1986).

Niacin toxicity may occur when pharmocological doses of niacin, especially the nicotinic acid form, are taken. The central nervous and cardiovascular systems, blood lipids, and blood sugar levels may all be affected.

So far, functional biochemical tests which reflect body stores of niacin are not available. Tests currently used reflect only recent dietary intakes of niacin, and therefore may not identify persons at risk to deficiency. The test regarded as the best index of niacin status is the measurement of the ratio of urinary excretion of N′-methyl-2-pyridone-5-carboxylamide to N′-methylnicotinamide. This test, and the measurement of niacin and its nucleotide in blood, are described below.

20.3.1   Urinary excretion of N′-methylnicotinamide and N′-methyl-2-pyridone-5-carboxylamide

The major end products of niacin metabolism in humans are N′-methylnicotinamide and N′-methyl-2-pyridone-5-carboxylamide (2-pyridone). Both are derived from either preformed niacin or niacin obtained from dietary tryptophan. Healthy adults excrete 20% to 30% of nicotinic acid as the N′-methylnicotinamide form, and 40% to 60% as 2-pyridone (deLange and Joubert, 1964). N′-methylnicotinamide excretion reaches

Subjects	Deficient	Low	Acceptable	High
Adults: (males and non-pregnant, nonlactating females)				
(mg/g creatinine)	< 0.5	0.5–1.59	1.6–4.29	≥ 4.3
(mg/6 hr)	< 0.2	0.2–0.59	0.6–1.59	≥ 1.6
Pregnant women (mg/g creatinine)				
1st trimester	< 0.5	0.5–1.59	1.6–4.29	≥ 4.3
2nd trimester	< 0.6	0.6–1.99	2.0–4.99	≥ 5.0
3rd trimester	< 0.8	0.8–2.49	2.5–6.49	≥ 6.5
All age groups 2-pyridone/N'-methyl-nicotinamide ratio		< 1.0	1.0–4.0	

Table 20.5: Interpretive guidelines for urinary N'-methylnicotinamide. From Sauberlich HE, Dowdy RP, Skala JH. (1974). Laboratory Tests for the Assessment of Nutritional Status. © CRC Press, Inc., Boca Raton, FL.

a minimum when clinical manifestations of niacin deficiency appear. The test is not appropriate for pregnant subjects, in whom elevated excretion levels of N'-methylnicotinamide occur as a result of alterations in pyridoxine metabolism (Table 20.5). As well, it should not be used for diabetic subjects, who excrete reduced amounts of urinary N'-methylnicotinamide. Excretion of 2-pyridone is more severely reduced in marginal niacin deficiency than that of N'-methylnicotinamide and may appear to fall to zero for several weeks before clinical signs of niacin deficiency appear (Goldsmith et al., 1952; Horwitt et al., 1956).

Some studies have used a nicotinamide load test involving the intramuscular administration of a 50-mg test dose of nicotinamide, followed by measurement of N'-methylnicotinamide in urine collected at the end of a four to five hour post-dose period. Gontzea et al. (1976) reported a 14% recovery of the test dose in well-nourished subjects over a three-hour period, compared with 8% for a rural population whose basal excretion of N'-methylnicotinamide was at the lower end of the normal range. Loading tests are impractical, however, for field surveys.

Unfortunately, excretion of both N'-methylnicotinamide and 2-pyridone in the urine is also reduced in subjects with generalized malnutrition, so these metabolites are not very specific indices of niacin deficiency (Sauberlich et al., 1974). Nevertheless, the ratio of 2-pyridone to N'-methylnicotinamide in urine is the preferred method of assessing niacin status (de Lange and Joubert, 1964). The ratio is relatively constant even after the administration of loading doses of tryptophan or niacin. Moreover, it is not affected by the duration of the urine collection period, making twenty-four-hour urine collections unnecessary. Instead, casual fasting urine samples can be used. Finally, the ratio is independent of age, so a single cutoff value can be used (Sauberlich et al., 1974). In normal healthy adults, ratios range from 1.3 to 4.0. Values below 1.0 indicate niacin deficiency. The interpretive guidelines suggested by ICNND are commonly used: < 1.0 = low; 1.0 to 4.0 = acceptable (Table 20.5).

Measurement of urinary excretion of N'-methylnicotinamide is technically simple, using either fluorometric methods (Clark, 1980) or HPLC (Shaikh and Pontzer, 1979). By contrast, measurement of 2-pyridone has, until recently, been more difficult and time consuming. The most widely used method involves removing interfering compounds by column chromatography, followed by determination of the absorption at 285 nm to 310 nm (Price, 1954). With the development of HPLC techniques, both urinary metabolites can now be readily measured with improved accuracy and sensitivity (Sandhu and Fraser, 1981).

20.3.2 Niacin in plasma, erythrocytes, and leukocytes

Concentrations of niacin compounds or derivatives in the plasma, erythrocytes, and leukocytes have also been investigated as potential indices of niacin nutriture. Results have been inconsistent. Levels in plasma are low and reflect dietary intake rather than body stores. Methods for the analysis of niacin in erythrocytes and leukocytes are presently unsatisfactory.

Measurement of whole blood concentrations of NAD(P) may be useful as an index of niacin status. The method is very sensitive and can be used on finger prick blood samples. As the coenzymes are extremely labile in whole blood, part of the analysis must be initiated ten to thirty seconds after taking the blood sample, a major disadvantage in field settings (Bender et al., 1982).

20.4 Summary

Thiamin

Beriberi, the classical syndrome of thiamin deficiency, is rare in Western countries except for persons with conditions such as alcoholism, chronic emesis, diarrhea, and marked anorexia. Thiamin is a component of the coenzyme thiamin pyrophosphate (TPP), which has a role in carbohydrate metabolism. Measurement of the erythrocyte activity of the transketolase enzyme, with and without added TPP, expressed as a ratio, is currently the most reliable test of thiamin status. The ratio, expressed as the 'activity coefficient' or percentage stimulation, provides a better measure of tissue stores of thiamin than static biochemical tests such as thiamin concentrations in whole blood, serum, erythrocytes, and urine. Thiamin in urine can be measured in both twenty-four-hour and casual urine specimens, concentrations reflecting dietary intakes, except at very low levels. Concentrations of thiamin in serum, erythrocytes, and whole blood are insensitive indices and are not recommended. Future methods for thiamin assessment may include measurements of thiamin pyrophosphate in erythrocytes.

Riboflavin

Riboflavin is a component of two coenzymes, flavin adenine dinucleotide (FAD) and flavin mononucleotide (FMN), which are essential for a number of oxidative enzyme systems involving electron transport. Classical signs of riboflavin deficiency (ariboflavinosis) generally occur in association with other nutrient deficiencies. Measurement of the activity of the enzyme glutathione reductase, with and without the added prosthetic group FAD, is the best method for assessing tissue riboflavin status in the absence of confounding factors. Urinary riboflavin excretion levels on casual or twenty-four-hour urine specimens reflect dietary intake and vary widely because concentrations are affected by many non-nutritional factors. Concentrations of riboflavin in serum, erythrocytes, or whole blood are insensitive indices of riboflavin status and are not recommended.

Niacin

The term 'niacin' refers to two compounds: nicotinamide and nicotinic acid. The former is a component of two coenzymes, nicotinamide adenine dinucleotide (NAD) and nicotinamide adenine dinucleotide phosphate (NADPH), both of which function in a variety of oxidation and reduction reactions. Pellagra, the syndrome of niacin deficiency, is rare in industrialized countries, but is prevalent where maize and sorghum are the dietary staples. No functional biochemical test of niacin status exists. At present, the best index is the measurement of the ratio of urinary excretion of N'-methylnicotinamide and N'-methyl-2-pyridone-5-carboxylamide (2-pyridone), two major end products of niacin metabolism in humans. In niacin deficiency, the ratio falls; values below 1.0 are indicative of niacin deficiency. Accurate and sensitive HPLC techniques can now be used for both urinary N'-methylnicotinamide and 2-pyridone analysis.

References

Bamji MS. (1981). Laboratory tests for the assessment of vitamin nutritional status. In: Briggs MH (ed). Vitamins in Human Biology and Medicine. CRC Press Inc., Boca Raton, FL, pp. 1–27.

Basu TK, Dickerson JW. (1976). The thiamin status of early cancer patients with particular reference to those with breast and bronchial carcinomas. Oncology 33: 250–252.

Basu TK, Patel DR, Williams DC. (1974). A simplified microassay of transketolase in human blood. International Journal for Vitamin and Nutrition Research. 44: 319–326.

Bates CJ, Prentice AM, Paul AA, Sutcliffe BA, Watkinson M, Whitehead RG. (1981). Riboflavin status in Gambian pregnant and lactating women and its implications for Recommended Dietary Allowances. American Journal of Clinical Nutrition 34: 928–935.

Bayoumi RA, Rosalki SB. (1976). Evaluation of methods of coenzyme activation of erythrocyte enzymes for detection of deficiency of vitamins B-1, B-2, and B-6. Clinical Chemistry 22: 327–335.

Bender DA. (1983). Effects of a dietary excess of leucine on the metabolism of tryptophan in the rat: a mechanism for the pellagragenic action of leucine. British Journal of Nutrition 50: 25–32.

Bender DA, Bender AE. (1986). Niacin and tryptophan metabolism: the biochemical basis of niacin requirements and recommendations. Nutrition Abstracts and Reviews (Series A) 56: 695–719.

Bender DA, Magboul BI, Wynick D. (1982). Probable mechanisms of regulation of the utilization of dietary tryptophan, nicotinamide and nicotinic acid as precursors of nicotinamide nucleotides in the rat. British Journal of Nutrition 48: 119–127.

Bessey OA, Horwitt MK, Love RH. (1956). Dietary deprivation of riboflavin and blood riboflavin levels in man. Journal of Nutrition 58: 367–383.

Brin M. (1967). Functional evaluation of nutritional status: thiamine. In: Albanese AA (ed). Newer Methods of Nutritional Biochemistry. Volume III. Academic Press, New York, pp. 407–445.

Brin M. (1980). Red cell transketolase as an indicator of nutritional deficiency. American Journal of Clinical Nutrition 33: 169–171.

Buttery JE, Milner CR, Chamberlain BR. (1982). The NADH-dependent transketolase assay: a note of caution. Clinical Chemistry 28: 2184–2185.

Cheng CH, Koch M, Shank RE. (1976). Leukocyte transketolase activity as an indicator of thiamin nutriture in rats. Journal of Nutrition 106: 1678–1685.

Chia CP, Addison R, McCormick DB. (1978). Absorption, metabolism and excretion of α-(amino acid) riboflavins in the rat. Journal of Nutrition 108: 373–381.

Clark BR. (1980). Fluorometric quantitation of picomole amounts of 1-methylnicotinamide and nicotinamide in serum. Methods of Enzymology 66: 5–8.

de Lange DJ, Joubert CP. (1964). Assessment of nicotinic acid status of population groups. American Journal of Clinical Nutrition 15: 169–174.

Garry PJ, Owen GM. (1976). An automated flavin adenine dinucleotide-dependent glutathione reductase assay for assessing riboflavin nutriture. American Journal of Clinical Nutrition 29: 663–674.

Garry PJ, Goodwin JS, Hunt WC. (1982). Nutritional status in a healthy elderly population: riboflavin. American Journal of Clinical Nutrition 36: 902–909.

Gatautis VJ, Naito HK. (1981). Liquid-chromatographic determination of urinary riboflavin. Clinical Chemistry 27: 1672–1675.

Glatzle D, Körner WF, Christeller S, Wiss O. (1970). Method for the detection of biochemical riboflavin deficiency. Stimulation of NADPH2-dependent glutathione reductase from human erythrocytes by FAD *in vitro*. Investigations on the vitamin B2 status in healthy people and geriatric patients. International Journal for Vitamin Research 40: 166–183.

Goldsmith GA, Sarett HP, Register UD, Gibbens J. (1952). Studies of niacin requirements in man. 1. Experimental pellagra in subjects on corn diets low in niacin and tryptophan. Journal of Clinical Investigation 31: 533–542.

Gontzea I, Rujinski A, Sutzesco P. (1976). Rapide évaluation biochimique de l'état de nutrition niacinique. Bibliotheca Nutritio et Diets. 23: 95–104.

Gopalan C, Krishnaswamy K. (1976). Effect of excess leucine on tryptophan-niacin pathway and pyridoxine (letter). Nutrition Reviews 34: 318–319.

Hatanaka Y, Ueda K. (1981). High incidence of subclinical hypovitaminosis of B-1 among university students found by a field study in Ehime, Japan. Medical Journal of Osaka University 31: 83–91.

Horwitt MK, Harvey CC, Rothwell WS, Cutler JL, Haffron D. (1956). Tryptophan-niacin relationships in man. Studies with diets deficient in riboflavin and niacin, together with observations on the excretion of nitrogen and niacin metabolites. Journal of Nutrition 60, Supplement 1: 43p.

ICNND (Interdepartmental Committee on Nutrition for National Defense) (1963). Manual for Nutrition Surveys. Second edition. US Government Printing Office, Washington, D.C.

Kawai C, Wakabayashi A, Matsumura T, Yui Y. (1980). Reappearance of beriberi heart disease in Japan. A study of 23 cases. American Journal of Medicine 69: 383–386.

Kjøsen B, Sein SH. (1977). The transketolase assay of thiamine in some diseases. American Journal of Clinical Nutrition 30: 1591–1596.

Kodicek E, Ashby DR, Muller M, Carpenter KJ. (1974). The conversion of bound nicotinic acid to free nicotinamide on roasting sweet corn. Proceedings of the Nutrition Society 33: 105A–106A.

Komindr S, Nichoalds GE. (1980). Clinical significance of riboflavin deficiency. In: Brewster MA, Naito HK (eds). Nutritional Elements and Clinical Biochemistry, Plenum Press, New York, pp. 22–28.

Leveille GA. (1972). Modified thiochrome procedure for the determination of urinary thiamin. American Journal of Clinical Nutrition 25: 273–274.

Lopez R, Schwartz JV, Cooperman JM. (1980). Riboflavin deficiency in an adolescent population in New York City. American Journal of Clinical Nutrition 33: 1283–1286.

Lossy FT, Goldsmith GA, Sarett HP. (1951). Study of test dose excretion of 5 B complex vitamins in man. Journal of Nutrition 45: 213–224.

McCormick DB. (1985). Vitamins. In: Textbook of Clinical Chemistry. WB Saunders, Philadelphia.

Nichoalds GE. (1981). Riboflavin. Clinics in Laboratory Medicine 1: 685–698.

Oldham HG. (1962). Thiamine requirements of women. Annals of the New York Academy of Sciences 98: 542–549.

Oldham HG, Davis MV, Roberts LJ. (1946). Thiamine excretions and blood levels of young women on diets containing varying levels of the B vitamins, with some observations on niacin and pantothenic acid. Journal of Nutrition 32: 163–180.

Pearson WN. (1962). Biochemical appraisal of nutritional status in man. American Journal of Clinical Nutrition 11: 462–474.

Plough IC, Bridgeforth EB. (1960). Relations of clinical and dietary findings in nutrition surveys. Public Health Reports 75: 699–706.

Powers HJ, Thurham DI. (1981). Riboflavin deficiency in man: effects on haemoglobin and reduced glutathione in erythrocytes of different ages. British Journal of Nutrition 46: 257–266.

Prentice AM, Bates CJ, Prentice A, Welch SG, Williams K, McGregor IA. (1981). The influence of G-6-PD activity on the response of erythrocyte glutathione reductase to riboflavin deficiency. International Journal for Vitamin and Nutrition Research 51: 211–215.

Price JM. (1954). The determination of N'-methyl-2-pyridone-5-carboxylamide in human urine. Journal of Biological Chemistry 211: 117–124.

Ramachandran M, Iyer GY. (1974). Erythrocyte glutathione reductase in iron deficiency anemia. Clinica Chimica Acta 52: 225–229.

Report of a Joint Food and Agriculture Organization / World Health Organization Expert Group. (1967). Requirement of vitamin A, thiamine, riboflavine and niacin. FAO Nutrition Meeting Report Series No. 41. Food and Agricultural Organization, Rome.

Roser RL, Andrist AH, Harrington WH, Naito HK, Lonsdale D. (1978). Determination of urinary thiamine by high-pressure liquid chromatography utilizing the thiochrome fluorescent method. Journal of Chromatography 146: 43–53.

Rutishauser IH, Bates CJ, Paul AA, Black AE, Mandel AR, Patnaik BK. (1979). Long term vitamin status and dietary intake of healthy elderly subjects. I. Riboflavin. British Journal of Nutrition 42: 33–42.

Sandhu JS, Fraser DR. (1981). Measurement of niacin metabolites in urine by high pressure liquid chromatography. A simple, sensitive assay of niacin nutritional status. International Journal for Vitamin and Nutrition Research 51: 139–144.

Sauberlich HE. (1984). Newer laboratory methods of assessing nutriture of selected B-complex vitamins. Annual Review of Nutrition 4: 377–407.

Sauberlich HE. (1985). Bioavailability of vitamins. Progress in Food and Nutrition Science 9: 1–33.

Sauberlich HE, Dowdy RP, Skala JH. (1974). Laboratory Tests for the Assessment of Nutritional Status. CRC Press Inc., Cleveland, Ohio.

Shaikh B, Pontzer NJ. (1979). Direct urinary assay method of N'-methylnicotinamide by soap chromatography. Journal of Chromatography 162: 596–600.

Sharda D, Bamji MS. (1972). Erythrocyte glutathione reductase activity and riboflavin concentration in experimental deficiency of some water soluble vitamins. International Journal for Vitamin and Nutrition Research 42: 43–49.

Sterner RT, Price WR. (1973). Restricted riboflavin: within-subject behavioral effects in humans. American Journal of Clinical Nutrition 26: 150–160.

Thurnham DI. (1972). Influence of glucose-6-phosphate dehydrogenase deficiency on the glutathione reductase test for ariboflavinosis. Annals of Tropical Medicine and Parasitology 66: 505–508.

Thurnham DI. (1981). Red cell enzyme tests of vitamin status: do marginal deficiencies have any physiological significance? Proceedings of the Nutrition Society 40: 155–163.

Tillotson JA, Baker EM. (1972). An enzymatic measurement of the riboflavin status in man. American Journal of Clinical Nutrition 25: 425–431.

Tillotson JA, Bashor MM. (1980). Fluorometric apoprotein titration of urinary riboflavin. Analytical Biochemistry 107: 214–219.

Tillotson JA, Sauberlich HE. (1971). Effect of riboflavin depletion and repletion on the erythrocyte glutathione reductase in the rat. Journal of Nutrition 101: 1459–1466.

Tucker RG, Mickelsen O, Keys A. (1960). The influence of sleep, work, diuresis, heat, acute starvation, thiamine intake and bed rest on human riboflavin excretion. Journal of Nutrition 72: 251–261.

Viteri FE. (1983). Vitamin deficiencies. In: Paige DM (ed). Manual of Clinical Nutrition. Nutrition Publications Inc., Pleasantville, New Jersey, pp. 331–337.

Waring PP, Fisher D, McDonnell J, McGown EL, Sauberlich HE. (1982). A continuous-flow (Auto Analyzer II) procedure for measuring erythrocyte transketolase activity. Clinical Chemistry 28: 2206–2213.

Warnock LG, Prudhomme CR, Wagner C. (1979). The determination of thiamin pyrophosphate in blood and other tissues, and its correlation with erythrocyte transketolase activity. Journal of Nutrition 108: 421–427.

Williams RR, Cline JK. (1936). Synthesis of vitamin B-1. Journal of the American Chemical Society 58: 1504–1505.

Chapter 21

Assessment of vitamin B-6 status

The term 'vitamin B-6' is the generic descriptor for all 3-hydroxy-2-methylpyridine derivatives that exhibit the biological activity of pyridoxine in rats. Vitamin B-6 is present in foods mainly as pyridoxal (the aldehyde), pyridoxine (the alcohol), and pyridoxamine (the amine) (Figure 21.1). These three dietary forms of vitamin B-6 are converted after absorption into pyridoxal phosphate or pyridoxamine phosphate, the coenzyme forms of vitamin B-6. These coenzymes catalyze a variety of enzyme systems involved primarily in protein, and to a lesser extent carbohydrate and lipid, metabolism.

Vitamin B-6 is widely distributed in foods, so frank dietary deficiencies are very rare. Good sources of vitamin B-6 in foods are meat, fish, and poultry, yeast, certain seeds, and bran. The adult human body has only a small body pool of this vitamin (20 to 30 mg), which is rapidly depleted when intakes of vitamin B-6 are deficient. Vulnerable population groups in industrialized countries at risk to suboptimal vitamin B-6 status include the elderly, adolescents, and pregnant and lactating women (Baker et al., 1979; Roepke and Kirksey, 1979; Schuster et al., 1981;

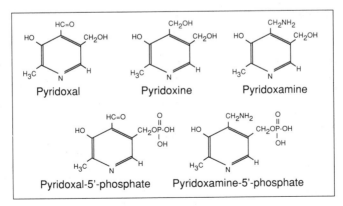

Figure 21.1: Structure of the various forms of vitamin B-6.

445

Driskell et al., 1985). Alterations in vitamin B-6 status have also
been associated with estrogen therapy, alcohol addiction, uremia, and
liver disease, and sometimes with the use of oral contraceptive agents.
The drugs isoniazid, cycloserine, penicillamine, and hydrocortisone also
interfere with vitamin B-6 metabolism. Therefore, these factors must be
considered when interpreting biochemical indices of vitamin B-6 status.

In the early stages, pyridoxine deficiency may cause fatigue and head-
aches. Later, microcytic hypochromic anemia, convulsions, and oral
lesions may develop (Sauberlich, 1981; Bapurao et al., 1982). Toxicity
of vitamin B-6 is low, daily doses of up to 1.0 g/day producing no
side effects (Haskell, 1978). Nevertheless, daily megadoses (2 to 6 g)
of vitamin B-6 have been associated with sensory neuropathy in some
studies (Schaumburg et al., 1983).

Biochemical assessment of vitamin B-6 status is essential, as the
clinical signs and symptoms of vitamin B-6 deficiency are nonspecific.
At present, no single index of vitamin B-6 status is recommended; at least
two indices are necessary, the choice depending on the objectives of the
assessment (Leklem and Reynolds, 1981). Details of the biochemical
indices most frequently used are given below.

21.1   Erythrocyte aminotransferase activities

Alanine aminotransferase (AlaAT) and aspartate aminotransferase (AspAT), also referred to as glutamate pyruvate transaminase (GPT) and glutamate oxaloacetate transaminase (GOT), respectively, both require pyridoxal phosphate as a coenzyme. They catalyze the following transamination reactions:

AlaAT

L-Alanine + α-ketoglutarate $\rightleftharpoons$ Pyruvate + L-glutamate

AspAT

L-Aspartate + α-ketoglutarate $\rightleftharpoons$ Oxaloacetate + L-glutamate

Both aminotransferase enzymes transfer the amino group from their
respective amino acid to α-ketoglutarate, forming L-glutamate and the
keto acid corresponding to the original amino acid.

The activity of the aminotransferase enzymes is greater in the erythrocytes than in the plasma. Consequently, the activities of the enzymes in erythrocytes are used as indices of vitamin B-6 nutriture. In
vitamin B-6 deficiency, the activity of these aminotransferase enzymes
falls, but the *in vitro* stimulation of the enzymes with added pyridoxal
phosphate increases. The activities are expressed in terms of activity
coefficients or percentage stimulation, as described for erythrocyte transketolase (Section 20.1.1). Unfortunately, chronic exposure to drugs and

diseases which affect the liver and heart cause alterations in erythrocyte aminotransferase activities and hence confound the interpretation of the results (Bamji, 1981).

To determine the activity coefficient (AC) or the percentage stimulation of erythrocyte (E) AlaAT, the red blood cell hemolysate is incubated with DL-alanine and α-ketoglutarate to yield the transamination product pyruvate, in the presence and absence of the *in vitro* addition of pyridoxal-5'-phosphate. The amount of pyruvate formed by the enzyme reaction is then measured spectrophotometrically.

$$\text{E AlaAT AC} = \frac{\mu\text{g pyruvate/mL/hr (with added pyridoxal-5'-phosphate)}}{\mu\text{g pyruvate/mL/hr (without added pyridoxal-5'-phosphate)}}$$

$$\text{Percentage stimulation} = (\text{activity coefficient} \times 100) - 100$$

The relationship of the activities of AlaAT and AspAT to other indices of vitamin B-6 status, including clinical manifestations of deficiency, has not been extensively evaluated. In general, results indicate that erythrocyte aminotransferase activities reflect long-term vitamin B-6 status and provide a gross index of vitamin B-6 deficiency (Bamji, 1981; Thurnham, 1981). They do not indicate the degree of deficiency because measurements of percentage stimulation for both the aminotransferase enzymes vary widely among normal healthy persons, as shown in Figure 21.2.

AlaAT is a more sensitive index of vitamin B-6 status in humans than AspAT because its activity changes more markedly during mild vitamin B-6 deficiency than AspAT. Furthermore, AlaAT activity is less prone to circadian variation than AspAT (Cinnamon and Beaton, 1970).

Schuster et al. (1981) measured the percentage stimulation of erythrocyte AlaAT to assess the vitamin B-6 status of low-income pregnant adolescent and adult women from the United States. The mean erythrocyte AlaAT percentage stimulation was elevated at the first clinic visit (34.8 ± 21%) and again in a subsample of thirty subjects at the 30th week of pregnancy (29.4 ± 14.5%). High values were also noted in pregnant Hispanic teenagers by Martner-Hewes et al. (1986). The clinical significance of these findings is uncertain. Relatively large supplements of vitamin B-6 are necessary to counteract the apparent biochemical B-6 deficiency during pregnancy. The latter may actually represent a normal physiological response and not a vitamin deficiency (Reynolds and Leklem, 1985). In general, measurement of the activity of AlaAT is not recommended for assessing the vitamin B-6 status of pregnant women, or those using oral contraceptive agents (Rose et al., 1973); estrogens increase the activity of AlaAT.

Despite the apparent advantages of using AlaAT for assessing the vitamin B-6 status of other nonpregnant population groups, its basal activity is about one-twentieth of that of AspAT, making it more difficult

Number of Subjects

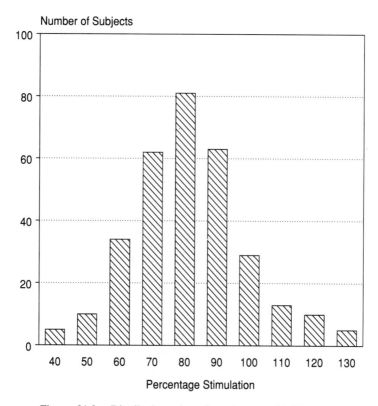

Figure 21.2: Distribution plot of erythrocyte AlaAT percentage stimulation in blood samples obtained from 312 male U.S. marine personnel. From Sauberlich HE. (1981). Vitamin B-6 status assessment: past and present. In: Leklem JE, Reynolds RD (eds). Methods in Vitamin B-6 Nutrition: Analysis and Status Assessment. Plenum Press, Figure 7, page 229 with permission.

to measure. Erythrocyte AlaAT is also much less stable during storage *in vitro* than AspAT. As a result, the erythrocyte AspAT test has also been used for population field surveys (Changbumrung et al., 1985).

At the present time the activities of the aminotransferase enzymes in erythrocytes which correspond either to optimal body stores of vitamin B-6, or to a borderline deficiency, are not well established. Hence, interpretive guidelines for erythrocyte AlaAT or AspAT activities are poorly defined; generally, those of Sauberlich et al. (1972) are used (Table 21.1). Vitamin B-6 status is classified as adequate if the percentage stimulation of erythrocyte AlaAT is $\leq 25\%$ (AC ≤ 1.25) or inadequate if the percentage stimulation is $> 25\%$ (AC $= > 1.25$). For erythrocyte AspAT, the cutoff point for percentage stimulation of erythrocytes designated as inadequate is $> 50\%$ (AC $= > 1.50$). Other investigators have used higher cutoff points ranging from $> 70\%$ (AC $= > 1.7$) to $> 100\%$ (AC

= > 2.0). More work is needed to establish interpretive guidelines for pregnant women and to validate current guidelines.

Colorimetry and coupled-enzyme spectrophotometry are commonly used to measure erythrocyte AlaAT and AspAT activities, and the *in vitro* stimulation effect of pyridoxal-5′-phosphate (Sauberlich, 1984). Both of these procedures lack specificity and sensitivity, suffer from severe matrix effects, and lack a suitable reference standard for quality control. Such methodological difficulties may be partly responsible for the discrepancies in the cutoff points used for the AC. To overcome some of these problems, automated methods based on a continuous flow procedure have been developed, as well as a freeze-dried erythrocyte pool for quality control (Skala et al., 1981).

The activities of AlaAT and AspAT have also been measured in leukocytes but large blood samples are required and the method of isolating the leukocytes is too tedious for routine use.

21.2 Plasma pyridoxal-5′-phosphate

Pyridoxal-5′-phosphate (PLP) is the major transport form of vitamin B-6 in plasma (Lumeng et al., 1978). Concentrations of plasma pyridoxal-5′-phosphate (PLP) are a direct measure of the active coenzyme form of vitamin B-6 and, in animals, reflect levels in the skeletal muscle (Lumeng et al., 1978). The latter is the largest store of vitamin B-6 in the body (Coburn et al., 1988). Hence, plasma PLP appears promising as an index of body stores of vitamin B-6 in normal healthy persons (Li and Lumeng, 1980); its use for individuals with clinical abnormalities or receiving medications is more limited.

Age- and sex-related changes in plasma PLP values have been noted. Male adults have higher plasma PLP concentrations than females; values decline with age in both males and females (Rose et al., 1976). These trends may be associated with changes in the mass of skeletal muscle mass, the major storage site for vitamin B-6 (Lee and Leklem, 1985). Pregnancy also influences plasma PLP concentrations; progressively lower levels during pregnancy may result from hemodilution caused by changes in plasma volume rather than result from vitamin B-6 deficiency. The fall in plasma PLP levels does not, however, exactly parallel increases in plasma volume (National Research Council, 1970). Furthermore, vitamin B-6 supplementation during pregnancy does not appear to arrest the fall in plasma PLP levels (Reynolds and Leklem, 1985).

Plasma PLP concentrations remain relatively stable when dietary intakes of vitamin B-6 are held constant, and change only slowly with alterations in dietary intake before reaching a new steady-state level; the change may take three to four weeks (Brown et al., 1975). Indeed, clinical signs of vitamin B-6 deficiency may be observed prior to measuring any changes in plasma PLP concentrations.

At present, there are no universally accepted guidelines for interpreting plasma PLP concentrations, and age-specific criteria have not been developed. Plasma PLP concentrations within the range of 8.7 to 15.7 ng/mL (52 to 94 nmol/L) have been reported for healthy U.S. adults consuming mixed diets (Li and Lumeng, 1980; Willett, 1985; Driskell et al., 1988). Plasma PLP levels associated with marginal vitamin B-6 status have ranged from values of 9.5 to 10.2 ng/mL (56.8 to 61.0 nmol/L) for adult males and 5.5 to 6.2 ng/mL (32.9 to 37.1 nmol/L) for adult females (Shultz and Leklem, 1981). Rose et al. (1976), however, suggested that values of < 8.5 ng/mL (50.8 ng/mL) indicated inadequate vitamin B-6 status. More data are urgently required to clearly define interpretive criteria for plasma PLP levels and to establish the effects of disease and drugs on this index.

Recent developments in methods for measuring plasma PLP concentrations include using cation-exchange HPLC or cation-exchange open column chromatography followed by fluorometric assay (Smith et al., 1983; Lui et al., 1985). Alternatively, sensitive enzymatic radiometric assays employing radioactive tyrosine and apodecarboxylase are used (Chabner and Livingston, 1970; Lui et al., 1985). Differences in sample extraction procedures markedly affect the accuracy and reproducibility of the enzyme assay. As newer, less time-consuming and more reliable and sensitive analytical techniques become available, plasma PLP levels may become the preferred index of vitamin B-6 status (Klasing and Pilch, 1985). The stability of pyridoxal-5'-phosphate in plasma is uncertain. Losses within one week have been reported when plasma is stored at $-20°C$; at $-80°C$, plasma PLP is stable for at least ten days (Camp et al., 1983). Pyridoxal-5'-phosphate in whole blood samples stored at $-20°C$ is stable for at least several months. Recent animal work suggests that PLP concentrations in erythrocytes may be a promising index of vitamin B-6 status, concentrations changing more rapidly over a wide range of intakes than plasma PLP concentrations. More work is required, however, to validate erythrocyte PLP as an index of vitamin B-6 status in humans.

21.3 Urinary vitamin B-6 excretion

Although vitamin B-6 is excreted in urine primarily as the metabolite 4-pyridoxic acid (Section 21.4), smaller amounts of free vitamin B-6 are also excreted as pyridoxal; pyridoxamine is also excreted in even smaller quantities. Consequently, urinary excretion of free vitamin B-6 has been investigated as an index of vitamin B-6 status. Several experimentally controlled depletion/repletion studies have demonstrated that urinary excretion generally reflects recent dietary intake of vitamin B-6 and not the state of tissue saturation. Furthermore, urinary excretion of free vitamin B-6 decreases proportionately with dietary intake only

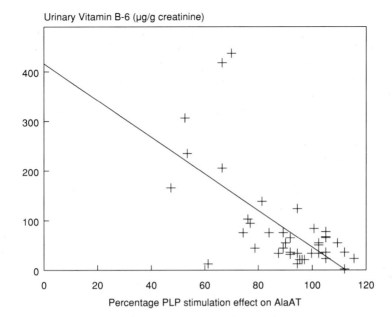

Figure 21.3: Relationship between urinary vitamin B-6 levels and percentage stimulation of erythrocyte AlaAT in forty-one samples from U.S. female marine personnel. From Sauberlich HE. (1981). Vitamin B-6 status assessment: past and present. In: Leklem JE, Reynolds RD (eds). Methods in Vitamin B-6 Nutrition: Analysis and Status Assessment. Plenum Press, Figure 4, page 226 with permission.

up to a critical point; beyond this stage, further reductions in dietary intake result in only small and variable changes in urinary vitamin B-6 excretion (Sauberlich, 1981). Drugs such as isoniazid, penicillamine, and cycloserine increase excretion of vitamin B-6 in the urine, confounding the use of urinary concentrations as an index of vitamin B-6 status.

Urinary vitamin B-6 concentrations have been used in several population studies (e.g. US Ten-State Nutrition Survey) because collection of urine specimens is relatively noninvasive and casual urine samples can be used. Morning fasting urine specimens are preferred to minimize variations associated with fluid intake and physical activity, and concentrations should be expressed per gram of creatinine. Values derived from such samples correlate with total twenty-four-hour urinary vitamin B-6 excretion. Results in Figure 21.3 confirm that erythrocyte AlaAT percent stimulation is related to vitamin B-6 levels in casual urine samples, when the concentrations are expressed in terms of creatinine. (Sauberlich, 1981).

	Vitamin B-6 Status	
Biochemical Measurement	Marginal or Inadequate	Acceptable
Tryptophan load (increased excretion)		
Xanthurenic acid (mg/day)	> 50	< 25
3-OH-kynurenine (mg/day)	> 50	< 25
Kynurenine (mg/day)	> 50	< 10
Quinolinic acid (μmol/day)	> 50	< 25
Urinary measurements		
Vitamin B-6 (μg/g creatinine)		
1–3 years	< 90	≥ 90
4–6 years	< 75	≥ 75
7–9 years	< 50	≥ 50
10–12 years	< 40	≥ 40
13–15 years	< 30	≥ 30
Adults	< 20	≥ 20
4-pyridoxic acid (mg/day)	< 0.5	≥ 0.8
Erythrocyte measurements		
E AlaAT AC	> 1.25	≤ 1.25
E AsPAT AC	> 1.5	≤ 1.5

Table 21.1: Tentative guidelines for evaluating the vitamin B-6 nutritional status of adults. The cutoff values used for the AlaAT and AsPAT indices will depend upon the methods used and the level of pyridoxal phosphate added in the in vitro stimulation assay. Reproduced with permission from Sauberlich HE, Dowdy RP, Skala JH. (1974). Laboratory Tests for the Assessment of Nutritional Status. © CRC Press, Inc., Boca Raton, FL.

Age- and sex-related differences in urinary vitamin B-6 per gram of creatinine are well recognized. Children have a markedly higher level of vitamin B-6 excretion, in terms of μg/g creatinine, than adults (Table 21.1). The mean excretion for females also tends to be higher than for males. Although the requirement for pyridoxine is known to be related to protein intake, the latter does not have a significant effect on urinary vitamin B-6 excretion. Age-specific interpretive guidelines for urinary vitamin B-6 excretion per gram of creatinine have been developed; the guidelines of Sauberlich et al. (1974) are presented in Table 21.1. Generally, urinary excretion of vitamin B-6 of less than 20 μg/g creatinine is indicative of marginal or inadequate pyridoxine intake in adults.

The analysis of free vitamin B-6 in urine is difficult. Microbiological assays using yeast, *Saccharomyces carlsbergensis* or *Saccharomyces uvarum*, are most commonly employed. High-performance liquid chromatography may be adopted in the future, provided that problems of sample extraction, sensitivity, and throughput can be resolved. Alternatively, radio-immuno assays or an enzyme-linked immunosorbent assay (ELISA) capable of analyzing large numbers of samples for any of the desired forms of vitamin B-6 may be developed (Sauberlich, 1984).

21.4   Urinary 4-pyridoxic acid excretion

4-Pyridoxic acid (2-methyl-3-hydroxy-4-carboxy-methylpyridine) is the major urinary metabolite of vitamin B-6 in humans. Approximately 40% to 60% of dietary vitamin B-6 is converted to this metabolite in adults, the percentage varying with age, and possibly with the composition of the diet. In experimentally controlled human studies, 4-pyridoxic acid excretion decreases during vitamin B-6 deficiency and increases during repletion (Kelsay et al., 1968; Lee and Leklem, 1985), demonstrating that concentrations reflect dietary intake of the vitamin.

Until recently, measurement of urinary 4-pyridoxic acid has been limited by analytical difficulties as well as the apparent necessity for twenty-four-hour urine samples. Schuster et al. (1984), however, noted a positive correlation between total 4-pyridoxic acid and 4-pyridoxic acid : creatinine ratios in the twenty-four-hour urine samples. Moreover, ratios of 4-pyridoxic acid : creatinine derived from the twenty-four-hour urine samples and casual urine samples taken the next day were similar. Hence 4-pyridoxic acid : creatinine measurements in casual urine samples are a valid alternative to the measurement of total 4-pyridoxic acid excretion in twenty-four-hour hour urine samples.

Both decreases (Shultz and Leklem, 1981) and increases in 4-pyridoxic acid excretion with age have been noted (Lee and Leklem, 1985). A decrease occurs with age in the number of binding sites available in the liver for the storage of vitamin B-6; this would produce an increase in the excretion of this vitamin.

Further work on 4-pyridoxic acid excretion and alternative indices (such as plasma PLP levels) is needed to establish the relationship between urinary 4-pyridoxic acid and vitamin B-6 status. Schuster et al. (1984) reported no correlation between these two biochemical indices of vitamin B-6 nutriture, whereas Lee and Leklem (1985) noted a positive relationship when a group of women received constant vitamin B-6 intakes of 2.3 mg/day, but not when they received 10.3 mg/day. Tentative guidelines for urinary excretion levels of 4-pyridoxic acid (mg/day) are shown in Table 21.1.

High-performance liquid chromatography is now the preferred method for analysis of 4-pyridoxic acid in urine. Sample preparation is minimal; urine samples are first treated with trichloroacetic acid to precipitate any protein and then injected directly into the HPLC system. 4-Pyridoxic acid is detected fluorometrically (Gregory and Kirk, 1979). 4-Pyridoxic

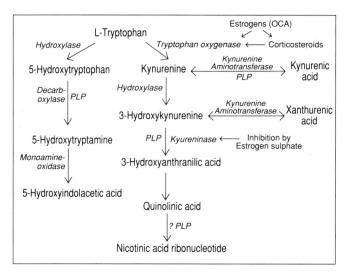

Figure 21.4: Tryptophan metabolic pathways. Reproduced with permission from Bamji MS. (1981). Laboratory tests for the assessment of vitamin nutritional status. In: Briggs MH (ed). Vitamins in Human Biology and Medicine. © CRC Press, Inc., Boca Raton, FL.

acid in urine samples stored at $-20°C$ is stable for at least twenty months (Arend and Brown, 1981).

21.5   Tryptophan load test

Vitamin B-6, as pyridoxal phosphate, is a coenzyme for kynureninase and kynurenine aminotransferase in the kynurenine pathway. Normally these enzymes act on kynurenine and 3-hydroxykynurenine to form anthranilic and 3-hydroxyanthranilic acids and the quinoline derivatives kynurenic and xanthurenic acids. In vitamin B-6 deficiency, the activities of kynureninase and kynurenine aminotransferase are reduced. As a result, 3-hydroxykynurenine and kynurenine accumulate, leading to increased formation and excretion of xanthurenic and kynurenic acids, as well as kynurenine, hydroxykynurenine, and quinolinic acid, particularly if preceded by an oral loading dose of tryptophan.

Of the metabolites excreted, xanthurenic acid is the most frequently determined after a tryptophan load because it is the most easily measured. Other factors which affect the urinary excretion of xanthurenic acid after a tryptophan load include protein intake, exercise, lean body mass, and the size of the tryptophan loading dose. Estrogen induces the enzyme tryptophan oxygenase (tryptophan pyrrolase) and hence the tryptophan load test is not appropriate for pregnant subjects and women taking oral contraceptive agents. Certain drugs (e.g. hydrocortisone) also interfere with the tryptophan load test by increasing the tryptophan oxygenase activity in the liver and hence urinary kynurenine excretion. Some drugs also interfere with the analytical procedures (e.g. sulfonamides and para-aminosalicylic acid). Colorimetric methods in association with ion-exchange chromatography are particularly affected (Price et al., 1965). Cancer patients also have increased urinary excretion of xanthurenic acid and other metabolites of tryptophan after a tryptophan load (Rose and Randall, 1973).

The L-isomer of tryptophan should be administered in human studies, as the D-isomeric form is not metabolized via the tryptophan-niacin pathway. For adults, a loading dose of 2 or 5 g of L-tryptophan is sufficient to cause an increased urinary excretion of metabolites of the kynurenine pathway. For infants and children, a loading dose of 100 mg/kg body weight is appropriate. The tryptophan can be given as a tablet or as a powder suspended in milk, with breakfast, to avoid side effects such as somnolence and nausea.

Urine collections over six- to eight-hour periods may suffice if xanthurenic acid is measured, as the majority of the xanthurenic acid is excreted during this period. Nevertheless, twenty-four-hour urine collections are preferred (Luhby et al., 1971). Urine samples must be acidified to a pH between 3 and 4 to reduce bacterial growth and to stabilize the metabolites. Samples should be frozen at $-15°C$. Tryptophan metabolites are stable for two to three months, if frozen, after which significant losses of 3-hydrokynurenine and 3-hydroxyanthranilic acid may occur. Table 21.1 presents the interpretive guidelines of Sauberlich et al. (1974) for urinary excretion levels of tryptophan metabolites for adults, after a 5 g L-tryptophan load.

Many methods have been used to measure xanthurenic acid in the urine. The most frequently used techniques employ thin layer or ion-exchange chromatography for the separation of xanthurenic acid, followed by colorimetry, spectrophotometry, or fluorometry. These methods are capable of analyzing many samples and are sensitive, specific, and reproducible (Brown, 1981).

21.6 Kynurenine load test

The kynurenine load test was developed particularly for use in pregnant women and subjects with disease or stress, when interpretation of the tryptophan load test is difficult (Section 21.5). Such a test bypasses the enzyme tryptophan oxygenase (tryptophan pyrrolase) (Figure 21.4). An oral dose of 200 mg of L-kynurenine sulfate produces modest and reproducible increases in the excretion of several urinary metabolites in normal subjects. Excretion levels of 3-hydroxykynurenine, kynurenine, and quinolinic acid are comparable to those seen after a 2.0-g tryptophan load (Table 21.1), although no increase in xanthurenic acid excretion occurs. This test has also been used in oral contraceptive

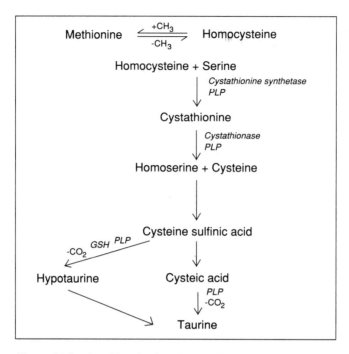

Figure 21.5: An abbreviated pathway of methionine metabolism showing the pyridoxal-5'-phosphate-dependent steps. Reproduced with permission from Bamji MS. (1981). Laboratory tests for the assessment of vitamin nutritional status. In: Briggs MH (ed). Vitamins in Human Biology and Medicine. © CRC Press, Inc., Boca Raton, FL.

users and postmenopausal women receiving small doses of estradiol (Brown, 1981).

21.7   Methionine load test

In vitamin B-6 deficiency states, elevated excretion levels of cystathionine also occur, which can be prevented with vitamin B-6 supplementation. Cystathionine is a metabolite of methionine which depends on vitamin B-6 for its synthesis and/or degradation. Figure 21.5 shows the PLP-dependent steps in an abbreviated pathway of methionine metabolism.

The urinary excretion of cystathionine and the ratio of cystathionine to cysteine sulfinic acid are both elevated in a vitamin B-6 deficient state, after a loading dose of 3 g L-methionine. Twenty-four-hour urine samples must be collected for the analysis (Park and Linkswiler, 1970; Linkswiler, 1974). In general, this test has been used in experimental studies of vitamin B-6 depletion and repletion, in pregnant women, in

adult men suffering from neuropathy, and in patients treated with isoni-
cotinic acid hydrazide (Park and Linkswiler, 1970; Krishnaswamy, 1972;
Shin and Linkswiler, 1974). The potential of this test as an index of
vitamin B-6 status in the general population is unknown. The analysis
of methionine metabolites in the urine requires an amino acid analyzer.

21.8 Summary

Several biochemical indices of vitamin B-6 status exist. The selection of
an appropriate index depends on the objectives and the characteristics of
the study group. Plasma pyridoxal-5'-phosphate (PLP) concentrations
provide a direct measure of the active coenzyme and reflect tissue
levels of vitamin B-6 in healthy, nonpregnant persons. Fasting blood
samples should be used. In contrast, urinary excretion levels of free
vitamin B-6 and 4-pyridoxic acid — and, to a lesser extent, erythrocyte
aminotransferase activities — reflect recent dietary intakes of vitamin B-6
rather than tissue levels. The tryptophan load test is a functional
biochemical test which is generally used in clinical settings to provide
an indirect measure of tissue vitamin B-6 status. At the present time, the
evaluation of vitamin B-6 status should include a combination of dietary
intake and at least two biochemical indices, one of which should be
plasma PLP. Future studies may include erythrocyte PLP concentrations,
as they appear to be a more sensitive index of tissue PLP levels than
plasma PLP.

References

Arend RA, Brown RR. (1981). Comparison of analytical methods for urinary 4-pyridoxic
  acid. American Journal of Clinical Nutrition 34: 1984–1985.

Baker H, Frank O, Thind IS, Jaslow SP, Louria DB. (1979). Vitamin profiles in elderly
  persons living at home or in nursing homes, versus profile in healthy young
  subjects. Journal of the American Geriatrics Society 27: 444–450.

Bamji MS. (1981). Laboratory tests for the assessment of vitamin nutritional status. In:
  Briggs MH (ed). Vitamins in Human Biology and Medicine. CRC Press Inc.,
  Boca Raton, Florida, pp. 2–27.

Bapurao S, Raman L, Tulpule PG. (1982). Biochemical assessment of vitamin B$_6$
  nutritional status in pregnant women with orolingual manifestations. American
  Journal of Clinical Nutrition 36: 581–586.

Brown RR. (1981). The tryptophan load test as an index of vitamin B$_6$ nutrition. In:
  Leklem JE, Reynolds RD (eds). Methods in Vitamin B-6 Nutrition. Analysis and
  Status Assessment. Plenum Press, New York–London, pp. 321–340.

Brown RR, Rose DP, Leklem JE, Linkswiler H, Anand R. (1975). Urinary 4-pyridoxic
  acid, plasma pyridoxal phosphate, and erythrocyte aminotransferase in oral contraceptive users receiving controlled intakes of vitamin B$_6$. American Journal of
  Clinical Nutrition 28: 10–19.

Camp VM, Chipponi J, Faraj BA. (1983). Radioenzymatic assay for direct measurement
  of plasma pyridoxal-5'-phosphate. Clinical Chemistry 29: 642–644.

Chabner ME, Livingston D. (1970). A simple enzymatic assay for pyridoxal phosphate. Analytical Biochemistry 34: 413–423.

Changbumrung S, Schelp FP, Habi IM, Hongtong K, Buavatana T, Supawan V, Migasena P. (1985). Pyridoxine status in preschool children in Northeast Thailand: a community study. American Journal of Clinical Nutrition 41: 770–775.

Cinnamon AD, Beaton JR. (1970). Biochemical assessment of vitamin B6 status in man. American Journal of Clinical Nutrition 23: 696–702.

Coburn SP, Lewis DLN, Fink WJ, Mahuren JD, Schaltenbrand WE, Costill DL. (1988). Human vitamin B-6 pools estimated through muscle biopsies. American Journal of Clinical Nutrition 48: 291–294.

Driskell JA, Clark AJ, Bazzarre TL, Chopin LF, McCoy H, Kenney MA, Moak SW. (1985). Vitamin B-6 status of Southern adolescent girls. Journal of the American Dietetic Association 85: 46–49.

Driskell JA, Chrisley BM, Thye FW, Reynolds LK. (1988). Plasma pyridoxal phosphate concentrations of men fed different levels of vitamin B-6. American Journal of Clinical Nutrition 48: 122–126.

Gregory JF 3rd, Kirk JR. (1979). Determination of urinary 4-pyridoxic acid using high performance liquid chromatography. America Journal of Clinical Nutrition 32: 879–883.

Haskell BE. (1978). Toxicity of vitamin B-6. In: Rechcigl M Jr. (ed). CRC Handbook Series in Nutrition and Food Science Section E. Nutritional Disorders. Volume I. Effect of Nutrient Excesses and Toxicities in Animals and Man. CRC Press Inc., West Palm Beach, Florida, pp. 43–45.

Kelsay J, Baysal A, Linkswiler H. (1968). Effect of vitamin B-6 depletion in the pyridoxal, pyridoxamine and pyridoxine content of the blood and urine of men. Journal of Nutrition 94: 490–494.

Klasing and Pilch. (1985). Suggested Measures of Nutritional Status and Health Conditions for the Third National Health and Nutrition Examination Survey. Life Sciences Research Office, Federation of American Societies for Experimental Biology, Bethesda, Maryland, pp. 23–34.

Krishnaswamy K. (1972). Methionine load test in pyridoxine deficiency. International Journal for Vitamin and Nutrition Research 42: 468–475.

Lee CM, Leklem JE. (1985). Differences in vitamin B6 status indicator responses between young and middle-aged women fed constant diets with two levels of vitamin B6. American Journal of Clinical Nutrition 42: 226–234.

Leklem JE, Reynolds RD. (1981). Recommendations for assessment of vitamin B-6 status. In: Leklem JE, Reynolds RD (eds). Methods in Vitamin B-6 Nutrition: Analysis and Status Assessment. Plenum Press, New York–London, pp. 389–392.

Li T-K, Lumeng L. (1980). Plasma PLP as an indicator of nutritional status: relationship to tissue vitamin B-6 content and hepatic metabolism. In: Leklem JE, Reynolds RD (eds). Methods in Vitamin B-6 Nutrition: Analysis and Status Assessment. Plenum Press, New York–London, pp. 289–296.

Linkswiler H. (1974). Tryptophan and methionine metabolism of adult females as affected by vitamin B_6 deficiency. Journal of Nutrition 104: 1348–1355.

Luhby AL, Brin M, Gorden M, Davis P, Murphy M, Spiegel H. (1971). Vitamin B_6 metabolism in users of oral contraceptive agents. I. Abnormal urinary xanthurenic acid excretion and its correction by pyridoxine. American Journal of Clinical Nutrition 24: 684–693.

Lui A, Lumeng L, Li T-K. (1985). The measurement of plasma vitamin B6 compounds: comparison of a cation-exchange HPLC method with the open-column chromatographic method and the L-tyrosine apodecarboxylase assay. American Journal of Clinical Nutrition 41: 1236–1243.

Lumeng L, Ryan MP, Li T-K. (1978). Validation of the diagnostic value of plasma pyridoxal-5′-phosphate measurements in vitamin B-6 nutrition of the rat. Journal of Nutrition 108: 545–553.

Martner-Hewes PM, Hunt IF, Murphy NJ, Swendseid ME, Settlage RH. (1986). Vitamin B-6 nutriture and plasma diamine oxidase activity in pregnant Hispanic teenagers. American Journal of Clinical Nutrition 44: 907–913.

National Research Council, Committee on Maternal Nutrition. (1970). Maternal Nutrition and the Course of Pregnancy. National Academy of Sciences, Washington, D.C.

Park YK, Linkswiler H. (1970). Effect of vitamin B_6 depletion in adult man on the excretion of cystathionine and other methionine metabolites. Journal of Nutrition 100: 110–116.

Price JM, Brown RR, Yess N. (1965). Testing the functional capacity of the tryptophanniacin pathway in man by analysis of urinary metabolites. Advances in Metabolic Disorders 2: 159–225.

Reynolds RD, Leklem, JE (1985). Implications on the role of vitamin B-6 in health and disease: a summary. In: Reynolds RD, Leklem JE (eds). Vitamin B-6: Its Role in Health and Disease. Alan R. Liss Inc., New York, pp. 481–489.

Roepke JL, Kirksey A. (1979). Vitamin B-6 nutriture during pregnancy and lactation. I. Vitamin B-6 intake, levels of the vitamin in biological fluids, and condition of the infant at birth. American Journal of Clinical Nutrition 32: 2249–2256.

Rose CS, György P, Butler M, Andres R, Norris AH, Shock NW, Tobin J, Brin M, Spiegel H. (1976). Age differences in vitamin B_6 status of 617 men. American Journal of Clinical Nutrition 29: 847–853.

Rose DP, Randall ZC. (1973). Influence of loading dose on the demonstration of abnormal tryptophan metabolism by cancer patients. Clinica Chimica Acta 47: 45–49.

Rose DP, Strong R, Folkard J, Adams PW. (1973). Erythrocyte amino transferase activities in women using oral contraceptives and the effect of vitamin B_6 supplementation. American Journal of Clinical Nutrition 26: 48–52.

Sauberlich HE. (1981). Vitamin B-6 status assessment: past and present. In: Leklem JE, Reynolds RD (eds). Methods in Vitamin B-6 Nutrition: Analysis and Status Assessment. Plenum Press, New York–London, pp. 203–239.

Sauberlich HE. (1984). Newer laboratory methods for assessing nutriture of selected B-complex vitamins. Annual Review of Nutrition 4: 377–407.

Sauberlich HE, Canham JE, Baker EM, Raica N, Herman YF. (1972). Biochemical assessment of the nutritional status of vitamin B_6 in the human. American Journal of Clinical Nutrition 25: 629–642.

Sauberlich HE, Dowdy RP, Skala JH. (1974). Laboratory Tests for the Assessment of Nutritional Status. CRC Press Inc., Cleveland, Ohio.

Schaumburg H, Kaplan J, Windebank A, Vick N, Rasmus S, Pleasure D, Brown MJ. (1983). Sensory neuropathy from pyridoxine abuse. A new megavitamin syndrome. New England Journal of Medicine 309: 445–448.

Schuster K, Bailey LB, Mahan CS. (1981). Vitamin B_6 status of low-income adolescent and adult pregnant women and the condition of their infants at birth. American Journal of Clinical Nutrition 34: 1731–1735.

Schuster K, Bailey LB, Cerda JJ, Gregory JF. (1984). Urinary 4-pyridoxic acid excretion in 24-hour versus random urine samples as a measurement of vitamin B_6 status in humans. American Journal of Clinical Nutrition 39: 466–470.

Shin HK, Linkswiler HM. (1974). Tryptophan and methionine metabolism of adult females as affected by vitamin B-6 deficiency. Journal of Nutrition 104: 1348–1355.

Shultz TD, Leklem JE. (1981). Urinary 4-pyridoxic acid, urinary vitamin B-6 and plasma pyridoxal phosphate as measures of vitamin B-6 status and dietary intake of adults. In: Leklem JE, Reynolds RD (eds). Methods in Vitamin B-6 Nutrition: Analysis and Status Assessment. Plenum Press, New York–London, pp. 297–320.

Skala JH, Waring PP, Lyons MF, Rusnak MG, Alletto JS. (1981). Methodology for determination of blood aminotransferases. In: Leklem JE, Reynolds RD (eds). Methods in Vitamin B-6 Nutrition: Analysis and Status Assessment. Plenum Press, New York–London, pp. 171–202.

Smith GP, Samson D, Peters TJ. (1983). A fluorimetric method for the measurement of pyridoxal and pyridoxal phosphate in human plasma and leucocytes, and its application to patients with sideroblastic marrows. Journal of Clinical Pathology 36: 701–706.

Thurnham DI. (1981). Red cell enzyme tests of vitamin status: do marginal deficiencies have any physiological significance? Proceedings of the Nutrition Society 40: 155–163.

Willett WC. (1985). Does low vitamin B-6 increase the risk of coronary heart disease? In: Reynolds RD, Leklem JE (eds). Vitamin B-6: Its Role in Health and Disease. Alan R Liss Inc., New York, pp. 337–346.

Chapter 22

Assessment of the status of folate and vitamin B-12

Deficiencies of the two related vitamins folic acid and vitamin B-12 cause megaloblastic anemia, an anemia characterized by abnormally large red-cell precursors (megaloblasts) in the bone marrow and larger than normal mature red cells (macrocytic cells) in the peripheral blood. These abnormalities in cell morphology arise because both vitamin B-12 and folic acid are involved in deoxyribonucleic acid (DNA) synthesis. Interference with DNA synthesis induces abnormal cell replication. Unlike folic acid, vitamin B-12 is also involved in synthesis of myelin in the nervous system, and hence B-12 deficiency may produce neurological disorders such as neuropathy and spinal cord dysfunction. In contrast to the hematological defects, these neurological abnormalities may not be reversible (Hughes-Jones, 1984).

Folate deficiency develops more rapidly than vitamin B-12 deficiency, because of differences in turnover rates. Inadequate dietary intake is a major factor associated with folate deficiency. In contrast, the amount of vitamin B-12 in omnivorous diets usually greatly exceeds the estimated daily requirements. Instead, vitamin B-12 deficiency is generally caused by defects in absorption or by a failure to secrete the gastric intrinsic factor necessary for the absorption of vitamin B-12.

Diagnosis of megaloblastic anemia can be confirmed by the presence of macro-ovalocytic erythrocytes in a peripheral blood film and megaloblasts in the bone marrow. It is essential to ascertain whether the megaloblastic anemia results from folic acid or vitamin B-12 deficiency by using biochemical assessment techniques. These techniques are discussed in the following sections.

22.1 Assessment of folate status

'Folate' is the term used as a generic descriptor for folic acid (pteroyl-monoglutamic acid) and related compounds which exhibit the biological

461

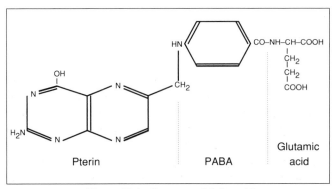

Figure 22.1: Structure of folic acid.

activity of folic acid. The pteroylmonoglutamic acid (PGA) molecule consists of a pteridine nucleus linked through a methylene bridge to para-aminobenzoic acid (PABA), and L-glutamic acid (Figure 22.1).

Folates are widely distributed in food, especially in liver, yeast, leafy vegetables, fruits, pulses, and nuts (Hoppner et al., 1972). Folates exist primarily in food as polyglutamates which contain from two to seven glutamate molecules linked in the form of a γ-polypeptide chain to PABA. The nutritional activity of these polyglutamates remains intact as long as the essential subunit structure of PGA is not broken. Heat, air, and ultraviolet light, cleave PGA, making it inactive (Herbert, 1987a). Consequently, diets based on thoroughly cooked foods are generally low in folate.

On average, approximately 70% of folate monoglutamates and 50% of folate polyglutamates are absorbed (Halsted, 1979). Absorption takes place primarily from the proximal third of the small intestine, and is by an active process. Before absorption, the polyglutamate forms of folate are deconjugated to the monoglutamate form by the enzyme pteroylpolyglutamate hydrolase (conjugase) on the luminal brush border. These monoglutamates are then taken up by the mucosal cells (Steinberg, 1984). Absorbed monoglutamates are then transported to the liver and peripheral tissues where the polyglutamyl coenzyme is resynthesized. Approximately half the body folate stores are in the liver (5 to 10 mg on average).

Folates function as coenzymes in their active form when they are involved in the transfer of single-carbon atom groups [e.g. formyl (CHO), methyl (CH_3), and formimino (CH=NH)], in amino-acid metabolism, and in purine and pyrimidine synthesis for the formation of nucleic acids (Blakley, 1977). As rapidly proliferating cells are especially sensitive to abnormalities in DNA synthesis, clinical manifestations of folate deficiency first appear in the hematopoietic system, and then in the epithelial cell surfaces and the gonads. Thus, one of the earliest signs of folate deficiency in humans is hypersegmentation of neutrophils, first in the bone marrow, and then in the peripheral blood. This is eventually followed by macrocytosis of the erythrocytes. Additional signs and symptoms associated with clinical folate deficiency include fatigue, anorexia, insomnia, glossitis, angular cheilosis, recurrent aphthous ulcers, and pallor of the skin and mucous membranes (Herbert, 1962; Waxman, 1973).

The prevalence of megaloblastic anemia resulting from primary folate deficiency is particularly high in pregnant and lactating women in developing countries such as India, where dietary intakes may be inadequate to meet their high requirements (Colman, 1977). Marginal folate status has also been reported in pregnant and lactating women from the United States (Bailey et al., 1980), in elderly persons (Wagner et al., 1981; Rosenberg et al., 1982), and adolescents of low socio-economic status (Bailey et al., 1982). In Canada, probably 5% to 10% of adults may be at moderate risk for folate deficiency; severe deficiency is uncommon (Beaton, 1981).

Secondary folate deficiency may also occur in association with a variety of conditions including malabsorption, some inborn errors of metabolism, alcoholism, and renal dialysis (Colman, 1977). Drugs such as the antimalarial drug pyrimethamine, and possibly some anticonvulsants, interfere with the metabolism of folate, whereas others apparently affect its absorption (e.g. sulfasalazine, aspirin, and perhaps cholestyramine). The effect of drugs such as oral contraceptive agents on folate status is uncertain (Martinez and Roe, 1977; Rhode et al., 1983). Some data suggest that suboptimal folate status during the periconceptual period may be associated with decreased birth weights (Baumslag et al., 1970) and a higher rate of occurrence of neural tube defects in infants (Laurence et al., 1981; Smithells et al., 1981; 1983). These later findings, however, require confirmation.

Generally, consumption of excess folate has not been accompanied by any adverse reactions and folate is considered to be a nontoxic vitamin (Preuss, 1978). Nevertheless, some (Milne et al., 1984), but not all (Keating et al., 1987), recent observations suggest that oral folate supplements may interfere with zinc absorption. Sleep, gastrointestinal disturbances, and behavioral changes were also reported in adults taking 15 mg folic acid daily for one month (Hunter et al., 1970), but not confirmed in a later double blind study (Hellström, 1971). Several methods are available for assessing the folate status of individuals and these are discussed in the following sections.

22.1.1 Red cell indices

The abnormal morphological changes in the peripheral blood and bone marrow are identical in folate and vitamin B-12 deficiency and occur when anemia is already apparent. They represent the final stages of chronic folate or vitamin B-12 deficiency. These abnormalities cannot be used to differentiate between these two vitamin deficiencies, but, if present, simply confirm megaloblastic anemia.

Macrocytosis can be tentatively diagnosed by identifying abnormally large red cells in a peripheral blood smear. Diagnosis is then confirmed by the presence of an elevated mean cell volume (MCV) (Section 17.3.1) and mean cell hemoglobin (MCH) (Section 17.3.3). Generally, if these tests are positive, a bone marrow biopsy is performed to ascertain whether megaloblasts exist in the bone marrow.

Macro-ovalocytic erythrocytes always occur when the anemia is severe, but their absence does not preclude folate deficiency (Giles, 1966). If megaloblastic anemia is confirmed, additional tests must be used to differentiate folate from vitamin B-12 deficiency. These tests are also used to estimate the prevalence of subclinical folate or vitamin B-12 deficiency states.

22.1.2   Serum folate concentrations

No polyglutamates are present in serum. The main folate derivative in serum is the reduced form — methyltetrahydrofolate. Serum folate concentrations fluctuate rapidly with recent changes in folate intakes and with temporary changes in folate metabolism, even when body stores remain stable. For example, serum folate values increase rapidly after the ingestion of folate-containing foods and supplements (Cooper and Lowenstein, 1964), and decrease rapidly on a folate-deficient diet, stabilizing at values below 3 ng/mL after only two to three weeks of negative folate balance (Herbert, 1962). Hence, serum folate levels reflect acute folate status but provide no information on the size of the folate tissue stores (Herbert, 1987b). If low serum folate values persist for more than a month, folate stores may be gradually reduced, resulting in a state of folate depletion. The latter is characterized by a fall in erythrocyte and liver folate concentrations (Herbert, 1987b,c). Abnormal hematological changes do not occur until after three to four months of folate deprivation. Most individuals with megaloblastic changes resulting from folate deficiency have low serum folate levels, but exceptions do occur. In vitamin B-12 deficiency uncomplicated by folate deficiency, serum folate levels are normal or raised.

Several non-nutritional factors affect serum folate concentrations. Alcohol ingestion results in an acute drop in serum folate levels, because reabsorption of folate is impaired by alcohol (Hillman et al., 1977). Hemolysis may produce misleadingly elevated serum folate values as the folate content of erythrocytes is much higher than plasma. Raised serum folate values have also been reported in patients with stagnant-loop syndrome, acute renal failure, and with active liver damage. Some (Martinez and

	Males		Females	
Age	No. of examined persons	% with low values	No. of examined persons	% with low values
6 mo–9 yr	294	2 ± 1.4	240	3 ± 2.1
10–19 yr	204	3 ± 1.3	210	12 ± 3.1
20–44 yr	362	18 ± 2.8	462	15 ± 3.1
45–74 yr	606	10 ± 2.5	532	9 ± 2.6

Table 22.1: Percentage of persons aged six months through seventy-four years with serum folate values < 3.0 ng/mL, by age and sex: NHANES II, 1976–1980. Value after the ± is the SEM of the percent. From Senti and Pilch (1985).

Roe, 1977), but not all (Rhode et al., 1983), investigators have reported low serum folate values in women taking oral contraceptives. Smoking lowers serum folate concentrations via its enhancing effect on erythropoiesis, which, in turn, increases folate requirements. In the NHANES II survey, significantly more women smokers had low serum folate concentrations (< 3.0 ng/mL; < 6.8 nmol/L) compared to nonsmoking women (Senti and Pilch, 1985).

Age-related trends in serum folate levels were documented in the NHANES II survey and are shown in Table 22.1. Percentages of persons in the NHANES II survey with low serum folate levels (i.e. < 3.0 ng/mL; < 6.8 nmol/L) were lowest in children aged six months to nine years (2%), followed by males aged ten to nineteen years (3%), and females aged forty-five to seventy-four years (9%) (Senti and Pilch, 1985).

The low prevalence of low serum folate levels may result from the consumption of folate-fortified infant formulas and breakfast cereals. Certainly, similar age-related trends during childhood were not observed in the Nutrition Canada Survey (Health and Welfare Canada, 1973), conducted at a time when folate was not added to breakfast cereals. Alternatively, age-related changes in folate metabolism may account for some of the trends observed (Senti and Pilch, 1985).

The interpretive guidelines (Table 22.3) are based on a comparison of serum folate concentrations with normal subjects and those with folate-deficient megaloblastic anemia (Herbert, 1964; WHO, 1972; Sauberlich, 1977). The most common cutoff point used for low serum folate concentrations is < 3 ng/mL (< 6.8 nmol/L) (Herbert, 1967; Sauberlich et al., 1974; Senti and Pilch, 1985). In the NHANES II survey, 18% of males and 15% of females aged twenty to forty-four years had serum folate concentrations below 3 ng/mL (Senti and Pilch, 1985). This level is now known to be indicative of negative folate balance, but not necessarily folate depletion, unless the negative balance persists (Herbert, 1987b,c). Hence, individuals may have normal biochemical function, and no evidence of tissue folate depletion, despite serum folate concentrations below this cutoff point. Methods of analysis for serum folate are discussed at the end of the following section.

22.1.3 Erythrocyte folate concentrations

Erythrocyte folate concentrations are less sensitive to short-term fluctuations in folate status than serum folate levels, and decrease only after several months of folate deprivation (Herbert, 1967). They correlate with liver folate levels (Wu et al., 1975) and reflect body folate stores. Consequently, erythrocyte folate concentrations are a more reliable index of folate status than serum folate and should be used in population studies to estimate the prevalence of subjects with depleted folate stores (Senti and Pilch, 1985). The latter are characterized by erythrocyte folate concentrations below 160 ng/mL (368 nmol/L). No evidence of biochemical or clinical impairment is evident at this stage.

When erythrocyte folate levels are below 120 ng/mL (280 nmol/L), biochemical function is affected, as indicated by an abnormal deoxyuridine (dU) suppression test, first in the bone marrow cells, and later in peripheral blood lymphocytes (Section 22.2.2). Hypersegmented neutrophils are also present at this stage, again at first in the bone marrow, and then in the peripheral blood (Section 22.1.5) (Herbert, 1987c). These changes characterize the second stage of folate depletion, folate-deficient erythropoiesis, sometimes referred to as 'subclinical' deficiency. There is no evidence of folate-deficiency anemia at this stage. The latter only occurs when erythrocyte folate values are less than 100 ng/mL (227 nmol/L), at which time liver folate concentrations are generally less than 1 μg/g (2.3 nmol/g). This is known as the third stage of folate depletion (folate-deficiency anemia), and is characterized by the appearance of macro-ovalocytic erythrocytes and a hemoglobin level below 13 g/dL (130 g/L) in men and below 12 g/dL (120 g/L) in women (Herbert, 1987c). Nearly all persons with folate-deficiency anemia have *low* erythrocyte (and serum) folate concentrations.

Low erythrocyte folate concentrations are not specific for folate deficiency. Low concentrations also occur in vitamin B-12 deficiency (Hoffbrand et al., 1966), although serum folate levels are normal or even raised. Hence to identify folate deficiency, both erythrocyte folate and serum vitamin B-12 concentrations should be measured. Secondary folate deficiency occurs in vitamin B-12 deficiency because vitamin B-12 is involved in the transport and storage of folate in cells (Cooper and Lowenstein, 1964; Herbert, 1964).

The interpretation of erythrocyte folate values is also confounded by the presence of other disease states. If patients have a raised reticulocyte count (e.g. when hemorrhage or hemolytic anemia is present), erythrocyte folate concentrations increase because reticulocytes tend to have higher

Sex and Age	Erythrocyte Folate		Serum Folate and Erythrocyte Folate	
	No. of examined persons	% with low values	No. of examined persons	% with low values
Male				
6 mo–9 yr	243	2 ± 1.6	241	2 ± 1.6
10–19 yr	178	5 ± 2.2	177	2 ± 1.1
20–44 yr	299	8 ± 2.5	298	5 ± 2.3
45–74 yr	503	8 ± 2.0	503	3 ± 1.2
Females				
6 mo–9 yr	201	2 ± 1.5	200	2 ± 1.5
10–19 yr	173	8 ± 2.8	173	2 ± 0.9
20–44 yr	389	13 ± 2.4	388	6 ± 2.3
45–74 yr	439	4 ± 0.8	439	2 ± 0.9

Table 22.2: Percentage of persons aged six months through seventy-four years with erythrocyte folate < 140 ng/mL, and with both low erythrocyte and low serum folate values < 3.0 ng/mL, by age and sex: NHANES II, 1976–1980. Value after the $\pm$ is the SEM of the percent. Conversion factor to SI units (nmol/L) = $\times$ 2.266. From Senti and Pilch (1985).

folate concentrations than older cells (Hoffbrand et al., 1966). Erythrocyte (and serum) folate values may also increase in iron deficiency (Omer et al., 1970a), although the magnitude of this effect, and the reason, is unknown. In such cases, a hidden folate deficiency may be present, as indicated by an abnormal deoxyuridine suppression test (Section 22.2.2) and hypersegmentation in the peripheral blood (Section 22.1.5) (Herbert, 1985; Herbert, 1987b,c).

Age-related trends in erythrocyte folate levels, comparable to those noted for serum folate, were observed in the NHANES II survey (Senti and Pilch, 1985) (Table 22.2). Median erythrocyte folate concentrations were relatively high for infants and young children, but declined in later childhood and adolescence. In females, pregnancy, oral contraceptive use, parity, and smoking tended to be associated with lower erythrocyte folate concentrations. In adults in the NHANES II survey, only 8% of the males and 13% of the females had erythrocyte folate concentrations below 140 ng/mL (322 nmol/L) (Senti and Pilch, 1985).

Cutoff points for classifying erythrocyte folate levels are based on data from subjects with biochemical and clinical manifestations associated with varying degrees of folate deficiency (Senti and Pilch, 1985). In the NHANES II survey, erythrocyte values between 140 and 160 ng/mL (322 and 368 nmol/L) were assumed to be low and suggestive of an individual at risk, whereas an erythrocyte concentration below a cutoff point of 140 ng/mL was selected as indicative of a deficiency; a summary appears

Folate Measurement	Deficient	Borderline	Acceptable
Serum (ng/mL)	< 3.0	3.0–6.0	> 6.0
Erythrocyte (ng/mL)	< 140	140–160	> 160

Table 22.3: Guidelines for the interpretation of folate concentrations. Conversion factor to SI units (nmol/L) = × 2.266. From Wagner C. (1984). Folic acid. In: Present Knowledge in Nutrition. Fifth edition. The Nutrition Foundation Inc., with permission.

in Table 22.3. This latter cutoff point has also been used in several other studies of folate status (Bailey et al., 1982; Bindra et al., 1987). Herbert (1987b,c) suggested that concentrations of less than 160 ng/mL (368 nmol/L) indicate a state of folate depletion, at which stage there is no evidence of biochemical or clinical functional deficit. Concentrations below a cutoff point of less than 120 ng/mL (280 nmol/L) indicate the second stage in the development of folate deficiency, known as folate-deficient erythropoiesis, when abnormal biochemical function (i.e. an abnormal dU suppression test (Section 22.2.2) and morphological defects in the peripheral blood (i.e. hypersegmented neutrophils) (Section 22.1.5) are apparent. Folate-deficiency anemia, as indicated by changes in red cell indices (Section 22.1.1), only occurs when erythrocyte folate concentrations fall to less than 100 ng/mL (227 nmol/L) (Herbert, 1987c).

Serum and erythrocyte folate concentrations can be assayed using either microbiological or radioisotope dilution techniques (Waddell et al., 1976). High-performance chromatography techniques have also been developed for the assessment of folate in biological samples (Lankelma et al., 1980) but are not routinely used owing to the large sample size required. The microbiological technique is the standard method for assessing total folate activity in serum, erythrocytes, tissues, and foods. *Lactobacillus casei* is the organism generally used because it responds to the greatest number of different folate derivatives, including those with up to three L-glutamic acid residues (Herbert, 1987a). The microbiological method cannot, however, be used for serum or erythrocyte samples containing antibiotics or methotrexate because these compounds interfere with bacterial growth.

Polyglutamate forms of folate are present in erythrocytes. Hence the hemolysate must first be incubated for a short period prior to the assay to ensure complete hydrolysis to the monoglutamate form by conjugase. In contrast, in serum the folate is unconjugated, making the incubation step unnecessary. The microbiological assay involves adding aliquots of diluted serum or erythrocyte hemolysates to the assay media which contain all the nutrients except folate required for the growth of *L. casei*. The growth response of the organism, estimated by measuring the increase in turbidity of the medium, is then proportional to the folate

Condition	Microbiological Assay	Radioisotope Dilution Assay
Acceptability	Widely accepted for both plasma (or serum) and erythrocyte	Serum values widely accepted
Cost of materials	Low	High
Initial equipment cost	Low	High
Personnel requirement	Must be well trained	Can be trained rapidly
Time and effort needed	24 hr, but few manipulations. Scrupulous attention to detail needed	Several hours, but many manipulations and more time needed to count and calculate data
Interferences	Antibiotics and other bacteriostatic agents invalidate the assay	Not affected by antibiotics. Folate analogues such as MTX interfere.

Table 22.4: A comparison of radioisotope dilution and microbiological assays for the determination of serum and erythrocyte folate concentrations. From Wagner C. (1984). Folic acid. In: Present Knowledge in Nutrition. Fifth edition. The Nutrition Foundation Inc., with permission.

concentration in the serum or red blood cell hemolysate. A number of commercial radioisotope dilution kits are available for measuring folate activity in serum and erythrocytes. The radioisotope dilution technique is rapid and not affected by antibiotics, tranquilizers, and/or antimitotic agents, all of which inhibit the growth of *L. casei*. The NHANES II adopted the Quanta-Count folate kit manufactured by Bio-Rad Laboratories, Richmond, California, USA (Senti and Pilch, 1985). The isotope dilution technique uses a binding protein derived from milk and ^{125}I-labeled folic acid or methyltetrahydrofolate (Waxman et al., 1971). The unlabeled folate present in the diluted serum or red cell hemolysate, competes on mixing with the labeled folate for the available binding sites on the binding protein. Both the unbound labeled and unlabeled folate are adsorbed onto charcoal which is subsequently removed by centrifugation. A sample of the supernatant, which contains the bound labeled folate, is then counted on a scintillation counter. The decrease in the radioactivity is proportional to the folate concentration in the sample.

A number of studies (Table 22.4) have compared radioisotope dilution and microbiological methods for measuring serum and erythrocyte folate

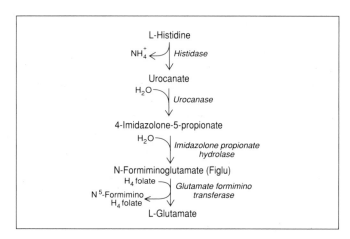

Figure 22.2: Pathway of histidine metabolism.

levels; correlations between results derived from the microbiological and radioisotope dilution assays are not always good. Table 22.4 summarises the findings of these studies (Wagner, 1984).

For both methods, quality control procedures must be rigorous. Samples should be assayed in duplicate and quality control pools included in each analytical run — a procedure adopted in the NHANES II survey (Senti and Pilch, 1985). Simultaneous radioisotope dilution assays for serum folic acid and vitamin B-12 are now available, some of which are semi-automated (Chen et al., 1982). The latter are also available for microbiological assays.

22.1.4   Formiminoglutamate excretion

Normally, histidine is converted to glutamic acid via the action of the enzyme formimino transferase and tetrahydrofolic acid (Figure 22.2). In folate deficiency this conversion is inhibited and, as a result, urinary excretion of formiminoglutamic acid (FIGLU) is increased, particularly if preceded by an oral loading dose of 2 to 15 g of L-histidine. The urine is usually collected over an eight-hour period (Wagner, 1984).

The sensitivity of the FIGLU test for folate deficiency is comparable to that of the erythrocyte folate assay. Unfortunately, the test is not specific to folate deficiency. Deficiency of vitamin B-12, or deficiency of the enzyme formimino transferase, also produces abnormally high urinary excretion of FIGLU after a histidine load. High urinary FIGLU excretion also occurs in patients with both liver and malignant diseases, or tuberculosis, regardless of the folate status (Herbert, 1967). In contrast, FIGLU excretion is normal in kwashiorkor and pregnancy, even when severe folate deficiency is present, and in persons with secondary folate deficiency arising from anticonvulsant drug therapy. The low specificity of the FIGLU test has prevented its widespread use.

Normal levels of FIGLU in urine excreted by folate-replete adults range between 0 and 15 µg/mL, whereas after a histidine load the concentration in urine rises to between 10 and 50 µg/mL (about 5 to 20 mg) in an eight-hour collection. In folate-deficient adults, FIGLU excretion after a histidine load usually exceeds 50 µg/mL.

22.1.5 Polymorphonuclear leukocyte lobe count

Usually, neutrophils have three to four segments, but in megaloblastic anemia, the number increases. Such hypersegmentation of neutrophils in the peripheral blood is a characteristic early feature of folate and vitamin B-12 deficiency, arising from inadequate tissue folate or vitamin B-12 concentrations (Colman, 1981). Hypersegmentation precedes the development of macrocytosis (Herbert, 1962). Unfortunately, no relationship exists between the severity of the megaloblastic anemia and the presence of hypersegmentation (Lindenbaum and Nath, 1980).

Neutrophil hypersegmentation also occurs in other conditions such as uremia, myeloproliferative disorders (e.g. myelogenous leukemia), and myelofibrosis and as a congenital lesion in approximately 1% of the population, even when vitamin B-12 and folate stores are adequate. The occasional cases of hypersegmentation of neutrophils in cases of iron deficiency probably result from the existence of a masked folate deficiency (Das et al., 1978). Neutrophil hypersegmentation is an unreliable index of folate deficiency in pregnancy when there is an underlying tendency to hyposegmentation. Herbert et al. (1975) noted no correlation between serum or erythrocyte folate concentrations and neutrophil lobe counts during pregnancy.

Neutrophil hypersegmentation can be evaluated in smears of peripheral blood, or in cells from the layer of white blood cells obtained at the interface of serum or plasma and the sedimented red cells (buffy coat). Several evaluation techniques are used, such as calculating the average number of lobes per neutrophil or the percentage of cells with five or more lobes. Abnormal hypersegmentation is taken when a lobe average of 3.5 lobes or more per cell is found, or when 5% or more of the cells have five or more lobes (Colman, 1981). Such methods are very time consuming. A more practical and less time-consuming approach involves examining smears for the existence of any six-lobed cells within a random sample of 100 cells. Six-lobed cells are a consistent feature of smears in nearly all persons with megaloblastic anemia (Lindenbaum and Nath, 1980). For persons with concomitant iron and folate deficiency, evaluation of neutrophil hypersegmentation is especially useful because it occurs even when macrocytosis is masked by a co-existing iron deficiency (Das and Herbert, 1978).

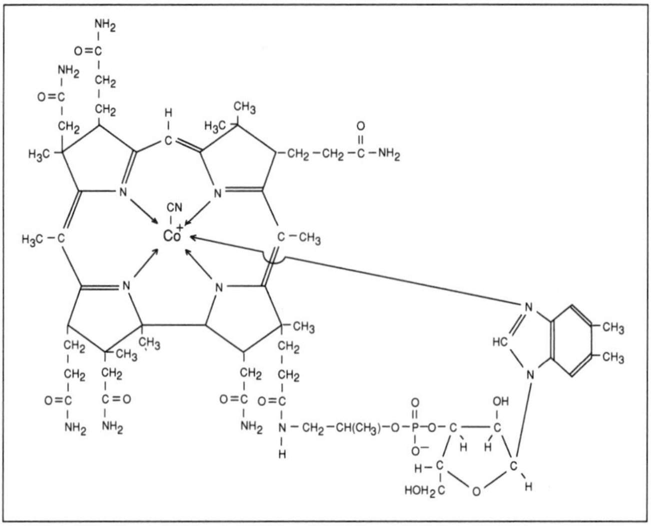

Figure 22.3: Structure of cyanocobalamin.

22.2 Assessment of vitamin B-12 status

The term 'vitamin B-12' is a generic descriptor for all corrinoids which exhibit the biological activity of cyanocobalamin. The latter was first isolated in the crystalline form in 1948 (Rickes et al., 1948; Smith, 1948). The cyanocobalamin molecule is made up of a planar group, consisting of a corrin ring with a cobalt atom at the center and a nucleotide set at right angles to the corrin ring (Figure 22.3). The nucleotide is made up of the base, 5,6-dimethylbenzimidazole, and a phosphorylated sugar (ribose-3-phosphate).

In nature, vitamin B-12 is produced almost entirely by bacterial synthesis. In the human this synthesis takes place in the colon and small intestine, although probably only the vitamin B-12 synthesized in the small intestine is absorbed (Albert et al., 1980). Plant products contain no vitamin B-12 unless they are contaminated by bacteria. The richest food sources of vitamin B-12 are the organ meats of liver and kidney. The vitamin is also found in shellfish, muscle meats, fish, and chicken; lesser amounts are found in dairy products (Gimsing and Nexø, 1983). Vitamin B-12 is fairly stable and not usually destroyed by cooking, although in an alkaline pH some loss may occur.

The main body storage site for vitamin B-12 is the liver; total body stores in healthy omnivorous subjects are about 2 to 4 mg. Loss of vitamin B-12 takes place via desquamation of epithelium and through excretion in the bile. Adult losses approximate 1 to 3 μg (about 0.1% of body stores) each day (Hughes-Jones, 1984). Absorption of vitamin B-12 takes place through receptor sites in the ileum, in the presence of an alkaline pH and calcium, and is mediated by a gastric intrinsic factor. The latter is a highly specific binding glycoprotein of molecular weight 45,000 to 60,000, which is synthesized and secreted by the parietal cells of the gastric mucosa. Absorption of small amounts of vitamin B-12 (generally 1% to 3% in normal diets) may also occur by simple diffusion (Herbert, 1987a).

There are two naturally occurring cobalamin-containing coenzymes: methylcobalamin, the main form in plasma, and 5'-deoxyadenosyl cobalamin, found in the liver, most body tissues, and foods. In humans, these coenzymes function in the folate-dependent methylation of homocysteine to methionine and in the conversion of methylmalonyl-coenzyme A to succinyl-coenzyme A. The latter is a common pathway for the degradation of certain amino acids and odd-chain fatty acids. Vitamin B-12 also has a link with nucleic acid metabolism via its role in the conversion of methyltetrahydrofolate to tetrahydrofolate. Consequently, deficiency of vitamin B-12, like folic acid, impairs the production of tetrahydrofolate, which is required for thymidine and thus DNA synthesis. Impaired DNA synthesis is responsible for the megaloblastic bone marrow, a characteristic of both vitamin B-12 and folic acid deficiencies. The role of cobalamin-containing coenzymes in the conversion of methylmalonyl-coenzyme A to succinyl-coenzyme A is probably associated with the neurological defects which may arise in vitamin B-12 deficiency, as well as in the accumulation of methylmalonic acid in the urine.

Clinical manifestations of vitamin B-12 deficiency occur in the hematopoietic, gastrointestinal, and neurological systems. Disturbances of the hematopoietic system include megaloblastic anemia whereas in the gastrointestinal tract, atrophic glossitis, papillary atrophy of the tongue, and sometimes diarrhea occur. Neuropathy and spinal cord dysfunction are now rarely seen because vitamin B-12 deficiency is usually diagnosed before the onset of these neurological disorders.

Dietary deficiency of vitamin B-12 is relatively rare and deficiency usually results from malabsorption. The latter accounts for >95% of the vitamin B-12 deficiency cases documented in the United States (Herbert, 1984). Nevertheless, nutritional deficiency has been described in persons adhering to diets which exclude animal products (Rose, 1976). Some infants, born to severely vitamin-B-12-deficient mothers, have also developed vitamin-B-12-responsive megaloblastic anemia at three to six months of age (Higginbottom et al., 1978).

A variety of disease states may cause malabsorption of vitamin B-12, and thus secondary vitamin B-12 deficiency. For example, in patients with pernicious anemia and gastrectomy, malabsorption of vitamin B-12 may result from a lack of intrinsic factor. Megaloblastic anemia may not appear until a long period after total gastrectomy (i.e. five to ten years), because of the capacity of the body to reutilize the vitamin. In subjects with intestinal lesions such as jejunal diverticulosis or anatomical abnormalities (e.g. fistulas and blind-loops), vitamin B-12 deficiency may develop because bacteria in the colon competitively utilize all the available vitamin B-12 (Cooke et al., 1963). Fish tape worm (*Diphyllobothriumlatum*) also sequesters vitamin B-12 and was a well-recognized cause of vitamin B-12 deficiency in Finland. Patients with tropical and nontropical (gluten-sensitive) sprue and regional ileitis may also develop vitamin B-12 deficiency, because of alterations in the brush border structure of the ileal mucosa, which contains the receptor for intrinsic factor. Some drugs, including para-aminosalicylic acid, colchicine, and excessive alcohol, also cause malabsorption of vitamin B-12, although the specific mechanisms are unclear (Hoffbrand, 1981).

Biochemical methods for assessing vitamin B-12 status are given below, together with tests for determining the cause of the vitamin B-12 deficiency.

22.2.1 Serum and erythrocyte vitamin B-12 concentrations

Of the vitamin B-12 in the serum, 20% is attached to the transport protein transcobalamin (TC) II and the remaining 80% is a mixture of glycoprotein B-12 binders, designated as TC I and TC III. The latter are mixtures of the same isoproteins, known collectively as haptocorrins or cobalophilins (Dolphin, 1982). Their function has not been clearly established. Human serum also contains a variable quantity of nonfunctional analogs of vitamin B-12. In early vitamin B-12 deficiency, when a negative balance exists, the amount of vitamin B-12 on the transport protein TC II falls with no concomitant decline in total serum vitamin B-12 concentrations. The latter decline only occurs when the percentage saturation of total TC II with vitamin B-12 falls to less than 5% (Herbert, 1987b). In the future, it may be possible to diagnose negative vitamin B-12 balance by measuring holo TC II levels in serum. Reduced percentage saturation of serum TC II may be the earliest index of developing vitamin B-12 deficiency (i.e. negative balance) (Herbert, 1985). If the negative balance persists, vitamin B-12 depletion will occur, as indicated by a fall in serum vitamin B-12 concentrations to values between 150 to 100 pg/mL; biochemical function, however, is normal (Table 22.6).

Assay of total serum vitamin B-12 is the normal routine biochemical test of vitamin B-12 status. In general, total serum vitamin B-12 concentrations reflect the liver vitamin B-12 content only when the latter falls below 0.6 µg/g (normal range = 0.6 to 1.5 µg/g wet weight). Moderately low values for serum vitamin B-12 (i.e. values between 150 and 200 pg/mL; 111 to 148 pmol/L) are not specific for vitamin B-12 deficiency; they sometimes occur in iron deficiency (Layrisse et al., 1959), in some patients with multiple myeloma (Hansen and Drivsholm, 1977), or megaloblastic anemia produced by folate deficiency. In pregnancy, vitamin B-12 is rapidly transferred to the fetal circulation, lowering the vitamin B-12 concentration in the maternal blood (Cooper, 1973). Very low serum vitamin B-12 concentrations, however, (i.e. below 100 to 80 pg/mL; 74 to 59 pmol/L) are almost always indicative of a vitamin B-12 deficiency state. At such low levels, biochemical function is affected, as indicated by an abnormal deoxyuridine suppression test (Section 22.2.2), and/or hypersegmented neutrophils (Section 22.1.5). Sometimes a clinical deficiency state, characterized by the appearance of macro-ovalocytic erythrocytes and a low hemoglobin level, also occurs.

Conversely, misleadingly normal or elevated serum vitamin B-12 concentrations occur in patients with myeloproliferative disorders and severe liver diseases, despite low tissue vitamin B-12 concentrations Such misleading levels are caused by an increase in the amounts of unsaturated TC I and TC III (Begley and Hall, 1975). Children with hereditary disorders of vitamin B-12 metabolism or transport will also have normal serum vitamin B-12 concentrations.

Each laboratory that analyzes serum vitamin B-12 should establish its own range of results for healthy persons, and those with vitamin B-12 deficiency, for its own assay method. In general, serum vitamin B-12 concentrations in normal healthy persons range from 200 to 900 pg/mL (148 to 682 pmol/L). According to Carmel and Herbert (1969), values below 100 pg/mL (74 pmol/L) almost always indicate a vitamin B-12 deficiency state and are associated with megaloblastic anemia, irrespective of the assay procedure, except in rare cases of transcobalamin I deficiency. The recent WHO Scientific Group on Nutritional Anemias (FAO/WHO Expert Group, 1988), however, recommended using a cutoff point below 80 pg/mL (59 pmol/L) as indicative of vitamin B-12 deficiency. Serum vitamin B-12 concentrations tend to decrease with age, perhaps a reflection of the increased incidence of gastritis with age (Doscherholmen et al., 1977). Healthy female adults appear to have higher serum vitamin B-12 concentrations than males (Fernandes-Costa et al., 1985).

Methodological problems may complicate the assay of serum vitamin B-12 levels. Normally, radioisotope dilution methods give higher results than the microbiological assays in which nonfunctional analogs of vitamin B-12 are poorly utilized (Dawson et al., 1980). The micro-organisms *Lactobacillus leichmanii, Euglena gracilis,* or *Ochromonas malhamensis* are used; all have relatively specific requirements for vitamin B-12 for growth and reproduction (Herbert et al., 1984).

The microbiological assay is based on the same principle as that for the analysis of serum or erythrocyte folate (Section 22.1.3) and has comparable limitations. For example, bacteriostatic substances in the blood, such as antibiotics or cancer chemotherapeutic agents, inhibit the growth of the micro-organism and interfere with the assay producing misleadingly low serum vitamin B-12 concentrations. Furthermore, long incubation times are necessary, making the procedure time consuming. In contrast, radioisotope dilution methods are very simple, less time consuming, and are not affected by antibiotics or cancer chemotherapeutic agents. The isotopic methods depend on the addition of radioactive cyanocobalamin which competes with serum vitamin B-12 for binding sites on an added cobalamin-binding protein. The latter may be pure intrinsic factor or impure intrinsic factor with its nonintrinsic factor blocked by a nonfunctional analog of vitamin B-12. By using one of these binding proteins, *true* B-12 rather than total B-12 (i.e. cobalamins plus noncobalamin analogs) is measured. This distinction is critical because in early vitamin B-12 deficiency, only that portion of total B-12 that is true B-12 may fall, whereas the vitamin B-12 analog levels may even rise. Most commercial radioassays available now utilize these two cobalamin-binding proteins. Herbert et al. (1984) concluded, however, that use of these two binding proteins is not essential, provided that each laboratory establishes its own range of results for the particular assay used, for healthy and vitamin-B-12-deficient subjects. Radioassays which measure serum folic acid and vitamin B-12 simultaneously are also available (Gutcho and Mansbach, 1977). Some of these radioassays can be semi-automated (Chen et al., 1982).

The use of erythrocyte assays for vitamin B-12 appears limited; variable results have been obtained, with a large overlap in values for normal and vitamin-B-12-deficient subjects (Omer et al., 1970b). Moreover, erythrocyte vitamin B-12 concentrations also tend to be low in folate deficiency (Harrison, 1971) because vitamin B-12 is necessary for the uptake of folate by red blood cells.

22.2.2 Deoxyuridine suppression test

This sensitive *in vitro* test is used to detect folate-deficient and/or vitamin-B-12-deficient erythropoiesis (Wickramasinghe and Longland, 1974; Herbert, 1987c) and was developed by Metz et al. (1968). Normal folate metabolism is necessary for methylation of deoxyuridine (dU) to thymidine. Therefore, in the presence of folate and/or vitamin B-12 deficiency, the incorporation of dU into bone marrow cells *in vitro* is impaired (Killmann, 1964). Bone marrow cells were originally used, limiting the test to clinical and research settings. The test has been modified, however, for use with lymphocytes (Das and Herbert, 1978) or whole blood (0.1 mL) (Das et al., 1980). Use of lymphocytes, although very time consuming, provides a measure of chronic folic acid or vitamin B-12 status rather than the acute status measured using bone marrow cells (Colman and Herbert, 1980). In cases of iron deficiency concurrent with folic acid or vitamin B-12 deficiency, an abnormal dU suppression test is evident first in the lymphocytes, and only later in the bone marrow cells (Das et al., 1978).

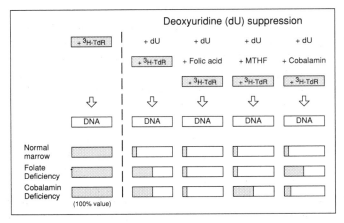

Figure 22.4: Deoxyuridine suppression test. Hatched bars represent ³H-thymidine (³H-TdR) radioactivity; results are expressed in percentage radioactivity incorporated into DNA, as compared with baseline 100% in the first column. The second column illustrates the normal value of < 10% as compared with values of > 20% in deficiency. Folate-deficient marrow is not corrected by cobalamin (column 5), whereas cobalamin-deficient marrow is not corrected by methyltetrahydrofolate (MTHF in column 4). For unexplained reasons, cobalamin-deficient marrow is always corrected more completely by folic acid than by cobalamin. From Carmel R (1983). Clinical and laboratory features of the diagnosis of megaloblastic anemia. In: Lindenbaum J (ed). Nutrition in Hematology. Churchill Livingstone Inc., by permission.

For the dU suppression test, normal bone marrow cells (or lymphocytes) are first pre-incubated with nonradioactive dU. The latter suppresses the ability of the marrow cells to incorporate subsequently added radioactive thymidine (³H-thymidine) into DNA. This suppression is reduced in patients with vitamin B-12 or folate deficiency (Herbert et al., 1973), and results in increased incorporation of the ³H-thymidine into DNA. For the test, pairs of bone marrow cultures, one with and one without nonradioactive dU, are pre-incubated prior to the addition of ³H-thymidine. The uptake of ³H-thymidine radioactivity for each culture is then counted on a scintillation counter and the results expressed as a percentage of the uptake without pre-incubation with dU. This percentage is called the 'dU-suppressed value'.

Elevated dU-suppression values (i.e. > 20%) will occur in both folate and vitamin-B-12-deficient bone marrow cultures (Figure 22.4). The test can be modified to distinguish between folate and vitamin B-12 deficiencies, by adding cobalamin or methyltetrahydrofolate to the bone marrow cultures (Figure 22.4). The uptake of ³H-thymidine radioactivity is then compared in the absence or presence of the *in vitro* addition of cobalamin or methyltetrahydrofolate (Wickramasinghe and Longland, 1974; Carmel, 1983). In this way, the vitamin which corrects the deficiency can be identified. This modification is especially useful in diagnosing early folate and vitamin B-12 deficiency before anemia is present (Wickramasinghe and Saunders, 1975; Das and Herbert, 1978). It is also used to diagnose vitamin B-12 and folate deficiency in the presence of concomitant iron deficiency, liver disease, myeloproliferative disorder, or hemoglobinopathy. Although these conditions do not confound the results of the dU suppression test, they may result in normal erythrocyte and serum folate and/or serum vitamin B-12 concentrations, despite the presence of vitamin B-12 and folate deficiency.

22.2.3 Methylmalonic acid excretion

Vitamin B-12 is required for normal methylmalonate metabolism. In vitamin B-12 deficiency, urinary excretion of methylmalonic acid is increased, and methylmalonic aciduria occurs (Cox and White, 1962). Folic acid is not involved in this pathway. Only rare congenital enzyme defects (e.g. methylmalonic aciduria) interfere with this test. The sensitivity of the test can be improved by administering a loading dose of L-valine (5 to 10 g) or isoleucine, precursors of methylmalonic acid. In normal subjects, 1.5 to 2 mg of methylmalonic acid is excreted per twenty-four hours, whereas in patients with vitamin B-12 deficiency, more than 300 mg per twenty-four hours may be excreted. The level of methylmalonic acid excretion is not necessarily related to the severity of the vitamin B-12 deficiency.

Gas-liquid chromatography is the most sensitive and reliable method for measuring methylmalonic acid (Cox and White, 1962). Unfortunately, this test is technically difficult, time-consuming, and requires twenty-four-hour urine samples. As a result, its use as a practical index of vitamin B-12 status in population studies is limited.

22.2.4 The Schilling and other tests for the cause of vitamin B-12 deficiency

Once vitamin B-12 deficiency has been diagnosed, it is essential to establish if malabsorption is the cause. This can be achieved by determining the absorption of a small oral dose (0.5 to 2 µg) of vitamin B-12 in the fasting state, often by measuring urinary excretion. This procedure is called the Schilling test (Schilling, 1953). For the test, a large flushing dose (1000 µg) of nonradioactive vitamin B-12 is administered parenterally one hour after the oral administration of radioactive B-12 (labeled with ^{57}Co or ^{58}Co) to the fasting patient. The purpose of the flushing dose is to saturate both tissue binding stores and circulating B-12 binding protein, and hence enhance the urinary excretion of the absorbed radioactive vitamin B-12. Most of the radioactivity appears in the urine within the first twenty-four hours when renal function is normal, but it is delayed with renal insufficiency. Hence urine should be collected preferably for a forty-eight-hour period. In patients with per-nicious anemia, generally less than 3.0% of the administered dose is excreted in the urine compared to more than 8.0% in normal healthy subjects.

If the results are abnormal, the test is generally repeated two to three days later, but with the addition of a commercial preparation of intrinsic factor with the oral radioactive dose. The urinary excretion should then be restored to near normal values if the low B-12 absorption arises from intrinsic factor deficiency. If, however, the vitamin B-12 deficiency is associated with intestinal disease or infestation with fish tapeworm, the test results will not be normalized by the addition of intrinsic factor. In such circumstances, further investigations must be undertaken.

Both stages of the Schilling test can be performed simultaneously, eliminating the two- to three-day delay and permitting a diagnosis of pernicious anemia even when urine collections are incomplete. The reliability of this combined method, however, has been questioned (Domstad et al., 1981). A further modification of this test, called the 'food Schilling test', involves using radioactive B-12 incorporated into foods such as eggs, chicken or egg albumin. In this way, the ability to absorb vitamin B-12 bound to food, rather than crystalline vitamin B-12, can be assessed. This approach is important for use with the elderly. A conventional Schilling test may appear normal in this age group, despite the existence of low serum vitamin B-12 concentrations, because they have adequate intrinsic factor to absorb free crystalline vitamin B-12, but not vitamin B-12 in foods (Doscherholmen et al., 1976).

Unfortunately, the Schilling test is not well standardized among lab-oratories; the timing of the flushing dose of vitamin B-12, the level of the isotope dose, and the duration of the urine collection may all vary (Chanarin and Waters, 1974). Furthermore, the flushing dose of parenterally administered vitamin B-12 is therapeutic and may subse-quently interfere with the diagnosis. As a result, alternative techniques which do not necessitate a flushing dose have been developed. These include measurement of plasma radioactivity, stool excretion, hepatic radioactivity, or whole body counting (one week post dose). Such methods are not widely used because they require specialized equip-ment. It is also necessary in the whole body counting and the stool excretion tests to ensure complete excretion of unabsorbed vita-min B-12.

In the future, screening tests for detecting early pernicious anemia may include radio-immunoassays for the presence of the intrinsic factor antibody in serum, saliva, or gastric juice (Gottlieb et al., 1965; Her-bert, 1985), or for detecting intrinsic factor in human urine (Grásbeck et al., 1966).

	Normal	Negative Folate Balance	Folate Depletion	Folate Deficient Erythro-poiesis	Folate Deficiency Anemia
Serum folate (ng/mL)	> 5	< 3	< 3	< 3	< 3
RBC folate (ng/mL)	> 200	> 200	< 160	< 120	< 100
dU suppression	Normal	Normal	Normal	Abnormal	Abnormal
Lobe average	< 3.5	< 3.5	< 3.5	> 3.5	> 3.5
Liver folate (μg/g)	> 3	> 3	< 1.6	< 1.2	< 1.0
Erythrocytes	Normal	Normal	Normal	Normal	Macro-ovalocytic
MCV	Normal	Normal	Normal	Normal	Elevated
Hemoglobin (g/dL)	> 12	> 12	> 12	> 12	< 12
Plasma clearance of intravenous folate	Normal	Normal	Normal	Increased	Increased

Table 22.5: Sequential stages in the development of folate deficiency. To convert folate ng/mL to SI units (nmol/L) or μg/g to SI units (nmol/g) multiply by 2.266. Modified from Herbert (1987c). © Am. J. Clin. Nutr. American Society for Clinical Nutrition.

22.3 Summary

Folate

Megaloblastic anemia associated with nutritional folate deficiency may occur in pregnant and lactating women in less industrialized countries. In industrialized countries, subclinical folate deficiency is more widespread, especially in pregnant and lactating women, and in the presence of certain diseases and drugs.

Folic acid, as a coenzyme, has an essential role in DNA synthesis. Hence, abnormal cell replication in the hematopoietic system, manifested by hypersegmented neutrophils, is one of the early morphological changes associated with folate deficiency. Later, macrocytes in the peripheral blood, and megaloblasts in the bone marrow, appear.

Serum and erythrocyte folate concentrations are the most frequently used biochemical indices of folate status. Serum levels reflect folate balance, fluctuate rapidly with recent changes in folate intakes, and provide no information on the size of tissue folate stores. The latter can be estimated by measuring erythrocyte folate concentrations, which fall in subjects in persistent negative folate balance. Concentrations of folate in erythrocytes, but not serum, also fall in vitamin B-12 deficiency. Consequently, both serum and erythrocyte folate concentrations must be measured to distinguish between folate and vitamin B-12 deficiency. A serum folate value of less than 3 ng/mL (6.8 nmol/L) is indicative of negative folate balance. If the negative balance persists, tissue folate

	Normal	Negative Vit. B-12 Balance	Vit. B-12 Depletion	Vit. B-12 Deficient Erythro-poiesis	Vit. B-12-Deficiency Anemia
HoloTC II (pg/mL)	> 30	< 20	< 20	< 12	< 12
TC II % sat.	> 5%	< 5%	< 2%	< 1%	< 1%
Holohap (pg/mL)	> 150	> 150	< 150	< 100	< 100
dU suppression	Normal	Normal	Normal	Abnormal	Abnormal
Hypersegmentation	No	No	No	Yes	Yes
TBBC* % sat.	> 15%	> 15%	> 15%	< 15%	< 10%
Hap % sat.	> 20%	> 20%	> 20%	< 20%	< 10%
RBC folate (ng/mL)	> 160	> 160	> 160	< 140	< 140
Erythrocytes	Normal	Normal	Normal	Normal	Macro-ovalocytic
MCV	Normal	Normal	Normal	Normal	Elevated
Hemoglobin	Normal	Normal	Normal	Normal	Low
TC II	Normal	Normal	Normal	Elevated	Elevated
Methylmalonate	No	No	No	?	Yes
Myelin damage	No	No	No	?	?

Table 22.6: Sequential stages in the development of vitamin B-12 deficiency. HoloTC II = holotranscobalamin II (i.e. transcobalamin II with attached cobalamin), TC II % Sat = percent of total TC II with attached cobalamin; Holohap = holohaptocorrin (i.e. haptocorrin or transcobalamin [I + III]) with attached cobalamin; TBBC % sat = percent of total B-12 binding capacity of plasma with attached B-12, Hap % sat = percent of total haptocorrin which has attached B-12. To convert B-12 pg/mL to SI units (pmol/L) multiply by 0.7378. Modified from Herbert (1987c). © Am. J. Clin. Nutr. American Society for Clinical Nutrition.

becomes depleted, and biochemical function is impaired as indicated by an abnormal dU suppression test. Hypersegmented neutrophils are also present. When tissue folate stores are severely depleted in the third and final stage of folate deficiency, macro-ovalocytic erythrocytes appear in the circulating blood and megaloblasts in the bone marrow. At this stage, abnormal red cell indices are apparent; mean red cell volume and mean cell hemoglobin are elevated and hemoglobin is low (i.e. < 13 g/dL in men; < 12 g/dL in women). Table 22.5 summarizes these sequential stages in the development of folate deficiency (Herbert, 1987c).

Vitamin B-12

In contrast to folate, dietary deficiencies of vitamin B-12 are relatively rare, usually arising from malabsorption. Early stages of vitamin B-12 deficiency, when negative balance occurs, can be detected by a reduction in the percentage saturation of serum TC II (Table 22.6). If the negative balance persists, vitamin B-12 depletion arises, indicated by a fall in serum vitamin B-12 concentrations to below 150 pg/mL, but normal biochemical function. When the latter is impaired, the dU suppression test is abnormal and/or hypersegmented neutrophils exist, as described for folate deficiency. Clinical deficiency of vitamin B-12 produces defects in the hematopoietic system, similar to those of folic acid deficiency. Macro-ovalocytic erythrocytes, abnormal red cell indices, and a low hemoglobin occur. Urinary excretion of methylmalonic acid also increases in vitamin B-12, but not folate-deficiency anemia. The role of vitamin B-12 in methylmalonate metabolism is probably responsible for the neurological disorders which only occur in vitamin B-12 deficiency. The Schilling test is often used to ascertain whether malabsorption is the cause of the vitamin-B-12 deficiency.

References

Albert MJ, Mathan VI and Baker SJ. (1980). Vitamin B-12 synthesis by human small intestinal bacteria. Nature 283: 781–782.

Bailey LB, Mahan CS, Dimperio D. (1980). Folacin and iron status in low-income pregnant adolescents and mature women. American Journal of Clinical Nutrition 33: 1997–2001.

Bailey LB, Wagner PA, Christakis GJ, Davis CG, Appledorf H, Araujo PE, Dorsey E, Dinning JS. (1982). Folacin and iron status and hematological findings in Black and Spanish-American adolescents from urban low-income households. American Journal of Clinical Nutrition 35: 1023–1032.

Baumslag N, Edelstein T, Metz J. (1970). Reduction of incidence of prematurity by folic acid supplementation in pregnancy. British Medical Journal 1: 16–17.

Beaton GH. (1981). Nutritional conditions in Canada. In: Nutrition in the 1980's: Constraints in our Knowledge. Alan R. Liss Inc., New York, pp. 221–235.

Begley JA, Hall CA. (1975). Measurement of vitamin B_{12} binding proteins of plasma II. Interpretation of patterns of disease. Blood 45: 287–293.

Bindra GB, Gibson RS, Berry M. (1981). Vitamin B-12 and folate status of East Indian immigrants living in Canada. Nutrition Research 7: 365–374.

Blakley RL. (1977). Folic acid biochemistry: present status and future direction. In: National Research Council, Food and Nutrition Board. Folic acid: Biochemistry and Physiology in relation to the Human Nutrition Requirement. National Academy of Sciences, Washington, D.C., pp. 3–24.

Carmel R. (1983). Clinical and laboratory features of the diagnosis of megaloblastic anemia. In: Lindenbaum J (ed). Nutrition in Hematology. Churchill Livingstone Inc., New York – Edinburgh, pp. 1–31.

Carmel R, Herbert V. (1969). Deficiency of vitamin B-12-binding alpha globulin in two brothers. Blood 33: 1–12.

Chanarin I, Waters DA. (1974). Failed Schilling tests. Scandinavian Journal of Haematology, 12: 245–248.

Chen IW, Silberstein EB, Maxon HR, Volle CP, Sohnlein BH. (1982). Semi automated system for simultaneous assays of serum vitamin B-12 and folic acid in serum evaluated. Clinical Chemistry 28: 2161–2165.

Colman N. (1977). Folate deficiency in humans. In: Draper HH (ed). Advances in Nutritional Research Volume 1. Plenum Publishing Co., New York, pp. 77–124.

Colman N. (1981). Laboratory assessment of folate status. Clinics in Laboratory Medicine 1: 755–796.

Colman N, Herbert V. (1980). Abnormal lymphocyte deoxyuridine suppression test. A reliable indicator of decreased lymphocyte folate levels. American Journal of Hematology 8: 169–174.

Cooke WT, Cox EV, Fone OJ, Meynell MJ, Gaddie R. (1963). The clinical and metabolic significance of jejunal diverticuli. Gut 4: 115–131.

Cooper BA. (1973). Folate and vitamin B_{12} in pregnancy. Clinical Haematology 2: 461–476.

Cooper BA, Lowenstein L. (1964). Relative folate deficiency of erythrocytes in pernicious anemia and its correction with cyanocobalamin. Blood 24: 502–521.

Cooper BA, Lowenstein L. (1966). Vitamin B-12-folate interrelationships in megloblastic anemia. British Journal of Haematology 12: 283–296.

Cox EV, White AM. (1962). Methylmalonic acid excretion: an index of vitamin B-12 deficiency. Lancet 2: 853–856.

Das KC, Herbert V. (1978). The lymphocyte as a marker of past nutritional status. Persistence of abnormal lymphocyte deoxyuridine (dU) suppression test and chromosomes in patients with past deficiency of folate and vitamin B-12. British Journal of Haematology 38: 219–233.

Das KC, Herbert V, Colman N, Longo DL. (1978). Unmasking covert folate deficiency in iron-deficient subjects with neutrophil hypersegmentation: dU suppression tests on lymphocytes and bone marrow. British Journal of Haematology 39: 357–375.

Das KC, Manusselis C, Herbert V. (1980). Simplifying lymphocyte culture and the deoxyuridine suppression test by using whole blood (0.1 mL) instead of separated lymphocytes. Clinical Chemistry 26: 72–77.

Dawson DW, Delamore IW, Fish DI, Flaherty TA, Gowenlock AH, Hunt LP, Hyde K, MacIver JE, Thornton JA, Waters HM. (1980). An evaluation of commercial radioisotope methods for the determination of folate and vitamin B-12. Journal of Clinical Pathology 33: 234–242.

Dolphin D (ed). (1982). B_{12}. Volume 1, Chemistry; Volume 2, Biochemistry and Medicine. John Wiley and Sons, New York.

Domstad PA, Choy YC, Kim EE, DeLand FH. (1981). Reliability of the dual-isotope Schilling test for the diagnosis of pernicious anemia or malabsorption syndrome. American Journal of Clinical Pathology 75: 723–726.

Doscherholmen A, McMahon J, Ripley D. (1976). Inhibitory effect of eggs on vitamin B-12 absorption: description of a simple ovalbumin [57]Co-vitamin B-12 absorption test. British Journal of Haematology 33: 261–272.

Doscherholmen A, Ripley D, Chang S, Ripley P, Chang S, Silvis SE. (1977). Influence of age and stomach functions on serum vitamin B-12 concentration. Scandinavian Journal of Gastroenterology 12: 313–319.

FAO/WHO (Food and Agricultural Organization/World Health Organization) Expert Group. (In Press). Requirements of vitamin A, iron, folate and vitamin B-12.

Fernandes-Costa F, Tonder S van, Metz J. (1985). A sex difference in serum cobalamin and transcobalamin levels. American Journal of Clinical Nutrition 41: 784–876.

Giles C. (1966). An account of 335 cases of megaloblastic anaemia of pregnancy and puerperium. Journal of Clinical Pathology 19: 1–11.

Gimsing P, Nexø E. (1983). The forms of cobalamin in biological materials. In: Hall CA (ed). The Cobalamins. Churchill-Livingstone, New York, pp. 7–30.

Gottlieb C, Lau KS, Wasserman LR, Herbert V. (1965). Rapid charcoal assay for intrinsic factor (IF), gastric juice unsaturated B-12 binding capacity, antibody to IF, and serum unsaturated B-12 binding capacity. Blood 25: 875–884.

Grásbeck R, Simons K, Sinkkonen I. (1966). Isolation of gastric intrinsic factor and its probable degradation product as their vitamin B_{12} complexes, from human gastric juice. Biochimica Biophysica Acta 127:47–58.

Gutcho S, Mansbach L. (1977). Simultaneous radioassay of serum in vitamin B-12 and folic acid. Clinical Chemistry 23: 1609–1614.

Halsted CH. (1979). The intestinal absorption of folates. American Journal of Clinical Nutrition 32: 846–855.

Hansen OP, Drivsholm A, Hippe E. (1977). Vitamin B-12 metabolism in myelomatosis. Scandinavian Journal of Haematology 18: 395–402.

Harrison RJ. (1971). Vitamin B-12 levels in erythrocytes in anemia due to folate deficiency. British Journal of Haematology 20: 623–628.

Health and Welfare Canada (1973). Nutrition Canada National Survey. Health and Welfare, Ottawa.

Hellström L. (1971). Lack of toxicity of folic acid given in pharmacological doses to healthy volunteers. Lancet 1: 59–61.

Herbert V. (1962). Experimental nutritional folate deficiency in man. Transactions of the Association of American Physicians 75: 307–320.

Herbert V. (1964). Studies of folate deficiency in man. Proceedings of the Royal Society of Medicine 57: 377–384.

Herbert V. (1967). Biochemical and hematological lesions in folic acid deficiency. American Journal of Clinical Nutrition 20: 562–568.

Herbert V. (1984). Vitamin B_{12}. In: Present Knowledge in Nutrition. Fifth edition. The Nutrition Foundation Inc, Washington, D.C., pp. 347–364.

Herbert V. (1985). Biology of disease: Megaloblastic anemia. Laboratory Investigation 52: 3–19.

Herbert V. (1987a). Recommended dietary intakes (RDI) of folate in humans. American Journal of Clinical Nutrition 45: 661–670.

Herbert V. (1987b). Making sense of laboratory tests of folate status: folate requirements to sustain normality. American Journal of Hematology 26: 199–207.

Herbert V. (1987c). The 1986 Herman Award Lecture. Nutrition Science as a continually unfolding story: the folate and vitamin B-12 paradigm. American Journal of Clinical Nutrition 46: 387–402.

Herbert V, Colman N, Palat D, Manusselis C, Drivas G, Block E, Akerkar A, Weaver D, Frenkel E. (1984). Is there a "gold" standard for human serum vitamin B_{12} assay? Journal of Laboratory and Clinical Medicine 104: 829–841.

Herbert V, Tisman G, Go LT, Brenner L. (1973). The dU suppression test using 125 I-UdR to define biochemical megaloblastosis. British Journal of Haematology 24: 713–723.

Herbert V, Colman N, Spivack M, Ocasio E, Ghanta V, Kimmel K, Brenner L, Freundlich J, Scott J. (1975). Folic acid deficiency in the United States: folate assays in a prenatal clinic. American Journal of Obstetrics and Gynecology 123: 175–179.

Higginbottom MC, Sweetman L, Nyhan WL. (1978). A syndrome of methylmalonic aciduria, homocystinuria, megaloblastic anemia and neurologic abnormalities in a vitamin B-12 deficient breast-fed infant of a strict vegetarian. New England Journal of Medicine 299: 317–323.

Hillman RS, McGuffin R, Campbell C. (1977). Alcohol interference with the folate enterohepatic cycle. Transactions of the Association of American Physicians 90: 145-156.

Hoffbrand AV. (1981). Megaloblastic anemias. In: Hoffbrand AV, Lewis SM (eds). Postgraduate Hematology. Appleton-Century-Crofts, New York, pp. 72–111.

Hoffbrand AV, Newcombe BFA, Mollin DL. (1966). Method of assay of red cell folate activity and the value of the assay as a test for folate deficiency. Journal of Clinical Pathology 19: 17–28.

Hoppner K, Lampi B and Perrin DE. (1972). The free and total folate activity in foods available on the Canadian market. Canadian Institute of Food Science and Technology Journal 5: 60–66.

Hughes-Jones NC. (1984). Lecture Notes on Haematology, Fourth edition. Blackwell Scientific Publications, Oxford, pp. 23–45.

Hunter R, Barnes J, Oakeley HF, Matthews DM. (1970). Toxicity of folic acid given in pharmacological doses to healthy volunteers. Lancet 1: 61–63.

Keating JN, Wada L, Stokstad ELR, King JC. (1987). Folic acid: effect on zinc absorption in humans and in the rat. American Journal of Clinical Nutrition 46: 835–839.

Killmann SA. (1964). Effect of deoxyuridine on incorporation of tritiated thymidine: difference between normoblasts and megaloblasts. Acta Medica Scandinavica 175: 483–488.

Kolhouse JF, Kondo H, Allen NC, Podell E, Allen RH. (1978). Cobalamin analogues are present in human plasma and can mask cobalamin deficiency because current radioradioisotope dilution assays are not specific enough for true cobalamin. New England Journal of Medicine 299: 785–792.

Lankelma J, Kleijn E van der, Jansen MJT. (1980). Determination of 5-methyltetrahydrofolic acid in plasma and spinal fluid by high-performance liquid chromatography, using on-column concentration and electrochemical detection. Journal of Chromatography 182: 35–45.

Laurence KM, James N, Miller MH, Tennant GB, Campbell H. (1981). Double-blind randomized controlled trial of folate treatment before conception to prevent recurrence of neural-tube defects. British Medical Journal 282: 1509–1511.

Lindenbaum J, Nath BJ. (1980). Megaloblastic anaemia and neutrophil hypersegmentation. British Journal of Haematology 44: 511–513.

Layrisse M, Blumenfeld N, Dugarte I, Roche M. (1959). Vitamin B-12 and folic acid metabolism in hookworm–infected patients. Blood 14: 1269-1279.

Martinez OB, Roe DA. (1977). Effect of oral contraceptives on blood folate levels in pregnancy. American Journal of Obstetrics and Gynecology 128: 255–261.

Metz J, Kelly A, Swett VC, Waxman S, Herbert V. (1968). Deranged DNA synthesis by bone marrow from vitamin B-12-deficient humans. British Journal of Haematology 14: 575–592.

Milne DB, Canfield WK, Mahalko JR, Sandstead HH. (1984). Effect of oral folic acid supplements on zinc, copper and iron absorption and excretion. American Journal of Clinical Nutrition 39: 535–539.

Omer A, Finlayson NDC, Shearman DJC, Samson RR, Girdwood RH. (1970a). Plasma and erythrocyte folate in iron deficiency and folate deficiency. Blood 35: 821–828.

Omer A, Finlayson NDC, Shearman DJC, Samson RR, Girdwood RH. (1970b). Erythrocyte vitamin B-12 activity in health, polycythemia, and in deficiency of vitamin B-12 and folate. Blood 35: 73–82.

Preuss HG. (1978). Effect of nutrient toxicities — excess in animals and man: folic acid. In: Recheigl M Jr (ed). CRC Handbook Series in Nutrition and Food. Section E: Nutritional Disorders. Volume I. Effect of Nutrient Excesses and Toxicities in Animals and Man. CRC Press Inc., West Palm Beach, Florida, pp. 61–62.

Rhode BM, Cooper BA, Farmer FA. (1983). Effect of orange juice, folic acid and oral contraceptives on serum folate in women taking a folate-restricted diet. Journal of the American College of Nutrition 2: 221–230.

Rickes EL, Brink NG, Koniuszy RF., Ward TR, Folkers K. (1948). Crystalline vitamin B_{12}. Science 107: 396-397.

Rose M. (1976). Vitamin-B-12 deficiency in Asian immigrants. Lancet 2: 681.

Rosenberg IH, Bowman BB, Cooper BA, Halsted CH, Lindenbaum J. (1982). Folate nutrition in the elderly. American Journal of Clinical Nutrition 36: 1060–1066.

Sauberlich HE, Dowdy RP, Skala JH. (1974). Laboratory Tests for the Assessment of Nutritional Status. CRC Press Inc., Cleveland, Ohio, pp. 49–57.

Sauberlich HE. (1977). Detection of folic acid deficiency in populations. In: Folic Acid: Biochemistry and Physiology in Relation to the Human Nutrition Requirement. National Research Council, Food and Nutrition Board, pp. 213–231.

Sauberlich HE. (1984). Newer laboratory methods for assessing nutriture of selected B-complex vitamins. Annual Review of Nutrition 4: 377–407.

Schilling RF. (1953). Intrinsic factor studies II. The effect of gastric juice on the urinary excretion of radioactivity after oral administration of radioactive vitamin B_{12}. Journal of Laboratory and Clinical Medicine 42: 860-866.

Senti FR, Pilch SM. (1985). Assessment of the folate nutritional status of the U.S. population based on data collected in the second National Health and Nutrition Examination Survey 1976–1980. Life Sciences Research Office, Federation of American Societies for Experimental Biology, Bethesda, Maryland.

Smith EL. (1948). Purification of antipernicious anaemia factors from liver. Nature 161: 638–639.

Smithells RW, Sheppard S, Schorah CJ, Seller MJ, Nevin NC, Harris R, Read AP, Fielding DW. (1981). Apparent prevention of neural tube defects by periconceptual vitamin supplementation. Archives of Disease in Childhood 56: 911–918.

Smithells RW, Nevin NC, Seller MJ, Sheppard S, Harris R, Read AP, Fielding DW, Walker S, Schorah CJ, Wild J. (1983). Further experience of vitamin supplementation for prevention of neural tube defect recurrences. Lancet 1: 1027–1031.

Steinberg SE. (1984). Mechanisms of folate homeostasis. American Journal of Physiology 246: G319–G324.

Waddell CC, Domstad PA, Pircher FJ, Lerner SR, Brown JA, Lawhorn BK. (1976). Serum folate levels. Comparison of microbiologic assay and radioisotope kit methods. American Journal of Pathology 66: 746–752.

Wagner PA, Bailey LB, Krista ML, Jerrigan JA, Robinson JD, Cerda JJ. (1981). Comparison of zinc and folacin status in elderly women from differing socio-economic backgrounds. Nutrition Research 1: 565–569.

Wagner C. (1984). Folic acid. In: Present Knowledge in Nutrition. Fifth edition. The Nutrition Foundation Inc., Washington, D.C., pp 332–346.

Waxman S. (1973). Metabolic approach to the diagnosis of megaloblastic anemias. Medical Clinics of North America 37: 315–334.

Waxman S, Schreiber C, Herbert V. (1971). Radioisotopic assay for measurement of serum folate levels. Blood 38: 219–228.

Wickramasinghe SN, Longland JE. (1974). Assessment of deoxyuridine suppression test in diagnosis of vitamin B_{12} or folate deficiency. British Medical Journal 3: 148–152.

Wickramasinghe SN, Saunders JE. (1975). Deoxyuridine suppression test. British Medical Journal 2: 87.

WHO (World Health Organization) (1972). Nutritional Anaemias. WHO Technical Report Series No. 503. World Health Organization, Geneva.

Wu A, Chanarin I, Slavin G, Levi AJ. (1975). Folate deficiency in the alcoholic — its relationship to clinical and hematological abnormalities, liver disease and folate stores. British Journal of Haematology 29: 469–478.

Chapter 23

Assessment of calcium, phosphorus, and magnesium status

Calcium, magnesium, and phosphorus are the major mineral components of the body. The distribution of these elements in the body compartments of a 70-kg reference man is shown in Table 23.1. All three minerals occur in combination with organic and inorganic compounds and as free ions. They have two major roles: structural components in bone and soft tissues, and regulatory agents in body fluids. Bone also serves as a reservoir for these minerals. Calcium and phosphorus exist in the bones mostly as calcium hydroxyapatite and octacalcium phosphate; more than half of the magnesium in bone is present within the apatite crystal structure.

The fractional absorption of calcium and magnesium is generally inversely related to dietary intake, whereas that of phosphorus is relatively constant. In adults consuming mixed North American diets, absorption of calcium and magnesium approximates 30% and 40%, respectively, compared to 60% to 70% for phosphorus. The vitamin D status of the individual affects the efficiency of absorption of calcium and possibly phosphorus, but has little or no effect on the absorption of magnesium. The absorption of calcium is influenced by many other dietary components such as phytate, dietary fiber, oxalate, lactose, and the amino acids lysine and arginine. Calcium, and to a lesser degree

Element	Mass Present	Percentage in the Skeleton	Percentage in Soft Tissues
Ca	1200 g	99%	1%
Mg	24 g	60%	40%
P	900 g	88%	12%

Table 23.1: Calcium, phosphorus, and magnesium distribution in an adult weighing 70 kg.

aluminium and strontium, can affect phosphorus absorption, but such effects are thought to be relatively unimportant in human nutrition. The factors influencing the absorption of magnesium are poorly understood. The kidney and the gastrointestinal tract are primarily responsible for regulating the total body content of magnesium. There is no regulation of phosphorus absorption. The gastrointestinal tract is the main site of regulation of calcium absorption, primarily via 1,25-$(OH)_2D$.

Calcium deficiency, characterized by demineralization of the skeleton (osteopenia), may occur slowly and insidiously as a result of a combination of co-existing dietary, genetic, endocrine, and age-related factors. Dietary factors are unimportant in the development of phosphorus and magnesium deficiencies. Instead, these deficiencies generally occur in association with disease states and/or drugs, or in patients receiving prolonged total parenteral nutrition deficient in phosphorus or magnesium.

23.1   Assessment of calcium status

Calcium is the most abundant mineral in the body, and more than 99% of body calcium is stored in bone (Table 23.1). The remainder, located in body tissues (10 g) and the extra-celluar fluids (900 mg), is involved in several metabolic processes, including enzyme activation, blood coagulation, muscle contractibility, nerve transmission, hormone function, and membrane transport. Intestinal calcium absorption is regulated primarily via vitamin D. Absorption is highest when dietary calcium intakes are low and/or requirements for calcium are high, as during periods of rapid growth, pregnancy, and lactation. Intestinal absorption of calcium decreases progressively with age (Avioli et al., 1965; Bullamore et al., 1970). Urinary excretion of calcium is also regulated in response to need. As a result of adaptive mechanisms, severe nutritional deficiency of calcium is rare.

Several other factors affect calcium absorption and retention, and hence calcium status. Diets high in protein increase the urinary excretion of calcium (hypercalciurea), which is only partly compensated by increased calcium absorption (Margen et al., 1974; Allen et al., 1979). The importance of this effect on the calcium status of persons consuming the normal, mixed high-protein North American diet is unclear. High-protein diets also have an elevated phosphorus content. High phosphorus intakes have a hypocalciuric effect, which may offset the hypercalciuric effect of the protein (Spencer et al., 1978; Hegsted et al., 1981). Several dietary components, such as phytates, oxalates, and dietary fiber, inhibit calcium absorption and hence may have a negative effect on calcium status. Other factors, including certain amino acids and lactose, enhance calcium absorption (Schuette and Linkswiler, 1984).

Calcium is not widely distributed in foods. Milk and milk products are excellent sources of readily available calcium. Leafy-green vegetables are also good sources, although absorption of calcium from these sources may be low. Meats, grains, and nuts are poor sources of calcium. Hence, if milk and milk products are not consumed regularly, intakes of available calcium may be inadequate. Inadequate calcium intakes during early life may limit peak adult bone mass (Heaney et al., 1982; Spencer et al., 1982). A larger peak adult bone mass reduces the subsequent risk of osteoporosis, a condition characterized by decreased bone mass and increased susceptibility to fractures. In adults over 35 years of age, the mass of mineralized bone decreases progressively at an average annual rate of about 1%. The bone loss is affected by non-nutritional risk factors such as lifestyle, body weight, smoking, alcohol abuse, certain diseases (e.g. hyperthyroidism) and drug treatments (e.g. glucocorticoids, aluminium-containing antacids), and some diuretics (Spencer et al., 1982). Nutritional factors, including calcium, protein, and phosphorus intakes, may also influence bone mineral losses (Anderson et al., 1977; Allen et al., 1979). Low calcium intakes have been linked with hypertension, although this association requires further confirmation (Kesteloot and Geboers, 1982).

More work is required to clarify the association between dietary calcium intake and osteoporosis. Epidemiological studies have not found a consistent relationship between calcium intake and bone density (Heaney et al., 1978; Matković et al., 1979). Results of calcium supplementation studies on postmenopausal bone loss have been negative (Freudenheim et al., 1986; Riis et al., 1987).

Excessive intakes of calcium are unlikely to cause hypercalcemia. Instead, the latter is normally the result of hyperparathyroidism or excessive intakes of vitamin D (Venugopal and Luckey, 1978). The U.S. Food and Drug Administration has concluded that calcium intakes up to 2500 mg per day are safe for healthy adults. Nevertheless, persons predisposed to the formation of kidney stones and milk alkali syndrome should avoid excessive intakes of calcium.

There is no satisfactory routine biochemical method for assessing calcium status, although serum ionized calcium appears promising and is described below. Several indirect, noninvasive, techniques can be used to measure bone mass in either the appendicular and/or the axial skeleton. Bone mass measurements provide an indirect assessment of bone calcium content, an index of body calcium stores.

23.1.1 Serum calcium concentrations

Serum calcium concentrations cannot be used as an index of calcium status because they are homeostatically controlled and remain remarkably constant under most conditions (Schuette and Linkswiler, 1984). Low levels of serum calcium only occur after prolonged periods of calcium deprivation, or following interference with calcium absorption.

Fifty percent of the calcium in plasma is ionized and physiologically active. It is this fraction that is under hormonal control. The remaining 50% is not ionized and is physiologically inert; of this, 40% to 50% is bound to protein, primarily albumin, and 5% to 10% is complexed with citrate, bicarbonate, and phosphate. Serum rather than plasma should be used for calcium analysis; most anticoagulants function by reacting with calcium.

If serum calcium concentrations are outside the normal range, pathological rather than nutritional problems should be suspected. For example, in cases of hypoparathyroidism, hypomagnesemia, and acute pancreatitis, serum calcium concentrations are low (hypocalcemia). Elevated serum calcium values (hypercalcemia) occur in association with hyperparathyroidism, hyperthyroidism, sarcoidosis, and when large areas of the body are immobilized (e.g. after spinal cord injury and bone fracture). In the latter, calcium from the rapidly atrophying bone is released into the circulating body fluids.

Serum calcium concentrations in normal healthy adults range from 8.8 to 10.6 mg/dL (2.20 to 2.64 mmol/L). Values decrease with age in men. Females have slightly lower concentrations (8.8 to 10.2 mg/dL; 2.20 to 2.54 mmol/L) than males (9.2 to 10.6 mg/dL; 2.30 to 2.64 mmol/L), associated with small differences in serum albumin content and the calcium-reducing effect of estrogens. Serum calcium decreases by 5% to 10% up to the end of the third trimester of pregnancy, after which concentrations rise. Serum calcium concentrations were determined in both the NHANES I survey (NCHS, 1979) and the Nutrition Canada National Survey (Health and Welfare Canada, 1973).

Serum calcium is used to identify vitamin D intoxication. Elevated serum calcium levels (hypercalcemia) invariably result from excess vitamin D (Section 18.2.4). Serum calcium is usually determined by flame atomic absorption spectrophotometry (AAS) (Zettner and Seligson, 1964). Earlier methods included flame photometry and the calcium oxalate titration procedure.

23.1.2 Serum ionized calcium concentrations

Serum ionized calcium, which makes up 50% of the calcium in plasma, is the physiologically active form of calcium in the blood. It can be measured using commercially available ion-specific electrodes (Wandrup and Kvetny, 1985). Serum ionized calcium concentrations, rather than total serum calcium concentrations, relate to disturbances in calcium metabolism. Reductions in ionized calcium concentrations occur in hypoparathyroidism and vitamin-D deficient rickets, and result in increased neuromuscular irritability. Elevated ionized calcium values suggest functional hypercalcemia, and occur in patients with hyperparathyroidism or receiving chronic renal hemodialysis. In such conditions, total serum calcium levels may be normal (Ladenson and Bowers, 1973b). Serum ionized calcium concentrations cannot be predicted from total serum calcium values because only a low correlation exists between ionized calcium and total serum calcium concentrations in healthy persons. Ladenson and Bowers (1973a) reported a mean serum ionized calcium concentration of 1.28 mmol/L (range 1.18 to 1.38 mmol/L) for eighty-six apparently healthy adults (nineteen to fifty years). This mean value corresponds closely to that obtained in some earlier studies (Oreskes et al., 1968; Li and Piechocki, 1971). In general, adult males have a higher mean serum ionized calcium concentration than females. Discrepancies exist for the reference values for serum ionized calcium in adults, some of which may be attributed to difficulties in collecting and handling serum samples anaerobically and to differences in the electrode systems used (Wandrup and Kvetny, 1985).

Several confounding factors affect the measurement of serum ionized calcium concentrations. These include high levels of magnesium and sodium, the presence of trypsin, triethanolamine, and heparin, and changes in pH of the sample (Ladenson and Bowers, 1973a). The confounding effects of magnesium and sodium can be eliminated by using calcium standards containing sodium and magnesium chloride in the same concentrations as those expected in the samples. Trypsin, triethanolamine, and heparin bind calcium and should be not be used. The effect of changes in pH of the blood during collection and storage on serum ionized calcium concentrations can be minimized by collecting and handling the serum samples anaerobically, and by adjusting the pH to 7.4 with CO_2 gas before the measurement (Schwartz, 1976). Fasting blood samples should be used to eliminate the effect of a recent meal on serum ionized calcium concentrations.

Wandrup and Kvetny (1985) recommend using whole-blood samples for ionized calcium measurements. Samples should be collected, and then stored anaerobically at 0°C to 4°C prior to the measurement.

23.1.3 Radiogrammetry

Radiogrammetry measures the thickness and the diameter of the cortex of the metacarpals or radius on standard anterio-posterior roentgenograms ('X-rays') of the hand. The X-rays can be taken in the field with portable equipment. A dial caliper or a digitizer is used to take the measurements, from which cortical bone volume can be calculated (Kimmel, 1984). Serial measurements can be used to monitor changes in cortical bone volume. No information on trabecular bone is obtained using this method (Cummings et al., 1985). Hence, although these measurements can be performed precisely, they do not accurately reflect the total amount of bone present, and correlations with the total mass of the skeleton, as determined by neutron activation, are poor. This method will not reliably detect bone loss of less than 20% in cross-sectional studies.

23.1.4 Single photon absorptiometry

Single photon absorptiometry is the most practical noninvasive method of measuring total bone mineral content of the limbs (Wahner et al., 1983). The method is based on the assumption that bone mineral content is inversely proportional to the amount of photon energy transmitted by the bone under study. The site most frequently selected for measurement by single photon absorptiometry is the lower radius, at approximately one-third of the distance from the styloid process to the olecranon. Bone mineral content of this site correlates well with that of the hip and with the total skeletal mineral and calcium content in healthy adults (Mazess, 1971), with errors ranging from 5% to 10%. Larger errors (10% to 15%) may arise when osteopenic subjects are used (Cohn et al., 1974a). Single photon absorptiometry is not suitable for measurements on the axial skeleton because the technique requires a uniform thickness of soft tissue surrounding the bone. The bone mineral content of the lower radius correlates only weakly with the amount of trabecular bone in the spine (Mazess, 1983). Hence, this method cannot be used to predict bone mineral content or density of the vertebrae, especially in patients with metabolic bone disease (Mazess et al., 1984a).

For single photon absorptiometry, the lower radius is exposed to a small amount of radiation (0.02 to 0.05 mGy; 2 to 5 mrad) from a mono-energetic photon source — usually ^{125}I or ^{241}Am. The quantity of bone mineral positioned in the beam path is inversely related to the amount of transmitted radiation, measured by a scintillation counter (Boyd et al., 1974). To standardize the measurements among individuals with different bone sizes, bone mineral content can be expressed as bone mineral per square centimeter of bone (i.e. as g/cm^2) (Harper et al., 1984). Alternatively, an index based on the ratio of bone mineral content to the width of the radius can be used (Mazess, 1971). The technique is fast, taking approximately five minutes. Precision and accuracy of the method range from 3% to 5%, and 2% to 4%, respectively (Mazess, 1971); values correlate well with those determined by conventional techniques. The method can be used to measure rate of bone loss in prospective longitudinal studies, if positioning errors are minimized.

Diagnosis of osteoporosis from measurements of total bone mineral content of the limbs of the appendicular skeleton by single photon absorptiometry is usually based on values which fall below the normal range of bone mass of healthy adults (Horsman et al., 1981). Such reference data have been derived from several studies in the United States on the bone mineral content of the midshaft and distal end of the radius (Mazess and Cameron, 1974; Hui et al., 1985). In the future, it may be possible to assess fracture risk using absolute levels of bone mass (Parfitt, 1984; Hayes and Gerhart, 1985).

23.1.5 Dual photon absorptiometry

Dual photon absorptiometry can be used to determine total bone mineral content of the axial skeleton, using the lumbar vertebrae sites, as well as the bone mineral content of the proximal femur. The method uses a radioisotope source that emits two gamma rays, usually [153]Gd with gamma rays at 44 and 100 KeV, enabling bone density to be assessed independently of soft-tissue thickness and composition. The technique takes approximately fifteen minutes with a radiation exposure to local tissues of 0.05 to 0.15 mGy (5 to 15 mrad). Precision and accuracy of the method are 2% to 3% and 4% to 6%, respectively (Kimmel, 1984). The lumbar vertebrae (L2 to L4) are the sites generally selected. The sternum interferes with the measurement if thoracic vertebrae are used. Calcification in the aorta, osteoarthritis of the spine, and vertebral compression fractures in the scanning area, may all confound the measurement. Diagnosis of osteoporosis from measurements by dual photon absorptiometry is generally based on levels of bone mass which are at least 20% less than the mean for comparable, healthy males or females (Mazess et al., 1984b).

The bone mineral content of the total skeleton is best predicted from measurements of the bone mineral content of both the appendicular and axial skeleton.

23.1.6 Computerized tomography

Although computerized tomography (CT) (Section 14.7.4) can be used to measure bone mass of both the appendicular and axial skeleton, the method is not feasible for survey studies. The equipment is not portable and the method involves a high radiation dose (2.0 to 2.5 mGy; 200 to 250 mrad) (Kimmel, 1984). Furthermore, precision is lower than that for dual-photon absorptiometry (3% to 5%) and accuracy is poor (12%); even small position changes markedly affect results because of the confounding effect of the bone marrow fat content (Mazess, 1983). The latter increases in the elderly and may result in misleadingly low CT measurements. Computerized tomography can be used to measure only trabecular bone, an advantage because some forms of osteoporosis are predominantly trabecular in character.

23.1.7 Neutron activation

This *in vivo* method assesses total body calcium content. As 99% of total body calcium is in the skeleton, and as calcium is a relatively constant fraction (38% to 39%) of bone mineral weight, measurement of total body calcium provides an estimate of total body bone mineral content, except in cases where extra-osseous deposits of calcium occur. The method is based on the conversion of a proportion of ^{48}Ca in the body to ^{49}Ca by exposing the body of the patient to a low neutron flux. The patient is then transferred to a whole-body counter where the gamma rays emitted by the ^{49}Ca are counted by sodium iodide detectors. The gamma ray count is proportional to the mass of total body calcium. Results of this technique correlate well with single photon absorptiometry of the lower radius (Mazess, 1983). The total radiation exposure using this method varies from 2.5 mSv to 25 mSv (0.25 rem to 2.5 rem) depending on the neutron source, a range considerably higher than photon absorptiometry and limiting the general applicability of the method. The preferred neutron source is ^{238}PuBe. The precision of repeated determinations of total body calcium by neutron activation over a four- to five-year period in healthy adults is estimated as 2.5%, suggesting that the method is suitable for studying longitudinal changes (Cohn et al., 1974b).

Harrison et al. (1979) have developed a calcium bone index (CaBI) in which total body calcium content is normalized for body size. This index may be used to distinguish between normal (with CaBI 1.0 ± 0.12) and osteoporotic (0.69 ± 0.10) subjects. Mild osteoporosis in patients who have not yet experienced any vertebral fractures can be detected.

23.2   Assessment of phosphorus status

Phosphorus is the second most abundant mineral in the body. About 85% of phosphorus in the adult body is present in the bones as calcium phosphate [$Ca_3(PO_4)_2$] and hydroxyapatite [$Ca_{10}(PO_4)_6(OH)_2$]. The remainder is in cells and extracellular fluids as inorganic phosphate and in combination with proteins, lipids, carbohydrates, and other compounds (Table 23.1). Phosphorus is an essential factor in all the energy-producing reactions of the cells.

Phosphorus is widely distributed in animal and plant foods. Protein-rich foods, such as meat, poultry, fish, eggs, milk, and milk products, are major sources of phosphorus in a mixed North American diet. Whole grain cereals, legumes, and nuts are also good sources. Dietary deficiency of phosphorus is rare because phosphorous intakes generally exceed requirements. Moreover, in the absence of disease, parathyroid and renal mechanisms function to conserve body phosphorus. The amount of dietary phosphorus absorbed depends on both the dietary intake and the food source. In healthy adults consuming a North American mixed diet, about 60% to 70% of dietary phosphorus is absorbed (Moon et al., 1974); maximal absorption (up to 90%) is achieved when phosphorus intakes are very low. Some sources of dietary phosphorus, for example phytic acid (inositol hexaphosphate) found in cereals, legumes, and nuts, are not absorbed in humans because the intestinal mucosa does not secrete a phytase enzyme, essential for the hydrolysis of phytic acid. Although vitamin D status is known to influence phosphorus absorption in certain animal species, a similar effect in humans is controversial (Avioli, 1984). Absorption of dietary phosphorus is reduced by excessive intakes of calcium, aluminium, and strontium, all cations that form insoluble phosphates in the intestine. Consequently, suboptimal phosphorus status may arise in persons taking prolonged and excessive intakes of the antacids aluminium hydroxide or aluminum carbonate (Lotz et al., 1968). Phosphorus depletion may also occur in patients receiving long-term total parenteral nutrition unsupplemented with phosphorus, and in patients with diabetic keto-acidosis treated with insulin without supplemental phosphate. Phosphorus depletion results in low intracellular levels of phosphoglycerate and other energy-rich phosphate esters, impairment of oxygen delivery, failure of muscle contractility, severe muscle weakness, and cardiac and respiratory failure.

Growing low-birthweight preterm infants fed human milk are also susceptible to suboptimal phosphorus status because the phosphate content of human milk is inadequate for their growth requirements. These infants may develop skeletal abnormalities, even in the presence of adequate vitamin D intakes (Harrison, 1984).

High phosphorus intakes may be associated with the consumption of commercially available foods containing phosphate additives (Bell et al., 1977). Animal studies have indicated that excessive dietary phosphorus, in relation to calcium, leads to increased bone resorption and bone loss (Anderson and Draper, 1972; Sie et al., 1974). A comparable effect in humans has not been clearly demonstrated (Spencer et al., 1965). Serum phosphorus is used most frequently to assess phosphorus status, as discussed below.

23.2.1 Serum phosphorus concentrations

Phosphorus in serum is largely present as inorganic phosphates, of which four fifths is the divalent anion HPO_4^{2-}, and one fifth is the monovalent anion, $H_2PO_4^-$. Very small amounts of trivalent phosphate, PO_4^{3-}, exist (Harrison, 1984). Nonhemolyzed samples must be used for serum or plasma phosphorus analysis because erythrocytes contain seventeen times more phosphorus than does plasma.

Serum phosphorus concentrations vary with age (Table 23.2), children having higher concentrations than adults. Normal adult values are reached by the third decade, after which male values decline progressively with age. In women, however, serum phosphorus values decline progressively between twenty and thirty-five years of age, increasing after aged forty years. Serum phosphorus concentrations were measured in the Nutrition Canada National Survey (Health and Welfare, 1973) and can be used, in association with serum calcium levels, for the assessment of rickets in children.

	Serum Phosphorus	
Subject Group	(mg/dL)	(mmol/L)
Prematurely born infants	7.9	2.5
Full-term infants (first month)	6.1	2.0
Children (one to ten years)	4.6	1.5
Adults	3.5	1.1

Table 23.2: Changes of average serum phosphorus concentrations with age. From Harrison HE. (1984). Phosphorus. In: Present Knowledge in Nutrition. Fifth edition. The Nutrition Foundation Inc., with permission.

Higher serum phosphorus values in children are necessary for adequate mineralization of the growing skeleton. The decrease in serum phosphorus which occurs with adulthood is probably a hormone-mediated effect. Seasonal variations in serum phosphorus concentrations in children have been described, levels rising during the summer and declining in winter.

Many confounding factors affect serum phosphorus concentrations. In the presence of rickets, for example, serum phosphorus values are reduced (hypophosphatemia), possibly because the active vitamin D metabolite, $1,25\text{-}(OH)_2D$, has an essential role in the efficacy of phosphorus absorption. Several other conditions associated with abnormalities of renal tubular function cause hypophosphatemia. These are listed in Table 23.3.

Persons with healing fractures tend to have higher serum phosphorus concentrations. In insulin-dependent diabetics, levels vary as insulin injections decrease phosphorus levels in the serum. Serum phosphorus concentrations are generally determined colorimetrically, by a modification of the molybdenum blue procedure of Fiske and Subbarow (1925).

23.3   Assessment of magnesium status

The adult human body contains approximately 24 g of magnesium, of which 60% is in the bone, the remainder being equally distributed between muscle and nonmuscular soft tissues (Table 23.1). Magnesium is also the second most abundant cation in the intracellular fluid. It has a role in many enzyme reactions, especially those involving energy metabolism, when it participates in phosphate-transfer reactions involving adenosine triphosphate and nucleotide triphosphates. Magnesium is also involved in protein synthesis, in the formation of cyclic adenosine monophosphate. In neuromuscular transmission and activity, magnesium acts synergistically, or in some cases antagonistically, with calcium (Shils, 1984).

Fanconi syndrome
    Cystinosis
    Tyrosinosis
    Heavy metal poisoning
    Nephrotoxic organic compounds
    Multiple myeloma
Renal tubular acidosis
Genetic primary hypophosphatemia
Acquired primary hypophosphatemia
    Connective tissue tumors

Table 23.3: Hypophosphatemia secondary to disorders of renal tubule reabsorption of phosphate. From Harrison HE. (1984). Phosphorus. In: Present Knowledge in Nutrition. Fifth edition. The Nutrition Foundation Inc., with permission.

Dietary magnesium deficiency in humans is rare. Magnesium is widely distributed in both plant and animal foodstuffs, especially in nuts, green vegetables, soybeans, chocolate, and whole grain cereals. Hard drinking water may also be an important source of dietary magnesium (Gibson et al., 1987). The amount of dietary magnesium absorbed is inversely related to intake, and can range from 25% on a high-magnesium diet to 75% on a low-magnesium diet (Graham et al., 1960). Little is known of the dietary factors modifying intestinal absorption of magnesium, but like calcium, urinary excretion of magnesium is regulated in response to need. Thus, when magnesium intake is severely restricted, urinary magnesium losses are reduced to very small amounts within four to six days (Shils, 1984).

Magnesium deficiency generally develops in association with certain clinical disease states (e.g. severe malabsorption, gastrointestinal disorders, alcoholism, regional enteritis, and cirrhosis), and in patients with severe burns (Broughton et al., 1968). It may also occur in patients with congestive heart failure or on long-term diuretic therapy (Wester and Dyckner, 1984). Prolonged treatment with certain drugs, such as gentamycin, can also result in magnesium deficiency. A familial disorder of magnesium metabolism, related specifically to the intestinal absorption of magnesium, has also been described (Strømme et al., 1969).

The signs and symptoms characterizing magnesium deficiency in humans are varied, and may include personality changes, spontaneous generalized muscle spasm, tremor, fasciculations, and Trousseau and Chvostek signs (Shils, 1964). Convulsions occur more frequently in magnesium-deficient infants than in adults. Magnesium deficiency has also been implicated as a factor in certain chronic diseases (e.g. cardiac arrhythmias, coronary heart disease, hypertension, and premenstrual

syndrome) (Johnson et al., 1979; Dyckner 1980; Abraham and Lubran, 1981; Cohen and Kitzes 1983; McCarron, 1983; Wester and
Dyckner, 1987; Anon, 1988), although these relationships remain controversial. The apparent magnesium depletion described in some of these
conditions may in fact be associated with a redistribution of magnesium in the body resulting from the disease process. The presence of
widespread chronic suboptimal magnesium status in the general population appears unlikely. Nevertheless, some adults in the United States
consuming self-selected diets were apparently in negative magnesium
balance on some of the metabolic-balance days during a year-long study
(Lakshmanan et al., 1984).   Subclinical magnesium deficiency may
also exist in pregnancy (Caddell et al., 1975) and lactation (Greenwald
et al., 1963).

Magnesium toxicity, arising from excessive intake of oral $MgSO_4$,
generally occurs only when kidney function is impaired (Venugopal and
Luckey, 1978). Diarrhea and dehydration may result. In cases of acute
magnesium toxicity via the parenteral route, nausea, depression, and
paralysis may occur. Magnesium toxicity arising from excessive dietary
magnesium intakes is unlikely.

Assessment of the magnesium status of an individual is difficult
because the tissue pool which is in equilibrium with the total body
magnesium content has not been identified (Elin, 1987a). Unfortunately,
different individual tissues become depleted in magnesium over varying
time periods and their magnesium contents are affected by many non-
nutritional factors.

23.3.1   Serum magnesium concentrations

Serum magnesium concentration is the most frequently used index
of magnesium status.   Serum magnesium appears to parallel tissue
levels in primary magnesium deficiency but not in diseases that affect
magnesium homeostasis (Dyckner and Wester, 1978). Only a very small
percentage of total body magnesium (0.3%) is present in the serum
(Alfrey et al., 1974). Of this, 55% is in the form of the free ion, 13% is
complexed, and 32% is bound nonspecifically to albumin and globulins
(Kroll and Elin, 1985). Serum, rather than plasma, is used because anticoagulants may be contaminated with magnesium (Caddell et al., 1974).

The mean serum magnesium concentration in adult humans is approximately 0.85 mmol/L (range 0.7 to 1.0 mmol/L) (Aikawa, 1981). A normal serum magnesium concentration does not preclude magnesium deficiency; only in severe cases of deficiency does hypomagnesemia consistently occur. For example, in five cases of cardiac arrhythmias subsequently dispelled by parenteral administration of magnesium, serum
magnesium concentrations were normal (Cohen and Kitzes, 1983).

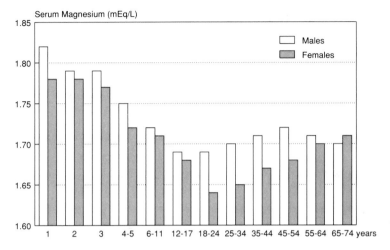

Figure 23.1: Variations in serum magnesium concentrations with age and sex. United States, 1971–1974. Conversion factor to SI units (mmol/L) = × 0.500. Data from Lowenstein and Stanton (1986).

Several confounding factors influence serum magnesium concentrations. Hemolysis affects serum magnesium levels because the magnesium concentration of erythrocytes is approximately three times that of serum. Slight diurnal variation in serum magnesium concentrations occurs; values are lower in the morning than the evening. Such trends are probably associated with food intake and physical activity level, although rhythmical changes in the function of the parathyroid gland may also play a part. Certainly, after strenuous exercise, serum magnesium concentrations fall (Stendig-Lindberg et al., 1987), partially as a result of a loss of magnesium in sweat (Bellar et al., 1975). Decreased serum magnesium concentrations also occur in late pregnancy as a result of physiological hemodilution (Chesley, 1972). There is a linear relationship between serum magnesium and albumin when the concentrations of the latter are high, or low, but not when serum albumin is within the normal range (Kroll and Elin, 1985). Hence, the presence of hypo- or hyper-albuminemia will confound the interpretation of serum magnesium concentrations.

When clinical signs and symptoms are suggestive of magnesium deficiency, a low serum magnesium concentration can be used to confirm the diagnosis. If, in these cases, the serum magnesium value appears normal, magnesium concentrations in leukocytes and twenty-four-hour urine samples should also be measured.

Serum magnesium concentrations were measured in the NHANES I survey (Lowenstein and Stanton, 1986) but not in the Nutrition Canada National Survey (Health and Welfare Canada, 1973). Concentrations in non-fasting blood samples for U.S. adults aged eighteen to seventy-four years ranged from 0.75 to 0.95 mmol/L; Caucasians had consistently higher serum magnesium concentrations than comparably aged persons of African descent. Values declined from aged one to eighteen years in males, after which levels remained fairly stable. In females, values decreased up to twenty-four years of age, and then increased until aged seventy-four years (Lowenstein and Stanton, 1986). Small sex differences were observed in adults aged eighteen and forty-five years; males had higher concentrations than females (Figure 23.1). Tables of selected percentiles, means, and standard deviations by race, age, and sex for persons in the NHANES I survey are available (Lowenstein and Stanton, 1986).

Serum magnesium can be readily measured using flame AAS. Other methods, less frequently used, include atomic emission spectrophotometry, compleximetry, chromatography, colorimetry, and fluorometry (Deuster et al., 1987).

23.3.2   Erythrocyte magnesium concentrations

Magnesium exists in erythrocytes in three forms: free, complexed, and protein-bound. Concentrations are about three times greater than in serum, approximating 2.5 mmol/L (Walser, 1967). Erythrocyte magnesium concentrations reflect chronic, rather than acute, magnesium status because of the long erythrocyte half-life (120 days). Decreases in erythrocyte magnesium concentrations are not observed until several weeks after the onset of a dietary deficiency. Erythrocyte magnesium concentrations do not correlate with other tissue pools of magnesium.

Concentrations of magnesium in erythrocytes are dependent on the age of the erythrocytes; the magnesium content slowly declines as they age (Elin et al., 1980). Consequently, concentrations of magnesium in nucleated erythrocytes and reticulocytes are greater (up to eight times) than in mature erythrocytes (Walser, 1967). Normally, the erythrocyte magnesium content is not seriously affected by the age distribution of cells in the erythrocyte pellet prepared for analysis (Deuster et al., 1987). In conditions in which the survival time of erythrocytes is reduced, such as during chronic renal failure, thalassemia, and sickle cell anemia, erythrocyte magnesium concentrations may be higher because magnesium-rich immature erythrocytes predominate. Erythrocyte magnesium content is also altered in several other clinical conditions such as hyperthyroidism (Rizek et al., 1965), chronic lymphatic leukemia (Rosner and Gorfien, 1968), and in women with premenstrual tension (Abraham and Lubran, 1981; Sherwood et al., 1986). There is also evidence that human erythrocyte magnesium concentrations are genetically controlled (Henrotte, 1982). All these effects may confound the interpretation of erythrocyte magnesium concentrations.

Both indirect and direct methods have been used for erythrocyte magnesium analysis (Deuster et al., 1987). The indirect methods involve measuring the magnesium concentration in whole blood and serum and calculating the content in erythrocytes by difference (Refsum et al., 1973; Abraham and Lubran, 1981; Lukaski et al., 1983). Deuster et al. (1987) concluded that such a procedure, using nitric acid to lyse erythrocytes, is reproducible, reliable, accurate, and much less time-consuming than the direct method. The latter involves separation of the erythrocytes from whole blood followed by digestion and analysis of the erythrocyte pellet. In both methods, magnesium concentrations are usually measured by flame AAS.

23.3.3 Leukocyte and mononuclear blood cell magnesium concentrations

Magnesium concentrations in leukocytes and in specific cell types appear promising as indices of body magnesium status. For instance, in experimental magnesium depletion in rats, changes in peripheral mononuclear blood cell magnesium concentrations (lymphocytes + monocytes) reflected those in cardiac and skeletal muscle (Ryan and Ryan, 1979). In humans, a correlation between the magnesium concentration of mononuclear blood cells and the magnesium balance of patients with chronic congestive heart failure has been documented. Such patients receive diuretics that increase urinary losses of magnesium (Ryan et al., 1981). The magnesium concentration of peripheral blood lymphocytes is also promising as an index of magnesium status (Cohen and Kitzes, 1983). Significant correlations of magnesium concentrations in lymphocytes and muscle have been noted in some patients with ischemic heart disease and mild arterial hypertension, as well as some healthy controls (Dyckner and Wetser, 1985). Nevertheless, more work is necessary before the validity of magnesium concentrations in leukocytes or specific cell types as indices of total body magnesium status can be firmly established. Care must be taken to ensure that the assay and units for reporting the results are standardized, enabling results among studies to be compared (Elin, 1987b).

The assay involves first removing the platelets from whole blood and then separating the leukocytes or mononuclear blood cells with a discontinuous Ficoll-Hypaque gradient. The separated cells are then washed, centrifuged to form a pellet, and lysed by sonication with distilled water. The lysate can be frozen until analysis with AAS. Lanthanum oxide should be added to the cell lysate before analysis to liberate the magnesium bound to cellular elements (Elin and Hosseini, 1985). The assay is often associated with large coefficients of variation (greater than 25%), arising from difficulties with the isolation of the different cell types. Standardizing the centrifugal force used to harvest the leukocytes or cell types after washing can reduce the coefficient of variation (Elin and Hosseini, 1985). The magnesium content of the leukocytes, like erythrocytes, may vary with cell age, contributing to large inter-individual differences in the measured magnesium concentrations of leukocytes. Large blood samples are required for harvesting the leukocytes or cell types, limiting the use of this assay in pediatric populations.

Three methods are used for quantifying the magnesium in leukocytes or mononuclear blood cell types (Elin, 1983; 1987b); these are: (a) magnesium per unit mass of protein, (b) magnesium concentration per cell, and (c) magnesium concentration per unit mass dry weight (Hossseini et al., 1983; Elin and Hosseini, 1985; Elin, 1987b). Elin and Hosseini (1985) reported a mean value of 70.7 ± 14.1 fg/cell for the magnesium content of mononuclear blood cells from twenty apparently healthy adult volunteers. This value falls within the range noted by others (Elin and Johnson, 1982). When results are reported per unit mass of protein, mean values range from 1.28 to 1.78 µg Mg/mg protein (Elin and Johnson 1982; Hosseini et al., 1983; Sjögren et al., 1986); for dry weight of cells mean values range from 31.0 to 43.4 mmol Mg/kg dry weight (Elin, 1987). The magnesium content of human blood leukocytes appears to be higher than that of mononuclear blood cells, possibly because leukocytes include neutrophils which may have a higher magnesium content than mononuclear blood cells (Rosner and Lee, 1972; Ross et al., 1980).

23.3.4 Urinary magnesium concentrations and magnesium load test

The major excretory route for absorbed magnesium is via the urine. Normal urinary magnesium excretion ranges from 120 to 140 mg/24 hr for persons on a mixed diet (Aikawa, 1981). Excretion is reduced in persons with low or depleted body stores of magnesium as a result of a compensatory conservation of magnesium by the kidneys (Heaton, 1969). Hence, urinary magnesium excretion has been used as an index of magnesium status, primarily in association with a magnesium load test. This test is regarded as the most reliable screening method for diagnosing magnesium deficiency (Holm et al., 1987), provided that renal function, fluid balance, and cardiovascular function are normal. It has been used to assess magnesium deficiency in infants, children with protein-energy malnutrition, postpartum U.S. women, alcoholics, patients with gastrointestinal disease, and patients who have had intestinal bypass operations for severe obesity (Thorén, 1962; Caddell, 1969; Caddell et al., 1975; Bøhmer and Mathiesen, 1982; Holm et al., 1987). An intravenous magnesium load test has also been used on patients with ischemic heart disease and acute myocardial infarction (Rasmussen et al., 1988). In most of these investigations, however, no other corroborating index of magnesium status, with the exception of serum magnesium, was measured. The increased retention of magnesium noted in some of these patients with acute illness may have been associated with alterations in the renal handling of magnesium, rather than a reduction in magnesium stores (Anonymous, 1988).

For the magnesium load test, basal urinary magnesium excretion is first determined on a timed preload urine collection. Three consecutive twenty-four-hour urine samples should be collected to counteract the effects of both diurnal and random day-to-day variation (Graham et al., 1960). A reduction in the urinary excretion of magnesium at night has been reported. Magnesium is then administered, generally over an eight-hour period, either intramuscularly for infants or intravenously for adults, at levels ranging from 0.25 (for infants) to 1.0 mmol/kg body weight. Parenteral administration is used to eliminate variability in intestinal absorption of magnesium. Following the load, the excretion of magnesium is measured over the subsequent twenty-four to forty-eight-hour period. Urine specimens should be collected with an acidifying agent in the container to prevent precipitation of magnesium compounds at high pH. The net retention of magnesium is calculated by comparing basal excretion data with net excretion after the load. Thorén (1963) recommended calculating retention over forty-eight hours, not twenty-four hours, to better distinguish normal and pathological magnesium retention.

The cutoff values used for net retention of magnesium associated with magnesium deficiency vary. Thorén (1963) claimed that magnesium retentions greater than 20% to 50% after an intravenous magnesium load indicate magnesium deficiency. Caddell et al. (1975) used 40% as their upper limit of normal for magnesium retention for postpartum U.S. women. Subjects with lower magnesium retention values (i.e. < 40%) had significantly higher plasma magnesium concentrations and correspondingly higher dietary magnesium intakes compared to their counterparts with retention values greater than 40%. More recently, Holm et al. (1987) showed that patients with magnesium retentions greater than 20% showed a significant decrease in magnesium retention after treatment with magnesium chloride. Consequently, these investigators recommend a cutoff value of greater than 20% magnesium retention as indicative of suboptimal magnesium status. More data are required on normal retentions of a magnesium load for different age groups.

23.3.5 Muscle magnesium concentrations

Magnesium concentrations of muscle have been used to assess magnesium status because muscle is a major tissue storage site for magnesium. Of the total body magnesium, approximately 27% is located in the muscle. Muscle magnesium concentrations were restored to normal levels after magnesium replacement therapy in patients with magnesium deficiency arising from long-term diuretic therapy for heart failure (Lim and

Jacob, 1972). Muscle specimens can be obtained by needle biopsy, but the procedure requires special skill and is too invasive for community surveys or routine clinical use. Concentrations of muscle magnesium do not correlate with serum magnesium (Lim and Jacob, 1972). Significant correlations between magnesium concentrations in muscle and those of mononuclear blood cells, however, have been noted in some, but not all, disease states. For example, in patients with Type I diabetes mellitus (Sjögren et al., 1986) or with mild arterial hypertension (Dyckner and Wester, 1984), magnesium concentrations in lymphocytes apparently reflected those in skeletal muscle. Such a relationship was not observed in patients with congestive heart failure (Dyckner and Wester, 1984); the reason for this discrepancy is unclear.

23.4 Summary

Calcium

Calcium, the most abundant mineral in the body, is stored primarily in the bones. The remainder is involved in enzyme activation, blood coagulation, muscle contractibility, nerve transmission, hormone function, and membrane transport. Several dietary components influence calcium absorption but severe nutritional deficiency of calcium is rare because calcium absorption and urinary excretion are regulated in response to need. Inadequate calcium intakes during early life may limit peak adult bone mass and hence increase the risk of osteoporosis in later life. Serum ionized calcium concentrations are more promising as an index of calcium status than total serum calcium levels, which are under strict homeostatic control. Measurements of the bone mass of the appendicular or axial skeleton are also performed as an indirect assessment of bone calcium content and hence body calcium stores. Generally, single or dual photon absorptiometry is used for the measurement of bone mineral content of the appendicular and axial skeleton, respectively. The bone mineral content is inversely related to the amount of transmitted radiation. Persons with osteoporosis have a bone mass which is at least 20% less than those of comparable healthy adults. Methods used less frequently include computerized tomography, radiogrammetry, and neutron activation measurements of total body calcium.

Phosphorus

Phosphorus is present in the bones, as well as in cells and extracellular fluids where it functions in all the energy-producing reactions of the cells. Dietary deficiency of phosphorus is rare, although cases associated with excessive intakes of antacids and prolonged total parenteral nutrition have occured. Serum phosphorus is the most frequently used index of phosphorus status, but it has a low specificity and sensitivity. Concentrations are affected by many confounding factors unrelated to phosphorus status, such as insulin injections or abnormalities of renal tubular function.

Magnesium

Approximately two thirds of the total body magnesium content is in the bone, the remainder being in the muscle and nonmuscular soft tissues and intracellular fluid. Magnesium is involved in energy metabolism, protein synthesis, and neuromuscular transmission and activity. Secondary deficiencies of magnesium develop in certain clinical disease states and/or during treatment with certain drugs. Nutritional deficiency is rare but suboptimal magnesium status may occur in pregnancy and lactation. Serum magnesium concentrations are most frequently used to assess magnesium status despite their low sensitivity and specificity. Erythrocyte magnesium concentrations reflect chronic magnesium status, decreasing only several weeks after the onset of a dietary deficiency. The age of the erythrocytes influences their magnesium concentration, confounding the interpretation in certain conditions. The magnesium concentrations of leukocytes and specific cell types (e.g. mononuclear cells) appear more promising as indices of magnesium status, reflecting muscle magnesium concentrations in rats. In persons with depleted body stores of magnesium, urinary excretion is low. Net retention of magnesium after a magnesium load test can be used to assess magnesium status in research studies. Basal urinary magnesium excretion is first determined, followed by the measurement of magnesium concentrations in two consecutive twenty-four-hour urine samples, post dose. The magnesium concentrations of muscle biopsy specimens may be determined in future studies of magnesium nutriture. Muscle comprises a major tissue storage site for magnesium, and concentrations appear to correlate with those of mononuclear blood cells.

References

Abraham GE, Lubran MM. (1981). Serum and red cell magnesium levels in patients with premenstrual tension. American Journal of Clinical Nutrition 34: 2364–2366.

Aikawa JK. (1981). Magnesium: its biological significance. CRC Press Inc., Boca Raton, Florida.

Alfrey AC, Miller NL, Butkus D. (1974). Evaluation of body magnesium stores. Journal of Laboratory and Clinical Medicine 84: 153–162.

Allen LH, Bartlett RS, Block GD. (1979). Reduction of renal calcium reabsorption in man by consumption of dietary protein. Journal of Nutrition 109: 1345–1350.

Anderson GH, Draper HH. (1972). Effect of dietary phosphorus on calcium metabolism in intact and parathyroidectomized adult rats. Journal of Nutrition 102: 1123–1132.

Anderson MP, Hunt RD, Griffiths HJ, McIntyre KW, Zimmerman RE. (1977). Long-term effect of low dietary calcim:phosphorus ratio on the skeleton of *Cebus albifrons* monkeys. Journal of Nutrition 107: 834–839.

Anonymous (1988). Magnesium deficiency and ischemic heart disease. Nutrition Reviews 46: 311–312.

Avioli LV, McDonald JE, Lee SW. (1965). The influence of age on the intestinal absorption of 47-Ca in postmenopausal osteoporosis. Journal of Clinical Investigation 44: 1960–1967.

Avioli LV. (1984). Calcium and osteoporosis. Annual Review of Nutrition 4: 471–491.

Bell RR, Draper HH, Tzeng DVM, Shin HK, Schmidt GR. (1977). Physiological responses of human adults to foods containing phosphate additives. Journal of Nutrition 107: 42–50.

Bellar GA, Maher JT, Hartley LH, Bass DE, Wacker WEC. (1975). Changes in serum and sweat magnesium levels during work in the heat. Aviation Space and Environmental Medicine 46: 709–712.

Bøhmer and Mathiesen, (1982). Magnesium deficiency in chronic alcoholic patients uncovered by an intravenous loading test. Scandinavian Journal of Clinical and Laboratory Investigation 42: 633–636.

Boyd RM, Cameron EC, McIntosh HW, Walker VR. (1974). Measurement of bone mineral content *in vivo* using photon absorptiometry. Canadian Medical Association Journal 111: 1201–1205.

Broughton A, Anderson IR, Bowden CH. (1968). Magnesium-deficiency syndrome in burns. Lancet 2: 1156–1158.

Bullamore JR, Wilkinson R, Gallagher JC, Nordin BEC, Marshall DH. (1970). Effect of age on calcium absorption. Lancet 2: 535–537.

Caddell JL. (1969). The effect of magnesium therapy on cardiovascular and electrocardiograph changes in severe protein-calorie malnutrition. Tropical and Geographic Medicine 21: 33-38.

Caddell JL, Erickson M, Byrne PA. (1974). Interference from citrate using the Titan Yellow method and two fluorometric methods for magnesium determination in plasma. Clinica Chimica Acta 50: 9–11.

Caddell JL, Saier FL, Thomason CA. (1975). Parenteral magnesium load tests in postpartum American women. American Journal of Clinical Nutrition 28: 1099–1104.

Chesley LC. (1972). Plasma and red blood cell volumes during pregnancy. American Journal of Obstetrics and Gynecology. 112: 440–450.

Cohen L, Kitzes R. (1983). Magnesium sulfate and digitalis-toxic arrhythmias. Journal of the American Medical Association 249: 2808–2810.

Cohn SH, Ellis KJ, Wallach J, Zanzi I, Atkins HL, Aloia JF. (1974a). Absolute and relative deficit in total skeletal calcium and radial bone mineral in osteoporosis. Journal of Nuclear Medicine 15: 428–435.

Cohn SH, Ellis KJ, Wallach J. (1974b). In vivo neutron activation analysis. Clinical potential in body composition analysis. American Journal of Medicine 57: 683–686.

Cummings SR, Kelsey JL, Nevitt MC, O'Dowd KJ. (1985). Epidemiology of osteoporosis and osteoporotic fractures. Epidemiologic Reviews 7: 178–208.

Deuster PA, Trostmann UH, Bernier LL, Dolev E. (1987). Indirect vs direct measurement of magnesium and zinc in erythrocytes. Clinical Chemistry 33: 529–532.

Dyckner T. (1980). Serum magnesium in acute myocardial infarction Relation to arrhythmias. Acta Medica Scandinavica 207: 59–66.

Dyckner T, Wester PO. (1978). The relation between extra- and intracellular electrolytes in patients with hypokalemia an/or diuretic treatment. Acta Medica Scandinavica 204: 269–282.

Dyckner T, Wester PO. (1984). Intracellular magnesium loss after diuretic administration. Drugs 28 (Supplement 1): 161–166.

Dyckner T, Wester PO. (1985). Skeletal muscle magnesium and potassium determinations: correlations with lymphocyte contents of magnesium and potassium. Journal of the American College of Nutrition 4: 619–625.

Elin RJ. (1983). The status of cellular analysis. Journal of the American College of Nutrition 4: 329–330.

Elin RJ. (1987a). Assessment of magnesium status. Clinical Chemistry 33: 1965–1970.

Elin RJ. (1987b). Status of the mononuclear blood cell magnesium assay. Journal of the American College of Nutrition 6: 105–107.

Elin RJ, Hosseini JM. (1985). Magnesium content of mononuclear blood cells. Clinical Chemistry 31: 377–380.

Elin RJ, Johnson E. (1982). A method for the determination of the magnesium content of blood mononuclear cells. Magnesium 1: 115–121.

Elin RJ, Utter A, Tan HK, Corash L. (1980). Effect of magnesium deficiency on erythrocyte aging in rats. American Journal of Pathology 100: 765–778.

Fiske CH, Subbarow Y. (1925). The colorimetric determination of phosphorus. Journal of Biological Chemistry 66: 375–400.

Freudenheim JL, Johnson NE, Smith EL. (1986). Relationships between usual nutrient intake and bone mineral content of women 35–65 years of age: longitudinal and cross-sectional analysis. American Journal of Clinical Nutrition 44: 863–876.

Gibson RS, Smit Vanderkooy PD, McLennan C, Mercer NJ. (1987). The contribution of tap water to mineral intakes of Canadian preschool children. Archives of Environmental Health 42: 165–169.

Graham LA, Caesar JJ, Burgen AS. (1960). Gastrointestinal absorption and excretion of Mg 28 in man. Metabolism 9: 646–659.

Greenwald JH, Dubin A, Cardon L. (1963). Hypomagnesemic tetany due to excessive lactation. American Journal of Medicine 35: 854–860.

Harper AB, Laughlin WS, Mazess RB. (1984). Bone mineral content in St. Lawrence Island Eskimos. Human Biology 56: 63–78.

Harrison HE. (1984). Phosphorus. In: Present Knowledge in Nutrition. Fifth edition. The Nutrition Foundation Inc., Washington, D.C., pp. 413–421.

Harrison JE, NcNeil KG, Hitchman AJ, Britt BA. (1979). Bone mineral measurements of the central skeleton by in vivo neutron activation analysis for routine investigation of osteopenia. Investigative Radiology 14: 27–34.

Hayes WC, Gerhart TN. (1985). Biomechanics of bone: applications for assessment of bone strength. In: Peck WA. (ed). Bone and Mineral Research. Elsevier Science Publishing Company, New York, pp. 259–294.

Health and Welfare Canada. (1973). Nutrition Canada National Survey. Health and Welfare, Ottawa.

Heaney RP, Recker RR, Saville PD. (1978). Menopausal changes in calcium balance performance. Journal of Laboratory and Clinical Medicine 92: 953–963.

Heaney RP, Gallagher JC, Johnston CC, Neer R, Parfitt AM, Whedon GD. (1982). Calcium nutrition and bone health in the elderly. American Journal of Clinical Nutrition 36: 986–1013.

Heaton FW. (1969). The kidney and magnesium homeostasis. Annals of the New York Academy of Sciences 162: 775–785.

Hegsted M, Schuette SA, Zemel MB, Linkswiler HM. (1981). Urinary calcium and calcium balance in young men as affected by level of protein and phosphorus intake. Journal of Nutrition 111: 553–562.

Henrotte JG. (1982). Genetic regulation of red blood cell magnesium content and major histocompatibility complex. Magnesium 1: 69–80.

Holm CN, Jepsen JM, Sjogaard G, Hessov I. (1987). A magnesium load test in the diagnosis of magnesium deficiency. Human Nutrition: Clinical Nutrition 41C: 301–306.

Horsman A, Nordin BEC, Aaron J, Marshall DH. (1981). Cortical and trabecular osteoporosis and their relation to fractures in the elderly. In: DeLuca HF, Frost HM, Jee WSS, Johnston CC Jr, Parfitt AM (eds). Osteoporosis: Recent Advances in Pathogenesis and Treatment. University Park Press, Baltimore, pp. 175–184.

Hosseini JM, Johnson E, Elin RJ. (1983). Comparison of two separation techniques for the determination of blood mononuclear cell magnesium content. Journal of the American College of Nutrition 4: 361–368.

Hui SL, Johnston CC Jr., Mazess RB. (1985). Bone mass in normal children and young adults. Growth 49: 34–43.

Johnson CJ, Peterson DP, Smith EK. (1979). Myocardial tissue concentrations of magnesium and potassium in men dying suddenly from ischaemic heart disease. American Journal of Clinical Nutrition 32: 967–970.

Karppanen H. (1986). Epidemiological aspects of magnesium deficiency in cardiovascular diseases. Magnesium-Bulletin 8: 199–203.

Kesteloot H, Geboers J. (1982). Calcium and blood pressure. Lancet 1: 813–815.

Kimmel PL. (1984). Radiologic methods to evaluate bone mineral content. Annals of Internal Medicine 100: 908–911.

Kroll MH, Elin RJ. (1985). Relationships between magnesium and protein concentrations in serum. Clinical Chemistry 31: 244–246.

Ladenson JH, Bowers GN. (1973a). Free calcium in serum. I. Determination with the ion-specific electrode, and factors affecting the results. Clinical Chemistry 19: 565–574.

Ladenson JH, Bowers GN. (1973b). Free calcium in serum. II. Rigor of homeostatic control, correlations with total serum calcium, and review of data on patients with disturbed calcium metabolism. Clinical Chemistry 19: 575–582.

Lakshmanan FL, Rao RB, Kim WW, Kelsay JL. (1984). Magnesium intakes, balances, and blood levels of adults consuming self-selected diets. American Journal of Clinical Nutrition 40: 1380–1389.

Lotz M, Zisman E, Bartter FC. (1968). Evidence for a phosphorus-depletion syndrome in man. New England Journal of Medicine 278: 409–415.

Li T-K, Piechocki JT. (1971). Determination of serum ionic calcium with an ion-selective electrode: Evaluation of methodology and normal values. Clinical Chemistry 17: 411–416.

Lim P, Jacob E. (1972). Magnesium deficiency in patients on long-term diuretic therapy for heart failure. British Medical Journal 3: 620–622.

Lowenstein FW, Stanton MF. (1986). Serum magnesium levels in the United States, 1971–1974. Journal of the American College of Nutrition 5: 399–414.

Lukaski HC, Bolonchuk WW, Klevay LM, Milne DB, Sandstead HH. (1983). Maximal oxygen consumption as related to magnesium, copper, and zinc nutriture. American Journal of Clinical Nutrition 37: 407–415.

Margen S, Chu J-Y, Kaufmann NA, Calloway DH. (1974). Studies in calcium metabolism. I. The calciuretic effect of dietary protein. American Journal of Clinical Nutrition 27: 584–589.

Matković V, Kostial K, Simonović I, Buzina R, Brodarec A, Nordin BE. (1979). Bone status and fracture rates in two regions of Yugoslavia. American Journal of Clinical Nutrition 32: 540–549.

Mazess RB. (1971). Estimation of bone and skeletal weight by direct photon absorptiometry. Investigative Radiology 6: 52–60.

Mazess RB. (1983). Errors in measuring trabecular bone by computed tomography due to marrow and bone composition. Calicified Tissue International 35: 148–152.

Mazess RB, Cameron JR. (1974). Bone mineral content of normal U.S. whites. In: Mazess RB (ed). Proceedings of the International Conference on Bone Mineral Measurement. Publication No. (NIH) 75–6. U.S. Government Printing Office, Washington, D.C., pp. 228–238.

Mazess RB, Peppler WW, Chesney RW, Lange TA, Lingren U, Smith E Jr. (1984a). Does bone measurement on the radius indicate skeletal status: concise communication. Journal of Nuclear Medicine 25: 281–288.

Mazess RB, Peppler WW, Chesney RW, Lange TA, Lingren U, Smith E Jr. (1984b). Total body and regional bone mineral by dual-photon absorptiometry in metabolic bone disease. Calcified Tissue International 36: 8–13.

McCarron DA. (1983). Calcium and magnesium nutrition in human hypertension. Annals of Internal Medicine 5: 800–805.

Moon WH, Malzer JL, Clark HE. (1974). Phosphorus balances of adults consuming several food combinations. Journal of the American Dietetic Association 64: 386–390.

Oreskes I, Hirsch C, Douglas KS, Kupfer S. (1968). Measurement of ionized calcium in human plasma with a calcium selective electrode. Clinica Chimica Acta 21: 303–313.

Parfitt AM. (1984). Age-related structural changes in trabecular and cortical bone: cellular mechanisms and biomechanical consequences. Calcified Tissue International 36: S123–S128.

Rasmussen HS, McNair P, Gøransson, Balslø, Larsen OG, Aurup. (1988). Magnesium deficiency in patients with ischemic heart disease with and without acute myocardial infarction uncovered by an intravenous loading test. Archives of Internal Medicine 148: 329–332.

Refsum HE, Mean HD, Strømme SB. (1973). Whole blood, serum and erythrocyte magnesium concentrations after repeated heavy exercise of long duration. Scandinavian Journal of Clinical and Laboratory Investigation 32: 123–127.

Riis B, Thomsen K, Christiansen C. (1987). Does calcium supplementation prevent postmenopausal bone loss? A double-blind, controlled clinical study. New England Journal of Medicine 316: 173–177.

Rizek JE, Dimich A, Wallach S. (1965). Plasma and erythrocyte magnesium in thyroid disease. Journal of Clinical Endocrinology and Metabolism 25: 350–358.

Ross R, Seelig M, Berger A. (1980). Isolation of leukocytes for magnesium determination. In: Cantin M, Seelig M (eds). Magnesium in Health and Disease. Spectrum Publications, New York, pp. 7–15.

Rosner F, Gorfien PC. (1968). Erythrocyte and plasma zinc and magnesium levels in health and disease. Journal of Laboratory and Clinical Medicine 72: 213–219.

Rosner F, Lee S. (1972). Zinc and magnesium content of leukocyte alkaline phosphatase isoenzymes. Journal of Laboratory and Clinical Medicine 79: 228–239.

Ryan MP, Ryan MF. (1979). Lymphocyte electrolyte alterations during magnesium deficiency in the rat. Irish Journal of Medical Science 148: 108–109.

Ryan MP, Ryan MF, Counihan TB. (1981). The effect of diuretics on lymphocyte magnesium and potassium. Acta Medica Scandinavica Supplement 647: 153–161.

Schuette SA, Linkswiler HM. (1984). Calcium. In: Present Knowledge in Nutrition. Fifth edition. The Nutrition Foundation Inc., Washington, D.C., pp. 410–412.

Schwartz HD. (1976). New techniques for ion-selective measurements of ionized calcium in serum after pH adjustment of aerobically handled sera. Clinical Chemistry 22: 461–467.

Sherwood RA, Rocks BF, Stewart A, Saxton RS. (1986). Magnesium and the premenstrual syndrome. Annals of Clinical Biochemistry 23: 667–670.

Shils ME. (1964). Experimental human magnesium depletion. I. Clinical observations and blood chemistry alterations. American Journal of Clinical Nutrition 15: 133–143.

Shils ME. (1984). Magnesium. In: Present Knowledge in Nutrition. Fifth edition. The Nutrition Foundation Inc., Washington, D.C., pp. 423–437.

Sie T-L, Draper HH, Bell RR. (1974). Hypocalcemia, hyperparathyroidism and bone resorption induced by dietary phosphate. Journal of Nutrition 104: 1195–1201.

Sjögren A, Floren CH, Nilsson A. (1986). Magnesium deficiency in IDDM related to level of glycosylated hemoglobin. Diabetes 35: 459–463.

Spencer H, Menczel J, Lewin I, Samachson J. (1965). Effect of high phosphorus intake on calcium and phosphorus metabolism in man. Journal of Nutrition 86: 125–132.

Spencer H, Kramer L, Osis D, Norris C. (1978). Effect of phosphorus on the absorption of calcium and on the calcium balance in man. Journal of Nutrition 108: 447–457.

Spencer H, Kramer L, Osis D. (1982). Factors contributing to calcium loss in aging. American Journal of Clincial Nutrition 36: 776–787.

Stendig-Lindberg G, Shapiro Y, Epstein Y, Galun E, Schonberger E, Graff E, Wacker WEC. (1987). Changes in serum magnesium concentration after strenuous exercise. Journal of the American College of Nutrition 6: 35–40.

Strømme JH, Nesbakken R, Normann T, Skorten F, Skyberg D, Johannessen R. (1969). Familial hypomagnesemia. Biochemical, histological and hereditary aspects studied in two brothers. Acta Paediatrica Scandinavica 58: 434–444.

Thorén L. (1963). Magnesium deficiency in gastrointestinal fluid loss. Acta Chirurgica Scandinavica Supplement 306: 1–65.

Thorén L. (1962). Magnesium deficiency; studies in two cases of acute fulminant ulcerative colitis treated by colectomy. Acta Chirurgica Scandinavica 124: 134–143.

Venugopal B, Luckey TD. (1978). Metal Toxicity in Mammals. Volume 2. Plenum Press, New York, pp. 41–100.

Wahner HW, Dunn WL, Riggs BL. (1983). Noninvasive bone mineral measurements. Seminars in Nuclear Medicine 13: 282–289.

Walser M. (1967). Magnesium metabolism. Review of Physiology Biochemistry and Pharmacology 59: 185–296.

Wandrup J, Ketny J. (1985). Potentiometric measurement of ionized calcium in anaerobic whole blood, plasma, and serum evaluated. Clinical Chemistry 31: 856–860.

Wester PO, Dyckner T. (1984). Problems with potassium and magnesium in diuretic-treated patients. Acta Pharmacologica et Toxicologica 54 (Supplement 1): 59–65.

Wester PO, Dyckner T. (1987). Magnesium and hypertension. Journal of the American College of Nutrition 6: 321–328.

Zettner A, Seligson D. (1964). Application of atomic absorption spectrophotometry in the determination of calcium in serum. Clinical Chemistry 10: 869–890.

Chapter 24

Assessment of trace-element status

Trace elements occur in the body in very small or 'trace' amounts, typically milligrams or micrograms per kilogram body weight; they generally constitute less than 0.01% of the body mass. Certain trace elements have been identified as essential for life, and these are listed in Table 24.1. They are considered essential when a deficient intake produces an impairment of function, and when supplementation with physiological levels of that element reverses the impaired function or prevents an impairment (Mertz, 1981a).

Trace elements differ in their properties and biological functions; many act primarily by forming metallo-enzymes. Deficiencies of trace elements produce multiple and diverse clinical signs and symptoms. Many of these symptoms were first identified in patients receiving total parenteral nutrition (TPN) unsupplemented with trace elements. Only some of the clinical manifestations of trace-element deficiencies have been explained in biochemical terms (Mertz, 1981b).

Essential in Humans and Animals	Essential in Some Animals	Possibly Essential in Some Animals
Chromium Cobalt Copper Fluorine Iodine Iron Manganese Molybdenum Selenium Zinc	Arsenic Lithium Nickel Silicon Vanadium	Bromine Cadmium Lead Tin

Table 24.1: The essential trace elements. Reproduced from Casey and Robinson (1983) Table 1, page 3 by courtesy of Marcel Dekker, Inc.

Trace-element deficiencies may arise from inadequate dietary intakes and/or decreased bioavailability, or may be associated with disease states in which decreased absorption, excessive excretion, and/or excessive utilization occur. Numerous interactions, both between trace elements (e.g. zinc and copper) and with other nutrients (e.g. zinc and vitamin A), have been identified, some producing suboptimal trace-element status in humans (Prasad et al., 1978a). Genetic defects in trace-element metabolism resulting in deficiency syndromes have been described for copper (Menkes' kinky hair syndrome), iron (congenital atransferrinemia), zinc (acrodermatitis enteropathica), and molybdenum (xanthine and sulfite oxidase deficiencies).

Some trace elements have a high toxicity; for example, the daily intake of selenium associated with the appearance of toxicity is only ten times the nutritional requirement. For others (e.g. trivalent chromium), toxicity after oral pharmacological doses has never been reported.

The biochemical indices currently used to assess trace-element status depend on measuring either: (a) the total quantity of the trace elements in various accessible tissues (e.g. hair, fingernails) and body fluids (e.g. whole blood or some fraction, urine, saliva, etc.), or (b) the activity of trace-element-dependent enzymes. The latter is the preferred biochemical method. Tests based on measurements of physiological or behavioral functions dependent on a specific trace element can also be used; unfortunately, such tests are not available for all the trace elements. In general, a combination of tests is recommended for each trace element; ideally, a combination which reflects total body trace-element content and/or tissue stores.

Major technological advances in the collection, preparation, and analysis of trace elements in biological samples have greatly improved the quality of analytical data on the trace-element content of biological tissues and fluids. Precautions introduced to avoid adventitious contamination include the use of: trace-element-free syringes and evacuated tubes fitted with siliconized needles; laminar flow hoods; 18-mega-ohm deionized water; ultrapure reagents; acid-washed glassware; and polyethylene materials for sample preparation and analysis (Casey and Robinson, 1983). The availability of standard reference materials with certified values for trace elements has also improved the accuracy of published trace-element analytical data.

Atomic absorption spectrophotometry (AAS) is the most widely used method for trace-element analysis in biological samples. Graphite furnace AAS is particularly suitable for analyzing the ultratrace elements such as chromium, nickel, and manganese. Several multi-element methods for trace-element analysis, including X-ray fluorescence, inductively coupled plasma spectroscopy, and instrumental neutron activation analysis (INAA), have been developed. Multi-element analytical methods are especially useful for investigating potential trace-element interactions.

For some (e.g. INAA), matrix effects are nonexistent, and treatment of the sample by ashing or digestion is usually unnecessary, reducing the risk of contamination. Efforts continue to reduce interferences (if present) and to increase both the precision and sensitivity of all of these methods.

For some of the trace elements (e.g. zinc and chromium), the most reliable method currently available for detecting marginal deficiency states is still supplementation, followed by an evaluation of improvement or reversal of a previously impaired trace-element-dependent function. This approach is time-consuming and tedious, and unsuitable for field use.

Frank and/or marginal nutritional deficiencies of chromium, copper, iodine, selenium, and zinc have been reported in certain population groups consuming self-selected diets. Consequently, these trace elements will be discussed in detail below. Iron has been considered earlier in Chapter 17. Trace elements with known toxic effects but which have not been demonstrated to be essential for humans (e.g. arsenic, lead, and cadmium) are not discussed (Table 24.1).

24.1 Assessment of chromium status

Estimates of the total adult body pool of chromium range from 4 to 6 mg; trivalent chromium is probably the only form present in biological tissues. To function physiologically, absorbed trivalent chromium is first converted to an organic biologically active form, the exact structure of which is unknown (Anderson, 1981). The biologically active molecule may contain nicotinic acid and glutathione or its constituent amino acids, in addition to chromium (Frieden, 1985). This organic chromium complex appears to have a role in glucose metabolism and insulin activity in humans, possibly by potentiating the action of insulin in cellular glucose uptake (Mertz, 1981a). It may also be involved in lipid and amino-acid metabolism (Roginski and Mertz, 1969; Abraham et al., 1980). At present, there is no known role of chromium in enzyme reactions.

Cases of a chromium-responsive deficiency syndrome have been reported in adults receiving long-term total parenteral nutrition (Jeejeebhoy et al., 1977; Freund et al., 1979; Brown et al., 1986). Clinical manifestations of chromium deficiency seen in these patients included impaired glucose tolerance, hyperglycemia, relative insulin resistance, peripheral neuropathy, and/or metabolic encephalopathy. Marginal nutritional deficiency states of chromium, confirmed by an improvement in glucose tolerance after chromium supplementation, have been described in malnourished children (Carter et al., 1968; Hopkins et al., 1968; Gürson and Saner, 1971), diabetics (Glinsmann and Mertz, 1966; Nath et al., 1979), the elderly (Levine et al., 1968; Offenbacher and Pi-Sunyer, 1980; Martinez et al., 1985), and in some apparently healthy individuals (Riales and

Albrink, 1981; Anderson et al., 1983a). Marginal chromium deficiency in humans appears to be associated not only with impaired glucose tolerance, but also with a lack of insulin sensitivity, and possibly with disturbances in lipid metabolism. As a result, suboptimal chromium status may be a risk factor in cardiovascular disease (Borel and Anderson, 1984).

Excellent food sources of chromium are brewers' yeast, nuts, asparagus, prunes, mushrooms, wine, and beer. Most meats, fresh fruits and vegetables, and cheeses are good sources of chromium. Cereals are poorer sources, their chromium content decreasing with refining and processing (Anderson, 1981). The absorption of trivalent chromium, the form of chromium in foods, is very poor (i.e. less than 1%). There is no evidence that oral pharmacological doses of trivalent chromium are toxic. High doses have been fed to rodents, fish, and cats (Schroeder et al., 1962) with no apparent toxic responses. Likewise, intravenous supplementation of 250 µg Cr per day to chromium-deficient, malnourished children produced no toxicity (Hopkins et al., 1968). In contrast, the toxicological effects of hexavalent chromium, which can penetrate biological membranes easily causing oxidative damage to cell contents, are well known. Hence workers exposed to industrial hexavalent chromium (e.g. chrome plate workers and welders) are potentially vulnerable. Toxic effects include contact dermatitis, skin ulcers, perforation of the nasal septum, bronchial asthma, and increased incidence of bronchogenic carcinoma (Langard, 1980).

Methods used for chromium analysis in biological samples include graphite furnace AAS, gas chromatography/mass spectrometry, and neutron activation analysis (Borel and Anderson, 1984). Standard reference materials, with certified chromium concentrations in the same range as the samples to be analyzed, should be routinely used. Chromium concentrations in several biological tissues and fluids have been investigated as potential indices of chromium status, and this work is discussed in the following sections. Further studies are needed, however, to establish the validity and precision of these indices. To date, the best method of identifying marginal chromium deficiency is a retrospective diagnosis based on an improvement in glucose tolerance after chromium supplementation at physiological levels.

24.1.1 Serum/plasma chromium concentrations

Chromium in serum exists largely as Cr^{3+}. It is bound competitively to transferrin, which transports chromium in the blood to body tissues. Methodological difficulties in measuring serum chromium concentrations accurately have discouraged the use of serum/plasma chromium as an index of chromium status. Indeed, until recently there has been no general agreement on the normal concentrations of chromium in serum or plasma. The reported values have declined dramatically in the last two

Authors and Year	Serum Chromium (ng/mL)
Schroeder et al., 1962	170–520
Hambidge, 1971	7.0
Versieck et al., 1978	0.16
Simonoff, 1984	8.51
Anderson et al., 1985	0.13

Table 24.2: Changes in the reported mean concentrations of chromium in serum. Conversion factor to SI units (μmol/L) = × 0.0192.

decades (Table 24.2). Early values are probably unreliable and may be associated with contamination and/or losses during sample preparation and analysis. Recent values for serum chromium range between 0.10 and 0.20 ng/mL, very close to the detection limits of modern atomic absorption spectrophotometers. Plasma chromium concentrations appear to be significantly higher than serum chromium values (Offenbacher et al., 1986).

Serum chromium concentrations are altered in seriously ill patients (Pekarek et al., 1975), hyperglycemic subjects (Liu and Morris, 1978; Donzelli et al., 1981), insulin-dependent diabetics (Vanderlinde et al., 1979; Rabinowitz et al., 1983), and during pregnancy (Davidson and Burt, 1973), although the changes observed have not always been consistent. Some of these inconsistencies may result from difficulty in measuring serum chromium, and hence the clinical significance of these changes is uncertain. Elevated serum chromium values have been reported in workers exposed to industrial hexavalent (Alsbirk et al., 1981) and trivalent (Randall and Gibson, 1987) chromium

To date, evidence that serum/plasma chromium reflects tissue chromium levels is equivocal. Earlier radioactive ^{51}Cr tracer studies suggested that chromium in the blood may not be in equilibrium with tissue levels or body stores (Mertz, 1969). In tannery workers exposed to industrial trivalent chromium, serum chromium levels were significantly and positively correlated with area of work, and with hair and urine chromium levels (Randall and Gibson, 1987, 1989). These findings suggest that serum chromium may provide an index of industrial exposure to trivalent chromium. The validity of serum chromium as an index of suboptimal chromium status remains uncertain.

24.1.2 Changes in serum chromium after a glucose load

Changes in serum chromium concentrations one hour after a glucose load have been advocated as an index of chromium status (Mertz, 1981b). The change is expressed as the ratio of the one-hour serum chromium to the fasting serum chromium and is termed the 'relative chromium response'.

This approach is based on the apparent increase in serum chromium values after a glucose load in normal subjects, but not in diabetic patients who are assumed to have a suboptimal chromium status. Increases in diabetic subjects were only observed after chromium supplementation (Glinsmann et al., 1966). These results suggest that subjects with adequate chromium stores release chromium from tissues after a glucose load, resulting in increased serum chromium concentrations. Unfortunately, such a response in healthy subjects has not been a consistent finding (Doisy et al., 1971; Davidson and Burt, 1973; Liu and Morris, 1978; Liu and Abernathy, 1982; Anderson et al., 1985). Hence, the relative chromium response cannot be considered a reliable index.

24.1.3 Whole blood and erythrocyte chromium concentrations.

Data on whole blood and erythrocyte chromium concentrations are limited. Physiological levels of chromium in erythrocytes appear to be twenty times higher than in plasma, facilitating chromium analysis (Manthey and Kübler, 1980; Rabinowitz et al., 1980). Nevertheless, reported erythrocyte chromium concentrations have a wide range, and there is a considerable overlap of values for diabetics and normal persons. Some investigators have suggested that erythrocyte chromium concentrations may serve as an index of industrial exposure to hexavalent chromium (Lewalter et al., 1985; Wiegand et al., 1985).

Whole blood chromium concentrations approximate 2.9 µg/mL (55.7 µmol/L) in normal healthy adults (Nomiyama et al., 1980; Zober et al., 1984). A few studies have attempted to use whole blood chromium concentrations as an index of industrial chromium exposure (Tola et al., 1977; Kiilunen et al., 1983; Rahkonen et al., 1983), but results are difficult to interpret because no unexposed control subjects were included in these studies. Whole blood chromium concentrations have been used infrequently in studies of suboptimal chromium status.

24.1.4 Urinary chromium concentrations

Urine is the major excretory route of absorbed chromium, accounting for about 95% of chromium excretion (Mertz, 1969). Hence, theoretically, urine may be a useful index of chromium status. Small amounts of absorbed chromium are also lost in the hair, perspiration, and bile (Doisy et al., 1971). Reported urinary chromium excretion values, like serum, have also decreased with improved sampling and analytical procedures and control of adventitious contamination (Veillon et al., 1982) (Table 24.3). Values accepted as accurate are less than 1 µg/day for normal healthy subjects.

It appears that urinary chromium concentrations reflect changes in chromium status induced by recent excessive dietary chromium intakes, not changes produced by chromium deficiency. Anderson et al. (1983b)

Authors and Year	Urinary Cr : Creatinine (ng/mg)
Davidson et al., 1974	1.65
Gürson and Saner, 1978	7.43
Anderson et al., 1982a	0.10

Table 24.3: Post-1966 data for urinary chromium : creatinine ratios in adults.

noted a five-fold increase in chromium excretion concomitant with a five-fold increase in dietary chromium intake as a result of supplementation with inorganic chromium. Confirmation of decreased urinary chromium concentrations in persons with moderate chromium deficiency is lacking, possibly because of analytical difficulties associated with measuring values near the detection limit.

In workers exposed to industrial chromium, urinary chromium concentrations were reportedly elevated immediately postshift, apparently falling to normal levels three days after exposure (Gylseth et al., 1977; Kiilunen et al., 1983). Studies using more sensitive analytical techniques, however, have documented elevated urinary chromium levels of workers exposed to industrial chromium after thirty-one (Welinder et al., 1983) and forty (Aitio et al., 1984) days of holiday and after 4.5 years of retirement (Welinder et al., 1983). In addition, in tannery workers exposed to trivalent chromium, urinary chromium : creatinine ratios were positively correlated with hair and serum chromium concentrations (Randall and Gibson, 1989). Hence, urinary chromium may reflect chromium exposure over a longer period than originally suggested by Gylseth et al. (1977).

Many confounding factors apparently affect chromium concentrations in urine, including hormones (Shapcott, 1979), diurnal variation (Gürson and Saner, 1978), certain constituents in the urine (e.g. salt) (Love, 1983), dietary intakes of glucose and sucrose (Kozlovsky et al., 1986), diabetes (Doisy et al., 1971; Vanderlinde et al., 1979; Rabinowitz et al., 1980), and trauma (Borel et al., 1984). In some of these studies, urinary chromium values are suspiciously high, and hence the importance of some of these confounding factors on urinary chromium values remains uncertain. Exercise also affects urinary chromium concentrations. Anderson et al. (1984) reported a nearly five-fold increase in urinary chromium concentrations in nine male runners, two hours after a six-mile run. Increases in serum glucose and glucagon also occurred (Anderson et al., 1982b). The elevated urinary chromium concentrations result from the mobilization of chromium induced by the increased uptake of glucose by exercising muscle.

Changes in urinary chromium excretion in normal healthy and diabetic subjects after a glucose load have also been inconsistent (Gürson and

Saner, 1978; Liu et al., 1979; Anderson et al., 1982a). Hence suboptimal chromium status cannot be detected by changes in urinary chromium excretion after an oral glucose tolerance test.

Urinary chromium concentrations, determined on casual urine samples rather than on twenty-four-hour urine samples, can be expressed in relation to creatinine excretion in an attempt to correct both for diurnal variation and for differences in urine volumes (Gürson and Saner, 1978; Anderson et al., 1983b) (Table 24.3). Daily output of endogenous creatinine correlates with muscle mass and is relatively constant in healthy adults, irrespective of diet or diuresis. Gürson and Saner (1978) reported comparable chromium : creatinine ratios calculated from four-hour fasting and corresponding twenty-four-hour urine samples. Elevated urinary chromium : creatinine ratios have been observed in tannery workers exposed to industrial trivalent chromium (Randall and Gibson, 1987).

In general, urinary chromium excretion, expressed either per twenty-four hours or as a chromium : creatinine ratio, appears more useful as an index of overexposure to chromium than as an index of suboptimal chromium status. Correlations of urinary chromium excretion with selected clinical parameters have produced inconclusive results (Anderson et al., 1983b), perhaps because even urinary chromium values in normal healthy persons are very low and approach the limits of detection for many analytical methods.

24.1.5 Hair chromium concentrations

Studies of hair as a biopsy material for assessing chromium status are limited. As hair is exposed to adventitious contamination, standardized procedures are essential for the collection and washing of hair samples prior to analysis. Several washing procedures have been investigated for hair chromium analysis. These include using nonionic and anionic detergents (sodium lauryl sulfate (SLS)), hexane-methanol, acetone, water, triton-X10, and a mixture of hexane and ethanol (Hambidge et al., 1972b; Kumpulainen et al., 1982). Kumpulainen et al. recommended two twenty-minute washes in SLS after a hexane rinse for hair chromium analysis.

Confounding factors known to affect trace-element concentrations in hair include hair color, hair beauty treatments, age, sex, pregnancy, season, geographical location, parity, smoking, and the presence of certain disease states (Section 15.1.1). To date, the effects of only some of these factors on hair chromium concentrations are known. For example, hair chromium concentrations are age dependent: values are high in infancy and decline with age (Hambidge and Baum, 1972), a trend also documented for the chromium levels of other tissues (Schroeder

Median Hair Cr (ng/g)

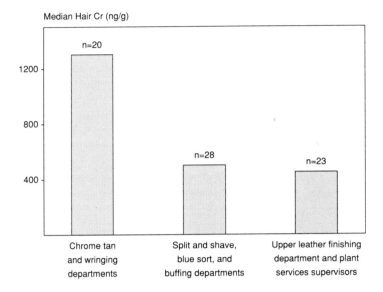

Figure 24.1: Hair chromium levels in relation to industrial exposure in a tannery. Conversion factor to SI units (nmol/g) = × 0.0192. From Randall JA, Gibson RS. (1989). Hair chromium as an index of chromium exposure of tannery workers. British Journal of Industrial Medicine 46: 172–176 with permission.

et al., 1962). Significantly higher hair chromium concentrations in nulliparous compared to parous women have been reported (Mahalko and Bennion, 1976; Shapcott et al., 1980; Saner, 1981) whereas lower hair chromium concentrations have been reported in female, but not male, diabetics (Rosson et al., 1979), and in persons with arteriosclerosis (Cote et al., 1979), compared to healthy controls.

Evidence that hair chromium concentrations may provide a chronic index of chromium status has accumulated from five sources: (a) hair chromium concentrations are low in persons with non-insulin-dependent diabetes, a disease associated with marginal chromium deficiency; (b) decreases in hair chromium concentrations with age apparently parallel those in tissue chromium (Schroeder et al., 1962); (c) low hair chromium concentrations were noted in a long-term TPN patient with a chromium-responsive deficiency syndrome (Jeejeebhoy et al., 1977); (d) hair chromium concentrations of tannery workers exposed to industrial trivalent chromium correlated positively with serum and urine chromium levels (Randall and Gibson, 1989); (e) a dose-effect relationship between area of work in the tannery and hair chromium concentrations of tannery workers has been documented (Figure 24.1) (Randall and Gibson, 1989). These findings suggest that hair chromium concentrations may be a useful index of chronic chromium status.

24.1.6   Oral glucose tolerance test

At present, the best method for diagnosing chromium deficiency is to demonstrate an improvement in glucose tolerance after chromium supplementation at physiological levels. The test involves taking a venipuncture blood sample after an overnight fast, to provide baseline data on fasting plasma glucose levels. A glucose load is then given orally, after which venipuncture blood samples for plasma glucose analysis are taken, at varying time intervals. Sometimes, blood is taken 30, 60, 90, and 120 minutes after the glucose drink (Levine et al., 1968; National Diabetes Data Group, 1979; Offenbacher and Pi-Sunyer, 1980), or at 45 and 90 minutes (Offenbacher et al., 1985). When the former intervals are used, the total areas under the curve for glucose are calculated using the formula

$$(A/2) + B + C + D + (E/2) = \text{Area Index Total (AIT)}$$

where A is the fasting value, and B, C, D, and E are the 30, 60, 90, and 120 minutes values, respectively (Vecchio et al., 1965). Alternatively, to facilitate screening in community studies, a single blood glucose level, at 90 (Anderson et al., 1985) or 120 (Glinsmann and Mertz, 1966; Martinez et al., 1985) minutes after the glucose load can be used. Plasma glucose can be analyzed by the glucose oxidase method (Raabo and Terkildsen, 1960) or by an oxygen consumption method (Kadish et al., 1969).

The level of the oral glucose load used for chromium supplementation studies has also varied. Oral loading doses of 75 g (Martinez et al., 1985; Offenbacher et al., 1985), as recommended by the National Diabetes Data Group (1979), 100 g (Offenbacher and Pi-Sunyer, 1980), or a load of 1 g of glucose per kilogram body weight (Anderson et al., 1985) have all been used. Such differences in glucose load apparently have little influence on blood glucose levels (National Diabetes Data Group, 1979), but higher glucose loads do have a greater effect on stimulating insulin secretion.

24.2   Assessment of copper status

The adult human body contains approximately 70 to 80 mg of copper, of which 24.7% is in the skeletal muscle, 15.3% in the skin, 14.8% in the bone marrow, 19% in the skeleton, 8.0 to 15% in the liver, and 8.0% in the brain. Copper is an essential component of many enzymes systems (Table 24.4), including some that catalyze oxido-reduction reactions.

Most of the clinical manifestations of copper deficiency are explicable in terms of changes in the activities of these cuproenzymes. For instance, a reduction in ceruloplasmin (ferroxidase) impairs the transport of iron to the erythropoietic sites, resulting in hypochromic anemia. Skeletal and

Enzyme	Functional Role	Known or Expected Consequence of Deficiency
Cytochrome c oxidase	Electron transport	Growth failure
Superoxide dismutase	Free-radical detoxification	Uncertain
Tyrosinase	Melanin production	Pigmentation failure
Dopamine β-hydroxylase	Catecholamine production	Neurological defects
Lysyl oxidase	Cross-linking of collagen and elastin	Vascular rupture
Ceruloplasmin	Ferroxidase; transport	Anemia
Unknown copper enzyme	Cross-linking of disulfide bonds of keratin	Pili torti

Table 24.4: Copper enzymes in humans. Modified after Anonymous (1987). Essentiality of copper in humans. Nutrition Reviews 42: 279–281 with permission.

vascular defects are caused by an impairment of collagen synthesis, arising from a deficiency of the cuproenzyme lysyl oxidase (O'Dell, 1976). Depigmentation is presumably associated with tyrosinase (monophenol mono-oxygenase) deficiency, an enzyme involved in melanin production. The central nervous system disturbances are probably the result of myelinization derangements, abnormal catecholamine concentrations associated with decreased activity of dopamine β-hydroxylase, and reduced activity of cytochrome c oxidase (Mason, 1979).

Copper deficiency in humans is rare, but it has been described in malnourished infants (Graham and Cordano, 1969), premature and/or low birth weight infants fed cow's milk (Al-Rashid and Spangler, 1971; Griscom et al., 1971; Ashkenazi et al., 1973), patients receiving prolonged TPN unsupplemented with copper (Karpel and Peden, 1972; Dunlap et al., 1974; Vilter et al., 1974), and in a woman receiving a normal diet supplemented with antacids (Anonymous, 1984a).

The earliest clinical manifestation of copper deficiency in humans is persistent neutropenia, usually followed by hypochromic anemia, scurvy-like bone changes, and osteoporosis (in infants) (Cordano et al., 1964; Al-Rashid and Spangler, 1971; Karpel and Peden, 1972). Some adults with sickle cell disease receiving prolonged zinc therapy, have developed hematological signs of copper deficiency (Prasad et al., 1978a). Clinical features of copper deficiency, with the exception of anemia, occur in infants with Menkes' kinky hair syndrome (KHS), an inherited disorder of copper metabolism in which there is an intracellular defect of copper utilization (Danks et al., 1972).

Most of the reports of copper deficiency in humans have resulted from inadequate dietary intakes of copper, often in association with prolonged diarrhea which prevents reabsorption of copper from the bile. The latter is the major excretory route for copper (Mason, 1979). Diseases associated with chronic loss of proteins, such as nephritic syndrome and protein-losing enteropathy, may also cause copper deficiency as a result of loss of ceruloplasmin and of copper bound to albumin. High intakes of fructose and sucrose appear to exacerbate the effects of copper deficiency (Fields et al., 1983; Reiser et al., 1983); the importance of this effect in humans is unknown.

Dietary intakes of copper for some population groups in the United States are below the Food and Nutrition Board (1980) safe and adequate range, but copper deficiency among the general population has not been described. Copper is widely distributed in foods; richest food sources are oysters, other shellfish, liver, kidney, nuts, and dried legumes (Solomons, 1980). Low copper intakes have been implicated as a risk factor in the development of cardiovascular disease by some (Klevay, 1975; Klevay et al., 1984; Aalbers and Houtman, 1985; Reiser et al., 1985), but not all (Shapcott et al., 1985), investigators.

Several cases of accidental copper toxicity in humans have been described, arising from ingestion of copper sulfate (Chuttanni et al., 1965), acidic drinks in prolonged contact with copper (Paine, 1968), or drinking water with an unusually high copper concentration (800 µg/L) (Salmon and Wright, 1971). Patients with Wilson's disease, a copper-related genetic defect, also exhibit symptoms of copper toxicity such as nausea, vomiting, diarrhea, acute hemolytic anemia, hepatic necrosis, hepatic central vein dilation, and jaundice (Zelkowitz et al., 1980). There is no evidence that high dietary copper intakes are a public health problem.

Methods used to assess copper status in humans include measurements of copper concentrations in blood and its components and in hair, and the measurement of the activities of certain copper enzymes. These methods are discussed below. An oral copper tolerance test (Section 24.5.8) cannot be used for copper; the dose required to increase plasma concentrations has a potent emetic effect.

24.2.1 Serum/plasma copper concentrations

There are two major forms of copper in plasma; one is firmly bound to ceruloplasmin, the other is reversibly bound to serum albumin. Plasma also contains the copper enzymes cytochrome c oxidase and monoamine oxidase, a small amount of free copper, and copper bound to amino acids. The function of the amino-acid-bound copper fraction is unknown.

Serum copper concentrations are at present routinely measured for the clinical assessment of severe copper deficiency, but are not sensitive and specific enough to be used as an index of copper status in apparently healthy individuals. Serum copper concentrations are influenced by many confounding factors unrelated to copper nutriture. For example, elevated serum copper concentrations (hypercupremia) occur in women taking oral contraceptive agents (Horwitt et al., 1975) and in pregnant women

Subject No.	Serum (µg/dL)	Plasma (µg/dL)	Percentage Difference
1	127	123	3
2	119	113	5
3	121	110	9
4	122	106	13
5	124	106	15
6	123	105	15
7	115	105	9
8	105	98	7
Mean ± SD	120± 7	108± 7	9± 4

Table 24.5: Copper concentrations of serum or citrated plasma prepared from single venipuncture samples of eight subjects. Plasma was prepared by adding 0.15 mL of 30% sodium citrate per 15 mL of whole blood. Percentage difference = [(serum − plasma)/serum] × 100. Conversion factor to SI units (µmol/L) = × 0.1574. From Smith JC Jr, Holbrook JT, Danford DE. (1985). Analysis and evaluation of zinc and copper in human plasma and serum. Journal of the American College of Nutrition 4: 627–638. With permission of John Wiley & Sons, Inc.

after the third month of pregnancy (Halsted et al., 1968; Hambidge and Droegemueller, 1974), probably resulting from mobilization of liver copper under the stimulus of estrogen. In conditions of infection or stress, serum copper concentrations also rise. This effect results from an increase in ceruloplasmin, mediated by leukocytic endogenous mediator (Pekarek et al., 1972). Serum copper values are also elevated in leukemia, Hodgkin's disease, various anemias, collagen disorders, hemochromatosis, and myocardial infarction (Mason, 1979).

Low serum copper concentrations (hypocupremia) are found in protein-energy malnutrition (Cordano et al., 1964), malabsorption syndromes (Sternlieb and Janowitz, 1964), ulcerative colitis, and the nephrotic syndrome (Cartwright et al., 1954). In Wilson's disease, the low serum copper levels are not related to copper deficiency but to defects in the hepatic storage of copper and in ceruloplasmin metabolism.

Concentrations of copper in serum and erythrocytes are comparable, so that slight hemolysis does not affect serum copper concentrations. Diurnal variation in serum/plasma copper concentrations in nonfasting subjects has been noted (Cartwright, 1950, Guillard et al., 1979); the highest levels in nonfasting subjects occur in the morning (Lifschitz and Henkin, 1971). Regular strenuous exercise may also affect serum/plasma copper concentrations (Lukaski et al., 1983).

Plasma copper concentrations appear to be consistently lower than corresponding serum copper values (Table 24.5), possibly as a result of water from erythrocytes diluting the plasma (Smith et al., 1985).

Age- and sex-related changes in serum/plasma copper levels are well documented. Newborn infants have low serum copper concentrations, which rise to the adult level by four months of age (Kirsten et al., 1985). Adult females tend to have higher levels than males (Cartwright, 1950). Serum copper levels were measured in subjects from three to seventy-four years of age in the Canada Health Survey (Health and Welfare Canada, 1981) and the NHANES II survey (Klasing and Pilch, 1985). Interpretive guidelines often used for normal serum copper concentrations for adults are 70 to 140 µg/dL for men (11.0 to 22.0 µmol/L) and 80 to 155 µg/dL (12.6 to 24.4 µmol/L) for women (Tietz, 1983), with a higher range for oral contraceptive users (216 to 300 µg/dL) (34.0 to 47.2 µmol/L) (Alpers et al., 1983). Decreases in plasma copper of approximately 11 µg/dL per week occur in patients receiving TPN solutions deficient in copper (Solomons et al., 1976).

Flame atomic absorption spectrophotometry (AAS) is the most widely used method for measuring serum copper. Generally, a direct technique is used involving sample dilution with deionized water (1 part plasma/serum to 1 part deionized water) (Smith et al., 1985; Osheim, 1983) or a signal enhancing mixture such as butanol/water (Meret and Henkin, 1971). In some instances, use of a 'high solids' burner head may be necessary (Boling, 1966). Sometimes, the protein in the blood sample is removed using an acid such as trichloroacetic acid (Kelson and Shamberger, 1978). This latter procedure may, however, introduce volume errors during the deproteinization step and adventitious contamination from the acid and is not recommended. Alternatively, for small pediatric samples, flameless AAS can be used.

24.2.2 Serum ceruloplasmin concentrations

Ceruloplasmin (MW 150,000) is the major copper-containing protein in the α_2-globulin fraction of human serum. It is a copper transport protein synthesized by the liver, and consists of a single-chain glycoprotein containing eight copper atoms per molecule. Ceruloplasmin is a ferroxidase that assists in iron transport by oxidizing intracellular Fe^{2+} to Fe^{3+}, which then can combine with transferrin. Serum ceruloplasmin concentrations, like serum copper, are elevated during pregnancy and lactation, in women taking oral contraceptive agents, and in association with malignancy, arthritis and inflammatory disease, myocardial infarction, liver disease, and a variety of infectious diseases (Mason, 1979).

Measurement of serum ceruloplasmin alone is not recommended as an index of copper status in cross-sectional surveys; the concentration of this metalloenzyme in the serum varies markedly among normal healthy individuals (Danks, 1980). Instead, it is preferable to measure serum ceruloplasmin concentrations prior to, and three to four days after, oral supplementation with copper at physiological levels. Following supplementation, serum ceruloplasmin concentrations will be elevated only in those subjects with copper deficiency (Danks, 1980). In patients with decreased ceruloplasmin produced by other causes, serum ceruloplasmin is unchanged after copper supplementation. This test has not been widely used. Serum ceruloplasmin can be assayed by measuring its enzymatic activity (Sunderman and Nomoto, 1970), or immunochemically by radial immunodiffusion.

24.2.3 Erythrocyte superoxide dismutase activity

Cytosolic superoxide dismutase (Cu,Zn-SOD) contains both copper and zinc, and is found in the cytosol of erythrocytes and other cells. It has a molecular weight of approximately 33,000 and contains 2 g-atoms each of copper and zinc. This Cu,Zn-SOD enzyme is important as a scavenger of O_2^-, a free radical which causes damage to membranes and biological structures (Anonymous, 1980). Cyanide inhibits the catalytic activity of Cu,Zn-SOD, a feature which distinguishes it from the manganese enzyme (Mn-SOD) (Anonymous, 1980).

Erythrocyte Cu,Zn-SOD activity is depressed during copper deficiency in several animal species, and in humans (Williams et al., 1975; Bettger et al., 1979; Paynter et al., 1979; Okahata et al., 1980), but is not affected by zinc status. Positive correlations between erythrocyte Cu,Zn-SOD activity and other parameters of copper status (e.g. serum copper and liver cytochrome c oxidase) have been observed (Bettger et al., 1979; Andrewartha and Caple, 1980). Erythrocyte Cu,Zn-SOD activity is a particularly sensitive index of copper depletion (Fischer et al., 1984); for example, in an experimental copper depletion study in male adults, erythrocyte Cu,Zn-SOD activity was reduced, despite there being no detectable decrease in serum copper or ceruloplasmin (Reiser et al., 1985).

Erythrocyte Cu,Zn-SOD activity has not been used as an index of copper status in noninstitutionalized subjects consuming self-selected diets. Such work is necessary to confirm the utility of this index in studies of the general population (Klasing and Pilch, 1985).

Several methods are available for measuring erythrocyte SOD activity (Marklund and Marklund, 1974; Misra and Fridovich, 1977). Some assays are very time-consuming, require large samples, and necessitate the removal of hemoglobin immediately after sample collection. The assay methods generally involve the inhibition of oxidation-reduction reactions which are catalyzed by the superoxide anion. The latter may be generated enzymatically by, for example, xanthine plus xanthine oxidase, which in turn reduces cytochrome c. The reduction of cytochrome c is followed spectrophotometrically (Marklund and Marklund, 1974). L'Abbé and Fischer (1986) have developed an automated method for determining Cu,Zn-SOD activity which is suitable for small samples.

24.2.4   Other copper-dependent enzymes

Other copper-dependent enzymes which may be useful indices of copper deficiency in humans include cytochrome c oxidase in leukocytes and/or the liver, and lysyl oxidase in the collagen connective tissue. In copper deficiency in rats, cytochrome c oxidase activity is decreased in many tissues, particularly in the liver and brain (Bettger et al., 1979). Further work is needed to establish the validity and feasibility of these enzymes as indices of copper deficiency in humans.

24.2.5   Hair copper concentrations

Concentrations of copper in hair appear to correlate with levels in the liver (Jacob et al., 1978), heart, and kidney (Klevay, 1981) of rats. The validity of hair copper concentrations as an index of copper status in humans, however, is much less certain. In human studies of two conditions in which copper accumulates in the liver—primary biliary cirrhosis (Epstein et al., 1980) and Wilson's disease (Rice and Goldstein, 1961; Gibbs and Walshe, 1965)—hair copper levels of patients were normal. Additionally, infants with copper deficiency, characterized clinically by neutropenia, and biochemically by concentrations of serum copper and ceruloplasmin below the limits of detectability, did not have lower hair copper levels than age- and sex-matched controls (Bradfield et al., 1980). Similarly, the copper content of the hair of children with Menkes' kinky hair syndrome is normal (Danks, 1980). In a more recent human study, hair copper concentrations did not correlate with the copper content of heart, muscle, liver, kidney, aorta, or rib (Aalbers and Houtman, 1985). It appears, therefore, that hair copper cannot be used as an index of copper status in humans.

Many studies have confirmed that gender (in adults), pregnancy, lactation, prematurity, hair color, race, and age all affect hair copper concentrations (Petering et al., 1971; Creason et al., 1975; Gibson and DeWolfe, 1980; Taylor, 1986). The marked rise in hair (and serum) copper concentrations during early infancy is presumably associated with the redistribution of tissue copper which occurs at this time, and not with changes in dietary copper intake (Gibson and DeWolfe, 1980) (Figure 24.2).

24.2.6   Other indices of copper status

Urinary copper is seldom used as an index of copper status; levels are very low in healthy subjects (10 to 60 μg/day) because copper is efficiently reabsorbed by the renal tubules. The main excretory route for copper is the biliary system. Urinary copper concentrations do decrease in persons receiving TPN copper-deficient solutions (Solomons, 1979), conserving body copper. Very limited data are available on copper concentrations in erythrocytes (Williams et al., 1977) and fingernails (Martin, 1964).

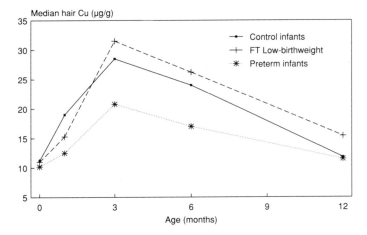

Figure 24.2: Changes in hair copper concentrations during infancy.
From Gibson RS. (1982). The trace metal status of some Canadian
full term and low birthweight infants at one year of age. Journal of
Radioanalytical Chemistry 70: 175–189 with permission.

Further studies are needed to ascertain their validity as indices of copper
status.

24.3 Assessment of iodine status

The adult human body contains about 15 to 20 mg iodine, of which 70%
to 80% is concentrated in the thyroid gland. Iodine occurs in the tissues
mainly as organically bound iodine; inorganic iodide is present in very
low concentrations. Iodine functions exclusively as a component of the
thyroid hormones, thyroxine (T_4) and 3,5,3'-triiodothyronine (T_3); their
structure is shown in Figure 24.3.

These hormones are required for normal growth and development and
for maintenance of a normal metabolic state. The thyroid hormones are
synthesized within the thyroid gland from thyroglobulin, an iodinated
glycoprotein contained in the colloid of the thyroid follicles. The

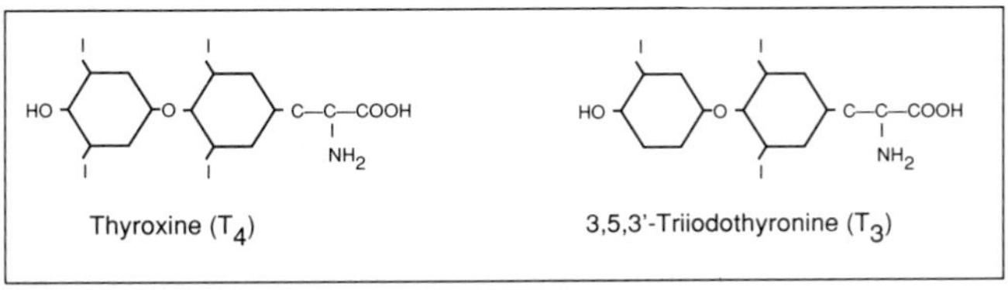

Figure 24.3: Structure of the thyroid hormones, thyroxine (T_4) and
3,5,3'-triiodothyronine (T_3).

hormones are transported in the plasma bound almost entirely to plasma proteins.

Iodine is present in foods largely as inorganic iodide. Seafoods are excellent food sources of iodine, but are eaten in small amounts in North America. Iodized salt, milk, and eggs are the major food sources of iodine in North America; meat and cereals comprise the secondary food sources. Vegetable products are generally low in iodine (Fisher and Carr, 1974). The iodine content of meat, milk, and eggs varies markedly with region, season, and the amount of iodine in the animal feed (Hemkin, 1979). In addition, many adventitious sources of iodine may contribute to the iodine content of foods. These include iodates used as dough conditioners, iodoform used in water as a disinfectant, iodophors used as sanitizers in the dairy industry, and iodine-containing food colors (e.g. erythrosine and rose bengal) (Vought et al., 1972; Dunsmore and Wheeler, 1977; Delange, 1985).

Goiter (thyroid enlargement) is the major consequence of chronic iodine deficiency. The estimated daily iodine requirement for U.S. adults for the prevention of goiter is 50 to 75 µg, or approximately 1 µg/kg body weight (Food and Nutrition Board, 1980). The activity of the thyroid is regulated through a negative feedback mechanism involving the thyroid-hypothalmus-pituitary axis. When dietary intakes of iodine are limited, thyroid hormone synthesis is inadequate and secretion declines. This stimulates the feedback mechanism, resulting in increased secretion of thyrotrophic hormone (TSH), which, in turn, promotes iodine uptake by the thyroid. If iodine intakes are limited for prolonged periods, the thyroid hypertrophies, producing an iodine-deficiency goiter (DeGroot et al., 1984). Endemic goiter is still very common world-wide. The World Health Organization has established a set of criteria which should be used to estimate thyroid gland size to standardize results among surveys (Thilly et al., 1980). Initially, the thyroid gland is diffusely and symmetrically enlarged, but as the severity of the iodine deficiency increases and the subject ages, the gland increases in size and palpable nodules occur. In some circumstances, gross enlargement of the thyroid can cause obstructive symptoms from compression of the trachea or esophagus.

In areas where endemic goiter exists and iodine deficiency is severe, endemic cretinism may occur. Geographical differences in the clinical manifestations of endemic cretinism are found. Clinical features always include mental deficiency and either a neurological syndrome consisting of hearing and speech defects and character-istic disorders of stance and gait or predominant hypothyroidism and stunted growth. In some areas (e.g. the Himalayas), a mixture of both syndromes occurs (Ibbertson et al., 1971), whereas in New Guinea, for example, the neurological syndrome predominates (Choufoer et al., 1965).

Cases of mild to moderate iodine deficiency, characterized by impairment of thyroid function, have been detected in newborn preterm infants in Europe and in neonates elsewhere (Kochupillai et al., 1986). Such transient impairment of thyroid function may be associated, in part, with the neuro-intellectual deficiencies frequently observed in preterm infants during their later development (Delange, 1985).

The most common cause of iodine deficiency is inadequate dietary intake of iodine; hypothyroidism may also develop from a number of diseases of the thyroid gland, or it may be secondary to pituitary or hypothalamic failure. Alternatively, thyroid function may be impaired after exposure to antithyroid compounds in foods and drugs; such substances are called goitrogens. Vegetables of the *Brassicaceae* family, especially cabbage, turnips, and rutabagas, contain an active antithyroid agent in a combined form (progoitrin). Other important goitrogens are linomarin, a cyanogenic glucoside of the cassava, disulfides of saturated and unsaturated hydrocarbons from organic sediments in drinking water, bacterial products of *Escherichia coli* in drinking water, and soyabeans (Matovinovic, 1984). Neonates, and to a lesser extent pregnant women, are more sensitive to the antithyroid action of dietary goitrogens than infants and children (Delange et al., 1982).

Under certain conditions, iodide in large doses blocks the synthesis of thyroid hormone, usually temporarily, after which hormone synthesis resumes. The phenomenon is known as the Wolff-Chaikoff effect (Wolff and Chaikoff, 1948). Occasionally, in 3% to 4% of otherwise healthy persons, the block persists and a goiter may develop.

The best method of preventing endemic goiter is to introduce the use of iodized salt, using potassium iodide or potassium iodate as the additive. In some countries (e.g. Papua New Guinea and Argentina), iodized oil, given either orally or (preferably) intramuscularly, has been used (Buttfield and Hetzel, 1969). Other countries have introduced iodized bread (Connolly et al., 1970) or iodized drinking water (Matovinovic and Ramalingaswami, 1960). Occasionally, when iodine has been given prophylactically in iodine-deficient areas, cases of hyperthyroidism or thyrotoxicosis (Jod-Basedow) have arisen. The precise mechanism of Jod-Basedow is unclear; the hyperthyroidism is generally mild and can be treated readily. Prolonged excessive intakes of iodine in normal persons markedly reduces the iodine uptake by the thyroid but goiter and hypothyroidism are rarely induced. Nevertheless, endemic goiter has been described in certain regions of Japan where seaweeds, rich in iodine, are dietary staples (Suzuki et al., 1965). Moreover some recent studies suggest that in some susceptible persons, high intakes of iodine may be associated with autoimmune thyroid disease (Boukis et al., 1983).

The most widely used method of assessing iodine status is to determine urinary iodine excretion in a twenty-four-hour urine specimen. This method is described below, together with the measurements of T_3, T_4, and TSH in serum and radioactive iodine uptake. Concentrations of iodine in the plasma are very low, difficult to measure, and apparently of no clinical use.

24.3.1 Urinary iodine excretion

Daily urinary excretion of iodine closely reflects iodine intake, and has been used as an index of iodine nutriture in many large-scale nutrition surveys (ICNND, 1963; Health and Welfare Canada, 1973); only a small fraction of iodine is excreted in the feces. Twenty-four-hour urine specimens are preferred, but they are not very practical for large-scale surveys. Consequently, nonfasting casual urine specimens are often obtained, and urinary excretion relative to creatinine determined, on the assumption that creatinine excretion is constant over time. The limitations of this assumption are discussed in Section 16.1.1. Sometimes, first-voided fasting morning urine specimens are collected as they are less affected by recent dietary intake. Casual urine samples are not appropriate for assessing the iodine status of individuals, but are probably adequate for population studies (Frey et al., 1973), if urinary creatinine concentrations are not affected by concomitant protein-energy malnutrition. Renal clearance must also be normal. Children have slightly higher urinary iodine : creatinine ratios than adults.

Casual urine specimens were analyzed for iodine content in the Nutrition Canada National Survey (Health and Welfare Canada, 1973); individuals with urinary iodine concentrations $< 50\,\mu\text{g/g}$ creatinine were considered at high risk. Median values for the different age groups ranged from 181 to $440\,\mu\text{g/g}$ of creatinine, and suggest that dietary intakes of iodine were adequate. The Pan American Health Organization technical group on endemic goiter suggests that urinary iodine excretion levels of less than 50 but more than $25\,\mu\text{g/g}$ of creatinine indicate moderate iodine deficiency; at such levels, adequate thyroid hormone formation may be impaired, as indicated by abnormal levels of thyroid hormones in the plasma. When average urinary iodine excretion levels are less than $25\,\mu\text{g/g}$ creatinine, endemic cretinism is a serious risk (Querido et al., 1974).

Urinary iodine in the ICNND surveys (ICNND, 1963) was assayed using the manual method of Zak et al. (1952), adapted by Benotti and Benotti (1963); automated methods have since been devised. A rapid, simple, and precise method for determining urinary iodine has been developed which involves destruction of organic matter by alkaline ashing before determining iodine by the Sandell and Kolthoff reaction (Aumont and Tressol, 1986). The method has a low detection limit, and can be used to determine iodine concentrations as low as $2\,\text{ng/g}$.

Variable	Brussels, Belgium	Ubangi, Zaire	
		Clinically euthyroid adults	Myxedematous cretins
Serum concentration			
T$_4$ (µg/dL)	8.1 ± 0.1	4.9 ± 0.2	0.50 ± 0.01
T$_3$ (ng/dL)	144 ± 3	166 ± 3	46 ± 3
TSH (µU/mL)	1.7 ± 0.1	18.6 ± 2.1	302.7 ± 20
Thyroid uptake of [131]I 24 hr (% dose)	46.4 ± 1.1	65.2 ± 0.9	28.3 ± 2.6

Table 24.6: Comparison of biochemical indices of iodine status in subjects in Brussels and in the Ubangi endemic goiter area, Zaire. Results are mean ± SEM. The differences for each variable between groups are significant (p< 0.001). Conversion factors to SI units: T$_4$ (nmol/L) = ×.12.87; T$_3$ (nmol/L = × 0.01536; TSH (mU/L) = × 1.00. Modified from Lagasse et al. (1982). Influence of the dietary balance of iodine-thiocyanate and protein on thyroid function in adults and young infants. In: Delange F, Iteke FB, Ermans AM (eds). Nutritional Factors involved in the Goitrogenic Action of Cassava. International Development Research Centre, Ottawa, pp. 84–86, with permission.

24.3.2 Serum/plasma thyroid-related hormone concentrations

Concentrations of T$_4$ and T$_3$ in serum range from 45 to 120 µg/L (58–154 nmol/L) and 0.65 to 2.2 µg/L (1.0–3.4 nmol/L) respectively (Alexander, 1984). Normally 99.8% of the T$_4$ and 99.5% of the T$_3$ are bound in serum to thyroxine-binding globulin, thyroxine-binding pre-albumin, and albumin. Measurements of T$_3$ and/or T$_4$ and serum TSH are routine screening procedures for detecting congenital hypothyroidism in neonates in Western countries. The hormones can be accurately and precisely measured (CV 5% to 8%) by sensitive and highly specific competitive radio-immunoassay methods available as commercial kits. These methods are expensive, however, and are not suitable for routine use in many developing countries.

In areas of endemic goiter, concentrations of serum T$_4$ are lower, but serum T$_3$ levels are often higher than normal values reported in non iodine-deficient areas. This replacement of T$_4$ by T$_3$ represents an iodine-sparing effect, because triiodothyronine (T$_3$) is a metabolically more active hormone and contains 25% less iodine (Pharoah et al., 1973). Serum TSH concentrations are notably higher in chronic severe iodine deficiency produced by the increased secretion of TSH by the pituitary. Such high concentrations may not be apparent in the presence of moderate iodine deficiency (Delange et al., 1982).

Table 24.6 presents a comparison of the serum concentrations of T$_4$, T$_3$, and TSH, together with thyroid uptake of ^{131}I in persons living in a severe endemic goiter area in Zaire, compared to Belgium controls. Serum TSH concentrations are higher in those persons living in Zaire, concentrations being particularly high in myxedematous cretins. Note the iodine-sparing effect evident in the clinically euthyroid adults with lower serum T_4, but elevated serum T_3 concentrations (Lagasse et al., 1982).

24.3.3 Radioactive iodine uptake

Measurement of uptake of radioactive ^{131}I is used as a test of thyroid function in clinical settings. The tracer is administered orally, and the thyroid uptake is determined by placing a gamma ray counter over the neck. To account for any nonthyroidal radioactivity in the neck, another area, such as the thigh, is also counted, and any counts obtained subtracted from those in the neck. In areas where iodine intakes are moderate (i.e. ranging from 100 to 300 µg/day), 20% to 50% of the radioactive ^{131}I dose is detected in the thyroid after twenty-four hours. In areas of iodine deficiency, the thyroidal uptake of ^{131}I is much faster and approaches 100% (Dunn, 1978). The uptake is also affected by variations in renal function because of differences in the amount of tracer excreted in the urine.

24.4 Assessment of selenium status

The selenium content of the human body varies. For U.S. adults it is about 15 mg (Schroeder et al., 1970), whereas for New Zealand adults, the amount is much lower (3 to 6 mg) (Stewart et al., 1978). Skeletal muscle contains the largest fraction of body selenium (Levander, 1985); liver contains a much smaller proportion. There is only one known selenium-containing enzyme in humans, glutathione peroxidase (GSHPx), which assists in protecting cellular components against oxidative damage (Levander, 1985). Selenium also affects the metabolism and toxicity of a variety of drugs and chemicals, and protects against the toxicity of silver, cadmium, and mercury (Levander and Cheng, 1980). More recently, selenium has been implicated in the immune response, although its mechanism of action is not yet known (Kiremidjian-Schumacher and Stotzky (1987).

Keshan's disease, a cardiomyopathy, is a naturally occurring selenium-responsive disease which mainly occurred in young children living in areas of China where the soil is low in selenium (Chen et al., 1980). Other interacting environmental factors, as yet unidentified, may also play a role in the development of Keshan's disease. The disease is characterized by heart enlargement, gallop rhythm, cardiogenic shock, electrocardiographic changes, and heart failure. Kashin-Beck disease, an endemic osteoarticular disorder, also occurs in the low-selenium regions of China. The biochemical role of selenium deficiency in this disease is unclear (Sokoloff, 1988). Selenium-responsive conditions have also been described in patients receiving long-term TPN unsupplemented with selenium (van Rij et al., 1979; Johnson et al., 1981; Stanley et al., 1982; Vinton et al., 1987) and in children with kwashiorkor (Schwarz, 1961).

The low selenium status in kwashiorkor, however, may not be a specific selenium deficiency (Mitchell Perry, 1978).

Important food sources of selenium are seafoods, liver, kidney, and muscle meats; fruits and vegetables are generally low in selenium. Grain products vary in their selenium content, depending on geographical location. Suboptimal selenium status arising from low dietary intakes has been documented in persons living in New Zealand (Robinson and Thomson, 1983), parts of Finland (Mutanen, 1984), and China (Chen et al., 1980). So far, low selenium intakes appear to have a detrimental effect on health only in China, for reasons which are unclear at the present time. Low selenium status has been linked with increased incidence of human cancers (Shamberger and Frost, 1969; Schrauzer et al., 1977; Willett et al., 1983; Clark, 1985; Salonen, 1986) and cardiovascular disease (Shamberger et al., 1979), although the evidence is equivocal (Ellis et al., 1984; Peleg et al., 1985; Virtamo et al., 1985; Salonen and Huttunen, 1986).

The margin between selenium deficiency and toxicity is narrower than for many other trace elements (Olson, 1986). Deleterious effects (nail changes, hair loss, and peripheral neuropathy) have been described in persons taking a selenium supplement in the form of a selenized yeast product containing 182 times more selenium than the stated level (Helzlsouer et al., 1985). Clinical manifestations of selenium toxicity have also been described in certain areas of China (Yang et al., 1983). The first signs of overexposure to selenium are invariably a garlic odor to the breath, a metallic taste in the mouth, nail changes, and, in severe cases, convulsions and paralysis. Other, more generalized effects, observed in high-selenium areas such as Venezuela, include pallor, lassitude, irritability, indigestion, and giddiness (Jaffé et al., 1972). The toxic dose is unknown, but in Japan a tentative maximum acceptable daily intake of 500 µg/day has been suggested (Sakurai and Tsuchiya, 1975). Olson (1986) suggested a maximum safe intake over extended periods of 5 µg/day per kilogram body weight for U.S. adults.

Uncertainties exist about the best index of selenium status. A combination of indices, which include selenium concentrations and, in some cases, glutathione peroxidase activity in whole blood or its components, is recommended. These indices are discussed below. As well, when assessing selenium status, the interactions of selenium with other nutrients (e.g. vitamins A, E , and polyunsaturated fat) and heavy metals (e.g. arsenic, cadmium, and lead) should also be considered.

24.4.1 Serum/plasma selenium concentrations

Serum selenium is mainly protein-bound and associated with α- and β-globulins and lipoproteins (Diplock, 1976). Selenium concentrations in plasma or serum respond to short-term changes in dietary selenium

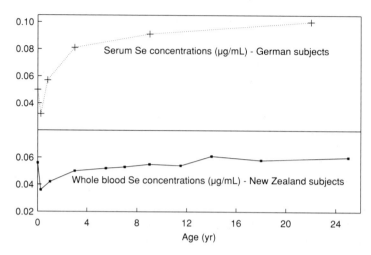

Figure 24.4: Effect of age on selenium concentrations in serum of German subjects and in whole blood of New Zealand subjects. Conversion factor to SI units (μmol/L) = × 12.66. From Thomson and Robinson (1980). © Am. J. Clin. Nutr. American Society for Clinical Nutrition.

intakes, and hence generally reflect the short-term or acute selenium status (Levander et al., 1981). Thus they can be used to monitor the selenium status of patients receiving total parenteral nutrition. In population groups with relatively constant dietary selenium intakes, serum/plasma selenium concentrations provide an index of selenium status. When large doses of organic forms of selenium have been ingested, however, plasma selenium concentrations may not reflect body selenium stores (Behne and Wolters, 1983; Levander et al., 1983a).

Data on factors affecting serum/plasma selenium concentrations are limited; measurements were not performed in the NHANES I or II or the Canada Health surveys. Serum/plasma selenium levels appear to be independent of sex in children (Lombeck et al., 1978; McKenzie et al., 1978) and adults (Kay and Knight, 1979; Lane et al., 1981; Lane et al., 1983), but may be dependent on race. The mean plasma selenium concentration of American negro adult males from Georgia, USA, was significantly lower than in white males (0.098 ± 0.020 μg/mL vs. 0.111 ± 0.020 μg/mL) (McAdam et al., 1984). These differences may be diet-related.

Age-related trends in serum selenium concentrations during infancy and childhood have been described (Lombeck et al., 1978; McKenzie et al., 1978) and attributed to changes in dietary selenium intakes (Figure 24.4). Values for German infants were high at birth and then declined to 30% to 50% of neonatal values by five to six months of age, after which they rose throughout the remainder of infancy (Figure 24.4) (Lombeck et al., 1978). This trend was ascribed to the low selenium content of the milk formulas used. In general, breast milk has a higher selenium content than commercial milk formulas, and exclusively breast-fed infants have significantly higher serum selenium concentrations than their formula-fed counterparts (Smith et al., 1982). Serum selenium values are relatively constant during adulthood (McAdam et al., 1984) until sixty years of age, after which values decline (Verlinden et al., 1983a; 1983b). This trend may also be diet-related.

Low plasma selenium concentrations have been observed in infants and young children with phenylketonuria and maple syrup urine disease, receiving formula diets low in selenium (Lombeck et al., 1975), and in premature infants (Gross, 1976). In the latter, plasma levels fell from 0.080 µg/mL (1.01 µmol/L) during the first week of life to 0.035 µg/mL (0.44 µmol/L) after seven to eight weeks, and were associated with hemolytic defects.

Although cardiovascular abnormalities develop in animal species on selenium-deficient diets, results of studies of the relationship between serum/plasma selenium status and cardiovascular disease in humans have been inconsistent. Significantly lower serum selenium concentrations have been documented in some but not all patients with congestive cardiomyopathy compared to healthy controls (Oster et al., 1983; Auzepy et al., 1987). Similarly, two out of three longitudinal Finnish studies have failed to find any significant relationship between low serum selenium levels and risk of coronary heart disease (Salonen et al., 1982; Miettinen et al., 1983; Virtamo et al., 1985).

Cutoff points for serum selenium concentrations, associated with selenium deficiency or toxicity, have not been defined in North America. A New Zealand TPN patient with a plasma selenium concentration of 0.009 µg/mL (0.11 µmol/L) developed clinical symptoms of selenium deficiency (i.e. muscle pain), which were reversed after selenium supplementation (van Rij et al., 1979). This low serum selenium concentration has been associated with selenium-responsive disease in other species. In the United States, plasma selenium concentrations in healthy adults range from 0.119 to 0.134 µg/mL (1.51–1.70 µmol/L) for areas where soil selenium levels are low or marginally adequate respectively (Snook et al., 1983; Levander and Morris, 1984). In the South Island of New Zealand, plasma selenium concentrations for healthy adults are frequently less than 0.050 µg/mL (< 0.63 µmol/L) (Thomson et al., 1982).

Serum/plasma selenium levels can be measured accurately and reliably using direct AAS with a Zeeman background correction (Pleban et al., 1982). Currently, however, the fluorometric determination, often as a semi-automated method (Watkinson, 1979), is most frequently used. Instrumental neutron activation analysis (Lombeck et al., 1978; Gibson et al., 1985) and electron capture gas chromatography (McCarthy

Area	Dietary Se Intake (µg/day)	Blood Se (µg/mL)	Hair Se (µg/g)	Urinary Se (µg/mL)
Low-Se area with Keshan's Disease	11	0.021	0.074	0.007
Low-Se area	–	0.027	0.16	–
Se-adequate area	116	0.091	0.36	0.026
High-Se area	750	0.44	3.7	0.14
High-Se area with chronic selenosis	4990	3.2	32.2	2.68

Table 24.7: Mean values of dietary intake, whole blood, hair, and urinary selenium concentrations in different areas of China. Conversion factors to SI units (µmol/L) = × 12.66; (nmol/g) = × 12.66. Adapted from Yang et al. (1983). © Am. J. Clin. Nutr. American Society for Clinical Nutrition.

et al., 1981) are very sensitive techniques and particularly suited for analyzing small samples. These techniques can also measure selenium in whole blood or its components, urine, and hair.

24.4.2 Whole blood selenium concentrations

Whole blood selenium concentrations, unlike serum selenium, are an index of long-term selenium status and do not fluctuate from day to day. Hence, low selenium concentrations in whole blood may reflect chronic dietary deficiencies of selenium. In a selenium depletion-repletion study of young adult men, for example, whole blood selenium concentrations were not altered after a six-week period on a low-selenium diet (19 to 24 µg Se per day) (Levander et al., 1981). Indeed, a response has only been observed after a period of months on a low-selenium diet (Thomson and Robinson, 1980).

Table 24.7 shows the relationship between dietary selenium intakes and whole blood (and hair and urine) selenium concentrations in population groups in China with high, normal, and deficient dietary intakes of selenium (Yang et al., 1983). In the United States, adults have whole blood selenium concentrations ranging from 0.19 to 0.25 µg/mL (2.4 to 3.2 µmol/L) (Allaway et al., 1968; Burk, 1984), whereas in New Zealand, where selenium intakes are low, whole blood selenium values for adults are in the range of 0.06 to 0.07 µg/mL (0.8 to 0.9 µmol/L) (Griffiths and Thomson, 1974). In Europe, whole blood selenium concentrations are lower than in North America, but higher than in New Zealand and Finland (Figure 24.5) (Brune et al., 1966; Allaway et al., 1968; Westermarck et al., 1977; Thomson and Robinson, 1980; Oster et al., 1983; Verlinden et al., 1983a; Wąsowicz and Zachara, 1987).

Many of the factors affecting serum/plasma selenium also influence whole blood selenium concentrations (Figure 24.4). For instance, low blood selenium concentrations have also been observed in children with

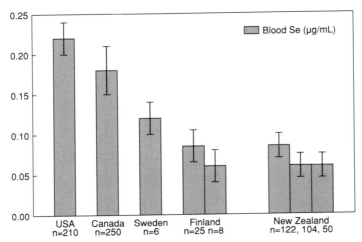

Figure 24.5: Whole blood selenium concentrations of healthy adults in selected countries. From Thomson and Robinson (1980). © Am. J. Clin. Nutr. American Society for Clinical Nutrition.

kwashiorkor (range 0.09 to 0.11 μg/mL) (1.1 to 1.4 μmol/L) (Levine and Olson, 1970), in children with phenylketonuria and maple syrup urine disease on special formula diets low in selenium (Lombeck et al., 1978) (range 0.010 to 0.027 μg/mL) (0.13 to 0.34 μmol/L), and in premature infants (Gross, 1976).

Patients with gastrointestinal cancers and juvenile neuronal ceroid lipofuscinosis also have low whole blood (and serum) selenium values (McConnell et al., 1975; Westermarck et al., 1982), perhaps as a consequence of the disease. Selenium supplementation has produced a positive clinical response in some of the patients with juvenile neuronal ceroid lipofuscinosis; transitory physical and mental improvements were observed (Westermarck et al., 1982). Chinese investigators have reported significantly lower whole blood selenium concentrations in patients with dilated cardiomyopathy compared to normal subjects (Bai-song et al., 1986).

24.4.3 Erythrocyte and platelet selenium concentrations

Erythrocyte selenium concentrations generally reflect long-term selenium status. Positive correlations between erythrocyte selenium concentrations and selenium intakes have been documented in individuals with relatively constant parenteral or enteral selenium intakes (Lane et al., 1982a). As well, consistent correlations between erythrocyte selenium values and signs of chronic toxicity or deficiency have observed. Only limited data are available on the effects of age, sex, and race on erythrocyte selenium concentrations (McAdam et al., 1984). In animal studies, erythrocyte selenium concentrations reflected the selenium content of muscle (and liver) of rats when relatively constant amounts of selenium were fed (Behne et al., 1981).

Selenium concentrations in platelets are markedly higher and fall more slowly than the corresponding concentrations in erythrocytes and plasma (Kasperek et al., 1982). Studies of platelet selenium concentrations as an index of selenium status in humans are limited.

24.4.4 Urinary selenium concentrations

Urine is the main excretory route for selenium, followed by the feces. Losses via the skin and expired air are small, except when intakes of selenium are toxic (Diplock, 1976). Daily urinary selenium excretion is closely related to plasma selenium (Robinson et al., 1978).

Urinary selenium levels have been more frequently used as an index of selenium toxicity and industrial exposure to selenium than as an index of selenium deficiency (Glover, 1967; Hojo, 1981). The proposed maximum allowable urinary selenium concentrations is 100 µg/L (Glover, 1967). The amount of selenium excreted in the urine depends on the recent dietary intake (Valentine et al., 1978; Thomson and Robinson, 1980), unless selenium intakes are very low. At such low intakes, no correlation between dietary intake and urinary selenium excretion occurs, presumably because urinary excretion reflects body stores rather than intake (Griffiths, 1973). Urinary selenium concentrations ranging from 0.9 to 3900 µg/L have been reported (Robberecht and Deelstra., 1984), although generally concentrations are less than 30 µg/L in nonexposed persons.

Twenty-four-hour urine collections are usually recommended for measuring urinary selenium levels (Thomson and Robinson, 1980), as urinary selenium excretion varies with time of day and the amount and nature of the diet (Valentine et al., 1978). Even so, some investigators suggest that urinary selenium concentrations, determined on casual urine specimens and expressed in relation to creatinine excretion (ng/g creatinine), are useful (Hojo, 1981). Wąsowicz and Zachara (1987) have reported significant positive correlations between urinary selenium : creatinine ratios and whole blood selenium concentrations in healthy Polish subjects.

Lower urinary excretion of selenium in females compared to males (Tsongas and Ferguson, 1978) and pregnant compared to nonpregnant females (Swanson et al., 1983) has been documented. Urinary selenium excretion levels are also lower in celiac, burn, and alcoholic patients (Robberecht and Deelstra, 1984), but it is not clear whether the lowered urinary selenium excretion is a cause or a consequence of the disease/condition. In some diseases/conditions, low urinary excretion levels may arise from reduced intakes of selenium and/or increased retention. The fluorometric method is most frequently used for measuring selenium concentrations in urine (Geahchan and Chambon, 1980).

Current data on the selenium metabolites in human urine are limited and rather inconsistent. Preliminary data on rats suggest that concentrations of urinary selenium metabolites may be promising indices of selenium status (Nahapetian et al., 1983); this requires further study.

24.4.5 Glutathione peroxidase activity

Glutathione peroxidase (GSHPx) is a selenium-containing enzyme which helps to protect the cell against lipid peroxidation damage. The activity of this selenoenzyme as a functional index of selenium status has been extensively investigated in erythrocytes and whole blood, and to a lesser extent in serum and platelets. GSHPx activity can only be used to assess selenium status in persons living in countries where dietary intakes of selenium are habitually low (e.g. New Zealand). In such circumstances, whole blood or erythrocyte selenium concentrations are often less than $0.1\,\mu g/mL$ ($1.27\,\mu mol/L$) (Thomson et al., 1977) and $0.14\,\mu g/mL$ ($1.77\,\mu mol/L$) (Rea et al., 1979) respectively, and correlate significantly with blood GSHPx activities. Above these concentrations, however, GSHPx activity in whole blood or erythrocytes tends to flatten out, and hence cannot be used to assess selenium status. Therefore, measurement of GSHPx activity in whole blood or erythrocytes as an index of selenium status in population groups with moderate or high-selenium intakes (e.g. the United States and Canada) is not recommended (Snook et al., 1983; McAdam et al., 1984). For example, in U.S. adults, GSHPx activity does not respond to relatively short-term periods of low selenium intake (19 to $24\,\mu g$ Se per day for six weeks) (Levander et al., 1981).

GSHPx activity tends to be affected by many other factors, such as age, ethnic background, sex, physical activity, exposure to antioxidants, iron-deficiency anemia, vitamin B-12 deficiency, and essential fatty acid deficiency (Ganther et al., 1976). These factors may have a greater effect when selenium intakes are adequate and hence the selenium requirement of the enzyme is met (Robinson and Thomson, 1983).

GSHPx activity in platelets has been investigated as an index of selenium status. Platelets contain more selenium than other tissues, and have a short half-life (about 1.5 weeks) (Kasperek et al., 1982), and hence, it is not surprising that GSHPx activity in platelets responds quickly to changes in selenium intakes (Thomson and Duncan, 1981; Levander et al., 1983a, 1983b; Thomson et al., 1988; Cohen et al., 1989). For example, higher GSHPx activity in platelets was noted in overseas visitors compared to New Zealand residents; the activity declined with exposure to the New Zealand low-selenium diet (Thomson and Duncan, 1981). Furthermore, in a selenium supplementation study of Finnish men with low selenium status, platelet enzyme activity nearly doubled after two weeks of supplementation (Levander et al., 1983b). Positive correlations between platelet GSHPx activity and selenium concentrations in human liver, as well as between GSHPx activities in platelets, human liver, and muscle tissue, have been demonstrated following four weeks of selenium supplementation (Thomson et al., 1988), confirming the validity of platelet GSHPx activity as an index of selenium status in humans.

In general, the assay for glutathione peroxidase is easier to perform than tissue selenium analysis. Nevertheless, no reference data for enzyme activity values are available for the interpretation of the results. Great care must be taken when handling and storing the tissue sample to avoid denaturing the enzyme. The enzyme assay has not been well standardized and results depend on the technique used. For example, differences in the choice of the substrate for the assay affect the enzyme activity (Ganther et al., 1976). One method involves modifications of the coupled enzyme assay of Paglia and Valentine (1967), in which glutathione peroxidase activity is measured by the oxidation of NADPH with cumen peroxide via glutathione reductase. Because hemoglobin interferes with the assay of glutathione peroxidase activity (Beilstein and Whanger, 1983), the absence of hemoglobin in platelets is an advantage.

Not all GSHPx activity is selenium-dependent; the distributions of the selenium-dependent and selenium-nondependent GSHPx varies among tissues and species, and has not been fully characterized (Robinson and Thomson, 1983).

24.4.6   Hair selenium concentrations

The clinical significance of hair selenium concentrations in human nutrition was unknown until Chinese workers studying Keshan's disease noted a close relationship between hair and whole blood selenium concentrations (Chen et al., 1980). The average hair selenium concentration in areas where Keshan's disease was endemic was 0.074 μg/g (0.94 nmol/g) compared to mean levels of 0.16 μg/g (2.03 nmol/g) in low-selenium areas without Keshan's disease, and 0.36 μg/g (4.56 nmol/g) in selenium-adequate areas (Table 24.7). Low hair selenium levels have also been reported in children with inborn errors of metabolism, treated with semisynthetic diets low in selenium (Lombeck et al., 1978), although none of the clinical features of Keshan's disease were observed.

Hair selenium concentrations can also be used as indices of over-exposure to selenium. Elevated hair selenium concentrations have been observed in persons living in seleniferous areas of China (Yang et al., 1983) (Table 24.7), in a child with acute selenium poisoning (Lombeck et al., 1986), and in U.S. adults after a six-week selenium supplementation study (100 μg Se/day) (Gallagher et al., 1984). Animal studies have also confirmed that hair selenium is a valid index of chronic selenium status. In rats fed a constant level of selenium, hair selenium concentrations reflected muscle or liver selenium content better than either plasma or erythrocyte selenium (Behne et al., 1981).

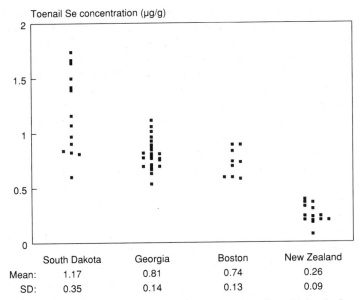

Figure 24.6: Toenail selenium concentrations in a high-selenium area (South Dakota), Georgia, and Boston, compared with a low-selenium area (New Zealand). Conversion factor to SI units (nmol/g) = × 12.66. From Morris et al. (1983) with permission.

The use of selenium-containing antidandruff shampoos in the United States and Europe may confound the interpretation of hair selenium concentrations, because the adventitious selenium from the shampoo is not removed during standardized hair washing procedures (Davies, 1982). The effect of hair color on human hair selenium concentrations has not yet been established.

24.4.7 Toenail selenium concentrations

Toenails may be a useful biopsy material of very long-term, retrospective, selenium status because selenium is incorporated into toenails as they grow. Toenail clippings probably reflect selenium status six to nine months prior to collection, depending on the nail length and growth rate. The collection of toenails, like hair, is noninvasive and simple, and selenium concentrations are relatively high (Hadjimarkos and Shearer, 1973). Nevertheless, studies on the use of toenail selenium concentrations as an index of selenium status are limited. Morris et al. (1983) reported that toenail selenium concentrations from a high-selenium area (South Dakota) were significantly higher than those from a low-selenium area (New Zealand) (Figure 24.6).

Bank et al. (1981) recommend cleaning nails before clipping with a scrubbing brush and a mild detergent, followed by mechanical scraping to remove any remaining soft tissue. More information is required on factors affecting toenail growth and the relationship between selenium concentration of toenails and body selenium stores before the validity of toenail selenium concentrations can be firmly established.

24.5 Assessment of zinc status

In an adult 70 kg male there is approximately 1.5 to 2.0 g of zinc, of which over 80% is found in muscle and bone. Zinc is a constituent of over 200 metallo-enzymes which participate in carbohydrate, lipid, and protein metabolism and nucleic acid synthesis and degradation (Prasad, 1985a). Hence, zinc is essential for many diverse functions including growth and development, reproduction, immune and sensory function, antioxidant protection, and the stabilization of membranes (Cousins, 1986).

The first cases of dietary zinc deficiency in humans were described in male dwarfs from the Middle East (Prasad et al., 1963). Typical clinical features, corrected by zinc supplementation, included growth retardation, delayed secondary sexual maturation (hypogonadism), poor appetite, mental lethargy, and skin changes. In North America and New Zealand, overt and severe nutritional zinc deficiency was first recognized in patients receiving either parenteral nutrition or enteral feedings without zinc supplements (Kay and Tasman-Jones, 1975; Arakawa et al., 1976). Later, secondary zinc deficiency was also documented in the presence of certain disease states such as cystic fibrosis, as well as in renal and liver diseases, and in association with burns and alcoholism. In such cases, zinc deficiency may arise from increased excretion of zinc in the urine (hyperzincuria) and/or loss of zinc via intestinal secretions and exudates (Aggett and Harries, 1979). Two genetic disorders, acrodermatitis enteropathica (Barnes and Moynahan, 1973). and sickle cell disease (Prasad and Cossack, 1982), are associated with suboptimal zinc status

Marginal nutritional zinc deficiency, characterized by a slowing of physical growth, poor appetite, and diminished taste acuity (hypogeusia), has also been identified in some apparently healthy infants and/or children in the United States (Hambidge et al., 1972a; Walravens and Hambidge, 1976; Walravens et al., 1983), Canada (Smit-Vanderkooy and Gibson, 1987; Gibson et al., 1989), Yugoslavia (Buzina et al., 1980), and China (Xue-Cun et al., 1985). Other groups susceptible to zinc deficiency include pregnant women (Solomons et al., 1986) and the elderly (Sandstead et al., 1982). In the latter, the presence of disease states, and/or the use of certain medications and supplements, may precipitate secondary zinc deficiency states (Aggett and Harries, 1979).

Nutritional deficiencies of zinc may arise from inadequate intakes and/or poor availability of dietary zinc associated with excessive intakes of dietary fiber, polyphosphates, iron, copper, and phytate, the latter in the presence of high dietary calcium levels (Solomons, 1982). Good sources of available dietary zinc are meat, liver, eggs, and seafood; zinc in whole grain cereals is less readily available.

Cases of toxicity from excess dietary intakes of zinc have not been reported. Nevertheless, pharmacological doses of zinc can interfere with the absorption of copper (Prasad et al., 1978a) and may also reduce serum HDL cholesterol levels (Hooper et al., 1980). High intakes of zinc also have a potentially detrimental effect on the immune system (Chandra, 1984). Consequently, excessive self-supplementation with zinc may have an adverse effect on health.

Diagnosis of zinc deficiency is hampered by the lack of a single, specific, and sensitive biochemical index of zinc status. A large number of indices have been proposed, but many are fraught with problems that affect their use and interpretation. The most reliable method for diagnosing marginal zinc deficiency at present is a positive response to zinc supplementation. Such an approach is time consuming, cumbersome, and impractical for community studies, and necessitates good compliance with follow-up visits. Therefore, a combination of biochemical and functional physiological indices is frequently used to evaluate zinc status and these are discussed below.

24.5.1 Serum/plasma zinc concentrations

Approximately 10% to 20% of the zinc in blood is in the plasma; the remainder is within the erythrocytes. Zinc is normally transported in the plasma bound principally to albumin, α_2-macroglobulin, and amino acids, especially histidine and cystine; a very small fraction also exists in the ionic form (Cousins, 1985).

Serum or plasma zinc is the most widely used index of zinc status. In persons with severe zinc deficiency, serum/plasma zinc concentrations are usually low. Decreases in serum/plasma zinc, for example, occur in patients receiving TPN unsupplemented with zinc (Arakawa et al., 1976), and in experimentally induced zinc deficiency (Hess et al., 1977; Prasad et al., 1978b; Gordon et al., 1982; Baer and King, 1984). Concentrations return to normal after zinc supplementation. Serum/plasma zinc concentrations are homeostatically controlled, so that in marginal zinc deficiency states values may be within the normal range (Fickel et al., 1986; Milne et al., 1987; Gibson et al., 1989). Furthermore, serum zinc concentrations are modified by a number of non-nutritional factors which confound their use as an index of zinc status (Halsted and Smith, 1970). For example, in acute infection or inflammation, serum/plasma zinc values are spuriously low because zinc is redistributed from the plasma to the liver (Beisel et al., 1976). This redistribution is mediated by leukocytic endogenous mediator which is liberated by phagocytizing cells during acute-phase response. Stress and myocardial infarction also modify serum zinc levels (Prasad, 1983). Other confounding factors include the presence of chronic disease states associated with hypoalbuminaemia, such as alcoholic cirrhosis and protein-energy malnutrition (Solomons, 1979). Decreases in serum/plasma zinc concentrations also occur in pregnancy (Hambidge and Droegemueller, 1974) and after the use of oral contraceptive agents (Halsted et al., 1968; Smith and Brown, 1976). Serum zinc changes in pregnancy have been partially attributed to changes in blood volume (hemodilution) (Swanson and King, 1982); this does not, however, explain the apparent decline in serum zinc concentrations (Breskin et al., 1983) which occur during the first trimester. Some (Hambidge et al., 1987), but not all (Yip et al., 1985), investigators noted a decline in serum zinc concentrations during iron therapy.

Serum/plasma zinc concentrations are also affected by hemolysis: erythrocytes have a high zinc content. Hemolysis may be particularly important in cases of zinc deficiency, when red cell fragility is increased (Bettger et al., 1978). Nevertheless, in the NHANES II survey, serum zinc levels of 'slightly' hemolyzed samples (by visual inspection) were not significantly different from those of nonhemolysed samples (Pilch and Senti, 1984).

Blood samples for serum or plasma zinc should be taken under carefully controlled, standardized conditions. Pilch and Senti (1984) reported serum zinc concentrations assayed from a large (n = 14,770), representative sample of children and adults (three to seventy-four years) during the NHANES II survey (1976–1980). Serum zinc levels were significantly elevated after an overnight fast, compared to levels of nonfasted individuals, and higher in the morning, regardless of fasting status, compared to the afternoon. Similar trends have been observed by others in serum (Markowitz et al., 1985) and in plasma (Jacobs Goodall et al., 1988). Pronounced changes in serum/plasma zinc associated with meals have been described in adults (Markowitz et al., 1985; Jacobs Goodall et al., 1988). Plasma zinc levels start to decline approximately one hour after a meal, the decline continuing for approximately two hours before reaching a plateau or reversing.

The length of time prior to separation of serum/plasma also affects zinc concentrations. Changes cannot be detected during the first hour, but longer intervals prior to separation are associated with progressively increasing serum and plasma zinc concentrations (English et al., 1988). An increase in serum/plasma zinc levels after venous occlusion has been reported by some (Walker et al., 1979; Juswigg et al., 1982), but not all (English et al., 1988), investigators. A 15% increase in plasma zinc levels was noted, however, when a sphygmomanometer instead of a tourniquet was used to maintain pressure above the diastolic pressure (English et al., 1988). English et al. concluded that the position of the subject did not affect plasma zinc values.

Age	Male Serum Zinc (µg/dL)	Female Serum Zinc (µg/dL)
3–8 years	85	84
9–19 years	95	90
20–44 years	96	86
45–64 years	88	83
65–74 years	84	81

Table 24.8: Median serum zinc levels of males and females in a reference population, by age: United States, 1976–1980. Data are for an 'a.m. nonfasting sample'. Conversion factor to SI units (µmol/L) = × 0.1530. From Pilch and Senti (1984).

Blood samples for zinc analysis must be taken carefully to avoid contamination from sources such as preservatives, evacuated tubes, and rubber stoppers. Trace-element-free evacuated tubes must be used. Ideally, preparation and analysis of serum/plasma zinc should be performed in a contamination-controlled environment. Certain anticoagulants (e.g. citrate, oxalate, and EDTA) efficiently chelate metallic ions, so that if used, plasma zinc values will be lower than if heparin were used as the anticoagulant (Danford and Chandler, 1983), provided the heparin is uncontaminated with zinc (Gervin et al., 1983). In general, if the blood collection and separation methods are performed under rigorously controlled conditions, values for serum and plasma zinc will probably be comparable (Kosman and Henkin, 1979; Makino, 1983). Some investigators prefer to use plasma because it is readily separated, less susceptible to platelet contamination, and not subject to contamination from a reaming instrument (Smith et al., 1985).

The NHANES II survey provides data for serum zinc concentrations in a reference population of apparently healthy U.S. persons. Observations from those persons with conditions known to affect serum zinc, other than nutritional deficiency, were excluded (Pilch and Senti, 1984). Data tables include mean, ± SD, and ±SEM, and selected percentiles according to age, sex, and race. Age- and sex-related trends in serum zinc concentrations were documented (Pilch and Senti, 1984). From adolescence onward, males had higher mean serum zinc levels than females (Table 24.8), the greatest differences being apparent in adults aged twenty to forty-four years. For both males and females, serum zinc values were low in childhood, reaching a peak in adolescence and young adulthood (Pilch and Senti, 1984) and declining with age in adults. Similar trends in serum zinc levels during infancy, childhood, and adulthood have been noted by others (Hambidge et al., 1972a; Kasperek et al., 1977; Butrimonvitz et al., 1978; Kirsten et al., 1985).

The cutoff point generally used to assess risk of zinc deficiency for both plasma and serum values is < 70 µg/dL (< 10.71 µmol/L), a value approximately two standard deviations below the adult mean. This value may only be appropriate for morning fasting blood samples. For nonfasting morning, and for afternoon samples, lower cutoff points of $< 65 \, \mu g/dL$ ($< 9.95 \, \mu mol/L$) and $< 60 \, \mu g/dL$ ($< 9.18 \, \mu mol/L$), respectively, have been recommended (Pilch and Senti, 1984).

Flame atomic absorption spectroscopy is most commonly used for serum zinc analysis, using a direct technique in which the sample is diluted with 4 to 9 parts of deionized water. A coefficient of variation of 5% is attainable for both zinc and copper using AAS (Smith et al., 1979). The trichloroacetic acid deproteinization technique, described in Section 24.2.1, is rarely used. Sometimes, the serum/plasma samples are ashed using a low-temperature asher, prior to analysis by flame AAS. For very small samples, flameless AAS can be used (Shaw et al., 1982).

Plasma copper/zinc ratios have sometimes been used in certain disease states (Bogden et al., 1977; Gray et al., 1982), particularly to monitor the response of patients to chemotherapy (Bogden, 1980). Such ratios are limited by the effects discussed for serum/plasma zinc and copper; their use appears limited in 'apparently' healthy subjects.

24.5.2 Erythrocyte zinc concentrations

Relatively few investigators have used erythrocytes as a biopsy material for assessing zinc status because the analysis is difficult and the response during experimentally induced zinc depletion-repletion studies has been equivocal (Prasad et al., 1978b; Baer and King, 1984). The half-life of erythrocytes is quite long (120 days), so that erythrocyte zinc concentrations will not reflect recent changes in body zinc stores. For example, in a human zinc depletion study, erythrocyte zinc concentrations declined by only 21% after feeding low-zinc diets for as long as ninety days (Buerk et al., 1973). Nishi (1980) reported age-related changes in erythrocyte zinc in Japanese subjects. Concentrations were very low during infancy ($18.7 \pm 6.1 \, \mu g/g$ Hb; one to six months), and increased gradually with age, reaching adult levels between eleven to fifteen years ($42.2 \pm 5.6 \, \mu g/g$ Hb).

Erythrocytes for zinc analysis are first washed with isotonic phosphate-buffered saline and then lysed with deionized water. A diluted aliquot of the erythrocyte lysate is analyzed for zinc via flame or flameless AAS (Whitehouse et al., 1982; Milne et al., 1985). Standard solutions containing the same inorganic constituents as erythrocytes should be used for flameless AAS to compensate for matrix effects. Hemoglobin is also determined concurrently on a sample of the erythrocyte lysate, enabling the zinc content to be expressed in terms of micrograms per gram of hemoglobin.

24.5.3 Leukocyte and neutrophil zinc concentrations

Leukocytes contain up to twenty-five times more zinc than erythrocytes, and early results suggested that leukocyte zinc was a more reliable index of zinc status than erythrocyte or plasma zinc (Prasad et al., 1978b; Meadows et al., 1981) and reflected levels of soft tissue zinc (Jones et al., 1981; Jackson et al., 1982). Specific cellular types of leukocytes (e.g. neutrophils and lymphocytes) have also been examined as potential indices of zinc status. Neutrophils have been selected because they have both a short half-life and a high zinc content. Indeed, in a human zinc depletion study, neutrophil zinc concentrations, but not plasma zinc, decreased significantly after only four weeks on a marginally zinc-deficient diet (Prasad and Cossack, 1982). Neutrophil zinc concentrations were also low in zinc-deficient sickle cell anemia patients and correlated with other biochemical indices of zinc status (Prasad and Cossack, 1982).

The separation of leukocytes and specific cellular types is difficult; contamination with zinc and/or platelets may occur. Milne et al. (1985) showed that the zinc content of leukocytes is a function of the type of separation used. Cell suspensions must be free of erythrocytes and platelets, as they both have a relatively high zinc content (Milne et al., 1985). Data are difficult to interpret because no consensus exists for the method used to express zinc concentrations in these two cell types. Results can be expressed on a mg/kg dry weight basis to eliminate the effects of variable cell water content, but results expressed as $ng/10^6$ cells are preferred (Nishi, 1980; Prasad and Cossack, 1982; Milne et al., 1985). When the latter is used, clump-free suspensions are essential; cell clumping results in an underestimate of the actual cell count.

The choice of the anticoagulant affects cell separation; EDTA is preferred (Milne et al., 1985). Cell types can be isolated from whole blood on discontinuous gradients of colloidal polyvinylpyrrolidone-coated silica ('Percoll'), recommended by Milne et al. (1985), or Ficoll-Hypaque (English and Anderson, 1974). Isolated cells are then digested with nitric acid and diluted with deionized water, prior to analysis via AAS. Flameless or flame AAS adapted for microsamples can be used. When flameless AAS is used, standard solutions simulating the sample matrix are required, to compensate for the matrix effects of the digested samples (Milne et al., 1985). In view of these methodological problems, the validity of leukocyte and neutrophil zinc as indices of zinc status remains uncertain. Relatively large volumes of blood are required, limiting the use of these indices in infants and children.

24.5.4 Urine zinc concentrations

In disease-free subjects, a decrease in urinary excretion of zinc occurs with the development of zinc deficiency. In cases of sickle cell disease and cirrhosis of the liver, however, hyperzincuria occurs, despite the presence of zinc deficiency (Prasad, 1983). Hyperzincuria is also present after injury, burns, and acute starvation, in certain renal diseases and infections, and after treatment with chlorothiazide. Hypertensive patients on long-term therapy with chlorothiazide may therefore be vulnerable to zinc deficiency (Prasad, 1983). Hence, the measurement of zinc in urine is helpful for diagnosing zinc deficiency only in apparently healthy persons. Levels of zinc in the urine usually range from 300 to 600 μg per day. In general, twenty-four-hour urine collections are preferred because diurnal variation in urinary zinc excretion occurs. Casual urine samples can be used, in which case zinc : creatinine ratios should be calculated (Zlotkin and Casselman, 1988).

24.5.5 Hair zinc concentrations

The available evidence suggests that low zinc concentrations in hair samples collected during childhood probably reflect a chronic suboptimal zinc status when the confounding effect of severe protein-energy malnutrition is absent (Hambidge et al., 1972a; Gibson, 1980; Smit-Vanderkooy and Gibson, 1987; Gibson et al., 1989). Hair zinc cannot be used in cases of very severe malnutrition and/or severe zinc deficiency, when the rate of growth of the hair shaft is diminished. In such cases, hair zinc concentrations may be normal or even high (Erten et al., 1978; Bradfield and Hambidge, 1980).

Low hair zinc concentrations were reported in the first documented cases of human zinc deficiency in young adult male dwarfs from the Middle East (Strain et al., 1966). Low hair zinc concentrations also characterize subjects with impaired taste acuity and/or those with low growth percentiles, two clinical features of marginal zinc deficiency in childhood (Hambidge et al., 1972a; Buzina et al., 1980; Xue-Cun et al., 1985; Smit-Vanderkooy and Gibson, 1987; Gibson et al., 1989). In some but not all of these cases of suboptimal zinc status, hair zinc concentrations have increased in response to zinc supplementation. The discrepancies may arise from variations in the dose, length of the zinc supplementation period, and confounding effects of season on hair zinc concentrations. Periods of six weeks or less are probably too short for a response in hair zinc, since the latter reflects only chronic changes in zinc status (Greger and Geissler, 1978; Lane et al., 1982b). Unfortunately, when studies are made over a longer term, seasonal changes in hair zinc concentrations must also be taken into account when interpreting the results (Hambidge et al., 1979; Gibson et al., 1989).

Standardized procedures for sampling, washing, and analyzing hair samples are essential in all studies (Section 15.1.1). Variations in hair zinc concentrations with hair color, hair beauty treatments, season, sex, age, anatomical site of sampling (scalp vs. pubic), and rate of hair growth have been described (Hambidge, 1982; Taylor, 1986; Klevay et al., 1987). The effects of these possible confounding factors must be considered in the interpretation of hair zinc concentrations.

Many investigators have failed to find any positive correlations between the zinc content of hair and serum/plasma zinc concentrations when conducting cross sectional (McBean et al., 1971) or relatively short-term (Lane et al., 1982b) longitudinal zinc depletion or zinc supplementation studies. These findings are not unexpected. The zinc content of the hair shaft reflects the quantity of zinc available to the hair follicles over an earlier time interval. For example, assuming a normal rate of hair growth, the zinc levels in the proximal 1 to 2 cm of hair reflect the zinc uptake by the follicles four to eight weeks prior to sample collection. Hence, positive correlations between hair zinc concentrations and other biochemical indices are only observed in chronic zinc deficiency. Unfortunately, very few long-term zinc depletion human studies have simultaneously examined hair, serum, and tissue zinc concentrations.

Clinical signs of marginal zinc deficiency in childhood, such as impaired growth and poor appetite (anorexia), are usually associated with hair zinc concentrations of less than 70 μg/g (1.07 μmol/g) (Hambidge et al., 1972a; Smit-Vanderkooy and Gibson, 1987). Therefore, this value is frequently used as the cutoff point for hair zinc concentrations indicative of suboptimal zinc status in children. The validity of hair zinc as a chronic index of suboptimal zinc status in adults is uncertain. Conflicting results have been obtained and no definitive conclusions can be drawn. Hair zinc analysis is most frequently performed by flame AAS, after ashing of the hair samples. Instrumental neutron activation analysis can also be used (Gibson and DeWolfe, 1979).

24.5.6 Salivary zinc concentrations

Concentrations of zinc in saliva have been investigated as an index of zinc status because zinc appears to be a component of gustin, an essential protein involved in taste acuity; the latter is impaired by marginal zinc deficiency (Henkin et al., 1971). Zinc concentrations in mixed saliva, parotid saliva, salivary sediment, and salivary supernatant have all been investigated, but their use as indices of zinc status is equivocal (Greger and Sickles, 1979; Freeland-Graves et al., 1981; Baer and King, 1984). Greger and Sickles noted changes in the zinc levels of salivary supernatant in response to slight variations in dietary zinc intakes, but no changes in salivary zinc concentrations were reported in experimentally induced zinc-deficient subjects (Baer and King, 1984) and in adults supplemented with zinc (Lane et al., 1982b).

Although the collection of saliva samples is quick and relatively noninvasive, the rate of flow and stimulation of saliva is difficult to control, and diurnal variation in zinc levels may occur (Warren et al., 1981). These problems, and the contradictory results observed, limit the use of salivary zinc as an index of zinc status (Greger and Sickles, 1979).

24.5.7   Zinc-dependent enzymes

Over 200 zinc metallo-enzymes have been identified. In humans, their response to zinc deficiency depends on the biopsy material sampled and their affinity to zinc. The activities of some zinc metallo-enzymes (e.g. carbonic anhydrase and dehydrogenases) decline only after the onset of clinical symptoms, and hence are not a sensitive index of marginal zinc status (Casey and Robinson, 1983). In contrast, the activities of alkaline phosphatase and carboxypeptidase decline rapidly after an inadequate zinc intake in experimental animals (Kirchgessner et al., 1976; Adeniyi and Heaton, 1980), although their response in humans is inconsistent (Nanji and Anderson, 1983). For example, no significant changes in the activity of serum alkaline phosphatase were observed during experimental zinc depletion in postmenopausal women (Milne et al., 1987), but activities fell, and subsequently rose, after zinc supplementation in a study of young men (Baer et al., 1985). Reduced activities of serum alkaline phosphatase were also observed in human zinc deficiency resulting from acrodermatitis enteropathica (Weismann and Høyer, 1978; 1985) and TPN (Ishikaza et al., 1981). Kasarskis and Schuna (1980) recommend taking serial measurements of serum alkaline phosphatase during zinc therapy for suspected marginal zinc deficiency, and calculating an alkaline phosphatase ratio as an index of marginal zinc deficiency. Measurements of alkaline phosphatase activity in neutrophils (Prasad, 1983; 1985b), leukocytes (Baer et al., 1985; Schilirò et al., 1987), and red cell membranes (Ruz et al., 1989) have been investigated as indices of body zinc status in humans, but more studies are needed before any definitive conclusions can be reached.

Other zinc metallo-enzymes which warrant further investigation as indices of zinc status in humans include δ-amino-levulinic acid dehydratase in erythrocytes (Faraji and Swendseid, 1983; Baer et al., 1985), angiotensin-1-converting enzyme (White et al., 1984; Reeves and O'Dell, 1985), and α-D-mannosidase in serum/plasma (Everett and Apgar, 1980; Apgar and Fitzgerald, 1987), nucleoside phosphorylase in whole, lysed cells (Prasad and Rabbani, 1981; Ballester and Prasad, 1983; Anonymous, 1984b), and ecto purine 5′nucleotidase in red cell membranes (Everett and Apgar, 1986).

24.5.8 Oral zinc tolerance test

A zinc tolerance test, also referred to as a plasma appearance test, measures the increase in plasma zinc from the fasting level after the oral ingestion of a pharmacological dose of zinc. Samples of plasma are collected after a twelve-hour fast and at hourly intervals post-dose for a five-hour period. Subjects must refrain from eating or drinking during the post-dose period. Generally, a fixed oral dose (e.g. 25 or 50 mg Zn as zinc acetate) is used, irrespective of body weight, although it may be preferable to give the dose on a per kilogram body weight basis (Freeland-Graves et al., 1988; Watson, 1988). The test is used as a measure of zinc status on the assumption that it reflects overall zinc absorption, which increases in zinc deficiency (Capel et al., 1982; Bales et al., 1986; Fickel et al., 1986). Variable results among subjects in any given group have been noted, making the test most useful when each subject serves as his or her own control (Abu-Hamdan et al., 1986).

Valberg et al. (1985) confirmed that the test does reflect zinc absorption. They compared results of the oral zinc tolerance test with those obtained by direct measurements of ^{65}Zn absorption and retention over a one-week period and obtained good agreement. The oral zinc tolerance test has also been used to assess the effects of different foods, meals, and vitamin mineral supplements (Solomons, 1982), disease processes (Crofton et al., 1983; Abu-Hamdan et al., 1986), and medications (Abu-Hamdan et al. 1986) on zinc absorption.

Figure 24.7 shows the plasma response of seven subjects to an oral load of 50 mg zinc, initially, after eight weeks on a zinc depleted diet, and after twelve days of zinc repletion. In all cases, the peak of the increase occurred at three hours post load. After the zinc depleted diet, the peak percentage increase of plasma zinc was significantly greater than that of the initial test, but generally not higher than that after zinc repletion (Fickel et al., 1986). This persistent elevation of the zinc tolerance curve after repletion markedly decreases the reliability of the zinc tolerance test as an index of zinc status. In addition, use of pharmacological doses of zinc limit the usefulness of the test. Such doses may be handled differently by the gastrointestinal tract than physiological levels of zinc. Parotid saliva does not respond to a zinc tolerance test and cannot be used as an alternative to plasma (Fickel et al., 1986).

24.5.9 Taste acuity tests

Diminished taste acuity (hypogeusia) is one of the features of marginal zinc deficiency in children (Hambidge et al., 1972a: Buzina et al., 1980; Gibson et al., 1989) and adults (Henkin, 1984; Larson Wright et al., 1981) and has been used as a functional index of zinc status. Several methods for testing taste acuity have been used (Bartoshuk, 1978), but for all

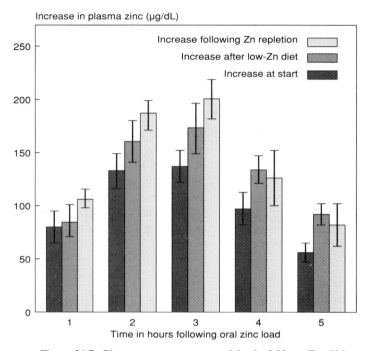

Figure 24.7: Plasma response to an oral load of 50 mg Zn. Values represent the mean (± SEM) increase of plasma zinc over the fasting level for 7 subjects. From Fickel et al. (1986). © Am. J. Clin. Nutr. American Society for Clinical Nutrition.

methods tests should preferably be performed midmorning, at least two hours after a meal, by the same person on each occasion.

The three-drop stimulus technique of Henkin et al. (1963) consists of presenting a single drop of each test solution, together with two single drops of distilled water, onto the anterior two-thirds of the tongue, in random order. The size of the stimulated area of the tongue should be controlled when using the three drop stimulus technique, because the the threshold is inversely related to the size; this variable is very difficult to control (Bartoshuk, 1978). Test solutions of varying concentrations for each of the four taste qualities are used: for salt (sodium chloride), for sweet (sucrose), for bitter (urea), and for sour (hydrochloric acid). Evaluation of taste acuity is generally based on the detection and recognition thresholds for each taste quality. The detection threshold is defined as the lowest concentration at which a taste can just be detected; the recognition threshold is the lowest concentration at which the quality of the taste stimulus can be recognized (Bartoshuk, 1978). The two thresholds are each determined for one taste quality before proceeding to the next. Several investigators have used this technique on young children

(Hambidge et al., 1972a; Buzina et al., 1980; Siegler et al., 1981; Watson et al., 1983), with varying degrees of success.

An alternative technique, which assesses only recognition thresholds and which is more suited to young children, was developed by Desor and Maller (1975). This method was adapted by Gibson et al. (1989) in their zinc supplementation study of Canadian boys with low height percentiles. Recognition taste thresholds for only one taste quality (salt) were determined to minimize potential problems with short attention span and distractions in children. Salt was selected because taste perception to moderately salty solutions was significantly altered during a zinc-depletion study of young adult men (Larson Wright et al., 1981). The concentrations of sodium chloride used for the Canadian children tested with this method were 10, 15, 20, and 25 mmol/L. Subjects rinse a small amount (10 mL) of each solution around in their mouths, expectorate it, and are then asked to identify the presented sample as salty or plain water. Salt solutions of increasing or decreasing concentrations are used, where appropriate, until the subjects correctly identify salt at one concentration and fail to do so at the next lower concentration. Only two out of ten judgements are allowed to be incorrect before moving to the next higher or lower salt concentration. The midpoint between these two concentrations is used as the recognition threshold for salt for each subject.

24.6 Summary

Chromium

Chromium, as an organic chromium complex, appears to have a role in glucose metabolism and insulin activity. It has not yet been identified as a constituent of any enzymes. Clinical manifestations of chromium deficiency include impaired glucose tolerance, hyperglycemia, relative insulin resistance, peripheral neuropathy, and/or metabolic encephalopathy. These disturbances have been reported in adults on long-term TPN, and respond to chromium supplementation. Marginal chromium deficiency states have also been reported in selected population groups, confirmed by an improvement in glucose tolerance after chromium supplementation at physiological levels. This approach is still the best method of diagnosing marginal chromium deficiency states. Alternative, less certain, methods include measurement of whole blood, erythrocytes, urine, hair, and serum chromium concentrations. Most of these methods have been used, with some success, for assessing overexposure to chromium, but not for identifying suboptimal chromium status. Difficulties have arisen in the analysis of chromium when concentrations in biological fluids and tissues are normal or low. Graphite furnace AAS is the analytical method most frequently used. So far, correlations of chromium concentrations in tissues and fluids with clinical parameters of suboptimal chromium status have produced inconsistent results.

Copper

Most of the clinical features of copper deficiency are associated with changes in the activities of cuproenzymes. Copper deficiency is rare in humans, although the hematological deficiency signs (e.g. neutropenia and hypochromic anemia), which occur first, have been described in premature and/or low-birthweight infants and some adults with sickle cell disease receiving prolonged zinc therapy. A few cases of copper toxicity have also been described, arising either accidentally or in patients with a copper-related genetic defect (Wilson's disease). Toxicity arising from high dietary intakes of copper has not been described.

Serum copper is most frequently used to assess copper status, despite its limited sensitivity and specificity. Superoxide dismutase (Cu,Zn-SOD) activity in erythrocytes is apparently more sensitive than serum copper and is a promising index. Nevertheless, its use as an index of copper status in the general population requires confirmation. Concentrations of copper in hair and urine are not valid indices of copper status. In cases of clinical copper deficiency, for example, hair copper levels are normal and urine copper concentrations are too low to measure accurately. In the future, alternative copper-dependent enzymes, such as cytochrome c oxidase in leukocytes and lysyl oxidase in collagen, may prove to be valid and feasible indices of copper status in humans.

Iodine

Iodine functions exclusively as a component of the thyroid hormones, thyroxine (T_4) and $3,5,3'$-triiodothyronine (T_3), which are required for normal growth and development and for maintenance of normal metabolism. Goiter (thyroid enlargement) is the major consequence of chronic iodine deficiency, and generally arises from prolonged inadequate intakes of iodine and/or exposure to goitrogens in foods and drugs. In areas where endemic goiter exists and iodine deficiency is severe, endemic cretinism may occur. Prolonged excessive intake of iodine in normal persons markedly reduces the iodine uptake by the thyroid. Goiter and hypothyroidism are rarely induced, although endemic goiter has been described in certain regions of Japan where seaweeds, rich in iodine, are dietary staples. Urinary iodine excretion closely reflects iodine intake and is the most widely used method of assessing iodine status. Urinary iodine excretion can be assessed in twenty-four-hour urine specimens (μg/day) or in casual samples, when it is expressed relative to creatinine excretion (μg/g creatinine). Concentrations of T_3 and/or T_4 and TSH in serum are routinely measured in neonates in Western countries to detect congenital hypothyroidism, using radio-immunoassay methods available as commercial kits. Uptake of radioactive ^{131}I is used as a test of thyroid function in clinical settings.

Selenium

Selenium, as a constituent of glutathione peroxidase (GSHPx), assists in protecting cellular components against oxidative damage. Selenium also has a role in the metabolism and toxicity of certain drugs and chemicals, and possibly in the immune system. Selenium-responsive conditions have occurred in patients on long-term TPN, and in young Chinese children with Keshan's disease. Suboptimal selenium status, without any apparent detrimental health effects, occurs in New Zealand and Finland. The margin between selenium deficiency and toxicity is relatively narrow, and naturally occurring selenium toxicity occurs in China and Venezuela. A combination of indices is currently recommended for the assessment of selenium status, which include selenium concentrations, and sometimes GSHPx activity, in blood and/or its components. Serum concentrations reflect dietary intakes of selenium for population groups with relatively stable selenium intakes. Cutoff points for serum selenium associated with selenium deficiency and toxicity in North America, and factors affecting serum selenium concentrations, are not yet clearly defined. Unlike serum, whole blood and erythrocyte selenium concentrations reflect long-term selenium status and hence are used to detect chronic deficiency or excess. As urine is the main excretory route for selenium, urinary selenium concentrations (in twenty-four-hour urine samples) are used as an index of toxicity, when levels reflect recent dietary intake. Hair selenium appears to be a promising index of chronic, not acute, selenium status in countries where selenium-containing antidandruff shampoos are not used. Alternatively, finger- and toenails have been investigated as indices of long-term selenium status because they are probably less affected by selenium-containing shampoos; more studies are required to establish their validity as indices of long-term selenium status. GSHPx activity in platelets, erythrocytes, and whole blood can only be used as a functional index of selenium status in countries where dietary intakes of selenium are habitually low. With moderate or high intakes, the GSHPx activity tends to flatten out and no correlations between whole blood or erythrocyte selenium concentrations are found. This enzyme assay, although easier to perform than tissue selenium analysis, is not well standardized and results are sometimes difficult to interpret.

Zinc

Zinc, as a constituent of over 200 metallo-enzymes, is essential for many diverse functions, including growth and development, normal reproduction, immune and sensory function, anti-oxidant protection, and the stabilization of membranes. Primary and secondary deficiencies of zinc are probably more prevalent in industrialized countries than those of chromium, copper, and selenium. Marginal zinc deficiency, characterized by slowing of physical growth, poor appetite, and diminished taste acuity, has been described in apparently healthy infants and children, arising from inadequate intakes and/or poor availability of dietary zinc. Toxicity from excess intakes from the diet has never been reported. Nevertheless, pharmacological doses of zinc supplements have produced hematological signs of copper deficiency, decreases in serum HDL cholesterol levels, and detrimental effects on the immune system.

No single, specific, and sensitive index of zinc status exists. A combination of biochemical and physiological functional indices is frequently used. Serum zinc concentrations are most frequently used, although their sensitivity and specificity are poor. Concentrations are usually low in severe zinc deficiency, but in marginal deficiency are often within the normal range. Many non-nutritional factors reduce the specificity and sensitivity of serum zinc. The validity of leukocyte and neutrophil zinc as indices of zinc status remains uncertain. Results have been inconsistent, perhaps because of difficulties with the separation and analysis. Urine zinc concentrations in casual and twenty-four-hour urine samples are only useful in disease-free subjects, when levels decrease as zinc deficiency develops. In the presence of certain diseases, however, hyperzincuria occurs, despite the presence of zinc deficiency. Hair zinc concentrations, measured during childhood, probably reflect chronic zinc status, provided that the effects of confounding factors such as age and season are taken into account, and the hair is sampled, washed, and analyzed by standardized procedures. Their validity as a chronic index of suboptimal zinc status in adults is less certain. Results of animal studies suggest that certain zinc-dependent enzymes may be promising as indices of zinc status, but these enzymes require more investigation in humans before their validity is established. Impaired taste acuity can be used as an additional physiological functional test of suboptimal zinc status, provided that it is used in association with other biochemical indices of zinc status. An oral zinc tolerance test has also been used, but results have been inconsistent.

References

Aalbers TG, Houtman JP. (1985). Relationship between trace elements and atherosclerosis. Science of the Total Environment. 43: 255–283.

Abraham AS, Sonnenblick M, Eini M, Shemesh O, Batt AP. (1980). The effect of chromium on established atherosclerotic plaques in rabbits. American Journal of Clinical Nutrition 33: 2294–2298.

Abu-Hamdan DK, Mahajan SK, Migdal SD, Prasad AS, McDonald FD. (1986). Zinc tolerance test in uremia. Annals of Internal Medicine 104: 50–52.

Adeniyi FA, Heaton FW. (1980). The effect of zinc deficiency on alkaline phosphatase (EC 3.1.3.1) and its isoenzymes. British Journal of Nutrition 43: 561–569.

Aggett PJ, Harries JT. (1979). Current status of zinc in health and disease states. Archives of Diseases of Childhood 54: 909–917.

Aitio A, Jarvisalo J, Kiilunen M, Tossavainen A, Vaittinen P. (1984). Urinary excretion of chromium as an indicator of exposure to trivalent chromium sulphate in leather tanning. International Archives of Occupational and Environmental Health 54: 241–249.

Allaway WH, Kubota J, Losée F, Roth M. (1968). Selenium, molybdenum, and vanadium in human blood. Archives of Environmental Health 16: 342–348.

Alexander NM. (1984). Iodine. In: Frieden E (ed). Biochemistry of the Essential Ultratrace Elements. Plenum Press, New York–London, pp. 33–53.

Alpers DH, Clouse RE, Stenson WF. (1983). Manual of Nutritional Therapeutics. Little Brown and Co., Boston.

Al-Rashid RA, Spangler J. (1971). Neonatal copper deficiency. New England Journal of Medicine 285: 841–843.

Alsbirk KE, Mogensen CE, Husted SE, Geday E. (1981). Liver and kidney function in stainless steel welders. Ugeskrift Laeger 143: 112–116.

Anderson RA. (1981). Nutritional role of chromium. Science of the Total Environment 17: 13–29.

Anderson RA, Bryden NA, Polansky MM. (1985). Serum chromium of human subjects: effects of chromium supplementation and glucose. American Journal of Clinical Nutrition 41: 571–577.

Anderson RA, Polansky MM, Bryden NA, Roginski EE, Patterson KY, Reamer C. (1982a). Effect of exercise (running) on serum glucose, insulin, glucagon and chromium excretion. Diabetes 31: 212–216.

Anderson RA, Polansky MM, Bryden NA, Roginski EE, Patterson KY, Veillon C, Glinsmann W. (1982b). Urinary chromium excretion of human subjects: effects of chromium supplementation and glucose loading. American Journal of Clinical Nutrition 36: 1184–1193.

Anderson RA, Polansky MM, Bryden NA, Roginski EE, Mertz W, Glinsmann W. (1983a). Chromium supplementation of human subjects: effect on glucose, insulin, and lipid variables. Metabolism 32: 894–899.

Anderson RA, Polansky MM, Bryden NA, Patterson KY, Veillon C, Glinsmann WH. (1983b). Effects of chromium supplementation on urinary Cr excretion of human subjects and correlation of Cr excretion with selected clinical parameters. Journal of Nutrition 113: 276–281.

Anderson RA, Polansky MM, Bryden NA. (1984). Acute effects on chromium, copper, zinc and selected clinical variables in urine and serum of male runners. Biological Trace Element Research 6: 327–336.

Andrewartha KA, Caple IW. (1980). Effects of changes in nutritional copper on erthyrocyte superoxide dismutase activity in sheep. Research in Veterinary Science 28: 101–104.

Anonymous (1980). Superoxide dismutase as an index of copper, zinc and manganese status. Nutrition Reviews 38: 326–327.

Anonymous (1984a). Conditioned copper deficiency due to antacids. Nutrition Reviews 42: 319–321.

Anonymous (1984b). Nucleoside phosphorylase: a zinc metalloenzyme and a marker of zinc deficiency. Nutrition Reviews 42: 279–281.

Anonymous (1987). Essentiality of copper in humans. Nutrition Reviews 45: 176–180.

Apgar J, Fitzgerald JA. (1987). Measures of zinc status in ewes given a low zinc diet throughout pregnancy. Nutrition Research 7: 1281–1290.

Arakawa T, Tamura T, Igarashi Y, Suzuki H, Sandstead HH. (1976). Zinc deficiency in two infants during total parenteral alimentation for diarrhea. American Journal of Clinical Nutrition 29:197–204.

Ashkenazi A, Levin S, Djaldetti M, Fishel E, Benvenisti D. (1973). The syndrome of neonatal copper deficiency. Pediatrics 52: 525–533.

Aumont G, Tressol JC. (1986). Improved routine method for the determination of total iodine in urine and milk. Analyst 111: 841–843.

Auzepy PH, Blondeau M, Richard CH, Pradeau D, Therond P, Thuong T. (1987). Serum selenium deficiency in myocardial infarction and congestive cardiomyopathy. Acta Cardiologica 42: 161–166.

Baer MT, King JC. (1984). Tissue zinc levels and zinc excretion during experimental zinc depletion in young men. American Journal of Clinical Nutrition 39: 556–570.

Baer MT, King JC, Tamura T, Margen S, Bradfield RB, Weston WL, Daugherty NA. (1985). Nitrogen utilization, enzyme activity, glucose intolerance and leukocyte chemotaxis in human experimental zinc depletion. American Journal of Clinical Nutrition 41: 1220–1235.

Bai-song N, Chun-sheng L, Li-hua C. (1986). Significance of low levels of blood and hair selenium in dilated cardiomyopathy. Chinese Medical Journal 99: 948–949.

Bales CW, Steinman LC, Freeland-Graves JH, Stone JM, Young RK. (1986). The effect of age on plasma zinc uptake and taste acuity. American Journal of Clinical Nutrition 44: 664–669.

Ballester OF, Prasad AS. (1983). Anergy, zinc deficiency, and decreased nucleoside phosphorylase activity in patients with sickle cell anemia. Annals of Internal Medicine 98: 180–182.

Bank HL, Robson J, Bigelow JB, Morrison J, Spell LH, Kantor R. (1981). Preparation of fingernails for trace element analysis. Clinica Chimica Acta 116: 179–190.

Barnes PM, Moynahan EJ. (1973). Zinc deficiency in acrodermatitis enteropathica: Multiple dietary intolerance treated with synthetic diet. Proceedings of the Royal Society of Medicine 66: 327–329.

Bartoshuk LM. (1978). The psycho-physics of taste. American Journal of Clinical Nutrition 31: 1068–1077.

Behne D, Hofer T, Wolters G, Wolters W, Bratter P, Gawlik D. (1981). Indicator parameters for the selenium status as studied in the rat. Dunckley JV (ed). Proceedings of New Zealand Workshop on Trace Elements in New Zealand. University of Otago, Dunedin, pp. 90–91.

Behne D, Wolters W. (1983). Distributions of selenium and glutathione peroxidase in the rat. Journal of Nutrition 113: 456–461.

Beilstein MA, Whanger PD. (1983). Distribution of selenium and glutathione peroxidase in blood fractions from humans, rhesus and squirrel monkeys, rats and sheep. Journal of Nutrition 113: 2138–2146.

Beisel WR, Pekarek RS, Wannemacher RW, Jr. (1976). Homeostatic mechanisms affecting plasma zinc levels in acute stress. In: Prasad AS (ed). Trace Elements in Human Health and Disease. Volume 1. Zinc and Copper. Academic Press, New York, pp. 87–106.

Benotti J, Benotti N. (1963). Protein-bound iodine, total iodine, and butanol-extractable iodine by partial automation. Clinical Chemistry 9: 408–416, 1963.

Bettger WJ, Fish TJ, O'Dell BL. (1978). Effects of copper and zinc status of rats on erythrocyte stability and superoxide dismutase activity. Proceedings of the Society of Experimental Biology and Medicine 158: 279–282.

Bettger WJ, Savage JE, O'Dell BL. (1979). Effects of dietary copper and zinc on erythrocyte superoxide dismutase activity in the chick. Nutrition Reports International 19: 893–900.

Bogden JD. (1980). Blood zinc in health and disease. In: Nriagu JO (ed). Zinc in the Environment, Part II: Health Effects. John Wiley and Sons, New York, pp. 137–169.

Bogden JD, Lintz DI, Joselow MM, Charles J, Salaki JS. (1977). Effect of pulmonary tuberculosis on blood concentrations of copper and zinc. American Journal of Clinical Pathology 67: 251–256.

Boling EA. (1966). A multiple slit burner for atomic absorption spectroscopy. Spectrochimica Acta 22: 425–431.

Borel JS, Anderson RA. (1984). Chromium. In: Frieden E (ed). Biochemistry of the Essential Ultratrace Elements. Plenum Press, New York, pp. 175–199.

Borel JS, Majerus TC, Polansky MM, Moser PB, Anderson RA. (1984). Chromium intake and urinary chromium excretion of trauma patients. Biological Trace Element Research 6: 317–326.

Boukis MA, Koutras A, Souvatzoglou A, Evangelopoulou A, Vrontakis M, Moulopoulos SD. (1983). Thyroid hormone and immunological studies in endemic goiter. Journal of Clinical Endocrinology and Metabolism 57: 859–862.

Bradfield RB, Cordano A, Baertl J, Graham GG. (1980). Hair copper in copper deficiency. Lancet 2: 343–344.

Bradfield RB, Hambidge KM. (1980). Problems with hair zinc as an indicator of body zinc status. Lancet [Letter] 1: 363.

Breskin MW, Worthington-Roberts BS, Knopp RH, Brown Z, Plovie B, Mottet NK, Mills JL. (1983). First trimester serum zinc concentrations in human pregnancy. American Journal of Clinical Nutrition 38: 943–953.

Brown RO, Forloines-Lynn S, Cross RE, Heizer WD. (1986). Chromium deficiency after long-term total parenteral nutrition. Digestive Diseases and Sciences 31: 661–664.

Brune D, Samsahl K, Wester P. (1966). A comparison between the amount of As, Au, Br, Cu, Fe, Mo, Se and Zn in normal and uremic human whole blood by means of neutron activation analysis. Clinica Chimica Acta 13: 285–291.

Buerk CA, Chandy MG, Pearson E, MacAuly A, Soroff HS. (1973). Zinc deficiency. Effect on healing and metabolism in man. Surgical Forum 24: 101–103.

Burk RF. (1984). Selenium. In: Present Knowledge in Nutrition. Fifth edition. The Nutrition Foundation Inc., Washington, D.C., pp. 519–527.

Burk RF Jr, Pearson WN, Wood RP, Viteri F. (1967). Blood-selenium levels and *in vitro* red blood cell uptake of 75-Se in kwashiorkor. American Journal of Clinical Nutrition 20: 723–733.

Butrimonvitz GP, Purdy WC. (1978). Zinc nutrition and growth in a childhood population. American Journal of Clinical Nutrition 31: 1409–1412.

Buttfield IH, Hetzel BS. (1969). Endemic goiter in New Guinea and the prophylactic program with iodinated poppyseed oil. In: Stanbury JB (ed). Endemic Goiter. PAHO/WHO, Scientific Publication No. 193. Washington, D.C., pp. 132–145.

Buzina R, Jusic M, Sapunar J, Milanovic N. (1980). Zinc nutrition and taste acuity in school children with impaired growth. American Journal of Clinical Nutrition 33: 2262–2267.

Capel ID, Spencer EP, Daivies AE, Levitt HN. (1982). The assessment of zinc status by the zinc tolerance test in various groups of patients. Clinical Biochemistry 15: 257–260.

Carter JP, Kattab A, Abd-el-Hadi K, Davis JT, Gholmy AE, Patwardhan VN. (1968). Chromium 3 in hypoglycemia and in impaired glucose utilization in kwashiorkor. American Journal of Clinical Nutrition 21: 195–202.

Cartwright GE. (1950). Copper metabolism in human subjects. In: McElroy WD, Glass B (eds). Symposium in Copper Metabolism. The Johns Hopkins Press, Baltimore, pp. 274–314.

Cartwright GE, Gubler CJ, Wintrobe MM. (1954). Studies on copper metabolism; copper and iron metabolism in the nephrotic syndrome. Journal of Clinical Investigation 33: 685–698.

Casey CE, Robinson MF. (1983). Some aspects of nutritional trace element research. In: Sigel H (ed). Metal Ions in Biological Systems Volume 16. Methods involving Metal Ions and Complexes in Clinical Chemistry. Marcel Dekker Inc., New York, pp. 1–26.

Chandra RK. (1984). Excessive intakes of zinc impairs immune responses. Journal of American Medical Association 252: 1443–1446.

Chen X, Yang G, Chen J, Chen X, Wen Z, Ge K. (1980). Studies on the relations of selenium and Keshan disease. Biological Trace Element Research 2: 91–107.

Choufoer JC, Rhijn M van, Querido A. (1965). Endemic goiter in Western New Guinea, II. Clinical picture, incidence and pathogenesis of endemic cretinism. Journal of Clinical Endocrinology and Metabolism 25: 385–402.

Chuttani HK, Gupta PS, Gulati S, Gupta DW. (1965). Acute copper sulfate poisoning. American Journal of Medicine. 39: 849–854.

Clark LC. (1985). The epidemiology of selenium and cancer. Federation Proceedings 44: 2584–2589.

Cohen HJ, Brown MR, Hamilton D, Lyons-Patterson J, Avissar N, Liegey P. (1989). Glutathione peroxidase and selenium deficiency in patients receiving home parenteral nutrition: time course for development of deficiency and repletion of enzyme activity in plasma and red blood cells. Americal Journal of Clinical Nutrition 49: 132–149.

Connolly RJ, Vidor GI, Stewart JC. (1970). Increase in thyrotoxicosis in endemic goitre area after iodation of bread. Lancet 1: 500-502.

Cordano A, Baertl JM, Graham GG. (1964). Copper deficiency in infancy. Pediatrics 34: 324–336.

Cote M, Munan L, Gagne-Billon M, Kelly A, Di Pietro O, Shapcott D. (1979). Hair chromium concentration and arteriosclerotic heart disease. In: Shapcott D, Hubert J (eds). Chromium in Nutrition and Metabolism. Elsevier/North Holland Biomedical Press, New York, pp. 223–228.

Cousins RJ. (1986). Towards a molecular understanding of zinc metabolism. Clinical Physiology and Biochemistry 4: 20–30.

Creason JP, Hinners TA, Bumgarner JE, Pinkerton C. (1975). Trace elements in hair, as related to exposure in metropolitan New York. Clinical Chemistry 21: 603–612.

Crofton RW, Glover SC, Ewan SWB, Aggett PJ, Mowat NAG, Mills CF. (1983). Zinc absorption in celiac disease and dermatitis herpetiformis: a test of small intestinal function. American Journal of Clinical Nutrition 38: 706–712.

Danford DE, Chandler DW. (1983) (Abst). Zinc estimation in clinical practice: Effect of anticoagulant choice on analyzed values. Federation Proceedings 42: 3102.

Danks DM. (1980). Copper deficiency in humans. In: Biological Roles of Copper. Ciba Foundation Symposium 79 (New Series). Excerpta Medica, New York, pp. 209–225.

Danks DM, Cambell PE, Stevens BJ, Mayne V, Cartwright E. (1972). Menke's kinky hair syndrome. An inherited defect in copper absorption with widespread effects. Pediatrics 50: 188–201.

Davidson IW, Burt RL. (1973). Physiologic changes in plasma chromium of normal and pregnant women: effect of a glucose load. American Journal of Obstetrics and Gynecology 116: 601–608.

Davidson IW, Burt RL, Parker JC. (1974). Renal excretion of trace elements: chromium and copper. Proceedings of the Society of Experimental Biology and Medicine 147: 720–725.

Davies TS. (1982). Hair analysis and selenium shampoos. Lancet 2: 935.

DeGroot L, Larsen PR, Rofetoff S, Stanbury JB. (1984). The Thyroid and Its Diseases. John Wiley and Sons, New York.

Delange F. (1985). Physiopathology of iodine nutrition. In: Chandra RK (ed). Trace Elements in Nutrition of Children. Nestlé Nutrition Workshop Series. Volume 8. Raven Press, New York, pp. 291–299.

Delange F, Iteke FB, Ermans AM. (1982). Nutritional factors involved in the goitrogenic action of cassava. International Development Research Centre, Ottawa, pp. 1-100.

Desor JA, Maller O. (1975). Taste correlates of disease states: cystic fibrosis. Journal of Pediatrics 87: 93–96.

Diplock AT. (1976). Metabolic aspects of selenium action and toxicity. CRC Critical Reviews in Toxicology 4: 271–329.

Doisy RJ, Streeten DHP, Souma ML, Kalafer ME, Rekant SI, Dalakos TG. (1971). Metabolism of chromium in human subjects — normal, elderly and diabetic subjects. In: Mertz W, Cornatzer WE (eds). Newer Trace Elements in Nutrition. Marcel Dekker Inc., New York pp. 155–168.

Donzelli GP, Vecchi C, Tucci PL, Poggini G, Galvan P. (1981) (Abst). Chromium, cholesterol, triglycerides and lipoproteins in diabetic men and women. Diabetologia 132: 265.

Dunn JT. (1978). Iodine deficiency in man. In: Rechcigl M (ed). Section E. Nutritional Disorders. Volume III. Effect of Nutrient Deficiencies in Man. CRC Handbook Series in Nutrition and Food. CRC Press Inc., Boca Raton, Florida, pp. 237–257.

Dunlap WM, James GW, Hume DM. (1974). Anemia and neutropenia caused by copper deficiency. Annals of Internal Medicine 80: 470–476.

Dunsmore DG, Wheeler SM. (1977). Iodophors and iodine in dairy products. 8. The total industry situation. Australian Journal of Dairy Technology 32: 166–171.

Ellis N, Lloyd B, Lloyd RS, Clayton BE. (1984). Selenium and vitamin E in relation to risk factors for coronary heart disease. Journal of Clinical Pathology 37: 200–206.

English JL, Anderson BR. (1974). Single step separation of red blood cells, granulocytes and mononuclear leucocytes on discontinuous gradients of Ficoll-Hypaque. Journal of Immunological Methods 5: 249–252.

English JL, Hambidge KM, Jacobs Goodall M, Nelson D. (1988). Evaluation of some factors that may affect plasma or serum zinc concentrations. In: Hurley LS, Keen CL, Lönnerdal B, Rucker RB (eds). Trace Elements in Man and Animals 6, Plenum Press, New York–London, pp. 459–460.

Epstein O, Boss AM, Lyon TDB, Sherlock S. (1980). Hair copper in primary biliary cirrhosis. American Journal of Clinical Nutrition 33: 965–967.

Erten J, Arcasoy A, Cavdar AO, Cin S. (1978). Hair zinc levels in healthy and malnourished children. American Journal of Clinical Nutrition 31: 1172–1174.

Everett G, Apgar J. (1980). An α-D-mannosidase in blood plasma as a possible indicator of zinc status. In: Brätter P, Schramel P (eds). Trace Element Analytical Chemistry in Medicine and Biology. Walter de Gruyter & Co., Berlin–New York, pp. 491–501.

Everett G, Apgar J. (1986). Comparison of four enzymes in zinc-deficient rats as possible indicators of marginal zinc status. Acta Pharmacologica et Toxicologica 59 (suppl VII): 163–165.

Faraji B, Swendseid ME. (1983). Growth rate, tissue zinc levels and activities of selected enzymes in rats fed a zinc-deficient diet by gastric tube. Journal of Nutrition 113: 447–455.

Fickel JJ, Freeland-Graves JH, Roby MJ. (1986). Zinc tolerance tests in zinc deficient and zinc supplemented diets. American Journal of Clinical Nutrition 43: 47–58.

Fields M, Ferretti RJ, Smith JC Jr, Reiser S. (1983). Effect of copper deficiency on metabolism and mortality in rats fed sucrose or starch diets. Journal of Nutrition 113: 1335–1345.

Fischer PWF, Giroux A, L'Abbé MR. (1984). Effect of zinc supplementation on copper status in adult man. American Journal of Clinical Nutrition 40: 743–746.

Fisher KD, Carr CJ. (1974). Iodide in Foods. Chemical Methodology and Sources of Iodine in the Human Diet. Life Sciences Research Office, Federation of American Societies for Experimental Biology, Washington, D.C.

Food and Nutrition Board (1980). Committee on Dietary Allowances, National Research Council, Ninth edition. National Academy of Sciences, Washington, D.C.

Freeland-Graves JH, Hendrickson PJ, Ebangit ML, Snowden JY. (1981). Salivary zinc as an index of zinc status in women fed a low-zinc diet. American Journal of Clinical Nutrition 34: 312–321.

Freeland-Graves JH, Steinman L, Bales C. (1988). Reply to Watson. American Journal of Clinical Nutrition 47: 336–344.

Freund H, Atamian S, Fischer JE. (1979). Chromium deficiency during total parenteral nutrition. Journal of the American Medical Association 241: 496–498.

Frey HMM, Rosenlund B, Torgersen JP. (1973). Value of single urine specimens in estimation of 24-hour urine iodine excretion. Acta Endocrinologica 72: 287–292.

Frieden E. (1985). New perspectives on the essential trace elements. Journal of Chemical Education 62: 917–923.

Gallagher ML, Webb P, Crounse R, Bray J, Webb A, Settle EA. (1984). Selenium levels in new growth hair and in whole blood during ingestion of a selenium supplement for six weeks. Nutrition Research 4: 577–582.

Ganther HE, Hafeman DG, Lawrence RA, Serfass RE, Hoekstra WG. (1976). Selenium and glutathione peroxidase in health and disease: a review. In: Prasad AS (ed). Trace Elements in Human Health and Disease. Volume 2. Essential and Toxic Elements. Academic Press, New York, pp. 165–234.

Geahchan A, Chambon P. (1980). Fluorometry of selenium in urine. Clinical Chemistry 26: 1272–1274.

Gervin CA, Gervin AS, Nichols W, Corrigan JJ Jr. (1983). Problems in the measurement of zinc using heparin as an anticoagulant. Life Sciences 33: 2643–2649

Gibbs K, Walshe JM. (1965). Copper content of hair in normal families and those with Wilson's disease. Journal of Medical Genetics 2: 181–184.

Gibson RS. (1980). Hair as a biopsy material for the assessment of trace element status in infancy. Journal of Human Nutrition 34: 405–416.

Gibson RS. (1982). The trace metal status of some Canadian full term and low birthweight infants at one year of age. Journal of Radioanalytical Chemistry 70: 175–189.

Gibson RS, DeWolfe MS. (1979). The zinc, copper, manganese, vanadium and iodine content of hair from 38 Canadian neonates. Pediatric Research 13: 959–962.

Gibson RS, DeWolfe MS. (1980). Changes in hair trace metal concentrations in some Canadian low birthweight infants. Nutrition Reports International 21: 341–349.

Gibson RS, Martinez OB, MacDonald AC. (1985). The zinc, copper, and selenium status of a selected sample of Canadian elderly women. Journal of Gerontology 40: 296–302.

Gibson RS, Smit-Vanderkooy PD, MacDonald AC, Goldman A, Ryan B, Berry M. (1989). A growth limiting mild zinc deficiency syndrome in some Southern Ontario boys with low growth percentiles. American Journal of Clinical Nutrition 49: 1266–1273.

Glinsmann WH, Mertz W. (1966). Effect of trivalent chromium on glucose tolerance. Metabolism 15: 510–521.

Glinsmann WH, Feldman FJ, Mertz W. (1966). Plasma chromium after glucose administration. Science 152: 1243–1245.

Glover JR. (1967). Selenium in human urine: a tentative maximum allowable concentration for industrial and rural populations. Annals of Occupational Hygiene 10: 3–14.

Gordon PR, Woodruff CW, Anderson HL, O'Dell BL. (1982). Effect of acute zinc depletion on plasma zinc and platelet aggregation in adult males. American Journal of Clinical Nutrition 35: 113–119.

Graham GG, Cordano A. (1969). Copper depletion and deficiency in the malnourished infant. Johns Hopkins Medical Journal 124: 139–150.

Gray BN, Walker C, Barnard R. (1982). Use of serum copper/zinc ratio in patients with large bowel cancer. Journal of Surgical Oncology 21: 230–232.

Greger JL, Geissler AH. (1978). Effect of zinc supplementation on taste acuity of the aged. American Journal of Clinical Nutrition 31: 633–637.

Greger JL, Sickles VS. (1979). Saliva zinc levels: potential indicators of zinc status. American Journal of Clinical Nutrition 32: 1859–1866.

Griffiths NM. (1973). Dietary intake and urinary excretion of selenium in some New Zealand women. Proceedings of the University of Otago Medical School. 51: 8–9.

Griffiths NM, Thomson CD. (1974). Selenium in whole blood of New Zealand residents. New Zealand Medical Journal 80: 199–202.

Griscom NT, Craig JN, Neuhauser EB. (1971). Systemic bone disease developing in small premature infants. Pediatrics 48: 883–895.

Gross S. (1976). Hemolytic anemia in premature infants: relationship to vitamin E, selenium, glutathione peroxidase and erythrocyte lipids. Seminars in Hematology 13: 187–199.

Guillard O, Piriou A, Gombert J, Reiss D. (1979). Diurnal variations of zinc, copper and magnesium in the serum of normal fasting adults. Biomedicine [Express] 31: 193–194.

Gürson CT, Saner G. (1971). Effect of chromium on glucose utilization in marasmic protein-calorie malnutrition. American Journal of Clinical Nutrition 24: 1313–1319.

Gürson CT, Saner G. (1978). The effect of glucose loading on urinary excretion of chromium in normal adults, in individuals from diabetic families and in diabetics. American Journal of Clinical Nutrition 31: 1158–1161.

Gylseth B, Gundersen N, Langøard S. (1977). Evaluation of chromium exposure based on a simplified method for urinary chromium determination. Scandinavian Journal of Work Environment and Health 3: 28–31.

Hadjimarkos DM, Shearer TR. (1973). Selenium content of human nails. New index for epidemiologic studies of dental caries. Journal of Dental Research 52: 389.

Halsted JA, Hackley BM, Smith JC Jr. (1968). Plasma-zinc and copper in pregnancy and after oral contraceptives. Lancet 2: 278–279.

Halsted JA, Smith JC, Jr. (1970). Plasma-zinc in health and disease. Lancet 1: 322–324.

Hambidge KM. (1971). Chromium nutrition in the mother and the growing child. In: Mertz W, Cornatzer WE (eds). Newer Trace Elements in Nutrition. Marcel Dekker, New York, pp. 169–194.

Hambidge KM. (1982). Hair analyses: worthless for vitamins, limited for minerals. American Journal of Clinical Nutrition 36: 943–949.

Hambidge KM, Baum JD. (1972). Hair chromium concentrations of human newborn and changes during infancy. American Journal of Clinical Nutrition 25: 376–379.

Hambidge KM, Droegemueller W. (1974). Changes in plasma and hair concentrations of zinc, copper, chromium and manganese during pregnancy. Journal of Obstetrics and Gynecology 44: 666–672.

Hambidge KM, Chavez MN, Brown RM, Walravens PA. (1979). Zinc nutritional status of young middle-income children and effects of consuming zinc-fortified breakfast cereals. American Journal of Clinical Nutrition 32: 2532–2539.

Hambidge KM, Franklin ML, Jacobs MA. (1972b). Hair chromium concentration: effect of sample washing and external environment. American Journal of Clinical Nutrition 25: 384–389.

Hambidge KM, Hambidge C, Jacobs M, Baum JD. (1972a). Low levels of zinc in hair, anorexia, poor growth, and hypogeusia in children. Pediatric Research 6: 868–874.

Hambidge KM, Krebs NF, Sibley L, English J. (1987). Acute effects of iron therapy on zinc status during pregnancy. Obstetrics and Gynecology 70: 593–596.

Health and Welfare Canada (1973). Nutrition Canada National Survey. Health and Welfare, Ottawa.

Health and Welfare Canada (1981). The Health of Canadians. Report of the Canada Health Survey. Ministry of Supply and Services, Ottawa.

Helzlsouer K, Jacobs R, Morris S. (1985)(abst). Acute selenium intoxication in the United States. Federation Proceedings 44: 7366.

Hemkin RW. (1979). Factors that influence the iodine content of milk and meat: a review. Journal of Animal Science 48: 981–985.

Henkin RI. (1984). Review. Zinc in taste function. A critical review. Biological Trace Element Research 6: 263–280.

Henkin RI, Gill JR, Bartler FC. (1963). Studies on taste thresholds in normal and in patients with adrenal cortical insufficiency: the role of adrenal cortical steriods and of serum sodium concentration. Journal of Clinical Investigation 42: 727–735.

Henkin RI, Schechter PJ, Hoye R, Mattern CFT. (1971). Idiopathic hypogeusia with dysgeusia, hyposmia, and dysosmia. A new syndrome. Journal of the American Medical Association 217: 434–440.

Hess FM, King JC, Margen S. (1977). Zinc excretion in young women on low zinc intakes and oral contraceptive agents. Journal of Nutrition 107: 1610–1620.

Hojo Y. (1981). Evaluation of the expression of urinary selenium level as ng Se/mg creatinine and the use of single-void urine as a sample for urinary selenium determinations. Bulletin of Environmental Contamination and Toxicology 27: 213–220.

Hooper PL, Visconti L, Garry PJ, Johnson GE. (1980). Zinc lowers high-density lipoprotein-cholesterol levels. Journal of the American Medical Association 244: 1960–1961.

Hopkins LL, Ransome-Kuti O, Majaj AS. (1968). Improvement of impaired carbohydrate metabolism by chromium (III) in malnourished infants. American Journal of Clinical Nutrition 21: 203–211.

Horwitt MK, Harvey CC, Dahm CH Jr. (1975). Relationship between levels of blood lipids, vitamins C, A, and E, serum copper compounds, and urinary excretions of tryptophan metabolites in women taking oral contraceptive therapy. American Journal of Clinical Nutrition 28: 403–412.

Ibbertson HK, Pearl M, McKinnon J, Tait JM, Lim T, Gill MB. (1971). Endemic cretinism in Nepal. In: Hetzel BS, Pharoah POD (eds). Institute of Human Biology, Papua New Guinea, pp. 71–88.

ICNND (Interdepartmental Committee on Nutrition for National Defense) (1963). Manual for Nutrition Surveys. Second edition. Superintendent of Documents. U.S. Government Printing Office, Washington, D.C.

Ishizaka A, Tsuchida F, Ishii T. (1981). Clinical zinc deficiency during zinc supplemented parenteral nutrition. Journal of Pediatrics 99: 339–340.

Jackson MJ, Jones DA, Edwards RH. (1982). Tissue zinc levels as an index of body zinc status. Clinical Physiology 2: 333–343.

Jacob RA, Klevay LM, Logan GM Jr. (1978). Hair as a biopsy material. V. Hair metal as an index of hepatic metal in rats: copper and zinc. American Journal of Clinical Nutrition 31: 477–480.

Jacobs Goodall M, Hambidge KM, Stall C, Pritts J, Nelson D. (1988). Daily variations in plasma zinc in normal adult women. In: Hurley LS, Keen CL, Lönnerdal B, Rucker RB (eds). Trace Elements in Man and Animals 6, Plenum Press, New York–London, pp. 491–492.

Jaffé WG, Ruphael MD, Mondragon MC, Cuevas MA. (1972). Clinical and biochemical studies on school children from a seleniferous zone. Archivos Latinoamericanos de Nutrición 22: 595–611.

Jeejeebhoy KN, Chu RC, Marliss EB, Greenberg GR, Bruce-Robertson A. (1977). Chromium deficiency, glucose intolerance, and neuropathy reversed by chromium supplementation in a patient receiving long-term parenteral nutrition. American Journal of Clinical Nutrition 30: 531–538.

Johnson RA, Baker SS, Fallon JT, Maynard EP, Ruskin JN, Wen Z, Ge K, Cohen HJ. (1981). An occidental case of cardiomyopathy and selenium deficiency. New England Journal of Medicine 304: 1210–1212.

Jones RB, Keeling PW, Hilton PJ, Thompson RP. (1981). The relationship between leukocyte and muscle zinc in health and disease. Clinical Science 60: 237–239.

Juswigg T, Bates R, Solomons NW, Pineda O, Milne DB. (1982). The effect of temporary venous occlusion on trace mineral concentrations in plasma. American Journal of Clinical Nutrition 36: 354–358.

Kadish AH, Litle RL, Sternberg JC. (1969). A new and rapid method for the determination of glucose by measurement of rate of oxygen consumption. Clinical Chemistry 14: 116–119.

Karpel JT, Peden VH. (1972). Copper deficiency in long-term parenteral nutrition. Journal of Pediatrics 80: 32–36.

Kasarskis EJ, Schuna A. (1980). Serum alkaline phosphatase after treatment of zinc deficiency in humans. American Journal of Clinical Nutrition 33: 2609–2612.

Kasperek K, Feinendegen LE, Lombeck I, Bremer HJ. (1977). Serum zinc concentrations during childhood. European Journal of Pediatrics 126: 199–202.

Kasperek K, Lombeck I, Kiem J, Iyengar GV, Wang YX, Feinendegen LE, Bremer HJ. (1982). Platelet selenium in children with normal and low selenium intake. Biological Trace Element Research 4: 29–34.

Kay RG, Knight GS. (1979). Blood selenium values in an adult Auckland population group. New Zealand Medical Journal 90: 11–13.

Kay RG, Tasman-Jones C. (1975). Acute zinc deficiency in man during intravenous alimentation. Australian and New Zealand Journal of Surgery 45: 325–330.

Kelson JR, Shamberger RJ. (1978). Methods compared for determining zinc in serum by flame atomic absorption spectroscopy. Spectroscopy 1. Clinical Chemistry 24: 240–244.

Kiilunen M, Kivistö H, Ala-Laurila P, Tossavainen A, Aitio A. (1983). Exceptional pharmacokinetics of trivalent chromium during occupational exposure to chromium lignosulfonate dust. Scandinavian Journal of Work Environment and Health 9: 265–271.

Kirchgessner M, Roth HP, Weigand E. (1976). Biochemical changes in zinc deficiency. In: Prasad AS (ed). Trace Elements in Human Health and Disease, Volume 1. Zinc and Copper. Academic Press, New York, pp. 189–225.

Kiremidjian-Schumacher L, Stotzky G. (1987). Review. Selenium and immune responses. Environmental Research 42: 277–303.

Kirsten GF, de V Heese H, De Villiers S, Dempster WS, Pocock F, Varkevisser H. (1985). Serum zinc and copper levels in the 1st year of life. South African Medical Journal 67: 414–418.

Klasing SA, Pilch SM. (1985). Suggested Measures of Nutritional Status and Health Conditions for the Third National Health and Nutrition Examination Survey. Life Sciences Research Office, Federation of American Societies for Experimental Biology, Bethesda, Maryland.

Klevay LM. (1975). Coronary heart disease: the zinc/copper hypothesis. American Journal of Clinical Nutrition 28: 764–774.

Klevay LM. (1981). Hair as a biopsy material. VI. Hair copper as an index of copper in heart and kidney of rats. Nutrition Reports International 23: 371–376.

Klevay LM, Inman L, Johnson LK, Lawler M, Mahalko JR, Milne DB, Lukaski HC, Bolonchuk W, Sandstead HH. (1984). Increased cholesterol in plasma in a young man during experimental copper depletion. Metabolism 33: 1112–1118.

Klevay LM, Bistrian BR, Fleming CR, Neumann CG. (1987). Hair analysis in clinical and experimental medicine. American Journal of Clinical Nutrition 46: 233–236.

Kochupillai N, Pandav CS, Godbole MM, Mehta M, Ahuja MMS. (1986). Iodine deficiency and neonatal hypothyroidism. Bulletin of the World Health Organization 64: 547–551.

Kosman DJ, Henkin RI. (1979). Plasma and serum zinc concentrations. [Letter]. Lancet 1: 1410.

Kozlovsky AS, Moser PB, Reiser S, Anderson RA. (1986). Effects of diets high in simple sugars on urinary chromium losses. Metabolism 35: 515–518.

Kumpulainen J, Salmela S, Vuori E, Leuto J. (1982). Effects of various washing procedures on the chromium content of human scalp hair. Analytica Chimica Acta 138: 361–364.

L'Abbé MR, Fischer PW. (1986). An automated method for the determination of Cu, Zn-superoxide dismutase in plasma and erythrocytes using an ABA-200 discrete analyzer. Clinical Biochemistry 19: 175–178.

Lagasse R, Bourdoux P, Courtois P, Hennart P, Putzeys G, Thilly C, Mafuta M, Yunga Y, Ermans AM, Delange F. (1982). Influence of the dietary balance of iodine-thiocyanate and protein on thyroid function in adults and young infants. In: Delange F, Iteke FB, Ermans AM (eds). Nutritional Factors involved in the Goitrogenic Action of Cassava. International Development Research Centre, Ottawa, pp. 84–86.

Lane HW, Barroso AO, Englert D, Dudrick SJ, MacFadyen BG Jr. (1982a). Selenium status of seven chronic intravenous hyperalimentation patients. Journal of Parenteral and Enteral Nutrition 6: 426–431.

Lane HW, Dudrick S, Warren DC. (1981). Blood selenium levels and glutathione peroxidase activities in university and chronic intravenous hyperalimentation subjects. Proceedings of the Society of Experimental Biology and Medicine 167: 383–390.

Lane HW, Warren DC, Squyres NS, Cotham AC. (1982b). Zinc concentrations in hair, plasma, and saliva and changes in taste acuity of adults supplemented with zinc. Biological Trace Element Research 4: 83–93.

Lane HW, Warren DC, Taylor BJ, Stool E. (1983). Blood selenium and glutathione peroxidase levels and dietary selenium of free-living and institutionalized elderly subjects. Proceedings of the Society for Experimental Biology and Medicine 173: 87–95.

Langard S. (1980). Chromium. In: Waldron HH (ed). Metals in the Environment. Academic Press, London, pp. 111–132.

Larson Wright A, King JC, Baer MT, Citron LJ. (1981). Experimental zinc depletion and altered taste perception for NaCl in young adult males. American Journal of Clinical Nutrition 34: 848–852.

Levander OA. (1985). Considerations on the assessment of selenium status. Federation Proceedings 44: 2579–2583.

Levander OA, Alfthan G, Arvilommi H, Gref CG, Huttunen JK, Kataja M, Koivistoinen P, Pikkarainen J. (1983b). Bioavailability of selenium to Finnish men as assessed by platelet glutathione peroxidase activity and other blood parameters. American Journal of Clinical Nutrition 37: 887–897.

Levander OA, Cheng L. (1980). Micronutrient interactions: vitamins, minerals and hazardous elements. New York Academy of Sciences 355: 1–372.

Levander OA, De Loach DP, Morris VC, Moser PB. (1983a). Platelet glutathione peroxidase activity as an index of selenium status in rats. Journal of Nutrition 113: 55–63.

Levander OA, Morris VC. (1984). Dietary selenium levels needed to maintain balance in North America adults consuming self-selected diets. American Journal of Clinical Nutrition 39: 809–815.

Levander OA, Sutherland B, Morris VC, King JC. (1981). Selenium balance in young men during selenium depletion and repletion. American Journal of Clinical Nutrition 34: 2662–2669.

Levine RJ, Olson RE. (1970). Blood selenium in Thai children with protein-calorie malnutrition. Proceedings of the Society for Experimental Biology and Medicine 134: 1030–1034.

Levine RA, Streeten DHP, Doisy RJ. (1968). Effects of oral chromium supplementation on the glucose tolerance of elderly human subjects. Metabolism 17: 114–125.

Lewalter J, Korallus U, Harzdorf CS, Weidemann H. (1985). Chromium bond detection in isolated erythrocytes: a new principle of biological monitoring of exposure to hexavalent chromium. International Archives of Occupational Environmental Health 55: 305–318.

Lifschitz MD, Henkin RI. (1971). Circadian variation in copper and zinc in man. Journal of Applied Physiology. 31: 88–92.

Liu VJ, Abernathy RP. (1982). Chromium and insulin in young subjects with normal glucose tolerance. American Journal of Clinical Nutrition 35: 661–667.

Liu VJK, Abernathy RP, Clikeman FM, Morris SJ. (1979) (Abst). Urinary chromium during a glucose tolerance test in college students. Federation Proceedings 38: 2047.

Liu VJK, Morris JS. (1978). Relative chromium response as an indicator of chromium status. American Journal of Clinical Nutrition 31: 972–976.

Lombeck I, Kasperek K, Harbisch HD, Becker K, Schumann E, Schröter W, Feinendegen LE, Bremer HJ. (1978). The selenium state of children. II. European Journal of Pediatrics 128: 213–223.

Lombeck I, Kasperek K, Feinendegen LE, Bremer HJ. (1975). Serum-selenium concentrations in patients with maple-syrup-urine disease and phenylketonuria under dieto-therapy. Clinica Chimica Acta 64: 57–69.

Lombeck I, Menzel H, Frosch D. (1986). Acute selenium poisoning of a 2-year-old child. European Journal of Pediatrics 146: 308–312.

Love AHG. (1983). Chromium — biological and analytical considerations. In: Burrows D (ed). Chromium — Metabolism and Toxicity. CRC Press Inc., Boca Raton, Florida, pp. 1–12.

Lukaski HC, Bolonchuk WW, Klevay LM, Milne DB, Sandstead HH. (1983). Maximal oxygen consumption as related to magnesium, copper, and zinc nutriture. American Journal of Clinical Nutrition 37: 407–415.

Mahalko JR, Bennion M. (1976). The effect of parity and time between pregnancies on maternal hair chromium concentration. American Journal of Clinical Nutrition 29: 1069–1072.

Makino T. (1983). A potential problem on comparison of plasma with serum for zinc content. [Letter]. Clinical Chemistry 29: 1313–1314.

Manthey J, Kübler W. (1980). High serum chromium levels after cardiac valve replacement: clinical significance and metabolic effects. American Journal of Cardiology 45: 940–944.

Marklund S, Marklund G. (1974). Involvement of the superoxide anion radical in the autoxidation of pyrogallol and a convenient assay for superoxide dismutase. European Journal of Biochemistry 47: 469–474.

Markowitz ME, Rosen JF, Mizruchi M. (1985). Circadian variations in serum zinc (Zn) concentrations: correlation with blood ionized calcium, serum total calcium and phosphate in humans. American Journal of Clinical Nutrition 41: 689–696.

Martin GM. (1964). Copper content of hair and nails of normal individuals and of patients with hepatolenticular degeneration. Nature (London) 202: 903–904.

Martinez OB, MacDonald AC, Gibson RS, Bourn DM. (1985). Dietary chromium and effect of chromium supplementation on glucose tolerance of elderly Canadian women. Nutrition Research 5: 609–620.

Mason KE. (1979). A conspectus of research on copper metabolism and requirements of man. Journal of Nutrition 109: 1979–2066.

Matovinovic J. (1984). Iodine. In: Present Knowledge of Nutrition. Fifth edition. The Nutrition Foundation Inc., Washington, D.C., pp. 587–606.

Matovinovic J, Ramalingaswami V. (1960). Therapy and prophylaxis of endemic goitre. In: Endemic Goitre. WHO Monograph Series No. 44. World Health Organization, Geneva.

McAdam PA, Smith DK, Feldman EB, Hames C. (1984). Effect of age, sex, and race on selenium status of healthy residents of Augusta, Georgia. Biological Trace Element Research 6: 3–9.

McBean LD, Mahloudji M, Reinhold JG, Halsted JA. (1971). Correlation of zinc concentrations in human plasma and hair. American Journal of Clinical Nutrition 24: 506–509.

McCarthy TP, Brodie B, Milner JA, Bevill RF. (1981). Improved method for selenium determination in biological samples by gas chromatography. Journal of Chromatography 225: 9–16.

McConnell KP, Broghamer WL Jr., Blotcky AJ, Hurt OJ. (1975). Selenium levels in human blood and tissues in health and in disease. Journal of Nutrition 105: 1026–1031.

McKenzie HM, Rea HM, Thomson CD, Robinson MF. (1978). Selenium concentration and glutathione peroxidase activity in blood of New Zealand infants and children. American Journal of Clinical Nutrition 31: 1413–1418.

Meadows NJ, Ruse W, Smith MF, Day J, Keeling PW, Scopes JW, Thompson RP, Bloxam DL. (1981). Zinc and small babies. Lancet 2: 1135–1137.

Meret S, Henkin RI. (1971). Simultaneous direct estimation by atomic absorption spectrophotometry of copper and zinc in serum, urine and cerebrospinal fluid. Clinical Chemistry 17: 369–373.

Mertz W. (1969). Chromium occurrence and function in biological systems. Physiological Reviews 49: 163–239.

Mertz W. (1981a). The essential trace elements. Science 213: 1332–1338.

Mertz W. (1981b). The scientific and practical importance of trace elements. Philosophical Transactions of the Royal Society of London Series B — Biological Sciences 294: 9–18.

Miettinen TA, Alfthan G, Huttunen JK, Pikkarainen J, Naukkarinen V, Mattila S, Kumlin T. (1983). Serum selenium concentration related to myocardial infarction and fatty acid content of serum lipids. British Medical Journal 287: 517–519.

Milne DB, Canfiled WK, Gallagher SK, Hunt JR, Klevay LM. (1987). Ethanol metabolism in post-menopausal women fed a diet marginal in zinc. American Journal of Clinical Nutrition 46: 688–693.

Milne DB, Ralston NVC, Wallwork JC. (1985). Zinc content of cellular components of blood: methods for cell separation and analysis evaluated. Clinical Chemistry 31: 65–69.

Misra HP, Fridovich I. (1977). Superoxide dismutase: a photochemical augmentation assay. Archives of Biochemistry and Biophysics 181: 308–312.

Mitchell Perry H Jr. (1978). Effect of nutrient deficiencies in man: Selenium. In: Rechcigl M Jr (ed). Section E: Nutritional Disorders, Volume III. Effect of Nutrient Deficiencies in Man. CRC Handbook Series in Nutrition and Food. CRC Press Inc., West Palm Beach, Florida, pp. 271–274.

Morris JS, Stampfer MJ, Willett W. (1983). Dietary selenium in humans. Toenails as an indicator. Biological Trace Element Research 5: 529–537.

Mutanen M. (1984). Dietary intake and sources of selenium in young Finnish women. Human Nutrition: Applied Nutrition 38C: 265–269.

Nahapetian AT, Janghorbani M, Young VR. (1983). Urinary trimethylselenonium excretion by the rat: effect of level and source of selenium-75. Journal of Nutrition 113: 401–411.

Nanji AA, Anderson FH. (1983). Relationship between serum zinc and alkaline phosphatase. Human Nutrition: Clinical Nutrition 37C: 461–462.

Nath R, Minocha J, Lyall V, Sunder S, Kuman V, Kapoor S, Dhar KL. (1979). Assessment of chromium metabolism in maturity onset and juvenile diabetes using chromium-51 and therapeutic response of chromium administration on plasma lipids, glucose tolerance and insulin levels. In: Shapcott D, Hubert J (eds).

Chromium in Nutrition and Metabolism. Elsevier/North Holland Biomedical Press, Amsterdam–New York–Oxford, pp. 213–221.

National Diabetes Data Group. (1979). Classification and diagnosis of diabetes mellitus and other categories of glucose intolerance. Diabetes 28: 1039–1057.

Nishi Y. (1980). Zinc levels in plasma, erythrocyte and leucocyte in healthy children and adults. Hiroshima Journal of Medical Sciences 29: 7–13.

Nomiyama H, Yotoriyama M, Nomiyama K. (1980). Normal chromium levels in urine and blood of Japanese subjects determined by direct flameless atomic absorption spectrophotometry, and valency of chromium in urine after exposure to hexavalent chromium. American Industrial Hygiene Association Journal 41: 98–102.

O'Dell BL. (1976). Biochemistry of Copper. Medical Clinics of North America 60: 687–703.

Offenbacher EG, Dowling HJ, Rinko CJ, Pi-Sunyer FX. (1986). Rapid enzymatic pretreatment of samples before determining chromium in serum or plasma. Clinical Chemistry 32: 1383–1386.

Offenbacher EG, Pi-Sunyer FX. (1980). Beneficial effect of chromium-rich yeast on glucose tolerance and blood lipids in elderly subjects. Diabetes 29: 919–925.

Offenbacher EG, Rinko CJ, Pi-Sunyer FX. (1985). The effects of inorganic chromium and brewer's yeast on glucose tolerance, plasma lipids, and plasma chromium in elderly subjects. American Journal of Clinical Nutrition 42: 454–461.

Okahata S, Nishi S, Hatano S, Kobayashi Y, Usui T. (1980). Changes in erythrocyte superoxide dismutase in a patient with copper deficiency. European Journal of Pediatrics 134: 121–124.

Olson OE. (1986). Selenium toxicity with emphasis on man. Journal of the American College of Toxicology 5: 45–70.

Osheim DL. (1983). Atomic absorption determination of serum copper: Collaborative study. Journal of the Association of Official Analytical Chemists 66: 1140–1142.

Oster O, Prellwitz W, Kasper W, Meinertz T. (1983). Congestive cardiomyopathy and the selenium content of serum. Clinica Chimica Acta 128: 125–132.

Paglia DE, Valentine WN. (1967). Studies on the quantitative and qualitative characterization of erythrocyte glutathione peroxidase. Journal of Laboratory and Clinical Medicine. 70: 158–169.

Paine CH. (1968). Food-poisoning due to copper. Lancet 2: 520.

Paynter DI, Moir RJ, Underwood EJ. (1979). Changes in activity of the Cu-Zn superoxide dismutase enzyme in tissues of the rat with changes in dietary copper. Journal of Nutrition 109: 1570–1576.

Pekarek RS, Hauer EC, Rafield EJ, Wannemacher RW Jr, Biesel WR. (1975). Relationship between serum chromium concentration and glucose utilization in normal and infected subjects. Diabetes 24: 350–353.

Pekarek RS, Powanda MC, Wannemacher RW Jr. (1972). The effect of leukocytic endogenous mediator (LEM) on serum copper and ceruloplasmin concentrations in the rat. Proceedings of the Society of Experimental Biology and Medicine 141: 1029-1031.

Peleg I, Morris S, Hames CG. (1985). Is serum selenium a risk factor for cancer? Medical Oncology and Tumor Pharmacotherapy 2: 157–163.

Petering HG, Yeager DW, Witherup SO. (1971). Trace metal content of hair. I. Zinc and copper content of human hair in relation to age and sex. Archives of Environmental Health 23: 202–207.

Pharoah POD, Lawton NF, Ellis SM, Williams ES, Ekins RP. (1973). The role of triiodothyronine (T$_3$) in the maintenance of euthyroidism in endemic goitre. Clinical Endocrinology 2: 193–199.

Pilch SM, Senti FR (eds). (1984). Assessment of the zinc nutritional status of the U.S. population based on data collected in the second National Health and Nutrition

Examination Survey, 1976–1980. Life Sciences Research Office, Federation of American Societies for Experimental Biology, Bethesda, Maryland.

Pleban PA, Munyani A, Beachum J. (1982). Determination of selenium concentration and glutathione peroxidase activity in plasma and erythrocytes. Clinical Chemistry 28: 311–316.

Prasad AS. (1983). Clinical, biochemical and nutritional spectrum of zinc deficiency in human subjects: an update. Nutrition Reviews 41: 197–208.

Prasad AS. (1985a). Clinical manifestations of zinc deficiency. Annual Review of Nutrition 5: 341–363.

Prasad AS. (1985b). Diagnostic approaches to trace element deficiencies. In: Chandra RK (ed). Trace Elements in Nutrition of Children. Nestlé Nutrition Workshop Series. Volume 8. Raven Press, New York, pp. 17–34.

Prasad AS, Brewer GJ, Schoomaker EB, Rabbani P. (1978a). Hypocupremia induced by zinc therapy in adults. Journal of the American Medical Association 240: 2166–2168.

Prasad AS, Cossack ZT. (1982). Neutrophil zinc: an indicator of zinc status in man. Transactions of the Association of American Physicians 95: 165–176.

Prasad AS, Miale A, Farid Z, Schulert A, Sandstead HH. (1963). Zinc metabolism in patients with the syndrome of iron deficiency anemia, hypogonadism and dwarfism. Journal of Laboratory and Clinical Medicine 61: 537–549.

Prasad AS, Rabbani P. (1981). Nucleoside phosphorylase in zinc deficiency. Transactions of the Association of American Physicians 94: 314–321.

Prasad AS, Rabbani P, Abbasi A, Bowersox E, Fox MRS. (1978b). Experimental zinc deficiency in humans. Annals of Internal Medicine 89: 483–490.

Querido A, DeLange F, Dunn JT, Fierro-Beñitez R, Ibbertson HK, Koutras DA, Perinetti H. (1974). Definitions of endemic goiter and cretinism, classification of goiter size and severity of endemias, and survey techniques. In: Dunn JT, Medeiros-Neto GA (eds). Report of the Fourth Meeting of the PAHO/WHO Technical Group on Endemic Goiter. PAHO/WHO. Scientific Publication No. 292. Washington, D.C., pp. 267–272.

Raabo E, Terkildsen TC. (1960). On the enzymatic determination of blood gluocse. Scandinavian Journal of Clinical and Laboratory Investigation 12: 402–405.

Rabinowitz MB, Levin SR, Gonick HC. (1980). Comparisons of chromium status in diabetic and normal men. Metabolism 29: 355–364.

Rabinowitz MB, Gonick HC, Levin SR, Davidson MB. (1983). Effects of chromium and yeast supplements on carbohydrate and lipid metabolism in diabetic men. Diabetes Care 6: 319–327.

Rahkonen E, Junttila ML, Kalliomaki PL, Olkinouora M, Koponen M, Kalliomaki K. (1983). Evaluation of biological monitoring among stainless steel welders. International Archives of Occupational Environmental Health 52: 243–255.

Randall JA, Gibson RS. (1987). Serum and urine chromium as indices of chromium status in tannery workers. Proceedings of the Society for Experimental Biology and Medicine 185: 16–23.

Randall JA, Gibson RS. (1989). Hair chromium as an index of chromium exposure of tannery workers. British Journal of Industrial Medicine 46: 172–176.

Rea HM, Thomson CD, Campbell DR, Robinson MF. (1979). Relation between erythrocyte selenium concentrations and glutathione peroxidase activities of New Zealand residents and visitors to New Zealand. British Journal of Nutrition 42: 201–208.

Reeves PG, O'Dell BL. (1985). An experimental study of the effect of zinc on the activity of angiotensin converting enzyme in serum. Clinical Chemistry 31: 581–584.

Reiser S, Ferretti RJ, Fields M, Smith JC., Jr. (1983). Role of dietary fructose in the enhancement of mortality and biochemical changes associated with copper deficiency in rats. American Journal of Clinical Nutrition 38: 214–222.

Reiser S, Smith JC Jr., Mertz W, Holbrook JT, Scholfield DJ, Powell AS, Canfield WK, Canary JJ. (1985). Indices of copper status in humans consuming a typical American diet containing either fructose or starch. American Journal of Clinical Nutrition 42: 242–251.

Riales R, Albrink MJ. (1981). Effect of chromium chloride supplementation on glucose tolerance and serum lipids including high-density lipoproteins of adult man. American Journal of Clinical Nutrition 34: 2670–2678.

Rice EW, Goldstein NP. (1961). Copper content of hair and nails in Wilson's disease (hepatolenticular degeneration). Metabolism 10: 1085–1087.

Rij AM van, Thomson CD, McKenzie JM, Robinson MF. (1979). Selenium deficiency in total parenteral nutrition. American Journal of Clinical Nutrition 32: 2076–2085.

Robberecht HJ, Deelstra HA. (1984). Selenium in human urine: concentration levels and medical implications. Clinica Chimica Acta 136: 107–120.

Robinson MF, Thomson CD. (1983). The role of selenium in the diet. Nutrition Abstracts and Reviews Series A. 53: 3–26.

Robinson MF, Rea HM, Friend GM, Stewart RDH, Snow PC, Thomson CD. (1978). On supplementing the selenium intake of New Zealanders. 2. Prolonged metabolic experiments with daily supplements of selenomethionine, selenite and fish. British Journal of Nutrition 39: 589–600.

Roginski EE, Mertz W. (1969). Effects of chromium (III) supplementation on glucose and amino acid metabolism in rats fed a low protein diet. Journal of Nutrition 97: 525–530.

Rosson JW, Foster KJ, Walton RJ, Monro PP, Taylor TG, Alberti KGMM. (1979). Hair chromium concentrations in adult insulin-treated diabetics. Clinica Chimica Acta 93: 299–304.

Ruz M, Cavan KR, Bettger WJ, Gibson RS. (1989). Indices of zinc status during experimental zinc deficiency in humans. Federation of the American Societies for Experimental Biology. New Orleans, p. A651 (Abstract).

Sakurai H, Tsuchiya K. (1975). A tentative recommendation for the maximum daily intake of selenium. Environmental Physiology and Biochemistry 5: 107–118.

Salmon MA, Wright T. (1971). Chronic copper poisoning presenting as pink disease. Archives of Disease in Childhood 46: 108–110.

Salonen JT. (1986). Selenium and human cancer. Annals of Clinical Research 18: 30–35.

Salonen JH, Huttunen JK. (1986). Selenium in cardiovascular disease. Annals of Clinical Research 18: 30–35.

Salonen JH, Alfthan G, Huttunen JK, Pikkarainen J, Puska P. (1982). Association between cardiovascular death and myocardial infarction and serum selenium in matched-pair longitudinal study. Lancet 2: 175–179.

Sandstead HH, Henriksen LK, Greger JL, Prasad AS, Good RA. (1982). Zinc nutriture in the elderly in relation to taste acuity, immune response, and wound healing. American Journal of Clinical Nutrition 36: 1046–1059.

Saner G. (1981). The effect of parity on maternal hair chromium concentrations and the changes during pregnancy. American Journal of Clinical Nutrition 34: 853–855.

Sargent T, Lim TH, Gensen RL. (1979). Reduced chromium retention in patients with hemochromatosis, a possible basis of hemochromatotic diabetes. Metabolism 28: 70–79.

Schilirò G, Russo A, Azzia N, Mancuso GR, Di Gregorio FD, Romeo MA, Fallico R, Sciacca S. (1987). Leucocyte alkaline phosphatase (LAP): A useful marker of zinc status in β-Thalassemic patients. American Journal of Pediatric Hematology/Oncology 9:149–152.

Schrauzer GN, White DA, Schneider CJ. (1977). Cancer mortality correlation studies. III. Statistical associations with dietary selenium intakes. Bioinorganic Chemistry 7: 23–31.

Schroeder HA, Balassa JJ, Tipton IH. (1962). Abnormal trace metals in man — chromium. Journal of Chronic Diseases 15: 941–964.

Schroeder HA, Frost DV, Balassa JJ. (1970). Essential trace metals in man: selenium. Journal of Chronic Diseases 23: 227–243.

Schwarz K. (1961). Development and status of experimental work on factor 3-selenium. Federation Proceedings 20: 666–673.

Sempos CT, Greger JL, Johnson NE, Smith EL, Seyedabadi FM. (1983). Levels of serum copper and magnesium in normotensives and untreated hypertensives. Nutrition Reports International 27: 1013–1020.

Shamberger RJ, Frost DV. (1969). Possible protective effect of selenium against human cancer. Canadian Medical Association Journal 100: 682.

Shamberger RJ, Willis CE, McCormak LJ. (1979). Selenium and heart disease. III — Blood selenium and heart mortality in 19 states. In: Hemphill DD (ed). Trace Substances in Environmental Health — XIII. University of Missouri Press, Columbia, pp. 59–63.

Shapcott D. (1979). The detection of chromium deficiency. In: Shapcott D, Hubert J (eds). Chromium Nutrition and Metabolism. Elsevier/North Holland Biomedical Press, New York, pp. 113–127.

Shapcott D, Cloutier D, Demers PP, Vobecky JS, Vobecky J. (1980). Hair chromium at delivery in relation to age and number of pregnancies. Clinical Biochemistry 13: 129–131.

Shapcott D, Vobecky JS, Vobecky J, Demers PP. (1985). Plasma cholesterol and the plasma copper/zinc ratio in young children. Science of the Total Environment. 42: 197–200.

Shaw JC, Bury AJ, Barber A, Mann L, Taylor A. (1982). A micromethod for the analysis of zinc in plasma or serum by atomic absorption spectrophotometry using graphite furnace. Clinica Chimica Acta 118: 229–239.

Siegler RL, Eggert JV, Udomkesmalee E. (1981). Diagnostic indices of zinc deficiency in children with renal diseases. Annals of Clinical and Laboratory Science 11: 428–433.

Simonoff M. (1984). Chromium deficiency and cardiovascular risk. Cardiovascular Research 18: 591–596.

Smit-Vanderkooy PD, Gibson RS. (1987). Food consumption patterns of Canadian preschool children in relation to zinc and growth status. American Journal of Clinical Nutrition 45: 609–616.

Smith JC Jr, Brown ED. (1976). Effects of oral contraceptive agents on trace element metabolism: a review. In: Prasad AS (ed). Trace Element in Human Health and Disease. Volume 1. Academic Press, New York, pp. 315–345.

Smith JC Jr, Butrimovitz GP, Purdy WC. (1979). Direct measurement of zinc in plasma by atomic absorption spectroscopy. Clinical Chemistry 25: 1487–1491.

Smith JC Jr, Holbrook JT, Danford DE. (1985). Analysis and evaluation of zinc and copper in human plasma and serum. Journal of the American College of Nutrition 4: 627–638.

Smith AM, Picciano MF, Milne RJA. (1982). Selenium intakes and status of human milk and formula fed infants. American Journal of Clinical Nutrition 35: 521–526.

Snook JT, Palmquist DL, Moxon AL, Cantor AH, Vivian VM. (1983). Selenium status of a rural (predominantly Amish) community living in a low-selenium area. American Journal of Clinical Nutrition 38: 620–630.

Sokoloff L. (1988). Kashin-Beck disease: current status. Nutrition Reviews 46: 113–119.

Solomons NW. (1979). On the assessment of zinc and copper nutriture in man. American Journal of Clinical Nutrition 32: 856–871.

Solomons NW. (1982). Biological availability of zinc in humans. American Journal of Clinical Nutrition 35: 1048–1075.

Solomons NW, Helitzer-Allen DL, Villar J. (1986). Zinc needs during pregnancy. Clinical Nutrition 5: 63–71.

Solomons NW, Layden TJ, Rosenberg IH, Vo-Khactu K, Sandstead HH. (1976). Plasma trace metals during total parenteral alimentation. Gastroenterology 70: 1022–1025.

Solomons NW. (1980). Zinc and copper in human nutrition. In: Karcioglu ZA, Sarper RM (eds). Zinc and Copper in Medicine. Charles C Thomas, Springfield, Illinois, pp. 224–275.

Stanley JC, Alexander JP, Nesbitt GA. (1982). Selenium, deficiency during total parenteral nutrition — a case report. The Ulster Medical Journal 51: 130–132.

Sternlieb I, Janowitz HD. (1964). Absorption of copper in malabsorption syndromes. Journal of Clinical Investigation 43: 1049–1055.

Stewart RDH, Griffiths NM, Thomson CD, Robinson MF. (1978). Quantitative selenium metabolism in normal New Zealand women. British Journal of Nutrition 40: 45–54.

Strain WH, Steadman LT, Lankau CA, Berliner WP, Pories WJ. (1966). Analysis of zinc levels in hair for the diagnosis of zinc deficiency in man. Journal of Laboratory and Clinical Medicine 68: 244–249.

Sunderman FW Jr, Nomoto S. (1970). Measurement of human serum ceruloplasmin by its *p*-phenylenediamine oxidase activity. Clinical Chemistry 16: 903–910.

Suzuki H, Higuchi T, Sawa K, Ohtaki S, Horuchi Y. (1965). "Endemic coast goitre" in Hokkaido, Japan. Acta Endocrinologica 50: 161–176.

Swanson CA, King JC. (1982). Zinc utilization in pregnant and nonpregnant women fed controlled diets providing the zinc RDA. Journal of Nutrition 112: 697–707.

Swanson CA, Reamer DC, Veillon C, King JC, Levander OA. (1983). Quantitative and qualitative aspects of selenium utilization in pregnant and nonpregnant women: an application of stable isotope methodology. American Journal of Clinical Nutrition 38: 169–180.

Taylor A. (1986). Usefulness of measurements of trace elements in hair. Annals of Clinical Biochemistry 23: 364–378.

Thilly CH, DeLange F, Stanbury JB. (1980). Epidemiologic surveys in endemic goiter and cretinism. In: Stanbury JB, Hetzel BS (eds). Endemic Goiter and Endemic Cretinism. John Wiley and Sons, New York.

Thomson CD, Duncan A. (1981). Glutathione peroxidase and selenium status. In: Howell JMcC, Gawthorne JM, White CL (eds). Trace Element Metabolism in Man and Animals (TEMA-4). Australian Academy of Science, Canberra, pp. 22–25.

Thomson CD, Rea HM, Doesburg VM, Robinson MF. (1977). Selenium concentrations and glutathione peroxidase activities in whole blood of New Zealand residents. British Journal of Nutrition 37: 457–460.

Thomson CD, Robinson MF. (1980). Selenium in human health and disease with emphasis on those aspects peculiar to New Zealand. American Journal of Clinical Nutrition 33: 303–323.

Thomson CD, Robinson MF, Campbell DR, Rea HM. (1982). Effect of prolonged supplementation with daily supplements of selenomethionine and sodium selenite on glutathione peroxidase (EC 1.11.1.9) activity in blood of New Zealand residents. American Journal of Clinical Nutrition 36: 24–31.

Thomson CD, Steven SM, Rij AM van, Wade CR, Robinson MF. (1988). Selenium and vitamin E supplementation: activities of glutathione peroxidase in human tissues. American Journal of Clinical Nutrition 48: 316–323.

Tietz NW (ed). (1983). Clinical Guide to Laboratory Tests. WB Saunders Co., Philadelphia, pp. 142–145.

Tola S, Kilpiö J, Virtamo M, Haapa K. (1977). Urinary chromium as an indicator of the exposure of welders to chromium. Scandinavian Journal of Work and Environmental Health 3: 192–202.

Tsongas TA, Ferguson SW. (1978). Selenium concentration in human urine and drinking water. In: Kirchgessner M (ed). Trace Element Metabolism in Man and Animals (TEMA-3). Institut fur Ernährungs Physiologie Technische Universität Munchen, Freising-Weihenstephan, FRG. pp. 320–321.

Valberg LS, Flanagan PR, Brennan J, Chamberlain MJ. (1985). Does the oral zinc tolerance test measure zinc absorption? American Journal of Clinical Nutrition 41: 37–42.

Valentine JL, Kang HK, Spivey GH. (1978). Selenium levels in human blood, urine, and hair in response to exposure via drinking water. Environmental Research 17: 347–355.

Vanderlinde RE, Kayne FJ, Komar G, Simmons MJ, Tsou JY, Lavine RL. (1979). Serum and urine levels of chromium. In: Shapcott D, Hubert J (eds). Chromium in Nutrition and Metabolism. Elsevier/North Holland Biomedical Press, Amsterdam–New York–Oxford, pp. 49–57.

Vecchio TJ, Oster HL, Smith DL. (1965). Oral sodium, tolbutamide and glucose tolerance tests. Archives of Internal Medicine 115: 161–166.

Veillon C, Patterson KY, Bryden NA. (1982). Chromium in urine as measured by atomic absorption spectrometry. Clinical Chemistry 28: 2309–2311.

Verlinden M, Sprundel M van, Auwera JC van der, Eylenbosch WJ. (1983a). The selenium status of Belgian population groups. I. Healthy adults. Biological Trace Element Research 5: 91–102.

Verlinden M, Sprundel M van, Auwera JC van der, Eylenbosch WJ. (1983b). The selenium status of Belgian population groups. II. Newborns, children, and the aged. Biological Trace Element Research 5: 103–113.

Versieck J, Hoste J, Barbier F, Steyaert H, De Rudder J, Michels H. (1978). Determination of chromium and cobalt in human serum by neutron activation analysis. Clinical Chemistry 24: 303–308.

Vilter RW, Bozian RC, Hess EV, Zellner DC, Petering HG. (1974). Manifestations of copper deficiency in patients with systemic sclerosis on intravenous hyperalimentation. New England Journal of Medicine 291: 188–191.

Vinton NE, Dahlstrom KA, Strobel CT, Ament ME. (1987). Macrocytosis and pseudoalbinism: manifestations of selenium deficiency. Journal of Pediatrics 111: 711–717.

Virtamo J, Valkeila E, Alfthan G, Punsar S, Huttunen JK, Karvonen MJ. (1985). Serum selenium and the risk of coronary heart disease and stroke. American Journal of Epidemiology 122: 276–282.

Vought RL, Brown FA, Wolff J. (1972). Erythrosine: an adventitious source of iodide. Journal of Clinical Endocrinology and Metabolism 34: 747–752.

Walker BE, Bone I, Mascie-Taylor BH, Kelleher J. (1979). Is plasma zinc a useful investigation? International Journal of Vitamin and Nutrition Research 49: 413–418.

Walravens PA, Krebs NF, Hambidge KM. (1983). Linear growth of low income preschool children receiving a zinc supplement. American Journal of Clinical Nutrition 38: 195–201.

Walravens PA, Hambidge KM. (1976). Growth of infants fed a zinc supplemented formula. American Journal of Clinical Nutrition 29:1114–1121.

Warren DC, Lane HW, Mares M. (1981). Variability of zinc concentrations in human stimulated parotid saliva. Biological Trace Element Research 3: 99–107.

Wąsowicz W, Zachara BA. (1987). Selenium concentrations in the blood and urine of a healthy Polish subpopulation. Journal of Clinical Chemistry and Clinical Biochemistry 25: 409–412.

Watkinson JH. (1979). The semi-automated fluorimetric determination of nomogram quantities of selenium in biological material. Analytica Chimica Acta 105: 319–325.

Watkinson JH. (1981). Changes of blood selenium in New Zealand adults with time and importation of Australian wheat. American Journal of Clinical Nutrition 34: 936–942.

Watson WS. (1988). Plasma zinc uptake and taste acuity. American Journal of Clinical Nutrition 47: 336.

Watson AR, Stuart A, Wells FE, Houston IB, Addison GM. (1983). Zinc supplementation and its effect on taste acuity in children with chronic renal failure. Human Nutrition: Clinical Nutrition 37C: 219–225.

Weismann K, Høyer H. (1978). Serum alkaline phosphatase activity in acrodermatitis enteropathica: an index of serum zinc level. Acta Dermato Venereologica 59: 89–90.

Weismann K, Høyer H. (1985). Serum alkaline phosphatase and serum zinc levels in the diagnosis and exclusion of zinc deficiency in man. American Journal of Clinical Nutrition 41: 1214–1219.

Welinder H, Littorin M, Gullberg B, Skerfving S. (1983). Elimination of chromium in urine after stainless steel welding. Scandinavian Journal of Work Environmental Health 9: 397–403.

Westermarck T, Raunu P, Kirjarinta M, Lappalainen L. (1977). Selenium content of blood and serum in adults and children of different ages from different parts of Finland. Acta Pharmacologica et Toxicologica 40: 465–475.

Westermarck T, Santavuori P, Marklund S, Pohja P, Salmi A. (1982). Studies on the effects of selenium administration to neuronal ceroid lipofuscinosis patients with special reference to reduced glutathione. In: Armstrong D, Kappong N, Rider-JA (eds). Ceroid Lipofuscinosis (Batten's disease). Elsevier Press, Amsterdam, 399–405.

White CL, Pschorr J, Jacob ICM, von Lutterotti N, Dahlheim H. (1984). Reduced plasma angiotensin I-converting enzyme and kininase activities in the plasma of zinc deficient rats. In: Mills CF, Bremner I, Chesters JK (eds). Trace Elements in Man and Animals 5. Commonwealth Agricultural Bureau, London, pp. 65–70.

Whitehouse RC, Prasad AS, Rabbani PI, Cossack ZT. (1982). Zinc in plasma, neutrophils, lymphocytes, and erythrocytes as determined by flameless atomic absorption spectrophotometry. Clinical Chemistry 28: 475–480.

Wiegand HJ, Ottenwalder H, Bolt HM. (1985). Die chrombestimmung in humanerythrozyten. Arbeitsmedizin Sozialmedizin Praventivmedizin 20: 1–4.

Willett WC, Morris JS, Pressel S, Taylor JO, Polk BF, Stampfer MJ, Rosner B, Schneider K, Hames CG. (1983). Prediagnostic serum selenium and risk of cancer. Lancet 2: 130–134.

Williams DM, Atkin CL, Frens DB, Bray PF. (1977). Menkes' Kinky hair syndrome: studies of copper metabolism and long term copper therapy. Pediatric Research 11: 823–826.

Williams DM, Lynch RE, Lee GR, Cartwright GE. (1975). Superoxide dismutase activity in copper-deficient swine. Proceedings of the Society of Experimental Biology and Medicine 149: 534–536.

Wolff J, Chaikoff IL. (1948). Plasma inorganic iodide as homeostatic regulator of thyroid function. Journal of Biological Chemistry 174: 555–564.

Xue-Cun C, Tai-An Y, Jin-Sheng H, Qiu-Yan M, Zhi-Min H, Li-Xiang L. (1985). Low levels of zinc in hair and blood, pica, anorexia, and poor growth in Chinese preschool children. American Journal of Clinical Nutrition 42: 694–700.

Yang GQ, Wang SZ, Zhou RH, Sun SZ. (1983). Endemic selenium intoxication of humans in China. American Journal of Clinical Nutrition 37: 872–881.

Yip R, Reeves JD, Lonnerdal B, Keen CL, Dallman PR. (1985). Does iron supplementation compromise zinc nutrition in healthy infants? American Journal of Clinical Nutrition 42: 683–687.

Zak B, Willard HH, Myers GB, Boyle AJ. (1952). Chloric acid method for determination of protein-bound iodine. Analytical Chemistry 24: 1345–1348.

Zelkowitz M, Verghese JP, Antel J. (1980). Copper and zinc in the nervous system. In: Karcioğlu ZA, Sarper RM (ed). Zinc and Copper in Medicine. Charles C. Thomas, Springfield, Illinois, pp. 418–463.

Zlotkin SH, Casselman C. (1988). Diurnal variation in urinary zinc excretion and the use of Zn/Cr ratio from random urine samples to monitor zinc status. Canadian Federation of Biological Societies, Quebec, (Abst).

Zober A, Kick K, Schaller KH, Schellmann B, Valentin H. (1984). Normal values of chromium and nickel in human lung, kidney, blood and urine samples. Zentralblatt für Bakteriologie Mikrobiologie und Hygiene 179: 80–95.

Chapter 25

Clinical assessment

Clinical assessment consists of a routine medical history and a physical examination to detect physical signs (i.e. observations made by a qualified examiner) and symptoms (i.e. manifestations reported by the patient) associated with malnutrition. These assessment procedures are normally used in community nutrition surveys and in clinical medicine. They are most useful during the advanced stages of nutritional depletion, when overt disease is present. Many of the critical physical signs are nonspecific and must therefore be interpreted in conjunction with laboratory, anthropometric, and dietary data before specific nutritional deficiencies can be identified.

Protein-energy malnutrition does occur among surgical patients in North America (Blackburn and Bistrian, 1976); cases of vitamin and mineral deficiencies among hospital patients are less common. Consequently, in clinical medicine, emphasis has been placed on identifying patients with protein and/or energy malnutrition, and subjects who are at high risk for developing these conditions. Nutritional support can then be directed specifically to the patients in need, and the effectiveness of the support evaluated.

25.1 Medical history

In clinical medicine, the medical history can be obtained by an interview with the patient and/or from the medical records. Two types of medical records are commonly used, the source-orientated medical record (SOMR) and the problem-orientated medical record (POMR) (Atwood et al., 1974). The organization of the former is based on the source of the information obtained during the course of the health care. The SOMR consists of patient identification data, admission notes, physician's orders, laboratory reports, medication records, consents, consultations, operating room records, progress notes, and flow sheets (Mason et al., 1982). The SOMR has been superseded by the POMR in many health care settings.

Nutrient intake
- Anorexia
- Actual intake
- Gastrointestinal tract malfunction affecting intake, digestion, or absorption

Underlying pathology with nutritional effects
- Chronic infections or inflammatory states
- Neoplasia
- Endocrine disorders
- Chronic illnesses: pulmonary disease, cirrhosis, or renal failure

End-organ effects
- Edema/ascites
- Weight changes
- Obesity
- Muscle mass relative to exercise status

Miscellaneous
- Catabolic medications or therapies: steroids, immunosuppressive agents, radiation, or chemotherapy
- Genetic background: body habitus of parents, siblings, and family
- Other medications: diuretics, laxatives
- Food allergies: food intolerances

Table 25.1: Example of information obtained from a medical history. Reproduced by permission from Cerra FB. (1984). Assessment of nutritional and metabolic status. Chapter 3. In: Pocket Manual of Surgical Nutrition, page 25. St Louis, 1984, The C.V. Mosby Co.

The POMR, unlike the SOMR, is organized according to a series of problems, identified during the data collection process. The POMR consists of a defined database, a complete problem list, the initial care plan, and progress notes, as well as flow sheets and a discharge summary (Fowler and Longabaugh, 1975). Use of either of these types of medical records ensures that all aspects of the care of the patient are noted in one place, as part of the total medical record.

The medical history generally includes a description of the patient, and relevant environmental, social, and family factors, as well as specific data on the medical history of the patient and his/her family. Such data are obtained by a variety of questions related to weight loss or gain, edema, anorexia, vomiting, diarrhea, and information on decreased or unusual food intake. Other information recorded includes: previous history of anemia and/or major surgery; presence of chronic illness; pica (ingestion of clay, starch, paint, etc.); presence of congenital conditions and inborn errors of metabolism; and the use of medications and/or dietary supplements. Details of food allergies and food intolerances are also obtained. An example of data obtained in a medical history is given in Table 25.1.

All of this information is used to establish whether a nutrient deficiency is primary, arising from inadequate dietary intake, or secondary in origin. In a secondary deficiency, the diet is potentially adequate but conditioning factors such as drugs, dietary components, and/or disease states interfere with the ingestion, absorption, transport, utilization, or excretion of the nutrient(s). Respondent bias may occur during the conduct of the medical history. In general, voluntary information given by the patient tends to be less biased than answers to specific questions on past medical history. Consequently, it is preferable to use open-ended questions to elicit such information.

In community surveys, the medical history component is obtained by administering a questionnaire in a household or site interview. Information on medications and dietary supplements should be collected directly from the container labels, by asking the subjects to show the interviewer, when possible, all drugs (prescription and over-the-counter) and supplements. In this way accurate data on type and dose may be obtained. Parents can be asked to supply additional information about their children, such as infant feeding history (e.g. breast vs. formula feeding; age of introduction of solid foods), histories of contagious diseases, immunization details, presence of parasites, weight and length of child at birth, etc. For female subjects, questions related to age at first menses, history of pregnancies and miscarriages, oral contraceptive use, and use of noncontraceptive estrogens are also frequently included.

Questions designed to quantify the consumption of tea, coffee, alcohol, the use of tobacco, and on the occurrence of fractures may also be included, as recommended for the NHANES III survey (Klasing and Pilch, 1985). Questions on the type and level of habitual physical activity and/or exercise may also be incorporated, as well as a physical fitness examination. An example of a medical history questionnaire used in the Nutrition Canada National Survey for persons aged six years and older is given in Appendix A25.1.

25.2 Physical examination

The physical examination, as defined by Jelliffe (1966), examines "those changes, believed to be related to inadequate nutrition, that can be seen or felt in superficial epithelial tissue, especially the skin, eyes, hair, and buccal mucosa, or in organs near the surface of the body (e.g. parotid and thyroid glands)". In community surveys, certain physical tests such as ankle jerks may also be included. An abbreviated list of physical signs indicative or suggestive of malnutrition is presented in Table 25.2. A detailed description and photographs of the physical signs recommended by the WHO Expert Committee on Medical Assessment of Nutritional Status (WHO, 1963) can be found in the Assessment of the Nutritional

Normal Appearance	Signs Associated with Malnutrition
Hair: Shiny; firm; not easily plucked	Lack of natural shine; hair dull and dry; thin and sparse; hair fine, silky, and straight; color changes (flag sign); can be easily plucked
Face: Skin color uniform with a smooth, pink, healthy appearance; not swollen	Skin color loss (depigmentation); skin dark over cheeks and under eyes (malar and supraorbital pigmentation); lumpiness or flakiness of skin of nose and mouth; swollen face; enlarged parotid glands; scaling of skin around nostrils (nasolabial seborrhea)
Eyes: Bright, clear, shiny; no sores at corners of eyelids; membranes are a healthy pink and are moist. No prominent blood vessels or mound of tissues or sclera	Eye membranes are pale (pale conjunctivae); redness of membranes (conjunctival injection); Bitot's spots; redness and fissuring of eyelid corners (angular palpebritis); dryness of eye membranes (conjunctival xerosis); cornea has dull appearance (corneal xerosis); cornea is soft (keratomalacia); scar on cornea; ring of fine blood vessels around cornea (circumcorneal injection)
Lips: Smooth, not chapped or swollen	Redness and swelling of mouth or lips (cheilosis); especially at corners of mouth (angular fissures and scars)
Tongue: Deep red in appearance; not swollen or smooth	Swelling; scarlet and raw tongue; magenta (purplish) color of tongue; smooth tongue; swollen sores; hyperemic and hypertrophic papillae; atrophic papillae
Teeth: No cavities; no pain; bright	May be missing or erupting abnormally; grey or black spots (fluorosis); cavities (caries)
Gums: Healthy; red; do not bleed; not swollen	'Spongy' and bleed easily; recession of gums
Face: Face not swollen	Thyroid enlargement (front of neck); parotid enlargement (cheeks become swollen)

Table 25.2: Physical signs indicative or suggestive of malnutrition. From Christakis G. (1973). Nutritional assessment in health programs. American Journal of Public Health 63 (Supplement): 1–82. With permission of American Public Health Association.

Status of the Community (Jelliffe, 1966). An example of the physical assessment form used in the Nutrition Canada National Survey is given in Appendix A25.2.

25.2.1 Limitations of the physical examination

The classical physical signs, listed in Table 25.2, are detected in the general population in Europe and North America less frequently than in populations living in less industrialized countries. They are also found

Normal Appearance	Signs Associated with Malnutrition
Skin: No signs of rashes, swellings, dark or light spots	Dryness of skin (xerosis); sandpaper feel of skin (follicular hyperkeratosis); flakiness of skin; skin swollen and dark; red swollen pigmentation of exposed areas (pellagrous dermatosis); excessive lightness or darkness of skin (dyspigmentation); black and blue marks resulting from skin bleeding (petechiae); lack of fat under skin
Nails: Firm, pink	Nails are spoon-shaped (koilonychia); brittle & ridged
Muscular & skeletal system: Good muscle tone; some fat under skin; can walk and run without pain	Muscles have 'wasted' appearance; baby's skull bones are thin and soft (craniotabes); round swelling of front and side of head (frontal and parietal bossing); swelling of ends of bones (epiphyseal enlargement); small bumps on both sides of chest wall (on ribs) — beading of ribs; baby's soft spot on head does not harden at proper time (persistently open anterior fontanelle); knock-knees or bow-legs; bleeding into muscle (musculo-skeletal hemorrhages); persons cannot get up or walk properly
Cardiovascular system: Normal heart rate and rhythm; no murmurs or abnormal rhythms; normal blood pressure for age	Heart rate above 100 (tachycardia); enlarged heart; abnormal rhythm; elevated blood pressure
Gastrointestinal system: No palpable organs or masses (in children, however, liver edge may be palpable)	Liver enlargement; enlargement of spleen (usually indicates other associated diseases)
Nervous system: Psychological stability; normal reflexes	Mental irritability and confusion; burning and tingling of hands and feet (paresthesia); loss of position and vibratory sense; weakness and tenderness of muscles (may result in inability to walk); decrease and loss of ankle and knee reflexes

Table 25.2 (continued)

in patients who enter hospital for surgery, and in those with certain disease states or conditions that result in secondary malnutrition. In clinical medicine the physical examination is conducted by a clinician, whereas in community surveys the physical examination can be undertaken by relatively junior personnel, provided that careful training in recognizing the critical signs, and ongoing supervision, is given. The physical examination as a technique for nutritional assessment has several limitations

	Examiner		
	1	2	3
Number of Examinations	1123	1127	589
Filiform papillary atrophy	4.1	1.1	11.2
Follicular hyperkeratosis	4.0	0.6	6.8
Swollen red gums	2.8	3.7	4.1
Angular lesions	0.4	0.4	1.2
Glossitis	0.6	0.4	0.5
Goiter	3.6	6.6	3.6

Table 25.3: The prevalence, as a percentage, of selected physical signs by three examiners, Texas Nutrition Survey, 1968-1969. From McGanity (1974) with permission.

which must be recognized (Christakis, 1973; McGanity, 1974). These are discussed in the following sections.

Nonspecificity of the physical signs

This is a major limitation, especially in mild or moderate deficiency states. Some physical signs may be produced by more than one nutrient deficiency (e.g. nasolabial seborrhea arises from deficiency of pyridoxine, riboflavin, or niacin; cheilosis and angular stomatitis are related to deficiencies of riboflavin and niacin; glossitis of the tongue occurs in deficiencies of riboflavin, niacin, folic acid, and vitamin B-12). Other physical signs may be caused by non-nutritional factors, such as eczema and other allergic manifestations (e.g. follicular hyperkeratosis) and the weather (e.g. Bitot's spots), or may be, in some cases, hereditary.

Multiple physical signs

Subjects with co-existing nutrient deficiencies (e.g. protein and zinc deficiency; riboflavin, niacin, and vitamin C) may exhibit multiple physical signs, confusing the diagnosis.

Signs may be two-directional

Signs may occur during the development of a deficiency and/or recovery. For example, an enlarged liver (hepatomegaly) occurs in protein-energy malnutrition and during its treatment.

Examiner inconsistencies

The recording of certain lesions may be subject to inconsistencies. For example, examiners with very limited experience may record lesions in subjects with mild or borderline evidence of the lesions. Other, more experienced, examiners may record only severe forms. Table 25.3 presents data for the prevalence (as a percentage) of some physical

Deficiency	Clinical Signs	Age (Years)		
		0–6	6–16	16+
Protein-energy	Abnormal hair (color, texture)	2.1	0.6	0.3
Iron or B vitamins	Filiform papillary atrophy	3.3	4.4	6.2
Vitamin A	Follicular hyperkeratosis	3.1	4.9	3.9
Vitamin D	Enlarged wrists	2.8	—	—
Vitamin C	Swollen, red gums	0.6	5.9	8.5
Riboflavin	Angular lesions of tongue	1.4	0.9	0.6
	Glossitis of tongue	0.4	2.0	8.3
Iodine	Visible enlargement of thyroid	1.1	5.4	5.5

Table 25.4: Variations in the percentage prevalence of clinical signs associated with nutritional deficiencies with age. From McGanity (1974) with permission.

signs recorded by three examiners in the 1968 Texas Nutrition Survey (McGanity, 1974). In this cross-sectional survey, the presence of filiform papillary atrophy ranged from 1.1% to 11.2%, according to the examiner. Generally, such inconsistencies are less when the physical signs are severe.

Examiner bias can be minimized by standardizing the criteria used to define the physical signs, and by training the examiners. The United States Interdepartmental Committee on Nutrition for National Defense (ICNND, 1963) held standardization sessions both before and at intervals during their surveys. In these sessions, each examiner recorded, independently, his clinical findings on 100 persons. Results were compared and any inconsistencies identified. Such standardization sessions will reduce inconsistencies in observations recorded by two or more examiners and/or the same examiner on different occasions.

Inconsistencies also arise if the physical lesions are graded during the physical examination. For most lesions, no attempt should be made to grade the severity of the physical signs, especially in the field. Instead, signs should simply be recorded as positive or negative, except in cases where objective measurements using instruments can be used (e.g. tendon jerks) (Jelliffe, 1966).

Variation in the pattern of physical signs

There is no universal set of signs and symptoms suitable for all ages and all countries. The pattern of physical lesions associated with specific nutrient deficiencies varies according to genetic factors, activity level, environment, dietary pattern, age, and the degree, duration, and speed of onset of malnutrition. Examples of the variations in the prevalence of physical signs of nutritional deficiencies with age are shown in Table 25.4.

All these limitations of the physical examination confound the diagnosis, making it essential to include laboratory tests to confirm the existence of specific nutrient deficiencies.

25.2.2 Classification and interpretation of physical signs

The World Health Organization has classified the most common physical signs into three groups: (1) signs indicating a probable deficiency of one or more nutrients; (2) signs indicating probable long-term malnutrition in combination with other factors, and (3) signs not related to nutritional status. Generally, in community surveys, only those signs in Group 1 should be sought in the physical examination.

	Risk Categories		
Clinical Signs	High	Moderate	Low
Protein-calorie malnutrition (1) Pretibial pitting, bilateral edema (2) Major weight deficit (less than 0.6 of median for age) (3) Minor weight deficit (between 0.8 and 0.6 of median for age) (4) Painless pluckability of hair			
0–5 yrs males and females	Sign 1 or 2	Sign(s) 3 or 3 + 4	Sign 4 or no signs
Vitamin C deficiency (1) Scorbutic rosary (2) Diffuse bleeding of gums (3) Purpura or petechiae and/or follicular hyperkeratosis — arms/back			
0–5 yrs males and females	Sign 1 or Signs 2 + 3	Signs 2 or 3	No signs
6+ yrs males and females	Signs 2 + 3	Sign 2 or 3	No signs
Rickets (Vitamin D deficiency) (1) Rachitic rosary (2) Craniotabes (3) Bowed legs (4) Delayed walking (more than 18 months)			
0–1 yr males and females	Combinations that include Signs 1 + 2	Other combin-ations that include 1 + 4	All other combinations
2–5 yrs males and females	Signs 1 + 3	Signs 1 + 4	All other combinations

Table 25.5: Examples of the use of combinations of clinical signs in the identification of nutrient deficiencies. From Health and Welfare Canada (1973). Reproduced with permission of the Minister of Supply and Services Canada.

To assist in the interpretation, the physical signs (and symptoms) are often combined into groups associated with a particular nutrient deficiency state. Generally, for any one subject, the greater the number of signs present within a specific group, the greater the probability that the subject has a specific nutrient deficiency. The major physical signs of specific nutrient deficiencies are well established, although their sensitivity and specificity varies. In the NHANES I survey, the major physical signs characteristic of a specific nutrient deficiency were assigned to one of three risk categories (high, moderate, and low), based on their specificity. Individuals with *one* of the physical signs in the high risk category would be considered at high risk of developing or having a specific nutrient deficiency. A similar approach was used for the Nutrition Canada National Survey (Health and Welfare Canada, 1973), although in the latter the risk categories were designated according to specified *combinations* of physical signs rather than a single sign characteristic of a specified nutrient deficiency. Examples of the combinations of the clinical signs for protein-energy malnutrition and deficiencies of vitamins C and D used in the Nutrition Canada National Survey are shown in Table 25.5

25.3 Summary

Clinical assessment consists of a routine medical history and a physical examination. Information for the medical history can be obtained by administering a questionnaire, or from medical records, and is used in the study of the etiology of the nutrient deficiency. In the physical examination, physical signs and symptoms related to inadequate nutrition are investigated. In industrialized countries, mild or moderate (but rarely severe) nutrient deficiencies generally occur, often concomitantly with certain disease states. Signs associated with such deficiencies are frequently not very specific, and may be two-directional, occurring during both deficiency and recovery, and/or multiple, co-existing with other nutrient deficiencies. Examiner inconsistencies may also be a source of error, but can be minimized by training examiners and standardizing the criteria used to define the signs. In most cases, signs should be recorded as positive or negative and not in terms of grades of severity. To assist in identifying specific nutrient deficiencies, signs (and symptoms) are grouped, combinations varying with age, race, country, etc. Generally, the greater the number of signs present within a specific group, the larger the probability that the individual has a specific nutrient deficiency. The signs within a group are often classified into three risk categories, designated as high, moderate, and low risk.

References

Atwood J, Mitchell PH, Yarnell SR. (1974). The POR: A system for communication. Nursing Clinics of North America 9: 229–234.

Blackburn GL, Bistrian BR. (1976). Nutritional care of the injured and/or septic patient. Surgical Clinics of North America 56: 1195–1224.

Cerra FB. (1984). Assessment of nutritional and metabolic status. Chapter 3. In: Pocket Manual of Surgical Nutrition. The C.V. Mosby Company, St Louis – Toronto – Princeton, pp. 24–48.

Christakis G. (1973). Nutritional assessment in health programs. American Journal of Public Health 63 (Supplement): 1–82.

Fowler DR, Longabaugh R. (1975). The problem-orientated record. Problem definition. Archives of General Psychiatry 32: 831–834.

Health and Welfare Canada (1973). Nutrition Canada National Survey. Health and Welfare, Ottawa.

ICNND (Interdepartmental Committee on Nutrition for National Defense) (1963). Manual for Nutrition Surveys. Second edition. Superintendent of Documents, US Government Printing Office, Washington, D.C.

Jelliffe DB. (1966). The Assessment of the Nutritional Status of the Community. WHO Monograph No. 53. World Health Organization, Geneva.

Klasing SA, Pilch SM. (1985). Suggested Measures of Nutritional Status and Health Conditions for the Third National Health and Nutrition Examination Survey. Life Sciences Research Office, Federation of American Societies for Experimental Biology, Bethesda, Maryland.

McGanity WJ. (1974). The clinical assessment of nutritional status. In: Hawkins WW (ed). Assessment of Nutritional Status. Miles Symposium II. Miles Laboratories Ltd., Rexdale, Ontario, pp. 47–64.

Mason M, Wenburg BG, Welsh PK. (1982). The Dynamics of Clinical Dietetics. Second edition. John Wiley and Sons, New York, pp. 66–77.

WHO (World Health Organization) (1963). WHO Expert Committee on Medical Assessment of Nutritional Status. WHO Technical Report Series No. 258. World Health Organization, Geneva.

Chapter 26

Nutritional assessment of hospital patients

The objectives of hospital nutritional assessment are: (a) to accurately define the nutritional status of the patient; (b) to define clinically relevant malnutrition; and (c) to monitor changes in nutritional status during nutritional support (Bozzetti, 1987). Clinically relevant malnutrition has been defined as "the state of altered nutritional status that is associated with an increased risk of adverse clinical events such as complications or death" (Dempsey and Mullen, 1987).

Nutritional assessment was introduced in clinical medicine during the 1970's, when protein and energy malnutrition of hospital patients in North America was first recognized (Blackburn et al., 1977). Initially, the precision, sensitivity, specificity, and predictive value of the measurements included in the nutritional assessment systems were rarely considered (Section 1.3); today, more attention is given to these criteria when selecting tests for the nutritional assessment system. Most of the routine tests assess protein-energy malnutrition because this is the type of malnutrition most prevalent in hospital patients at the present time. Table 26.1 presents a list of those tests most frequently used for hospital patients. Tests include dietary, anthropometric, biochemical, and functional indices of nutritional status, all of which have been discussed in earlier chapters. The identification of patients at risk to protein-energy malnutrition is difficult because many of the indices measured in the laboratory and listed in Table 26.1 are modified by non-nutritional factors.

Studies have identified certain high-risk disease states and medical conditions for which the associated risk of secondary protein-energy malnutrition is high; these are outlined in Table 26.2. Nutrition screening is routinely applied to these high risk patients in many hospitals, to identify individuals with subtle or early protein-energy malnutrition; appropriate nutritional support can then be implemented to improve

Anthropometric Measurements		
Height (cm)	HT:	....
Weight (kg)	WT:	....
Usual weight (kg)	US-WT:	....
Sex (m/f)	SEX:	....
Ideal body weight (kg)	IBW:	....
Weight as a percentage of IBW (%)	%IBW:	....
Weight as a percentage of usual weight (%)	%US-WT:	....
Triceps skinfold (mm)	TSF:	....
Arm circumference (cm)	AC:	....
Arm muscle circumference (cm)	AMC:	....
Triceps skinfold as % of standard	%TSF:	....
Arm muscle circumference as % of standard	%AMC:	....
Laboratory Determinations		
Serum albumin (g/dL)	ALB:	....
Total iron binding capacity (μg/dL)	TIBC:	....
Serum transferrin (mg/dL)	TRANS:	....
Lymphocyte count (%)	LYMPH:	....
White blood cell count (No./mm^3)	WBC:	....
Total lymphocyte count (No./mm^3)	TLC:	....
24-hour urinary urea nitrogen (g)	UUN:	....
24-hour urinary creatinine (mg)	UCR:	....
Creatinine height index as % of standard (%)	CHI:	....
Diet and Nutrition Status		
Protein intake (g)	PRO:	....
Caloric intake (kJ)	CAL:	....
Nitrogen balance (g)	N-BAL:	....
Obligatory nitrogen loss (g)	N-OBG:	....
Net protein utilization (apparent)	NPU:	....
Basal energy expenditure (kJ/day)	BEE:	....
Caloric intake as % of BEE (%)	%BEE:	....
Skin test results (mm)	ST:	....

Table 26.1: Nutritional and metabolic variables commonly measured in a complete nutritional assessment. From Blackburn GL, Bistrian BR, Maini BS, Schlamm HT, Smith MF. (1977). Nutritional and metabolic assesment of the hospitalized patient. Journal of Parenteral and Enteral Nutrition 11: 115S–121S. © Am. Soc. for Parenteral and Enteral Nutrition, 1977.

their nutritional status. Evidence suggests that the latter is an important determinant of postoperative morbidity and mortality.

Numerous protocols have been developed to assess the nutritional status of these high risk hospital patients. Some of these protocols are based on single anthropometric, biochemical, or immunological measurements. In others, measurements have been aggregated to form multi-parameter indices, or alternatively are based exclusively on clinical assessment. Examples of these protocols are discussed in the following sections.

General Category	Clinical Examples
Body weight aberrations	20% over ideal body weight; 10% under ideal body weight; more than 10% change in usual body weight in last 6 months; inappropriate weight for height in children; deviation from normal weight gain in pregnancy
Increased metabolic needs	Fever; infection; hyperthyroidism; burns; recent surgery or soft tissue trauma; skeletal trauma; growth; corticosteroid therapy
Increased nutrient losses	Draining fistulas; open wounds; draining abscesses; effusions; chronic blood losses; chronic renal dialysis; exudative enteropathies; burns
General chronic diseases	Diabetes mellitus; hypertension; hyperlipidemia; coronary artery disease; chronic lung disease; chronic renal disease; chronic liver disease; circulatory problems or heart failure; carcinoma; mental retardation; psychosis; epilepsy; rheumatoid arthritis; peptic ulcer; prolonged comatose state
Diseases or surgery of the gastrointestinal tract	Congenital malformations; pancreatic insufficiency; malabsorption states; blind loop syndrome; severe diarrhea; gastrointestinal fistula; resection of stomach or small bowel; intestinal bypass
Medications	Insulin or other hypoglycemic agents; vitamin-mineral supplements; corticosteroids; anticoagulants; monamine oxidase inhibitors; diuretics; antacids; ethanol; oral contraceptive agents; tricyclic antidepressants; phenylhydantoin

Table 26.2: Conditions associated with an increased risk of protein-energy malnutrition. Modified from Hooley (1986) with permission.

26.1 Methods based on a single index

Many of the variables listed in Table 26.1 have been used as single 'nutritional assessment' indices. The relative value and clinical importance of these indices, used individually, have not been firmly established. Some of these indices are relatively insensitive (Section 1.3); for example, serum albumin and transferrin have relatively long half-lives and hence they respond slowly to nutritional depletion and repletion (Shetty et al., 1979). Furthermore, the indices may be affected by non-nutritional factors which limit their specificity and sensitivity (Section 1.3); for example, patients with hepatic disease and nephrosis also have reduced serum albumin and transferrin levels. Similarly, infection, immune suppression, trauma, and zinc deficiency interfere with the interpretation of delayed cutaneous hypersensitivity (Golden et al., 1978). As well, the indices often have wide confidence limits, restricting their use for individual patients (Collins et al., 1979).

For some of these nutritional parameters, investigators have attempted to quantify their clinical relevance by correlating these single measurements of nutritional status with subsequent outcome such as postoperative infections, morbidity, and/or mortality. For example, Mullen et al. (1979) correlated pre-operative serum albumin, serum transferrin, skinfold thickness, and delayed cutaneous hypersensitivity to postoperative morbidity and mortality in 64 consecutive patients. Kaminski et al. (1977) demonstrated a relationship between serum transferrin and hospital mortality, and MacLean et al. (1975) and Meakins et al. (1977) correlated delayed cutaneous hypersensitivity to postoperative infections, septicemia, and death. The existence of such correlations, however, does not necessarily indicate that the predictive value of the index is high. Predictive value is the best measure of the clinical usefulness of any index of nutritional status. It measures the ability of a test to correctly predict the presence or absence of nutrition-associated complications such as postoperative infection, septicemia, death, etc. The predictive value of any specific test is not constant but depends on the sensitivity, specificity, and the prevalence of disease (Section 1.3). Unfortunately, very few studies of the clinical importance of single nutritional assessment parameters have analyzed their data in terms of sensitivity, specificity, predictive value, and outcome. Baker et al. (1982b) compared the ability of three individual nutritional indices (serum albumin above or below 3.0 g/dL; serum transferrin above or below 200 mg/dL; and delayed cutaneous hypersensitivity — present or absent), to predict infection in 59 surgical patients. Their results suggested that none of these single nutritional parameters unambiguously distinguished patients who were at high risk for infection from those who were at low risk. Clearly, the predictive value of these single indices is uncertain.

Dempsey and Mullen (1987) reviewed data on the use of single nutritional assessment parameters, using mortality as the outcome measure. They calculated sensitivity, specificity, and predictive value from these data (Table 26.3) and concluded, for example, that mortality could be correctly predicted by serum albumin in 81% of individuals in similar populations whereas for serum transferrin the predictive value was 48%. Interstudy comparisons must be made with caution, however, because of differences in research design, study populations, and disease prevalence.

Abnormal values for more than one parameter frequently occur in hospital patients and no single parameter is completely satisfactory with regard to sensitivity and specificity. In an effort to increase sensitivity and specificity, and hence predictive value, recent studies have investigated the use of multi-parameter indices of nutritional status. Two examples are discussed in Section 26.2 and 26.3.

Parameter	n	SE	SP	PV
Weight loss	46	0.86	0.69	0.72
Serum albumin	3019	0.69	0.82	0.81
Serum transferrin	229	0.77	0.39	0.48
Anergy	1738	0.52	0.86	0.82
Total lymphocyte count	857	0.76	0.62	0.63
Creatinine height index	225	0.65	0.58	0.60

Table 26.3: Single nutritional assessment parameters as predictors of mortality. Abbreviations: n = number of subjects, SE = sensitivity, Sp = specificity, PV = predictive value. Modified from Dempsey DT, Mullen JL. (1987). Prognostic value of nutritional indices. Journal of Parenteral and Enteral Nutrition 11: 109S–114S. © Am. Soc. for Parenteral and Enteral Nutrition, 1987.

26.2 Prognostic nutritional index

The Prognostic Nutritional Index (PNI) was developed by Mullen and associates (1979) to identify those nutritional indices most highly correlated with clinically relevant malnutrition. They examined a series of nutritional assessment indices, measured on admission, in a group of nonemergency surgical patients ($n = 161$). The indices measured included weight, weight loss history (i.e. percentage weight loss), serum albumin, serum transferrin, total protein, midarm muscle circumference, triceps skinfold, total lymphocyte count, delayed hypersensitivity reactivity (assessed using mumps, *Candida*, and streptokinase-streptodornase antigens), as well as selected demographic data (e.g. age, sex, race), and diagnosis. After nutritional assessment, all patients underwent a major surgical procedure and their clinical course was monitored for objective complications until discharge or death. Discriminant function analysis and stepwise multiple regression procedures were used to select those parameters most highly correlated with surgical outcome. Four indices were incorporated into a Prognostic Nutritional Index: serum albumin, serum transferrin, triceps skinfold and delayed cutaneous hypersensitivity. The PNI indicates the risk, expressed as a percentage, of postoperative morbidity and mortality in an individual patient.

$$\text{PNI(\%)} = 158 - (16.6 \times \text{ALB}) - (0.78 \times \text{TSF}) - (0.2 \times \text{TFN}) - (5.8 \times \text{DCH})$$

where ALB = serum albumin concentrations (g/dL); TSF = triceps skinfold (in mm); TFN = transferrin (g/dL); DCH = delayed hypersensitivity (grade of reactivity to any of three antigens — 0 : nonreactive; 1 : < 5 mm reactivity; 2 : > 5 mm reactivity).

The validity of this model was then tested prospectively using a heterogenous group of patients undergoing major nonemergency gastrointestinal surgery (n = 100) (Buzby et al., 1980). In these studies, the

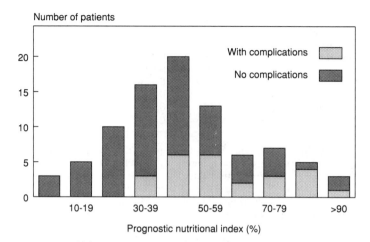

Figure 26.1: Distribution of gastrointestinal surgical patients with and without complications as a function of the prognostic nutritional index (PNI). From Mullen (1981). Reproduced with permission from Clinical Consultations in Nutritional Support, Vol. 1, No. 1, 1981, Medical Directions, Inc., Chicago, IL.

PNI was calculated before surgery, and patients were classified according to the risk of complications (low risk PNI < 40%; intermediate risk PNI 40% to 50%; high risk PNI > 50%). Patients were then followed until discharge or death, and monitored for postsurgical complications by an observer not involved in the patient care and with no knowledge of the predicted outcome. The accuracy of the PNI model for predicting the occurrence of complications was assessed by comparing the predicted risk of complications with the actual occurrences. The results, shown in Figure 26.1, demonstrate that the incidence of complications and death generally increased with an increase in PNI; those patients identified as high risk by the PNI did indeed have a significantly increased risk of complications, sepsis, and mortality, compared to those identified as low risk.

In terms of sensitivity, specificity, and predictive value, when the cutoff point for an abnormal PNI was taken as > 50%, the index predicted mortality with a sensitivity of 86%, a specificity of 69%, and had a predictive value of 72%. Changing the cutoff point of the PNI from > 50% to > 40%, increased the sensitivity to 93%, but, as expected, decreased the specificity to 44% and lowered the predictive value for mortality to 51%.

The use of the PNI model for the prospective identification of patients who would benefit from pre-operative support has also been tested using both prospective nonrandomized and randomized intervention studies in adult surgical patients (Mullen et al., 1980) and patients with gastrointestinal cancer (Mullen et al., 1982), respectively. In both studies, those patients classified as high risk on the basis of a PNI > 50% benefitted from pre-operative support, as indicated by a significant reduction in mortality when compared to those patients with a PNI < 50%.

Nevertheless, several limitations of the PNI have been identified. Subsequent studies have failed to show that the PNI predicts the outcome of patients with acute abdominal trauma (Jones et al., 1983). In addition, it may not be appropriate for predicting survival in patients who do not undergo surgery. Furthermore, the PNI does not give information about the type of nutritional abnormalities. The indices selected for inclusion in the PNI have also been criticized because they are not independent of one another (e.g. serum albumin and transferrin), an assumption of stepwise multiple regression procedures (Chatterjee and Price, 1977). Moreover, the indices selected may be affected by non-nutritional factors, as discussed in Section 26.1. Hence, it becomes very difficult to separate the effects of actual nutrient deficiency from those of the disease process on the basis of the measurements (Baker et al., 1982b).

26.3 Hospital prognostic index

A hospital prognostic index (HPI), based on serum albumin, delayed hypersensitivity response to recall skin antigens, clinical status (i.e. septic or not septic), and presence or absence of cancer, was developed by Harvey et al. (1981) from a retrospective study of 282 adult medical and surgical patients. A discriminant function equation was developed:

$$\text{HPI} = (0.91 \times \text{ALB}) - (1.00 \times \text{DCH}) - (1.44 \times \text{SEP}) + (0.98 \times \text{DX}) - 1.09$$

where: ALB = serum albumin (g/dL); DCH = delayed cutaneous hypersensitivty (1 : positive response to one or more antigens; 2 : negative response to all antigens); SEP = sepsis (1 : present; 2 : not present); DX = diagnosis (1 : cancer; 2 : no cancer);

The equation has an overall predictive value for subsequent hospital mortality of 72%, a sensitivity of 74%, and a specificity of 66%. Serum albumin was the best single predictor of mortality, anergy, and sepsis; an initial serum albumin below 2.2 g/dL was associated with a greater than 75% chance of anergy, sepsis, and death during hospitalization. An improvement in delayed hypersensitivity response was the most accurate predictor of an improved prognosis (overall predictive value 86%, sensitivity 93%, specificity 63%). The HPI has not been widely used; its prognostic accuracy in well-nourished patients and in patients (well nourished and malnourished) with other diseases has not been established.

26.4   Cluster analysis

Cluster analysis is a statistical method that has been used to group patients on the basis of selected clinical, physiological, and therapeutic variables into different nutritional states, termed 'clusters'. Patients can then be classified according to cluster in an effort to identify those at high-risk. In the cluster analysis of Nazari et al. (1981), nutritional assessment indices were used to define four different nutritional states, each associated with different clinical presentation and course:

- **Cluster I:** Only minor variations from normal occur in values for all indices. This nutritional pattern is shown by most (96%) of the controls (noncancer patients admitted for minor surgery) and some cancer patients. The lowest incidence of postoperative infection occurred in patients belonging to this cluster. Moreover, those cancer patients undergoing radical operations who fell into this cluster showed the lowest mortality rate.

- **Cluster II:** The nutritional state of patients in this cluster was similar to an adult kwashiorkor-like syndrome, with impaired delayed cutaneous hypersensitivity and reductions in the visceral protein compartment (with the exception of ceruloplasmin) but with normal body weight. Patients with this nutritional pattern had the highest mortality rate (42%), the highest incidence of palliative procedures, and a high incidence of postoperative sepsis. Consequently cluster II patients are at high risk.

- **Cluster III:** The nutritional state of patients in this cluster represents a mixed marasmus-kwashiorkor-like pattern with mild visceral protein depletion, decrease in some immunological parameters (C3 and lymphocytes), and some modifications of anthropometric measurements. Patients in this group had an increased risk of postoperative infections and a mortality rate between that of cluster I and clusters II and IV.

- **Cluster IV:** The nutritional condition of patients in this cluster IV was characterized by a pronounced increase in acute phase proteins (ceruloplasmin, C3, transferrin, and retinol-binding protein). Patients in this group suffered a 40% mortality rate.

Cluster analysis has also been used to assess plasma amino acids as prognostic indicators of human sepsis (Cerra et al., 1979). The plasma amino-acid profile changes with time as the septic process proceeds. Differences in certain amino-acid levels between survivors and nonsurvivors have been noted.

The cluster analysis approach appears to have the potential to identify patients at risk to nutritionally based postoperative complications. Nevertheless, further studies utilizing various patient populations are necessary

HISTORY

Weight loss in past 6 months: ......kg % loss ......
Change in past 2 weeks: increase ☐ no change ☐ decrease ☐

Dietary changes: no changes ☐ changes ☐ duration...wk
If changes indicate type:
suboptimal solid diet ☐ full liquid diet ☐
hypocaloric liquids ☐ starvation ☐

Gastrointestinal symptoms (persisting for more than 2 weeks) none ☐
    nausea ☐ vomiting ☐ diarrhea ☐ anorexia ☐

Functional capacity none ☐ dysfunction ☐ duration ...
    working suboptimally ☐ ambulatory ☐ bedridden ☐

Disease and its relation to nutritional requirements
Primary diagnosis ....
....

Metabolic demand:
    no stress ☐ low stress ☐ modest stress ☐ high stress ☐

PHYSICAL
For each trait specify: 0 = normal, 1 = mild, 2 = moderate, 3 = severe
loss of subcutaneous fat (triceps, chest) ... ankle edema...
muscle wasting (quadriceps, deltoids) ... sacral edema ... ascites ...

SGA rating well moderately severely
(select one) nourished ☐ nourished ☐ malnourished ☐

Table 26.4: Components of subjective global assessment. Modified from Detsky AS, Baker JP, Mendelson RA, Wolman SL, Wesson DE, Jeejeebhoy KN. (1987). What is subjective global assessment of nutritional status? Journal of Parenteral and Enteral Nutrition 11: 8–13. © Am. Soc. for Parenteral and Enteral Nutrition, 1987.

to establish the sensitivity, specificity, and predictive value of this technique.

26.5 Subjective global assessment

The usefulness of performing objective measurements of nutritional assessment in hospital patients has been questioned in view of the confounding effects of the disease process on many of the measurements. The subjective global assessment (SGA) method (Table 26.4) is an alternative method of nutritional assessment based exclusively on a carefully performed medical history and physical examination. No anthropometric or laboratory indices are included.

Five features are emphasized in the medical history component: (1) weight change, (2) changes in dietary intake, (3) presence of gastrointestinal symptoms, (4) functional capacity or energy level (bedridden to full capacity), and (5) the metabolic demands of the patient's underlying disease state. Both the extent of the weight loss and the rate and pattern of weight loss are considered. Dietary intake is classified as normal or abnormal, with the duration and degree of abnormal intake being recorded. The presence of gastro-intestinal symptoms, classified as anorexia, nausea, vomiting, and diarrhea, is also noted if they persist on a daily basis for more than two weeks. Intermittent diarrhea or vomiting is not included, although vomiting that occurs secondary to obstruction, once or twice daily, is recorded. The fourth feature of the medical history concerns the functional capacity or energy level of the patient, noted in relation to both degree of dysfunction (i.e. bedridden to full capacity) and duration. The final feature of the history considers the metabolic demands or stress associated with the underlying disease state of the patient, and categorizes the degree of stress as high, moderate, or low.

The physical examination of the SGA also emphasizes five features: (1) loss of subcutaneous fat, (2) muscle wasting, (3) presence of edema in the ankles, (4) presence of edema in the sacral region, and (5) presence of ascites. Each of these features is classified as normal (0), mild (1+), moderate (2+), or severe (3+). The presence of co-existing disease states such as congestive heart failure and neurological deficits is also taken into consideration when grading edema and muscle wasting respectively.

Physicians assign a SGA rank for each patient's nutritional status, based on the features emphasized in the history and physical examination. The SGA rank is assigned on the basis of subjective weighting, using particularly the variables weight loss, poor dietary intake, loss of subcutaneous tissue, and muscle wasting. A rigid scoring system based on a numerical weighting is not used. The SGA rank can be one of three categories: (1) well nourished, (2) moderate or suspected malnutrition, and (3) severe malnutrition. A more detailed description of the method of rating can be found in Detsky et al. (1987).

The interobserver reproducibility of the SGA ratings appears high. In a study of fifty-nine general surgical patients, two examiners agreed on the nutritional status, as indicated by a SGA rating, in 81% of the cases (Baker et al., 1982a); with gastrointestinal surgical patients, the percentage agreement was 91% (Detsky et al., 1987). The SGA technique also appears valid, based on the presence of: (a) significant correlations with objective nutritional assessment (i.e. anthropometric and laboratory measurements), and with three measures of hospital morbidity (the incidence of infection, the use of antibiotics, and the length of stay in hospital) (Baker et al., 1982a); (b) the absence of any significant differences between the number of patients classified as malnourished on the basis of SGA compared to objective assessment techniques (Detsky et al., 1984); and (c) the ability of SGA to statistically predict the tendency to develop an infection (Baker et al., 1982b). Nevertheless, not all investigators concur with these findings (Pettigrew et al., 1984). To detect less advanced cases of protein malnutrition, inclusion of some objective indices is probably advisable.

26.6 The prognostic value of nutritional assessment indices

All of the considerations discussed in relation to the design of nutritional assessment systems in Section 1.3 are also applicable when selecting and evaluating hospital nutritional assessment indices. Such considerations include study objectives, sampling protocols, validity, precision, random and systematic measurement errors, accuracy, sensitivity, specificity, and predictive value. The ideal nutritional indices are those that are accurate markers of nutritional status, accurate predictors of outcome, and easily monitored during nutritional repletion (Bozzetti, 1987).

For the adequate evaluation of any nutritional assessment protocol, it must be tested on well-nourished subjects and on patients (well-nourished and malnourished) with other diseases. This approach is essential to establish the effects of nutritional and non-nutritional factors on the test result (Dempsey and Mullen, 1987). Moreover, in addition to correlating the test measurements with clinical outcomes such as morbidity and/or mortality, the predictive value of the protocol in identifying high-risk patients should also be assessed. It is essential to recognize that the predictive value of any test is not constant: it is dependent on the prevalence of disease and on the sensitivity and specificity of the test, as discussed in Section 1.3, which in turn depend on the study population and outcome used to assess efficacy. Hence, it is not surprising that discrepancies in the predictive value for the PNI, for example, have been reported for relatively well-nourished and more severely malnourished population groups (Dempsey and Mullen, 1979).

The sensitivity and specificity can be affected by the cutoff point of the nutritional parameter used. For example, when the cutoff point is raised (e.g. from $< 2.0\,g/dL$ to $< 3.5\,g/dL$ for serum albumin), the sensitivity in predicting mortality increases from 20% to 82%, but specificity falls from 99% to 80%. This effect is shown in Figure 26.2. The ideal test has a high specificity and a high sensitivity. Hence to identify the ideal test, the sensitivity and specificity of a test must always be determined.

26.7 Summary

The objectives of nutritional assessment of hospital patients are to accurately define the nutritional status of the patient, to define clinically

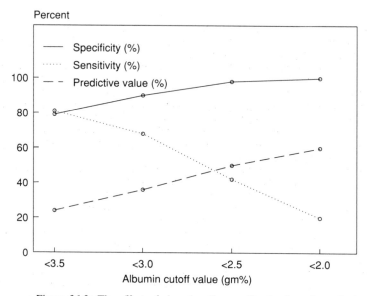

Figure 26.2: The effect of changing the cutoff point for serum albumin on the sensitivity, specificity, and predictive value of albumin
as a test for predicting postoperative mortality. From Dempsey DT,
Mullen JL. (1987). Prognostic value of nutritional indices. Journal
of Parenteral and Enteral Nutrition 11: 109S–114S. © Am. Soc.
for Parenteral and Enteral Nutrition, 1987.

relevant malnutrition, and to monitor changes in nutritional status during nutritional support. Generally, nutritional assessment is routinely
applied to high-risk patients using single or multiple indices. The sensitivity, specificity, and predictive value of single indices such as serum
transferrin, serum albumin, and delayed cutaneous hypersensitivity are
low because of the confounding effects of non-nutritional factors. To
increase their predictive value, multi-parameter indices have been developed. The prognostic nutritional index (PNI) incorporates serum albumin,
serum transferrin, triceps skinfold thickness, and delayed hypersensitivity, and appears promising for predicting complications, sepsis, and
mortality in certain patients, and for identifying those who would benefit from pre-operative support. The hospital prognostic index (HPI),
based on serum albumin and delayed cutaneous hypersensitivity, has not
been widely used. Cluster analysis groups patients on the basis of selected clinical, physiological, and therapeutic variables, in an effort to
identify high-risk surgical patients. As interpretation of many of the
laboratory indices is confounded by the effects of the disease process,
an approach based exclusively on a medical history and physical examination has been developed. This technique, called subjective global
assessment, is able to provide a valid and reproducible prediction of
morbidity in surgical patients. All of the multi-parameter nutritional

assessment indices must be tested in well nourished subjects, and in well-nourished and malnourished patients with other diseases, before their sensitivity, specificity, and predictive value can be firmly established.

References

Baker JP, Detsky AS, Wesson DE, Wolman SL, Stewart S, Whitewell J, Langer B, Jeejeebhoy KN. (1982a). Nutritional Assessment. A comparison of clinical judgement and objective measurements. New England Journal of Medicine 306: 969–972.

Baker JP, Detsky AS, Whitewell J, Langer B, Jeejeebhoy KN. (1982b). A comparison of the predictive value of nutritional assessment techniques. Human Nutrition: Clinical Nutrition 36C: 233–241.

Blackburn GL, Bistrian BR, Maini BS, Schlamm HT, Smith MF. (1977). Nutritional and metabolic assessment of the hospitalized patient. Journal of Parenteral and Enteral Nutrition 1: 11–22.

Bozzetti F. (1987). Nutritional assessment from the perspective of a clinician. Journal of Parenteral and Enteral Nutrition 11: 115S–121S.

Buzby GP, Mullen JL, Matthews DC, Hobbs CL, Rosato EF. (1980). Prognostic nutritional index in gastrointestinal surgery. American Journal of Surgeons 39: 160–167.

Cerra FB, Siegel JH, Border JR, Peters DM, McMenamy RR. (1979). Correlations between metabolic and cardiopulmonary measurements in patients after trauma, general surgery, and sepsis. Journal of Trauma 19: 621–629.

Chatterjee S, Price B. (1977). Regression Analysis by Example. John Wiley and Sons, New York.

Collins JP, McCarthy ID, Hill GL. (1979). Assessment of protein nutriture in surgical patients — the value of anthropometrics. American Journal of Clinical Nutrition 32: 1527–1530.

Dempsey DT, Mullen JL. (1987). Prognostic value of nutritional indices. Journal of Parenteral and Enteral Nutrition 11: 109S–114S.

Detsky AS, Baker JP, Mendelson RA, Wolman SL, Wesson DE, Jeejeebhoy KN. (1984). Evaluating the accuracy of nutritional assessment techniques applied to hospitalized patients: methodology and comparisons. Journal of Parenteral and Enteral Nutrition 8: 53-159.

Detsky AS, McLaughlin JR, Baker JP, Johnston N, Whittaker S, Mendelson RA, Jeejeebhoy KN. (1987). What is subjective global assessment of nutritional status? Journal of Parenteral and Enteral Nutrition 11: 8–13.

Golden MHN, Harland PSEG, Golden BE, Jackson AA. (1978). Zinc and immune competence in protein-energy malnutrition. Lancet 1: 1226–1228.

Harvey KB, Lyle L, Moldawer LL, Bistrian BR, Blackburn GL. (1981). Biological measures for the formulation of a hospital prognostic index. American Journal of Clinical Nutrition 34: 2013–2022.

Hooley R. (1986). The nutrition history and physical assessment. In: Krey SH, Murray RL (eds). Dynamics of Nutrition Support. Assessment, Implementation, Evaluation. Appleton-Century-Crofts, Norwalk, Connecticut, pp. 53-81.

Jones TN, Moore EE, Van Way CW. (1983). Factors influencing nutritional assessment in abdominal trauma patients. Journal of Parenteral and Enteral Nutrition 7: 115–116.

Kaminski MV Jr, Fitzgerald MJ, Murphy RJ, Pagast P, Hoppe MC, Winborn AL, Pluta J. (1977). Correlation of mortality with serum transferrin and anergy. Journal of Parenteral and Enteral Nutrition 1: 27 (Abstract).

MacLean LD, Meakins JL, Taguchi K, Buignan JP, Phillon KS, Gordon J. (1975). Host resistance in sepsis and trauma. Annals of Surgery 182: 207–217.

Meakins JL, Pietsch JB, Bubenick O, Kelly R, Rode H, Gordon J, MacLean LD. (1977). Delayed hypersensitivity: indicator of acquired failure of host defenses in sepsis and trauma. Annals of Surgery 186: 241–250.

Mullen JL. (1981). Nutritional assessment: its role in nutritional and metabolic support. Clinical Consultations in Nutritional Support. 1: 3–9.

Mullen JL, Buzby GP, Matthews DC, Smale BF, Rosato EF. (1980). Reduction of operative morbidity and mortality by combined preoperative and postoperative nutritional support. Annals of Surgery 192: 604–613.

Mullen JM, Brenner U, Dienst C, Brenner U, Pichlmai H. (1982). Preoperative parenteral feeding in patients with gastrointestinal carcinoma. Lancet 1: 68–71.

Mullen JL, Buzby GP, Waldman MT, Gertner MH, Hobbs CL, Rosato EF. (1979). Prediction of operative morbidity and mortality by preoperative nutritional assessment. Surgical Forum 30: 80–82.

Nazari S, Cominciolli V, Dionigi R, Comodi I, Dionigi P, Capelo A, Bonoldi AP, Bonacasa R, Cozzi M. (1981). Cluster analysis of nutritional and immunological indicators for identification of high-risk surgical patients. Journal of Parenteral and Enteral Nutrition 5: 307–316.

Pettigrew RA, Charlesworth PM, Formilo RW, Hill GL. (1984). Assessment of nutritional depletion and immune competence: a comparison of clinical examination and objective measurements. Journal of Parenteral and Enteral Nutrition 8: 21–24.

Shetty DS, Jung RT, Watrasiewicz KE, James WPT. (1979). Rapid-turnover transport proteins: an index of subclinical protein-energy. Lancet 2: 230–232.

Appendix A

FOOD BALANCE SHEET

Metric tons unless otherwise specified

Population _____

Date _____

Commodity	Domestic Production	Change in Stocks	Foreign Trade		Gross Supplies	Utilization						Per Capita Daily Availability		
			Gross Ex-ports	Gross Im-ports		Seed	Feed	Ind. Non-food	Waste	Proces-sing Loss	Available for Human Consumption	Grams	Calories	Protein (grams)

Appendix A2.1: Forms for calculating a national food balance. From Food and Agriculture Organization of the United Nations (1980) with permission.

σ_a^2/σ_r^2	Number of Measurements per Subject										
	1	2	3	4	5	6	7	8	10	12	14
0.00	1.00	1.00	1.00	1.00	1.00	1.00	1.00	1.00	1.00	1.00	1.00
0.25	0.89	0.94	0.96	0.97	0.98	0.98	0.98	0.98	0.99	0.99	0.99
0.50	0.82	0.89	0.93	0.94	0.95	0.96	0.97	0.97	0.98	0.98	0.98
1.00	0.71	0.82	0.87	0.89	0.91	0.93	0.94	0.94	0.95	0.96	0.97
1.50	0.63	0.76	0.82	0.85	0.88	0.89	0.91	0.92	0.93	0.94	0.95
2.00	0.58	0.71	0.77	0.82	0.85	0.87	0.88	0.89	0.91	0.93	0.94
2.50	0.53	0.67	0.74	0.78	0.82	0.84	0.86	0.87	0.89	0.91	0.92
3.00	0.50	0.63	0.71	0.76	0.79	0.82	0.84	0.85	0.88	0.89	0.91
3.50	0.47	0.60	0.68	0.73	0.77	0.79	0.82	0.83	0.86	0.88	0.89
4.00	0.45	0.58	0.65	0.71	0.75	0.77	0.80	0.82	0.85	0.87	0.88
4.50	0.43	0.55	0.63	0.69	0.73	0.76	0.78	0.80	0.83	0.85	0.87
5.00	0.41	0.53	0.61	0.67	0.71	0.74	0.76	0.78	0.82	0.84	0.86

Appendix A6.1: Attenuation factors for simple correlation coefficients. (σ_a^2 = intra-subject variation, σ_r^2 = inter-subject variation.) For example, if the ratio of intra- to inter-subject variances for a given nutrient is 2.5, and three twenty-four-hour recalls are used to estimate the intake, the observed correlation coefficient between the estimated intake and a biochemical measurement is 74% of the true correlation. From Anderson (1986). Guidelines for Use of Dietary Data. Life Sciences Research Office, Federation of American Societies for Experimental Biology.

σ_a^2/σ_r^2	Number of Measurements per Subject										
	1	2	3	4	5	6	7	8	10	12	14
0.00	1.00	1.00	1.00	1.00	1.00	1.00	1.00	1.00	1.00	1.00	1.00
0.25	0.80	0.89	0.92	0.94	0.95	0.96	0.97	0.97	0.98	0.98	0.98
0.50	0.67	0.80	0.86	0.89	0.91	0.92	0.93	0.94	0.95	0.96	0.97
1.00	0.50	0.67	0.75	0.80	0.83	0.86	0.88	0.89	0.91	0.92	0.93
1.50	0.40	0.57	0.67	0.73	0.77	0.80	0.82	0.84	0.87	0.89	0.90
2.00	0.33	0.50	0.60	0.67	0.71	0.75	0.78	0.80	0.83	0.86	0.88
2.50	0.29	0.44	0.55	0.62	0.67	0.71	0.74	0.76	0.80	0.83	0.85
3.00	0.25	0.40	0.50	0.57	0.63	0.67	0.70	0.73	0.77	0.80	0.82
3.50	0.22	0.36	0.46	0.53	0.59	0.63	0.67	0.70	0.74	0.77	0.80
4.00	0.20	0.33	0.43	0.50	0.56	0.60	0.64	0.67	0.71	0.75	0.78
4.50	0.18	0.31	0.40	0.47	0.53	0.57	0.61	0.64	0.69	0.73	0.76
5.00	0.17	0.29	0.38	0.44	0.50	0.55	0.58	0.62	0.67	0.71	0.74

Appendix A6.2: Attenuation factors for simple linear regression coefficients (σ_a^2 = intra-subject variation, σ_r^2 = inter-subject variation). For example, if the ratio of the intra- to inter-subject variance is equal to 2.0, and three measurements are taken of the dietary intake, then the regression coefficient of a biological variable on the estimated value of the dietary factor is 60% of the true coefficient. From Anderson (1986). Guidelines for Use of Dietary Data. Life Sciences Research Office, Federation of American Societies for Experimental Biology.

Age	Sex	Weight (kg)	Protein (g/d)[c]	Ca (mg/d)	Mg (mg/d)	Minerals Fe (mg/d)	I (μg/d)	Zn (mg/d)
Months								
0–2	Both	4.5	11[d]	350	30	0.4[e]	25	2[f]
3–5	Both	7.0	14[d]	350	40	5.0	35	3
6–8	Both	8.5	17[d]	400	50	7.0	40	3
9–11	Both	9.5	18	400	50	7.0	45	3
Years								
1	Both	11	19	500	55	6	55	4
2–3	Both	14	22	500	70	6	65	4
4–6	Both	18	26	600	90	6	85	5
7–9	M	25	30	700	110	7	110	6
7–9	F	25	30	700	110	7	95	6
10–12	M	34	38	900	150	10	125	7
10–12	F	36	40	1000	160	10	110	7
13–15	M	50	50	1100	210	12	160	9
13–15	F	48	42	800	200	13	160	8
16–18	M	62	55	900	250	10	160	9
16–18	F	53	43	700	215	14	160	8
19–24	M	71	58	800	240	8	160	9
19–24	F	58	43	700	200	14	160	8
25–49	M	74	61	800	250	8	160	9
25–49	F	59	44	700	200	14[g]	160	8
50–74	M	73	60	800	250	8	160	9
50–74	F	63	47	800	210	7	160	8
75+	M	69	57	800	230	8	160	9
75+	F	64	47	800	220	7	160	8
Pregnancy (additional)								
1st Trimester			15	500	15	6	25	0
2nd Trimester			20	500	20	6	25	1
3rd Trimester			25	500	25	6	25	2
Lactation (additional)			20	500	80	0	50	6

Appendix A8.1: Recommended Nutrient Intakes for Canadians [a,b] — Protein and Minerals. [a] Recommended intakes of energy and of certain nutrients are not listed because of the nature of the variables upon which they are based. [b] Recommended intakes during periods of growth are taken as appropriate for individuals representative of the mid-point in each age group. All recommended intakes are designed to cover individual variations in essentially all of a healthy population subsisting upon a variety of common foods available in Canada. [c] The primary units are grams per kilogram of body weight. The figures shown here are only examples. [d] Assumption that the protein is from breast milk or is of the same biological value as that of breast milk and that between 3 and 9 months adjustment for the quality of the protein is made. [e] It is assumed that breast milk is the source of iron up to 2 months of age. [f] Based on the assumption that breast milk is the source of zinc for the first 2 months. [g] After the menopause the recommended intake is 7 mg/day. From Health and Welfare Canada (1983). Reproduced with permission of the Minister of Supply and Services Canada.

Age	Sex	Weight (kg)	Fat-soluble Vitamins			Water-soluble Vitamins		
			Vit. A (RE/d)[b]	Vit. D (μg/d)[c]	Vit. E (mg/d)[d]	Vit. C (mg/d)	Folacin (μg/d)[e]	Vit. B-12 (μg/d)
Months								
0–2	Both	4.5	400	10.0	3	20	50	0.3
3–5	Both	7.0	400	10.0	3	20	50	0.3
6–8	Both	8.5	400	10.0	3	20	50	0.3
9–11	Both	9.5	400	10.0	3	20	55	0.3
Years								
1	Both	11	400	10.0	3	20	65	0.3
2–3	Both	14	400	5.0	4	20	80	0.4
4–6	Both	18	500	5.0	5	25	90	0.5
7–9	M	25	700	2.5	7	35	125	0.8
7–9	F	25	700	2.5	6	30	125	0.8
10–12	M	34	800	2.5	8	40	170	1.0
10–12	F	36	800	2.5	7	40	180	1.0
13–15	M	50	900	2.5	9	50	150	1.5
13–15	F	48	800	2.5	7	45	145	1.5
16–18	M	62	1000	2.5	10	55	185	1.9
16–18	F	53	800	2.5	7	45	160	1.9
19–24	M	71	1000	2.5	10	60	210	2.0
19–24	F	58	800	2.5	7	45	175	2.0
25–49	M	74	1000	2.5	9	60	220	2.0
25–49	F	59	800	2.5	6	45	175	2.0
50–74	M	73	1000	2.5	7	60	220	2.0
50–74	F	63	800	2.5	6	45	190	2.0
75+	M	69	1000	2.5	6	60	205	2.0
75+	F	64	800	2.5	5	45	190	2.0
Pregnancy (additional)								
1st Trimester			100	2.5	2	0	305	1.0
2nd Trimester			100	2.5	2	20	305	1.0
3rd Trimester			100	2.5	2	20	305	1.0
Lactation (additional)			400	2.5	3	30	120	0.5

Appendix A8.2: Recommended Nutrient Intakes for Canadians[a] — Vitamins. For nutrients not shown, the following amounts are recommended: thiamin, 0.4 mg/1000 kcal (0.48 mg/5000 kJ); riboflavin, 0.5 mg/1000 kcal (0.6 mg/5000 kJ); niacin, 7.2 NE/1000 kcal (8.6 NE/5000 kJ); vitamin B-6, 15 μg, as pyridoxine, per gram of protein; phosphorus, same as calcium. [a] Recommended intakes during periods of growth are taken as appropriate for individuals representative of the mid-point in each age group. All recommended intakes are designed to cover individual variations in essentially all of a healthy population subsisting upon a variety of common foods available in Canada. [b] One retinol equivalent (RE) corresponds to the biological activity of 1 μg of retinol, 6 μg of β-carotene or 12 μg of other carotenes. [c] Expressed as cholecalciferol or ergocalciferol. [d] Expressed as d-α-tocopherol equivalents, relative to which β and γ tocopherol and α-tocotrienol have activities of 0.5, 0.1 and 0.3 respectively. [e] Expressed as total folate. From Health and Welfare Canada (1983). Reproduced with permission of the Minister of Supply and Services Canada.

Age (yr)	Wt. (kg)	Ht. (cm)	Protein (g/d)	Minerals					
				Ca (mg/d)	P (mg/d)	Mg (mg/d)	Fe (mg/d)	Zn (mg/d)	I (μg/d)
Infants									
0–0.5	6	60	kg×2.2	360	240	50	10	3	40
0.5–1.0	9	71	kg×2.0	540	360	70	15	5	50
Children									
1–3	13	90	23	800	800	150	15	10	70
4–6	20	112	30	800	800	200	10	10	90
7–10	28	132	34	800	800	250	10	10	120
Males									
11–14	45	157	45	1200	1200	350	18	15	150
15–18	66	176	56	1200	1200	400	18	15	150
19–22	70	177	56	800	800	350	10	15	150
23–50	70	178	56	800	800	350	10	15	150
51+	70	178	56	800	800	350	10	15	150
Females									
11–14	46	157	46	1200	1200	300	18	15	150
15–18	55	163	46	1200	1200	300	18	15	150
19–22	55	163	44	800	800	300	18	15	150
23–50	55	163	44	800	800	300	18	15	150
51+	55	163	44	800	800	300	10	15	150
Pregnant (additional)			30	400	400	150	b	5	25
Lactating (additional)			20	400	400	150	b	10	50

Appendix A8.3: Recommended Daily Dietary Allowances for Protein and Minerals [a], Revised 1980. Designed for the maintenance of good nutrition of practically all healthy people in the U.S.A. [a] The allowances are intended to provide for individual variations among most normal persons as they live in the United States under usual environmental stresses. Diets should be based on a variety of common foods in order to provide other nutrients for which human requirements have been less well defined. [b] The increased requirement during pregnancy cannot be met by the iron content of habitual American diets nor by the existing iron stores of many women; therefore the use of 30–60 mg of supplemental iron is recommended. Iron needs during lactation are not substantially different from those of nonpregnant women, but continued supplementation of the mother for 2–3 months after parturition is advisable in order to replenish stores depleted by pregnancy. From: Food and Nutrition Board, Committee on Dietary Allowances (1980). Reproduced with permission of the National Academy Press, Washington, D.C.

Age (yr)	Wt. (kg)	Ht. (cm)	Fat-soluble Vitamins			Water-soluble Vitamins						
			Vit. A [c] (μg RE)	Vit. D [d] (μg)	Vit. E [e] (mg)	Vit. C (mg)	Thiamin (mg)	Riboflavin (mg)	Niacin [f] (NE)	Vit. B-6 (mg)	Folacin [g] (μg)	Vit. B-12 (μg)
Infants												
0–0.5	6	60	420	10	3	35	0.3	0.4	6	0.3	30	0.5 [h]
0.5–1.0	9	71	400	10	4	35	0.5	0.6	8	0.6	45	1.5
Children												
1–3	13	90	400	10	5	45	0.7	0.8	9	0.9	100	2.0
4–6	20	112	500	10	6	45	0.9	1.0	11	1.3	200	2.5
7–10	28	132	700	10	7	45	1.2	1.4	16	1.6	300	3.0
Males												
11–14	45	157	1000	10	8	50	1.4	1.6	18	1.8	400	3.0
15–18	66	176	1000	10	10	60	1.4	1.7	18	2.0	400	3.0
19–22	70	177	1000	7.5	10	60	1.5	1.7	19	2.2	400	3.0
23–50	70	178	1000	5	10	60	1.4	1.6	18	2.2	400	3.0
51+	70	178	1000	5	10	60	1.2	1.4	16	2.2	400	3.0
Females												
11–14	46	157	800	10	8	50	1.1	1.3	15	1.8	400	3.0
15–18	55	163	800	10	8	60	1.1	1.3	14	2.0	400	3.0
19–22	55	163	800	7.5	8	60	1.1	1.3	14	2.0	400	3.0
23–50	55	163	800	5	8	60	1.0	1.2	13	2.0	400	3.0
51+	55	163	800	5	8	60	1.0	1.2	13	2.0	400	3.0
Pregnant (additional)			200	5	2	20	0.4	0.3	2	0.6	400	1.0
Lactating (additional)			400	5	3	40	0.5	0.5	5	0.5	100	1.0

Appendix A8.4: Recommended Daily Dietary Allowances for Vitamins, Revised 1980. [c] retinol equivalent. 1 retinol equivalent = 1 μg retinol or 6 μg β-carotene. [d] As cholecalciferol. 10 μg cholecalciferol = 400 IU of vitamin D. [e] α-tocopherol equivalents. 1 mg d-α tocopherol = 1 α-TE. [f] 1 NE (niacin equivalent) is equal to 1 mg of niacin or 60 mg of dietary tryptophan. [g] The folacin allowances refer to dietary sources as determined by *Lactobacillus casei* assay after treatment with enzymes (conjugases) to make polyglutamyl forms of the vitamin available to the test organism. [h] The recommended dietary allowance for vitamin B-12 in infants is based on average concentration of the vitamin in human milk. The allowances after weaning are based on energy intakes (as recommended by the American Academy of Pediatrics) and consideration of other factors, such as intestinal absorption. From: Food and Nutrition Board, Committee on Dietary Allowances (1980). Reproduced with permission of the National Academy Press, Washington, D.C.

Age [a] (yrs)	Activity level	Energy [b] (MJ)	(kcal)	Protein [c] (g)	Calcium (g)	Iron (mg)
Boys						
1		5.0	1200	30	600	7
2		5.75	1400	35	600	7
3–4		6.5	1560	39	600	8
5–6		7.25	1740	43	600	10
7–8		8.25	1980	49	600	10
9–11		9.5	2280	57	700	12
12–14		11.0	2640	66	700	12
15–17		12.0	2880	72	600	12
Girls						
1		4.5	1100	27	600	7
2		5.55	1300	32	600	7
3–4		6.25	1500	37	600	8
5–6		7.0	1680	42	600	10
7–8		8.0	1900	47	600	10
9–11		8.5	2050	51	700	12 [d]
12–14		9.0	2150	53	700	12 [d]
15–17		9.0	2150	53	600	12 [d]
Men						
18–34	Sedentary	10.5	2510	63	500	10
	Moderately active	12.0	2900	72	500	10
	Very active	14.0	3350	84	500	10
35–64	Sedentary	10.0	2400	60	500	10
	Moderately active	11.5	2750	69	500	10
	Very active	14.0	3350	84	500	10
65–74	Sedentary	10.0	2400	60	500	10
75 +	Sedentary	9.0	2150	54	500	10
Women						
18–54	Most occupations	9.0	2150	54	500	12 [d]
	Very active	10.5	2500	62	500	12 [d]
55–74	Sedentary	8.0	1900	47	500	10
75 +	Sedentary	7.0	1680	42	500	10
	Pregnancy	10.0	2400	60	1200 [e]	13
	Lactation	11.5	2750	69	1200	15

Appendix A8.5: Recommended daily amounts of food energy, protein, calcium and iron for population groups in the United Kingdom. [a] Since the recommendations are average amounts, the figures for each age range represent the amounts recommended at the middle of the range. Within each age range, younger children will need less, and older children more than the amount recommended. [b] Megajoules (10^6 joules). Calculated from the relation 1 kilocalorie = 4.184 kilojoules, i.e., 1 MJ = 240 kilocalories. [c] Recommended amounts have been calculated as 10% of the recommendations for energy. [d] This intake may not be sufficient for 10% of girls and women with large menstrual losses. [e] For the third trimester only. From Department of Health and Social Security (1981). Recommended Intakes of Nutrients for the United Kingdom. Second Impression. Reproduced with the permission of the Controller of Her Majesty's Stationery Office.

Age[a] (yrs)	Activity level	Thia-min (mg)	Ribo-flavin (mg)	Nicotinic acid equiv. (mg)[b]	Vit. C (mg)	Vit. A (μg)[c]	Vit. D (μg)[d]
Boys							
1		0.5	0.6	7	20	300	10
2		0.6	0.7	8	20	300	10
3–4		0.6	0.8	9	20	300	10
5–6		0.7	0.9	10	20	300	–
7–8		0.8	1.0	11	20	400	–
9–11		0.9	1.2	14	25	575	–
12–14		1.1	1.4	16	25	725	–
15–17		1.2	1.7	19	30	750	–
Girls							
1		0.4	0.6	7	20	300	10
2		0.5	0.7	8	20	300	10
3–4		0.6	0.8	9	20	300	10
5–6		0.7	0.9	10	20	300	–
7–8		0.8	1.0	11	20	400	–
9–11		0.8	1.2	14	25	575	–
12–14		0.9	1.4	16	25	725	–
15–17		0.9	1.7	19	30	750	–
Men							
18–34	Sedentary	1.0	1.6	18	30	750	–
	Moderately active	1.2	1.6	18	30	750	–
	Very active	1.3	1.6	18	30	750	–
35–64	Sedentary	1.0	1.6	18	30	750	–
	Moderately active	1.1	1.6	18	30	750	–
	Very active	1.3	1.6	18	30	750	–
65–74	Sedentary	1.0	1.6	18	30	750	–
75 +	Sedentary	0.9	1.6	18	30	750	–
Women							
18–54	Most occupations	0.9	1.3	15	30	750	–
	Very active	1.0	1.3	15	30	750	–
55–74	Sedentary	0.8	1.3	15	30	750	–
75 +	Sedentary	0.7	1.3	15	30	750	–
	Pregnancy	1.0	1.6	18	60	750	10
	Lactation	1.1	1.8	21	60	1200	10

Appendix A8.6: Recommended daily amounts of vitamins for population groups in the United Kingdom. [a] Since the recommendations are average amounts, the figures for each age range represent the amounts recommended at the middle of the range. Within each age range, younger children will need less, and older children more than the amount recommended. [b] 1 nicotinic acid equivalent = 1 mg available nicotinic acid or 60 mg tryptophan. [c] 1 retinol equivalent = 1 μg retinol or 6 μg β-carotene or 12 μg other biologically active carotenoids. [d] No dietary sources may be necessary for children and adults who are sufficiently exposed to sunlight, but during the winter children and adolescents should receive 10 μg (400 IU) daily by supplementation. Adults with inadequate exposure to sunlight, for example those who are housebound, may also need a supplement of 10 μg daily. From Department of Health and Social Security (1981). Recommended Intakes of Nutrients for the United Kingdom. Second Impression. Reproduced with the permission of the Controller of Her Majesty's Stationery Office.

Disclaimer: The information in Appendix A10.1 and A11.1 is provided for the information of readers; it should not be taken as an endorsement by the author or publisher of the listed products, manufacturers, or suppliers. No significance should be attached to the absence from this list of any product, manufacturer, or supplier. A more extensive guide to equipment for nutritional assessment may be obtained from: Nutrition Services Section, Division of Health Assessment and Screening, Illinois Department of Public Health.

- **Portable Length/Stature Measuring Board.** Model: PE-A-1-M-101 Company: Perspective Enterprises, Inc., 7622 Sprinkle Rd., Kalamazoo, Michigan 49001. Tel: (616)-327-0869. Description: Portable board, designed primarily for use in international surveys. Constructed of plywood and hardwood. Weight: approximately 20 pounds.

- **Recumbent Infant Length Board.** Model: PE-RILB-122 (12 inches wide) Company: Perspective Enterprises 7622 Sprinkle Road, Kalamazoo, Michigan 49001. Tel: (616) 327-0869. Description: This length board is constructed of plywood and has a clear plexiglass footboard. Calibration: $1/_{16}$th inch and 0.2 centimeters up to 39 inches and 100 centimeters. Dimension: $43 1/_2$ inch long by 12 inches wide by 8 inches high. Weight: 12 pounds.

- **Infantometer.** Model: 98-702 Company: Pfister Import-Export, Inc., 450 Barell Avenue Carlstadt, New Jersey 07072. Description: This infantometer is specifically designed for post-neonate growth studies. It has a measuring range of 300 mm to 940 mm.

- **Harpenden Portable Stadiometer.** Model: 98-603 Company: Seritex, Inc., 450 Barell Avenue, Carlstadt, New Jersey 07072. Tel: (201) 939-4606. Description: This instrument is a portable form of the 'Harpenden' standard Stadiometer. Range of 850 mm to 2060 mm. Easy to erect, free-standing unit. Measures to the nearest millimeter. Dimensions: Base 120 cm x 36 cm x 7.5 cm. Weight (including base): 20.5 kg.

- **Wall Mounted Measuring Board (Height).** Model: PE-WM-103 Company: Perspective Enterprises 7622 Sprinkle Road, Kalamazoo, Michigan 49001 Tel: (616) 327-0869. Description: This device permanently attaches to the wall and is constructed of $3/_4$ inch laminated wood to prevent warping. Its clear plexiglass sliding head piece is spring-loaded to remain in place. Measures subjects up to 75 inches (190.5 cm). Dimensions: 48 inches by 10 inches wide by $3/_4$ inch thick. Weight: 8 pounds.

- **'Handi-Stat' Measuring Device Kit.** Model: PE-RA-108 Company: Perspective Enterprises, Inc., 7622 Sprinkle Road, Kalamazoo, Michigan 49001. Tel: (616) 327-0869. Description: Right angle piece with tape. Calibration: $1/_{16}$th inch and millimeters. Weight: 10–12 oz. Suitable for those wishing to manufacture their own measuring equipment.

- **Microtoise Modified Tape Measure.** Company: CMS Weighing Equipment Ltd., 18 Camden High Street, London, N.W.1 UK. Tel: (01)-387 2060.

Appendix A10.1: Anthropometric equipment — length and height

- **Portable Infant Weighing Scale.** Model: MP 25: Infant weighing pack 800 Company: CMS Weighing Equipment Ltd., 18 Camden High Street, London, N.W.1. UK. Tel: (01)-387 2060, or ITAC Corporation, P.O. Box 1742, Silver Springs, Maryland 20902. Tel: (301) 593-8007. Weight: 1.5 kg net weight.

- **Pediatric Scale.** Model No. 62449 (kg) Company: American Hospital Supply, 1250 Waukegan Road, McGaw Park, Illinois 60085. Tel: 1-800-322-6870; (312) 689-8800. Calibration 20 gram increments.

- **Detector, Dual Reading Scale.** Model No. 62408-WHI Company: American Hospital Supply, 1250 Waukegan Road, McGaw Park, Illinois 60085. Tel: 1-800-322-6870; (312) 689-8800. Capacity 160 kilograms.

- **Standard Weights for Calibration.** Company: Ricelake Bearing Co., 230 W. Coleman St., Ricelake, Wisconsin 54868. Tel: 1-800-472-6703. Weights 5, 10, 20, 25, 30, 50 pounds. (recommended to use two smaller weights rather than one large weight.)

- **Metropolitan Height and Weight Tables.** Company: Metropolitan Life Insurance Company, Health and Safety Education Division, One Madison Ave., New York, N.Y., 10010.

Appendix A10.1: (cont.) Anthropometric equipment — weight

- **Harpenden Skinfold Caliper.** Company: Hemco Corporation 455 Douglas Ave, Holland, Michigan 49423. Tel: (616) 396-4604 or CMS Weighing Equipment Ltd., 18 Camden High Street, London N.W.1, UK. Tel: (01)-387 2060.

- **Lange Skinfold Caliper.** Company: Cambridge Scientific Industries, Inc., P.O. Box 265, Cambridge, Maryland 21613. Tel: (301) 376-3124.

- **Holtain Skinfold Caliper.** Company: Holtain Ltd., Crosswell, Crymych, Dyfed SA41 3UF, UK. Tel: (023) 979656.

- **McGaw Skinfold Caliper.** Company: Ross Laboratories, Division of Abbott Laboratories, Columbus, Ohio 43216. Tel: (614) 227-3706.

- **Elbow breadth Frame Gauge.** Company: Metropolitan Life Insurance Company, Health and Safety Education Division, One Madison Ave., New York, N.Y., 10010.

- **Insertion Circumference Tape.** Company: Ross Laboratories, Division of Abbott Laboratories, Columbus, Ohio 43216. Tel: (614) 227-3706. Measures up to 22 inches (56 cm). Can be used for arm and head circumference.

Appendix A11.1: Skinfold calipers and insertion tapes

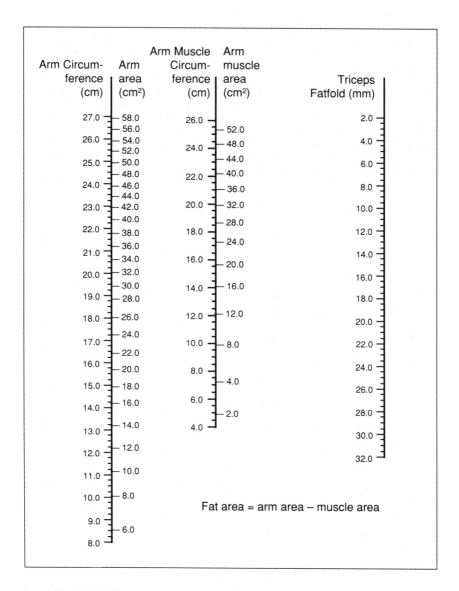

Appendix A11.2: Nomogram for the determination of arm muscle circumference and arm muscle area for children. From Gurney and Jelliffe (1973). © Am. J. Clin. Nutr. American Society for Clinical Nutrition.

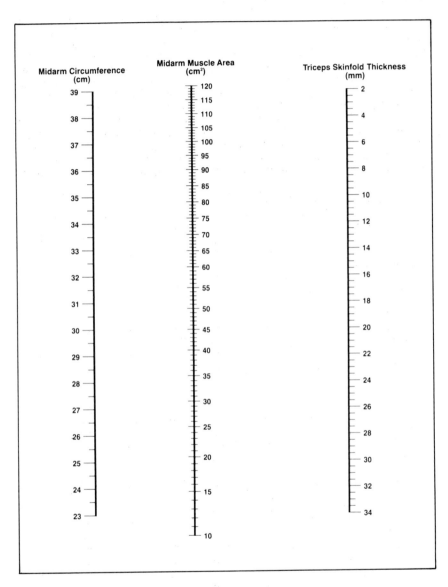

Appendix A11.3: Nomogram for the determination of arm muscle area for adults. Adapted from Gurney and Jelliffe (1973). © Am. J. Clin. Nutr. American Society for Clinical Nutrition.

Skinfold		17–19	20–29	Age (yrs) 30–39	40–49	50+	17–72
				Males			
Biceps	c	1.1066	1.1015	1.0781	1.0829	1.0833	1.0997
	m	0.0686	0.0616	0.0396	0.0508	0.0617	0.0659
Triceps	c	1.1252	1.1131	1.0834	1.1041	1.1027	1.1143
	m	0.0625	0.0530	0.0361	0.0609	0.0662	0.0618
Subscapular	c	1.1312	1.1360	1.0978	1.1246	1.1334	1.1369
	m	0.0670	0.0700	0.0416	0.0686	0.0760	0.0741
Suprailiac	c	1.1092	1.1117	1.1047	1.1029	1.1193	1.1171
	m	0.0420	0.0431	0.0432	0.0483	0.0652	0.0530
Biceps + Triceps	c	1.1423	1.1307	1.0995	1.1174	1.1185	1.1356
	m	0.0687	0.0603	0.0431	0.0614	0.0683	0.0700
Biceps + Subscapular	c	1.1457	1.1469	1.0753	1.1341	1.1427	1.1498
	m	0.0707	0.0709	0.0445	0.0680	0.0762	0.0759
Biceps + Suprailiac	c	1.1247	1.1259	1.1174	1.1171	1.1307	1.1331
	m	0.0501	0.0502	0.0486	0.0539	0.0678	0.0601

Skinfold		16–19	20–29	Age (yrs) 30–39	40–49	50+	16–68
				Females			
Biceps	c	1.0889	1.0903	1.0794	1.0736	1.0682	1.0871
	m	0.0553	0.0601	0.0511	0.0492	0.0510	0.0593
Triceps	c	1.1159	1.1319	1.1176	1.1121	1.1160	1.1278
	m	0.0648	0.0776	0.0686	0.0691	0.0762	0.0775
Subscapular	c	1.1081	1.1184	1.0979	1.0860	1.0899	1.1100
	m	0.0621	0.0716	0.0567	0.0505	0.0590	0.0669
Suprailiac	c	1.0931	1.0923	1.0860	1.0691	1.0656	1.0884
	m	0.0470	0.0509	0.0497	0.0407	0.0419	0.0514
Biceps + Triceps	c	1.1290	1.1398	1.1243	1.1230	1.1226	1.1362
	m	0.0657	0.0738	0.0646	0.0672	0.0710	0.0740
Biceps + Subscapular	c	1.1241	1.1314	1.1120	1.1031	1.1029	1.1245
	m	0.0643	0.0706	0.0581	0.0549	0.0592	0.0674
Biceps + Suprailiac	c	1.1113	1.1112	1.1020	1.0921	1.0857	1.1090
	m	0.0537	0.0568	0.0528	0.0494	0.0490	0.0577

Appendix A11.4: Parameters for linear regression equations for the estimation of body density $\times$ $10^3\,\text{kg/m}^3$ from the logarithm of the skinfold thickness: density = $c - m \times$ log skinfold. From Durnin JVGA, Womersley J. (1974). Body fat assessed from total body density and its estimation from skinfold thickness: measurements on 481 men and women aged 16 to 72 years. British Journal of Nutrition 32: 77–97. Reproduced with permission of Cambridge University Press.

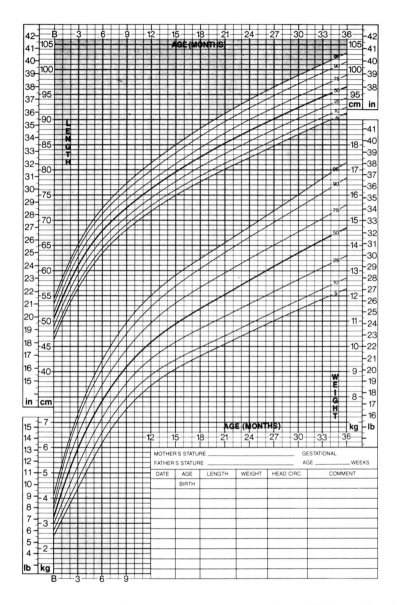

Appendix A12.1: Physical growth NCHS percentiles - Boys: Birth to thirty-six months — Weight for age and length for age. Adapted from Hamill PVV, Drizd TA, Johnson CL, Reed RB, Roche AF, Moore WM. (1979). Physical growth: National Center for Health Statistics percentiles. Am. J. Clin. Nutr. 32: 607–629. Data from the National Center for Health Statistics (NCHS) Hyattsville, Maryland. Reproduced with permission of Ross Laboratories.

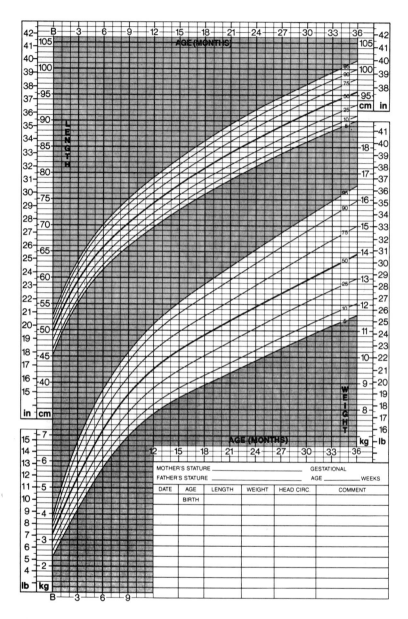

Appendix A12.2: Physical growth NCHS percentiles—Girls: Birth to thirty-six months—weight for age and length for age. Adapted from Hamill PVV, Drizd TA, Johnson CL, Reed RB, Roche AF, Moore WM. (1979). Physical growth: National Center for Health Statistics percentiles. Am. J. Clin. Nutr. 32: 607–629. Data from the National Center for Health Statistics (NCHS) Hyattsville, Maryland. Reproduced with permission of Ross Laboratories.

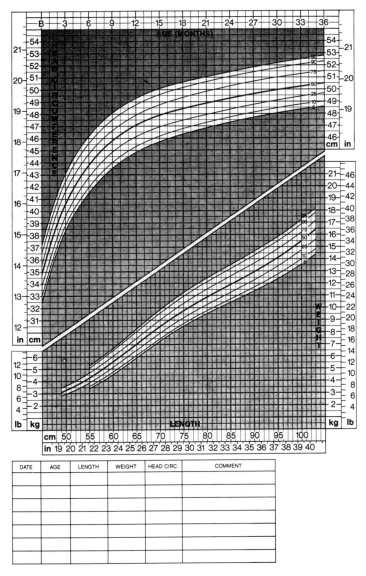

DATE	AGE	LENGTH	WEIGHT	HEAD CIRC.	COMMENT

Appendix A12.3: Physical growth NCHS percentiles—Boys: Birth to thirty-six months—head circumference for age and weight for length. Adapted from Hamill PVV, Drizd TA, Johnson CL, Reed RB, Roche AF, Moore WM. (1979). Physical growth: National Center for Health Statistics percentiles. Am. J. Clin. Nutr. 32: 607–629. Data from the National Center for Health Statistics (NCHS) Hyattsville, Maryland. Reproduced with permission of Ross Laboratories.

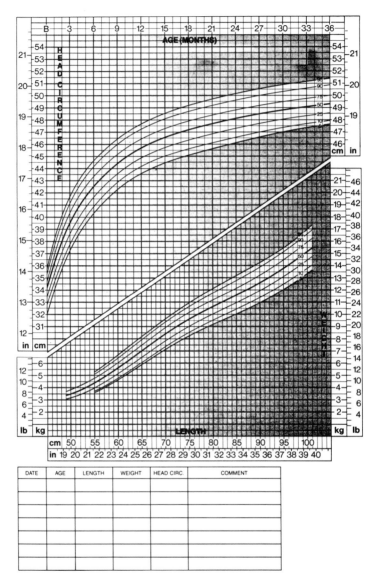

DATE	AGE	LENGTH	WEIGHT	HEAD CIRC.	COMMENT

Appendix A12.4: Physical growth NCHS percentiles — Girls: Birth to thirty-six months — head circumference for age and weight for length. Adapted from Hamill PVV, Drizd TA, Johnson CL, Reed RB, Roche AF, Moore WM. (1979). Physical growth: National Center for Health Statistics percentiles. Am. J. Clin. Nutr. 32: 607–629. Data from the National Center for Health Statistics (NCHS) Hyattsville, Maryland. Reproduced with permission of Ross Laboratories.

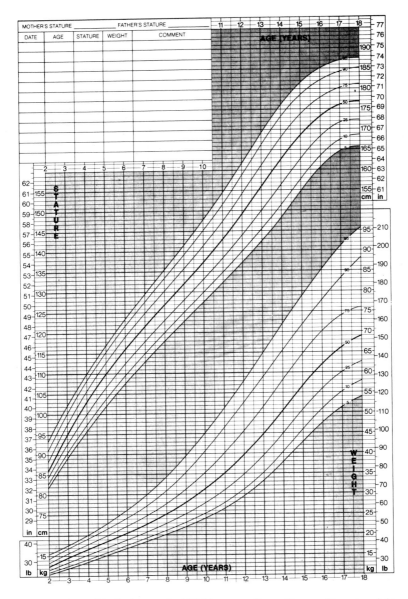

Appendix A12.5: Physical growth NCHS percentiles—Boys: Two to eighteen years—stature for age and weight for age. Adapted from Hamill PVV, Drizd TA, Johnson CL, Reed RB, Roche AF, Moore WM. (1979). Physical growth: National Center for Health Statistics percentiles. Am. J. Clin. Nutr. 32: 607–629. Data from the National Center for Health Statistics (NCHS) Hyattsville, Maryland. Reproduced with permission of Ross Laboratories.

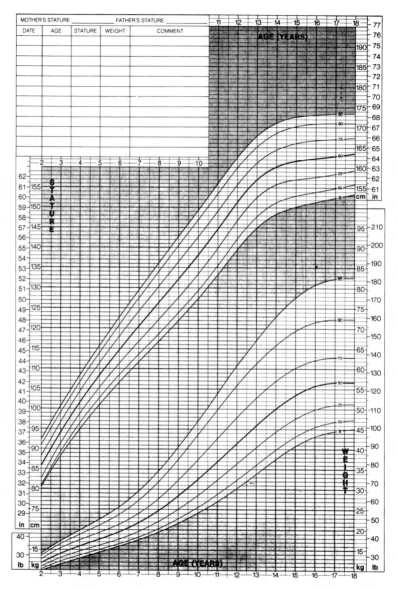

Appendix A12.6: Physical growth NCHS percentiles—Girls: Two to eighteen years—stature for age and weight for age. Adapted from Hamill PVV, Drizd TA, Johnson CL, Reed RB, Roche AF, Moore WM. (1979). Physical growth: National Center for Health Statistics percentiles. Am. J. Clin. Nutr. 32: 607–629. Data from the National Center for Health Statistics (NCHS) Hyattsville, Maryland. Reproduced with permission of Ross Laboratories.

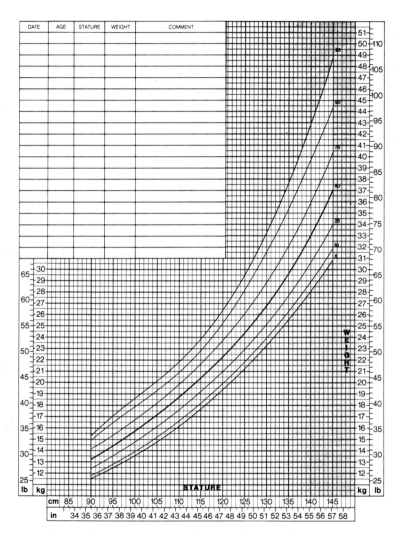

Appendix A12.7: Physical growth NCHS percentiles — Boys: Prepubescent — weight for stature. Adapted from Hamill PVV, Drizd TA, Johnson CL, Reed RB, Roche AF, Moore WM. (1979). Physical growth: National Center for Health Statistics percentiles. Am. J. Clin. Nutr. 32: 607–629. Data from the National Center for Health Statistics (NCHS) Hyattsville, Maryland. Reproduced with permission of Ross Laboratories.

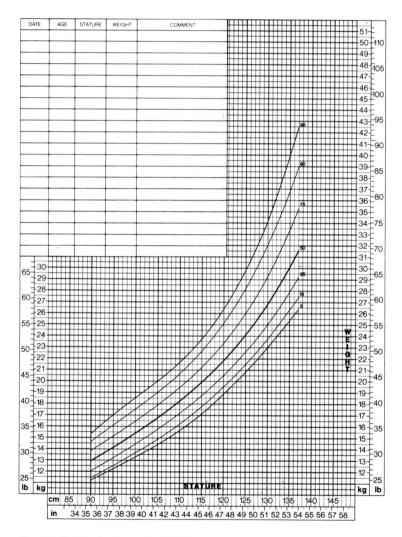

Appendix A12.8: Physical growth NCHS percentiles — Girls: Prepubescent — weight for stature. Adapted from Hamill PVV, Drizd TA, Johnson CL, Reed RB, Roche AF, Moore WM. (1979). Physical growth: National Center for Health Statistics percentiles. Am. J. Clin. Nutr. 32: 607–629. Data from the National Center for Health Statistics (NCHS) Hyattsville, Maryland. Reproduced with permission of Ross Laboratories.

Range	Constant	Linear	Quadratic	Cubic
	Fels portion of reference curves			
Length for age				
0.0–9.0 mo	46.18240	4.012570	−0.2554490	0.0078997 cm
9.0–24.0 mo	67.36300	1.334100	−0.0421583	0.0010158 cm
24.0–36.0 mo	81.31730	0.755023	0.0035529	−0.0005901 cm
Weight for age				
0.0–6.0 mo	2.49740	0.462056	0.0481125	−0.0045889 kg
6.0–18.0 mo	6.01058	0.543800	−0.0344885	0.0009736 kg
18.0–36.0 mo	9.25227	0.136684	0.0005621	−0.0000236 kg
Weight for length				
49.0–72.0 cm	2.50836	0.068177	0.0126871	−0.0002594 kg
72.0–90.0 cm	7.63160	0.240094	−0.0052124	0.0001500 kg
90.0–103.0 cm	11.13930	0.198252	0.0028879	−0.0000207 kg
	NCHS portion of reference curves			
Stature for age				
24.0–138.0 mo	79.60170	0.725005	−0.0039456	0.0000149 cm
138.0–168.0 mo	133.05600	0.406485	0.0011516	0.0000272 cm
168.0–204.0 mo	147.02200	0.549084	0.0036017	−0.0001626 cm
204.0–215.99 mo	163.87000	0.176161	−0.0139606	0.0002574 cm
Weight for age				
24.0–96.0 mo	10.22710	0.110605	0.0005027	−0.0000036 kg
96.0–156.0 mo	19.46770	0.127619	−0.0002664	0.0000234 kg
156.0–204.0 mo	31.22840	0.348780	0.0039524	−0.0000675 kg
204.0–215.99 mo	49.61660	0.261986	−0.0057606	0.0000334 kg
Weight for stature				
55.0–80.0 cm	2.88221	0.311757	−0.0033999	0.0000333 kg
80.0–115.0 cm	9.07104	0.204144	−0.0009046	0.0000465 kg
115.0–145.0 cm	17.10380	0.311893	0.0039831	−0.0000277 kg

Appendix A12.9: Polynomial equations for normalized growth reference curves. I. Equations for males: 3rd percentile. Data from Dibley et al. (1987). © Am. J. Clin. Nutr. American Society for Clinical Nutrition.

Range	Constant	Linear	Quadratic	Cubic
	Fels portion of reference curves			
Length for age				
0.0–9.0 mo	50.48490	4.381550	−0.3120880	0.0105514 cm
9.0–24.0 mo	72.33180	1.327970	−0.0271990	0.0004485 cm
24.0–36.0 mo	87.64530	0.814752	−0.0070155	0.0000610 cm
Weight for age				
0.0–6.0 mo	3.26804	1.087950	−0.0677657	0.0022657 kg
6.0–18.0 mo	7.84554	0.519450	−0.0269840	0.0007380 kg
18.0–36.0 mo	11.46850	0.190655	−0.0004155	−0.0000134 kg
Weight for length				
49.0–72.0 cm	3.14986	0.148592	0.0094768	−0.0002056 kg
72.0–90.0 cm	9.07905	0.258223	−0.0047102	0.0001330 kg
90.0–103.0 cm	12.97630	0.217885	0.0024692	0.0001044 kg
	NCHS portion of reference curves			
Stature for age				
24.0–138.0 mo	85.59310	0.837795	−0.0053379	0.0000234 cm
138.0–168.0 mo	146.37400	0.532432	0.0026593	−0.0000599 cm
168.0–204.0 mo	163.12200	0.530131	−0.0027360	−0.0000523 cm
204.0–215.99 mo	176.22200	0.129924	−0.0083808	0.0001434 cm
Weight for age				
24.0–96.0 mo	12.34240	0.202445	−0.0011641	0.0000118 kg
96.0–156.0 mo	25.29640	0.218676	0.0013895	0.0000071 kg
156.0–204.0 mo	44.95150	0.462032	0.0026664	−0.0000630 kg
204.0–215.99 mo	66.30610	0.282610	−0.0064044	0.0000620 kg
Weight for stature				
55.0–80.0 cm	4.31260	0.371447	−0.0063312	0.0000877 kg
80.0–115.0 cm	11.01220	0.219333	0.0002466	0.0000313 kg
115.0–145.0 cm	20.33360	0.351685	0.0035349	0.0001044 kg

Appendix A12.10: Polynomial equations for normalized growth reference curves. II. Equations for males: 50th percentile. Data from Dibley et al. (1987). © Am. J. Clin. Nutr. American Society for Clinical Nutrition.

Range	Constant	Linear	Quadratic	Cubic
	Fels portion of reference curves			
Length for age				
0.0–9.0 mo	54.78620	4.752200	−0.3688450	0.0132042 cm
9.0–24.0 mo	77.30550	1.321630	−0.0123304	−0.0001137 cm
24.0–36.0 mo	93.97200	0.874997	−0.0174451	0.0006937 cm
Weight for age				
0.0–6.0 mo	4.20915	1.459100	−0.1242120	0.0054670 kg
6.0–18.0 mo	9.67299	0.558989	−0.0258067	0.0006445 kg
18.0–36.0 mo	13.77840	0.218043	−0.0026054	0.0001068 kg
Weight for length				
49.0–72.0 cm	4.09354	0.188963	0.0087391	−0.0001934 kg
72.0–90.0 cm	10.70900	0.283963	−0.0046087	0.0001132 kg
90.0–103.0 cm	14.98740	0.228093	0.0015048	0.0001335 kg
	NCHS portion of reference curves			
Stature for age				
24.0–138.0 mo	91.57670	0.950895	−0.0067335	0.0000319 cm
138.0–168.0 mo	159.69200	0.658332	0.0041671	−0.0001471 cm
168.0–204.0 mo	179.22200	0.511316	−0.0090677	0.0000578 cm
204.0–215.99 mo	188.57400	0.083111	−0.0028269	0.0000383 cm
Weight for age				
24.0–96.0 mo	15.48740	0.219986	−0.0008413	0.0000190 kg
96.0–156.0 mo	34.05010	0.394048	0.0032588	−0.0000164 kg
156.0–204.0 mo	65.88070	0.607904	0.0003054	−0.0000378 kg
204.0–215.99 mo	91.58540	0.376078	−0.0051351	−0.0000178 kg
Weight for stature				
55.0–80.0 cm	6.58687	0.352637	−0.0034583	0.0000293 kg
80.0–115.0 cm	13.69970	0.234726	−0.0012581	0.0000890 kg
115.0–145.0 cm	24.18850	0.473620	0.0080837	0.0001033 kg

Appendix A12.11: Polynomial equations for normalized growth reference curves. III. Equations for males: 97th percentile. Data from Dibley et al. (1987). © Am. J. Clin. Nutr. American Society for Clinical Nutrition.

Range	Constant	Linear	Quadratic	Cubic
	Fels portion of reference curves			
Length for age				
0.0–9.0 mo	45.78290	3.673230	−0.2372120	0.0077933 cm
9.0–24.0 mo	65.30910	1.297190	−0.0267922	0.0004660 cm
24.0–36.0 mo	80.31150	0.807980	−0.0058217	−0.0001846 cm
Weight for age				
0.0–6.0 mo	2.30235	0.545715	0.0131161	−0.0022140 kg
6.0–18.0 mo	5.57059	0.463994	−0.0267363	0.0007730 kg
18.0–36.0 mo	8.62425	0.156261	0.0010919	−0.0000898 kg
Weight for length				
49.0–72.0 cm	2.60988	0.063004	0.0115431	0.0002316 kg
72.0–90.0 cm	7.34790	0.226503	−0.0044345	0.0001374 kg
90.0–101.0 cm	10.78920	0.200373	0.0029828	0.0000891 kg
	NCHS portion of reference curves			
Stature for age				
24.0–60.0 mo	78.46090	0.769969	−0.0057907	0.0000299 cm
60.0–132.0 mo	100.07100	0.469370	−0.0025593	0.0000298 cm
132.0–156.0 mo	131.72600	0.564490	0.0038804	−0.0002117 cm
156.0–192.0 mo	144.58200	0.384879	−0.0113642	0.0001323 cm
192.0–215.99 mo	149.88200	0.081058	0.0029247	−0.0000738 cm
Weight-for-age				
24.0–84.0 mo	9.58878	0.162168	−0.0015879	0.0000142 kg
84.0–144.0 mo	16.66390	0.124691	0.0009632	0.0000031 kg
144.0–192.0 mo	28.27710	0.273485	0.0015167	−0.0000370 kg
192.0–215.99 mo	40.80420	0.163173	−0.0038148	0.0000316 kg
Weight for stature				
55.0–85.0 cm	3.03896	0.276098	−0.0022693	0.0000201 kg
85.0–108.0 cm	9.82301	0.194286	−0.0004578	0.0000538 kg
108.0–137.0 cm	14.70370	0.258573	0.0032529	0.0000169 kg

Appendix A12.12: Polynomial equations for normalized growth reference curves. IV. Equations for females: 3rd percentile. Data from Dibley et al. (1987). © Am. J. Clin. Nutr. American Society for Clinical Nutrition.

Range	Constant	Linear	Quadratic	Cubic
	Fels portion of reference curves			
Length for age				
0.0–9.0 mo	49.86440	3.937460	−0.2629990	0.0088478 cm
9.0–24.0 mo	70.44870	1.353500	−0.0241086	0.0003396 cm
24.0–36.0 mo	86.47300	0.859488	−0.0088254	0.0000322 cm
Weight for age				
0.0–6.0 mo	3.22751	0.768817	−0.0124130	−0.0008575 kg
6.0–18.0 mo	7.20834	0.527256	−0.0278471	0.0007522 kg
18.0–36.0 mo	10.82520	0.183875	−0.0007680	0.0000071 kg
Weight for length				
49.0–72.0 cm	3.29545	0.103651	0.0119637	−0.0002558 kg
72.0–90.0 cm	8.89598	0.248036	−0.0056861	0.0001813 kg
90.0–101.0 cm	12.57560	0.219539	0.0041029	−0.0000204 kg
	NCHS portion of reference curves			
Stature for age				
24.0–54.0 mo	84.48720	0.877385	−0.0085419	0.0000727 cm
54.0–132.0 mo	105.08300	0.561061	−0.0020022	0.0000171 cm
132.0–156.0 mo	144.78300	0.560961	0.0020009	−0.0001642 cm
156.0–192.0 mo	157.12800	0.373200	−0.0098243	0.0000982 cm
192.0–215.99 mo	162.41300	0.047711	0.0007829	−0.0000218 cm
Weight for age				
24.0–84.0 mo	11.79630	0.219662	−0.0026279	0.0000293 kg
84.0–144.0 mo	21.84090	0.220578	0.0026431	−0.0000142 kg
144.0–192.0 mo	41.53190	0.384808	0.0000940	−0.0000392 kg
192.0–215.99 mo	55.88760	0.123101	−0.0055462	0.0000702 kg
Weight for stature				
55.0–85.0 cm	4.30208	0.364667	−0.0062945	0.0000836 kg
85.0–108.0 cm	11.83410	0.212702	0.0012290	0.0000202 kg
108.0–137.0 cm	17.62160	0.301222	0.0026197	0.0001213 kg

Appendix A12.13: Polynomial equations for normalized growth reference curves. V. Equations for females: 50th percentile. Data from Dibley et al. (1987). © Am. J. Clin. Nutr. American Society for Clinical Nutrition.

Range	Constant	Linear	Quadratic	Cubic
	Fels portion of reference curves			
Length for age				
0.0–9.0 mo	53.92920	4.211020	−0.2900550	0.0099537 cm
9.0–24.0 mo	75.59030	1.408800	−0.0213041	0.0002101 cm
24.0–36.0 mo	92.63780	0.911461	−0.0118516	0.0002430 cm
Weight for age				
0.0–6.0 mo	3.91945	1.154260	−0.0635733	0.0017658 kg
6.0–18.0 mo	8.93781	0.582092	−0.0317886	0.0009303 kg
18.0–36.0 mo	12.95290	0.221049	0.0017017	−0.0000907 kg
Weight for length				
49.0–72.0 cm	3.93902	0.201926	0.0074638	−0.0001782 kg
72.0–90.0 cm	10.36410	0.262530	−0.0048288	0.0001548 kg
90.0–101.0 cm	14.42780	0.239142	0.0035295	0.0001393 kg
	NCHS portion of reference curves			
Stature for age				
24.0–54.0 mo	90.57840	0.973526	−0.0108372	0.0000110 cm
54.0–132.0 mo	112.99900	0.620169	−0.0009413	0.0000046 cm
132.0–156.0 mo	157.83700	0.557600	0.0001392	−0.0001174 cm
156.0–192.0 mo	169.67600	0.361401	−0.0083141	0.0000649 cm
192.0–215.99 mo	174.93900	0.015085	−0.0013058	0.0000269 cm
Weight for age				
24.0–84.0 mo	14.43850	0.322835	−0.0043837	0.0000540 kg
84.0–144.0 mo	29.69450	0.380152	0.0053389	−0.0000449 kg
144.0–192.0 mo	62.02150	0.535709	−0.0027463	−0.0000206 kg
192.0–215.99 mo	79.12800	0.129558	−0.0057152	0.0000649 kg
Weight for stature				
55.0–85.0 cm	6.58206	0.363970	−0.0060986	0.0000885 kg
85.0–108.0 cm	14.40260	0.237072	0.0018687	0.0000269 kg
108.0–137.0 cm	21.17150	0.365772	0.0037270	0.0003322 kg

Appendix A12.14: Polynomial equations for normalized growth reference curves. VI. Equations for females: 97th percentile. Data from Dibley et al. (1987). © Am. J. Clin. Nutr. American Society for Clinical Nutrition.

Day	Jan	Feb	Mar	Apr	May	Jun	July	Aug	Sept	Oct	Nov	Dec
1	000	085	162	247	329	414	496	581	666	748	833	915
2	003	088	164	249	332	416	499	584	668	751	836	918
3	005	090	167	252	334	419	501	586	671	753	838	921
4	008	093	170	255	337	422	504	589	674	756	841	923
5	011	096	173	258	340	425	507	592	677	759	844	926
6	014	099	175	260	342	427	510	595	679	762	847	929
7	016	101	178	263	345	430	512	597	682	764	849	932
8	019	104	181	266	348	433	515	600	685	767	852	934
9	022	107	184	268	351	436	518	603	688	770	855	937
10	025	110	186	271	353	438	521	605	690	773	858	940
11	027	112	189	274	356	441	523	608	693	775	860	942
12	030	115	192	277	359	444	526	611	696	778	863	945
13	033	118	195	279	362	447	529	614	699	781	866	948
14	036	121	197	282	364	449	532	616	701	784	868	951
15	038	123	200	285	367	452	534	619	704	786	871	953
16	041	126	203	288	370	455	537	622	707	789	874	956
17	044	129	205	290	373	458	540	625	710	792	877	959
18	047	132	208	293	375	460	542	627	712	795	879	962
19	049	134	211	296	378	463	545	630	715	797	882	964
20	052	137	214	299	381	466	548	633	718	800	885	967
21	055	140	216	301	384	468	551	636	721	803	888	970
22	058	142	219	304	386	471	553	638	723	805	890	973
23	060	145	222	307	389	474	556	641	726	808	893	975
24	063	148	225	310	392	477	559	644	729	811	896	978
25	066	151	227	312	395	479	562	647	731	814	899	981
26	068	153	230	315	397	482	564	649	734	816	901	984
27	071	156	233	318	400	485	567	652	737	819	904	986
28	074	159	236	321	403	488	570	655	740	822	907	989
29	077		238	323	405	490	573	658	742	825	910	992
30	079		241	326	408	493	575	660	745	827	912	995
31	082		244		411		578	663		830		997

Appendix A12.15: Decimals of a Year. From Tanner (1978) with permission.

Age (yrs)	Percentiles for Stature (cm)						
	5	10	25	50	75	90	95
	Male children						
0.0–0.5	56.5	56.5	61.2	65.2	67.1	70.0	78.9
0.5–1.0	64.8	68.3	69.6	73.4	76.4	78.5	79.4
1.0–1.5	71.4	72.9	74.9	77.9	80.8	82.8	86.5
1.5–2.0	80.4	82.7	83.5	83.9	85.3	87.8	91.9
2.0–2.5	83.0	84.2	85.8	88.2	90.1	90.7	91.6
3	88.6	90.4	93.3	95.2	97.5	100.4	103.9
4	92.7	94.4	98.5	101.9	105.0	108.6	112.1
5	98.7	102.0	104.8	107.4	113.0	114.6	115.6
6	101.7	105.4	110.3	115.5	117.9	121.3	121.4
7	111.8	113.6	114.2	118.5	122.7	125.6	126.8
8	116.5	119.2	121.9	126.6	131.0	132.0	134.3
9	115.6	117.9	125.3	130.8	140.1	143.4	145.7
10	123.8	129.0	132.7	137.1	139.6	144.8	148.5
11	128.6	131.3	136.2	139.0	145.5	147.6	149.3
12	135.9	136.7	142.8	147.8	152.6	159.2	166.1
13	140.0	141.3	147.6	151.9	160.8	163.3	164.4
14	146.9	147.8	151.4	158.9	164.5	172.0	174.1
15	151.8	152.4	161.4	165.9	171.5	173.8	175.5
16	157.9	161.1	165.5	172.3	176.0	179.0	180.0
17	160.3	162.8	167.0	173.4	178.2	182.4	185.4
18	160.8	163.3	166.2	171.1	178.1	180.9	184.3
19	164.3	165.5	168.7	173.1	180.8	183.7	183.7
	Male adults						
20–29	163.7	165.3	170.5	174.7	178.9	183.8	189.6
30–39	161.8	164.9	168.0	172.9	178.1	182.7	184.6
40–49	160.2	162.6	167.6	171.9	176.4	181.1	184.5
50–59	161.2	162.3	166.8	171.8	175.9	179.8	182.0
60–69	158.9	160.3	164.5	168.3	172.6	176.3	178.1
70+	157.0	159.9	163.0	167.6	171.0	174.2	176.9

Appendix A12.16: Percentiles for stature (cm) of male Canadians by age. From Nutrition Canada (1980). Anthropometry Report — Height, Weight and Body Dimensions. Bureau of Nutritional Sciences, Health Protection Branch, Health and Welfare, Ottawa. Reproduced with permission of the Minister of Supply and Services Canada.

Age	Percentiles for Stature (cm)						
(yrs)	5	10	25	50	75	90	95
	Female children						
0.0–0.5	52.5	56.0	60.1	62.0	63.5	65.5	67.5
0.5–1.0	65.4	67.0	69.5	73.0	75.0	78.3	78.3
1.0–1.5	71.5	74.1	76.6	78.6	79.9	82.8	86.2
1.5–2.0	70.7	75.7	81.3	83.4	86.5	86.6	87.1
2.0–2.5	81.4	81.8	83.5	87.7	88.4	91.2	92.7
3	84.7	86.0	90.1	94.0	96.5	99.7	100.7
4	94.5	95.6	99.7	102.3	104.5	106.8	108.3
5	101.4	102.5	103.0	105.5	111.2	114.1	117.6
6	104.5	107.7	111.4	114.4	116.3	118.7	119.9
7	104.6	108.0	113.3	116.0	121.3	125.3	126.6
8	114.2	117.3	120.7	125.6	128.8	134.4	136.4
9	120.0	122.9	127.5	130.3	132.6	136.0	140.9
10	129.3	130.6	133.9	137.6	141.7	142.7	146.5
11	130.0	132.4	139.2	142.9	148.2	151.2	153.5
12	135.5	137.3	141.3	145.5	153.9	158.6	161.8
13	145.1	146.4	151.1	154.4	160.4	163.7	166.7
14	147.4	148.2	152.3	157.1	160.5	165.3	168.2
15	150.9	154.2	154.9	158.8	161.0	165.7	167.7
16	149.7	152.5	155.9	160.5	164.4	169.2	171.2
17	153.2	153.3	156.0	159.9	162.9	164.9	166.9
18	146.0	153.2	157.1	159.8	165.6	167.4	167.5
19	149.0	155.0	156.3	160.7	163.0	163.9	167.9
	Female adults						
20–29	150.9	153.0	157.1	160.3	165.4	169.2	170.9
30–39	149.2	150.9	155.5	160.4	164.5	167.7	170.2
40–49	149.6	151.9	154.8	159.1	163.8	168.7	169.5
50–59	148.6	150.0	155.3	159.1	163.9	167.8	171.9
60–69	147.3	149.4	152.9	156.0	160.9	165.4	166.7
70+	144.0	146.3	149.9	155.2	158.7	162.5	164.1

Appendix A12.17: Percentiles for stature (cm) of female Canadians by age. From Nutrition Canada (1980). Anthropometry Report—Height, Weight and Body Dimensions. Bureau of Nutritional Sciences, Health Protection Branch, Health and Welfare, Ottawa. Reproduced with permission of the Minister of Supply and Services Canada.

Age	Percentiles for Weight (kg)						
(yrs)	5	10	25	50	75	90	95
				Male children			
0.0–0.5	4.4	4.8	6.2	7.2	8.2	9.7	10.9
0.5–1.0	7.6	7.8	8.7	9.9	10.6	11.8	12.3
1.0–1.5	8.5	9.3	9.6	10.3	11.3	12.6	13.5
1.5–2.0	10.6	11.0	11.6	12.2	13.2	13.9	15.1
2.0–2.5	11.0	11.3	11.9	12.7	13.2	14.0	14.2
3	12.8	13.2	13.8	14.5	15.8	17.0	17.8
4	13.5	14.4	15.2	16.8	18.2	19.7	22.5
5	14.9	15.2	17.2	18.5	21.1	22.9	23.8
6	17.1	17.5	18.7	20.2	22.5	24.5	25.3
7	18.5	18.8	20.7	21.9	24.4	26.0	27.3
8	20.4	21.4	23.3	24.9	27.5	32.5	35.8
9	19.1	19.8	23.8	28.3	35.5	39.8	43.0
10	25.6	26.4	27.3	30.4	33.3	39.5	44.9
11	27.2	27.6	30.4	33.0	38.0	45.1	45.1
12	29.7	31.2	33.0	37.6	44.2	51.1	54.8
13	32.1	33.0	36.9	43.8	49.5	53.8	58.6
14	34.7	37.4	42.4	46.2	54.8	58.7	63.2
15	41.2	42.9	48.9	54.7	58.8	63.4	67.5
16	43.9	48.4	51.6	59.2	69.0	81.2	81.2
17	46.5	49.6	56.2	60.6	74.8	80.9	82.2
18	48.3	48.3	58.0	62.4	69.0	77.6	80.1
19	53.5	56.0	59.6	69.3	75.6	78.8	97.5
				Male adults			
20–29	56.2	57.7	62.0	71.5	78.7	91.9	102.1
30–39	54.0	59.8	65.4	74.6	81.6	88.8	96.6
40–49	57.3	60.4	67.3	74.4	83.3	90.3	92.3
50–59	55.3	59.0	65.1	74.2	82.2	88.0	93.8
60–69	49.7	57.9	63.6	72.5	82.1	88.1	92.1
70+	52.4	56.6	60.6	68.7	77.6	84.7	89.1

Appendix A12.18: Percentiles for weight (kg) of male Canadians by age. From Nutrition Canada (1980). Anthropometry Report—Height, Weight and Body Dimensions. Bureau of Nutritional Sciences, Health Protection Branch, Health and Welfare, Ottawa. Reproduced with permission of the Minister of Supply and Services Canada.

Age	Percentiles for Weight (kg)						
(yrs)	5	10	25	50	75	90	95
	Female children						
0.0–0.5	4.1	4.3	5.8	6.5	7.1	8.6	11.0
0.5–1.0	7.3	7.7	8.5	9.1	10.1	11.0	11.7
1.0–1.5	8.7	9.0	10.0	10.4	11.0	11.9	12.0
1.5–2.0	9.4	9.4	10.7	11.8	12.4	13.0	13.0
2.0–2.5	10.4	11.1	11.6	11.9	12.9	13.2	14.4
3	10.7	11.1	12.0	13.8	15.8	16.2	17.4
4	13.9	14.4	15.2	16.2	17.4	18.4	19.7
5	15.0	15.8	16.3	17.3	19.8	22.3	22.5
6	16.5	17.7	19.4	20.1	22.3	23.9	26.4
7	16.8	17.0	18.5	20.0	23.5	26.4	27.1
8	18.8	19.8	22.9	24.8	29.0	30.8	31.1
9	21.4	23.2	25.5	28.0	30.2	35.5	37.1
10	24.1	24.5	27.8	31.0	38.7	44.1	44.2
11	26.8	28.7	31.2	36.2	40.8	48.7	55.7
12	27.0	31.2	34.7	40.3	44.9	54.1	59.5
13	34.1	36.0	40.4	45.1	52.7	60.1	62.8
14	33.5	36.5	41.4	47.0	51.7	59.5	64.1
15	41.0	42.7	47.8	50.8	53.8	62.8	67.2
16	43.7	46.7	49.7	52.5	57.0	65.6	71.4
17	42.0	43.5	49.0	52.0	56.1	63.2	65.6
18	38.3	41.7	48.5	55.9	60.0	68.3	74.2
19	45.4	47.8	49.0	52.0	56.6	65.6	67.6
	Female adults						
20–29	42.0	46.0	50.9	58.2	65.8	73.2	82.1
30–39	44.8	47.4	52.0	58.1	63.1	72.3	83.9
40–49	46.2	47.6	53.8	59.9	68.9	77.2	82.6
50–59	47.3	50.4	56.4	63.4	72.7	84.0	90.3
60–69	44.4	55.1	57.3	62.9	72.4	79.3	86.5
70+	43.7	48.3	58.0	63.8	72.0	76.3	79.9

Appendix A12.19: Percentiles for weight (kg) of female Canadians by age. From Nutrition Canada (1980). Anthropometry Report—Height, Weight and Body Dimensions. Bureau of Nutritional Sciences, Health Protection Branch, Health and Welfare, Ottawa. Reproduced with permission of the Minister of Supply and Services Canada.

Height	Percentiles for Weight (kg) for Height						
(cm)	5	10	25	50	75	90	95
				Male children			
<60	4.1	4.1	4.8	5.8	6.9	33.3	33.3
60–62	6.1	6.1	6.2	6.2	6.2	6.2	6.2
62–64	6.7	6.7	7.0	7.0	9.7	9.7	9.8
64–66	7.3	7.3	7.3	7.7	7.8	7.8	7.8
66–68	4.0	6.5	7.2	7.3	9.1	10.0	10.0
68–70	7.7	7.7	8.5	8.5	8.7	8.7	10.0
70–72	8.3	8.3	8.3	9.1	9.3	10.1	10.1
72–74	8.5	9.0	9.1	9.4	9.4	10.4	10.4
74–76	8.5	8.5	9.2	10.6	12.5	13.0	13.0
76–78	9.1	9.9	10.0	10.0	10.8	11.2	11.2
78–80	9.7	10.0	10.3	11.3	11.7	11.8	21.9
80–82	10.1	10.1	11.0	11.9	12.4	12.7	12.7
82–84	10.4	10.9	11.0	12.2	13.2	13.2	13.2
84–86	11.6	11.7	11.9	12.2	12.9	13.9	13.9
86–88	11.0	11.3	11.6	12.5	13.1	14.9	14.9
88–90	11.9	12.4	12.8	12.8	13.7	13.9	14.1
90–92	13.0	13.0	13.0	13.7	14.0	14.5	14.5
92–94	13.4	13.9	14.1	15.1	15.5	15.5	15.7
94–96	13.4	13.5	13.8	14.2	14.7	15.9	16.4
96–98	14.6	14.6	15.2	15.6	16.1	16.7	16.8
98–100	13.3	14.3	14.6	15.8	16.5	17.0	17.7
100–102	15.1	15.8	16.3	16.4	22.0	22.0	22.0
102–104	15.2	16.1	17.3	17.8	18.2	18.6	19.4
104–106	16.5	16.9	17.0	17.5	18.2	19.4	20.2
106–108	17.0	17.1	17.3	18.1	19.2	19.7	19.7
108–110	16.7	17.4	18.0	18.3	18.9	19.5	19.8
110–112	15.5	17.2	18.7	19.5	20.8	21.1	21.2
112–114	17.1	17.5	18.5	20.2	22.5	23.1	23.1
114–116	18.8	18.8	19.1	20.2	21.1	21.9	22.7
116–118	18.7	18.8	20.5	22.2	23.4	25.0	25.3
118–120	20.5	20.7	20.8	22.0	23.4	25.3	25.5
120–122	20.2	20.2	21.3	22.9	24.5	26.2	26.2
122–124	21.5	22.6	23.3	23.3	24.6	26.0	29.2
124–126	23.0	23.3	23.3	25.2	25.8	27.1	28.3
126–128	22.7	22.8	24.5	26.9	27.3	29.3	29.6
128–130	23.5	23.8	24.7	27.0	28.2	29.5	36.4
130–132	24.0	25.4	26.9	27.2	30.4	35.8	35.8
132–134	25.6	26.3	27.5	28.2	29.4	33.0	34.3
134–136	26.9	26.9	27.6	30.3	31.2	36.2	36.9
136–138	28.5	28.9	30.2	30.5	33.0	33.2	34.8
138–140	28.2	29.5	30.5	31.7	35.1	38.4	43.0
140–142	31.3	32.0	32.4	35.5	35.7	39.9	44.1
142–144	31.2	31.2	32.5	35.0	38.3	44.2	44.2

Appendix A12.20: Percentiles for weight (kg) for height in Canadian male children from birth to nineteen years of age. From Nutrition Canada (1980). Anthropometry Report—Height, Weight and Body Dimensions. Bureau of Nutritional Sciences, Health Protection Branch, Health and Welfare, Ottawa. Reproduced with permission of the Minister of Supply and Services Canada.

Height	Percentiles for Weight (kg) for Height						
(cm)	5	10	25	50	75	90	95
				Male children (cont.)			
144–146	31.7	32.4	35.5	36.9	39.8	41.2	44.4
146–148	34.2	34.5	35.8	40.8	45.1	45.1	46.8
148–150	33.3	33.7	35.6	38.1	44.4	46.9	55.4
150–152	34.5	35.0	39.5	41.3	45.8	49.3	51.1
152–154	36.2	39.5	42.1	44.0	51.0	52.9	54.9
154–156	40.7	41.7	43.7	44.5	46.3	51.4	58.7
156–158	41.8	43.1	44.6	45.0	49.0	52.7	56.9
158–160	38.7	40.0	42.1	45.3	51.3	52.5	54.4
160–162	38.9	39.0	47.2	50.5	53.8	55.0	56.5
162–164	44.5	46.7	48.3	49.5	56.1	61.1	62.9
164–166	46.2	49.0	51.2	55.4	58.5	66.1	68.0
166–168	48.6	48.9	54.8	58.1	60.8	67.5	81.8
168–170	50.9	53.5	55.6	57.0	60.5	69.7	78.2
170–172	52.0	52.7	52.8	57.3	60.1	66.2	66.7
172–174	54.3	55.2	56.8	64.1	81.2	81.2	81.2
174–176	54.2	55.4	59.7	62.3	65.6	87.0	87.3
176–178	49.6	57.2	59.7	68.1	74.2	80.7	81.2
178–180	60.5	60.5	66.0	68.9	75.7	77.6	79.0
180–182	62.3	62.3	68.8	73.7	77.6	90.0	103.5
182–184	51.8	51.8	77.1	78.8	82.2	82.2	84.0
184–186	59.3	64.6	68.1	77.3	79.5	102.5	102.5
186–188	65.2	67.6	68.6	68.6	74.2	82.9	82.9
				Female children			
<60	3.5	3.5	4.1	4.3	5.5	7.1	8.5
60–62	5.3	5.4	5.8	6.7	34.0	34.0	34.0
62–64	5.4	5.8	5.8	6.6	7.1	7.6	7.9
64–66	6.1	6.1	6.1	6.6	7.2	7.4	8.6
66–68	6.4	6.4	6.8	7.7	8.0	8.8	11.6
68–70	7.2	8.2	8.6	8.6	8.6	8.6	8.7
70–72	7.8	7.8	8.3	9.1	9.4	9.4	9.7
72–74	9.0	9.0	9.2	9.2	9.7	11.7	11.7
74–76	8.6	8.6	8.7	10.0	10.0	11.9	11.9
76–78	9.1	9.1	9.3	9.8	10.3	10.9	10.9
78–80	10.0	10.1	10.2	10.6	10.7	12.4	12.4
80–82	10.4	10.7	10.7	11.0	11.6	11.6	11.7
82–84	10.4	10.4	11.1	11.9	12.2	12.2	12.8
84–86	10.7	10.7	10.7	11.6	12.4	12.9	13.0
86–88	11.2	11.2	12.0	12.0	12.4	13.0	13.0
88–90	11.8	11.8	11.8	12.2	13.2	13.4	14.2
90–92	11.2	12.5	12.8	13.2	14.0	15.3	16.2
92–94	11.1	11.1	11.1	13.7	14.0	14.4	14.9
94–96	12.0	12.0	12.0	14.2	15.5	16.2	16.2

Appendix A12.20: (cont.) Percentiles for weight (kg) for height in Canadian male and female children from birth to nineteen years of age. From Nutrition Canada (1980). Anthropometry Report — Height, Weight and Body Dimensions. Bureau of Nutritional Sciences, Health Protection Branch, Health and Welfare, Ottawa. Reproduced with permission of the Minister of Supply and Services Canada.

Height (cm)	Percentiles for Weight (kg) for Height (cm)						
	5	10	25	50	75	90	95
	Female children (cont.)						
96–98	14.0	14.0	15.5	15.6	16.1	16.2	16.8
98–100	14.4	14.4	15.7	15.9	16.2	16.4	16.7
100–102	13.9	14.5	15.0	16.1	17.0	18.6	21.9
102–104	14.5	14.8	16.0	16.3	17.2	17.5	18.1
104–106	16.1	16.2	16.6	17.1	17.8	18.4	18.8
106–108	15.2	15.2	16.8	17.3	18.9	20.8	20.8
108–110	16.8	17.3	17.5	19.4	19.5	20.0	20.0
110–112	15.7	17.5	18.7	19.5	21.4	22.3	22.3
112–114	18.1	18.3	18.4	19.5	21.0	23.3	23.9
114–116	18.6	18.7	19.5	20.2	22.2	22.4	22.5
116–118	17.7	18.5	19.8	20.5	21.9	22.1	23.0
118–120	18.8	19.5	20.0	21.2	22.6	24.1	26.5
120–122	20.5	22.1	23.2	23.5	25.5	26.5	26.6
122–124	22.1	23.0	23.7	24.1	26.0	27.6	28.0
124–126	22.0	22.0	22.4	23.9	25.7	26.6	27.4
126–128	22.4	24.0	25.2	26.9	29.5	30.4	33.2
128–130	23.5	23.8	26.2	28.1	29.1	33.8	36.2
130–132	24.1	24.6	25.6	30.1	30.3	32.7	37.1
132–134	24.0	25.0	27.0	30.1	32.0	41.7	41.7
134–136	24.5	24.5	25.2	27.0	34.6	37.3	38.6
136–138	25.4	27.2	30.2	30.8	33.0	37.1	49.3
138–140	26.9	27.8	29.7	31.7	37.1	44.9	44.9
140–142	28.9	30.0	31.1	33.8	35.7	38.9	38.9
142–144	28.8	31.1	34.1	37.6	44.2	45.5	50.8
144–146	30.4	31.3	34.1	39.0	40.9	46.1	52.0
146–148	32.5	33.5	37.2	38.3	42.8	53.3	54.6
148–150	36.0	38.7	39.7	40.8	47.0	52.7	57.0
150–152	35.9	40.2	40.4	42.6	48.4	53.7	54.5
152–154	33.5	36.9	39.6	43.0	51.2	53.7	62.4
154–156	38.0	41.0	43.0	50.8	52.8	56.2	65.7
156–158	40.3	41.0	46.4	49.0	51.8	60.2	65.5
158–160	42.6	45.4	48.5	51.2	58.5	67.6	70.1
160–162	42.5	45.8	47.8	52.0	54.4	59.5	66.9
162–164	45.2	49.4	51.5	53.5	59.5	65.6	65.6
164–166	47.1	48.9	50.4	54.0	60.2	65.6	68.4
166–168	49.6	52.1	56.1	59.4	61.2	71.3	73.7
168–170	47.0	51.2	53.1	57.7	61.2	65.0	66.3
170–172	47.1	47.1	56.5	63.8	72.5	81.0	81.0
172–174	50.2	59.6	59.6	59.9	62.3	65.2	65.2
174–176	55.5	55.5	57.6	57.6	57.6	63.5	69.4
176–178	54.6	56.3	56.3	61.3	67.2	67.2	67.2

Appendix A12.20: (cont.) Percentiles for weight (kg) for height in Canadian female children from birth to nineteen years of age. From Nutrition Canada (1980). Anthropometry Report — Height, Weight and Body Dimensions. Bureau of Nutritional Sciences, Health Protection Branch, Health and Welfare, Ottawa. Reproduced with permission of the Minister of Supply and Services Canada.

| Height | Percentiles for Weight (kg) for Height (cm) | | | | | | |
(cm)	5	10	25	50	75	90	95
				Males			
152–154	44.2	46.1	46.1	54.3	56.3	64.4	64.4
154–156	52.7	57.1	57.7	58.1	61.6	69.8	69.8
156–158	50.3	51.9	54.3	63.5	68.2	76.9	81.4
158–160	49.4	51.5	52.8	60.0	66.4	77.6	78.5
160–162	49.5	56.4	60.4	69.5	77.1	81.3	81.8
162–164	52.5	55.7	58.0	63.4	66.9	74.3	78.6
164–166	47.6	50.4	61.6	70.0	75.9	82.0	85.5
166–168	56.8	58.5	60.6	67.0	74.3	81.0	87.9
168–170	55.1	59.8	63.4	69.0	77.9	84.5	90.4
170–172	53.3	57.2	66.2	72.8	80.3	87.2	94.6
172–174	58.6	63.0	69.5	76.9	82.9	88.5	93.8
174–176	60.3	61.5	66.9	75.1	82.3	88.2	91.9
176–178	58.2	60.4	65.7	75.7	84.6	89.0	93.3
178–180	62.5	66.2	71.9	79.0	83.4	89.1	91.9
180–182	69.2	71.1	73.6	79.4	84.4	88.5	95.2
182–184	65.9	66.8	73.7	85.1	97.1	104.3	104.3
184–186	68.5	72.2	76.0	84.0	94.5	102.2	105.3
186–188	67.0	69.6	79.4	92.0	92.3	92.5	94.7
188–190	73.3	74.4	77.8	86.8	93.7	101.9	105.6
190 +	73.7	79.6	79.6	104.7	104.7	104.7	104.7
				Females			
<140	25.4	33.5	44.0	44.8	52.6	52.8	99.5
140–142	45.5	45.5	45.5	52.1	60.3	60.3	60.3
142–144	43.9	43.9	51.9	70.3	72.6	72.6	83.7
144–146	41.2	45.3	47.0	47.0	61.7	66.6	81.4
146–148	40.0	40.0	44.2	49.4	63.2	75.0	75.0
148–150	43.6	45.4	49.9	59.5	73.0	88.0	89.4
150–152	42.1	46.7	50.6	55.9	63.0	72.5	74.5
152–154	41.0	44.4	47.3	59.4	67.5	78.6	85.0
154–156	41.2	44.8	53.1	58.3	66.2	74.7	80.0
156–158	46.3	48.5	53.1	57.7	68.0	75.4	81.6
158–160	45.0	49.0	52.7	58.5	66.4	77.3	82.8
160–162	48.7	49.2	54.1	61.0	69.8	80.5	87.6
162–164	48.9	50.2	55.0	60.0	68.9	78.8	87.8
164–166	50.7	55.0	56.8	62.7	67.2	79.1	86.1
166–168	49.9	53.3	58.4	63.4	69.1	82.5	84.2
168–170	52.8	52.8	59.9	65.6	70.7	75.6	89.3
170–172	54.4	56.5	59.7	65.2	70.2	80.0	84.1
172–174	60.7	60.7	63.1	69.5	75.5	84.8	88.8
174–176	57.0	63.6	63.6	65.1	69.5	71.1	71.1

Appendix A12.21: Percentiles for weight (kg) for height (cm) in Canadian adults. From Nutrition Canada (1980). Anthropometry Report—Height, Weight and Body Dimensions. Bureau of Nutritional Sciences, Health Protection Branch, Health and Welfare, Ottawa. Reproduced with permission of the Minister of Supply and Services Canada.

Height		Weight Percentiles (kg)						
in	cm	5	10	20	50	80	90	95
Males (18–24 yr)								
62	157.5	38.5	43.1	48.5	58.9	69.4	74.8	79.4
63	160.0	40.8	45.3	50.8	61.2	71.6	77.1	81.6
64	162.6	43.1	47.6	53.1	63.5	73.9	79.4	83.9
65	165.1	45.4	49.9	55.3	65.8	76.2	81.6	86.2
66	167.6	47.6	52.2	57.6	68.0	78.5	83.9	88.4
67	170.2	49.4	54.0	59.4	69.8	80.3	85.7	90.2
68	172.7	51.7	56.2	61.7	72.1	82.5	88.0	92.5
69	175.3	54.0	58.5	63.9	74.4	84.8	90.2	94.8
70	177.8	55.8	60.3	65.8	76.2	86.6	92.1	96.6
71	180.3	58.0	62.6	68.0	78.5	88.9	94.3	98.9
72	182.9	60.3	64.9	70.3	80.7	91.2	96.6	101.1
73	185.4	62.6	67.1	72.6	83.0	93.4	98.9	103.4
74	188.0	64.9	69.4	74.8	85.3	95.7	101.1	105.7
Females (18–24 yr)								
57	144.8	30.8	35.4	40.8	51.7	62.6	68.0	72.6
58	147.3	32.2	36.7	42.2	53.1	63.9	69.4	73.9
59	149.9	33.6	38.1	43.5	54.4	65.3	70.7	75.3
60	152.4	34.9	39.5	44.9	55.8	66.7	72.1	76.6
61	154.9	36.3	40.8	46.3	57.1	68.0	73.5	78.0
62	157.5	37.6	42.2	47.6	58.5	69.4	74.8	79.4
63	160.0	39.0	43.5	49.0	59.9	70.7	76.2	80.7
64	162.6	40.4	40.8	50.3	61.2	72.1	77.6	82.1
65	165.1	41.7	46.3	51.7	62.6	73.5	78.9	83.4
66	167.6	43.1	48.1	53.1	63.9	74.8	80.3	84.8
67	170.2	44.4	49.0	54.4	65.3	76.2	81.6	86.2
68	172.7	45.8	50.3	55.8	66.7	77.6	83.0	87.5
Males (25–34 yr)								
62	157.5	41.3	46.3	52.2	63.9	75.7	81.6	86.6
63	160.0	43.1	48.1	54.0	65.7	77.5	83.4	88.4
64	162.6	45.4	50.3	56.2	68.0	79.8	85.7	90.7
65	165.1	48.1	53.1	59.0	70.7	82.5	88.4	93.4
66	167.6	49.9	54.9	60.8	72.6	84.4	90.2	95.2
67	170.2	52.1	57.1	63.0	74.8	86.6	92.5	97.5
68	172.7	54.4	59.4	65.3	77.1	88.9	94.8	99.8
69	175.3	56.2	61.2	67.1	78.9	90.7	96.6	101.6
70	177.8	58.5	63.5	69.4	81.2	93.0	98.9	103.9
71	180.3	60.8	65.8	71.7	83.4	95.2	101.1	106.1
72	182.9	63.0	68.0	73.9	85.7	97.5	103.4	108.4
73	185.4	65.3	70.3	76.2	88.0	99.8	105.7	110.7
74	188.0	67.6	72.6	78.5	90.2	102.0	107.9	112.9

Appendix A12.22: Percentiles for weight by age and height for U.S. adults aged eighteen to seventy-four years from the NHANES I survey (1971–1974). Data from NCHS (1979).

Height		Weight Percentiles (kg)						
in	cm	5	10	20	50	80	90	95
Females (25–34 yr)								
57	144.8	29.5	34.9	41.3	53.5	65.8	72.1	77.6
58	147.3	30.8	36.3	42.6	54.9	67.1	73.5	78.9
59	149.9	32.7	38.1	44.4	56.7	68.9	75.3	80.7
60	152.4	34.0	39.5	45.8	58.0	70.3	76.6	82.1
61	154.9	35.8	41.3	47.6	59.9	72.1	79.4	83.9
62	157.5	37.6	43.1	49.4	61.7	73.9	80.3	85.7
63	160.0	39.0	44.4	50.8	63.0	75.3	81.6	87.1
64	162.6	40.4	45.8	52.2	64.4	76.6	83.0	88.4
65	165.1	42.2	47.6	54.0	66.2	78.5	84.8	90.2
66	167.6	44.0	49.4	55.8	68.0	80.3	86.6	92.1
67	170.2	45.4	50.8	57.1	69.4	81.6	88.0	93.4
68	172.7	47.2	52.6	59.0	71.2	83.4	89.8	95.2
Males (35–44 yr)								
62	157.5	44.4	49.0	54.4	64.8	75.3	80.7	85.3
63	160.0	46.7	51.2	56.7	67.1	77.5	83.0	87.5
64	162.6	49.0	53.5	58.9	69.4	79.8	85.3	89.8
65	165.1	51.2	55.8	61.2	71.7	82.1	87.5	92.1
66	167.6	53.5	58.0	63.5	73.9	84.4	89.8	94.3
67	170.2	56.2	60.8	66.2	76.6	87.1	92.5	97.1
68	172.7	58.5	63.0	68.5	78.9	89.3	94.8	99.3
69	175.3	60.8	65.3	70.7	81.2	91.6	97.1	101.6
70	177.8	63.0	67.6	73.0	83.4	93.9	96.1	103.9
71	180.3	65.8	70.3	75.7	86.2	96.6	102.0	106.6
72	182.9	67.6	72.1	77.6	88.0	98.4	103.9	108.4
73	185.4	70.3	74.8	80.3	90.7	101.1	106.6	111.1
74	188.0	72.6	77.1	82.5	93.0	103.4	108.8	113.4
Females (35–44 yr)								
57	144.8	30.4	36.3	43.5	56.7	69.8	77.1	83.0
58	147.3	32.2	38.1	45.4	58.5	71.7	78.9	84.8
59	149.9	34.0	39.9	47.2	60.3	73.5	80.7	86.6
60	152.4	35.8	41.7	49.0	62.1	75.3	82.5	88.4
61	154.9	37.6	43.5	50.8	63.9	77.1	84.4	90.2
62	157.5	39.0	44.9	52.2	65.3	78.5	85.7	91.6
63	160.0	40.8	46.7	54.0	67.1	80.3	87.5	93.4
64	162.6	42.6	48.5	55.8	68.9	82.1	89.3	95.2
65	165.1	44.4	50.3	57.6	70.7	83.9	91.2	97.1
66	167.6	45.8	51.7	59.0	72.1	85.3	92.5	98.4
67	170.2	47.6	71.7	60.8	73.9	87.1	94.3	100.2
68	172.7	49.4	55.3	62.6	75.7	88.9	96.1	102.0

Appendix A12.22: (Cont.) Percentiles for weight by age and height for U.S. adults aged eighteen to seventy-four years from the NHANES I survey (1971–1974). Data from NCHS (1979).

Height		Weight Percentiles (kg)						
in	cm	5	10	20	50	80	90	95
Males (45–54 yr)								
62	157.5	45.4	50.3	55.8	66.7	77.6	83.0	88.0
63	160.0	47.6	52.6	58.0	68.9	79.8	85.3	90.2
64	162.6	49.4	54.4	59.9	70.7	81.6	87.1	92.1
65	165.1	51.2	56.2	61.7	72.6	83.4	88.9	93.9
66	167.6	53.1	58.0	63.5	74.4	85.3	90.7	95.7
67	170.2	55.3	60.3	65.8	76.6	87.5	93.0	98.0
68	172.7	57.1	62.1	67.6	78.5	89.3	94.8	99.8
69	175.3	59.0	63.9	69.4	80.3	91.2	96.6	101.6
70	177.8	61.2	66.2	71.7	82.5	93.4	98.9	103.9
71	180.3	63.5	68.5	73.9	84.8	95.7	101.1	106.1
72	182.9	65.3	70.3	75.7	86.6	97.5	102.9	107.9
73	185.4	67.6	72.6	78.6	88.9	99.8	105.2	110.2
74	188.0	69.4	74.4	79.8	90.7	101.6	107.0	112.0
Females (45–54 yr)								
57	144.8	33.1	39.0	45.8	58.5	71.2	78.0	83.9
58	147.3	34.9	40.8	47.6	60.3	73.0	79.8	85.7
59	149.9	36.3	42.2	49.0	61.7	74.4	81.2	87.1
60	152.4	38.1	44.0	50.8	63.5	76.2	83.0	88.9
61	154.9	39.5	45.4	52.2	64.9	77.6	84.4	90.2
62	157.5	41.3	47.2	54.0	66.7	79.4	86.2	92.1
63	160.0	42.6	48.5	55.3	68.0	80.7	87.5	93.4
64	162.6	44.4	49.9	57.1	69.8	82.5	89.3	95.2
65	165.1	46.3	52.2	59.0	71.7	84.4	91.2	97.1
66	167.6	47.6	53.5	60.3	73.0	85.7	92.5	98.4
67	170.2	49.4	55.3	62.1	74.8	87.5	94.3	100.2
68	172.7	50.8	56.7	63.5	76.2	88.9	95.7	101.6
Males (55–64 yr)								
62	157.5	43.5	48.1	54.0	64.9	75.7	81.6	86.2
63	160.0	45.4	49.9	55.8	66.7	77.6	83.4	88.0
64	162.6	48.1	52.6	58.5	69.4	80.3	86.2	90.7
65	165.1	50.3	54.9	60.8	71.7	82.5	88.4	93.0
66	167.6	52.6	57.1	63.0	73.9	84.8	90.7	95.2
67	170.2	54.9	59.4	65.3	76.2	87.1	93.0	97.5
68	172.7	57.1	61.7	67.6	78.5	89.3	95.2	99.8
69	175.3	59.4	63.9	69.8	80.7	91.6	97.5	102.0
70	177.8	61.7	66.2	72.1	83.0	93.9	99.8	104.3
71	180.3	64.4	68.9	74.8	85.7	96.6	102.5	107.0
72	182.9	66.2	70.7	76.6	87.5	98.4	104.3	108.8
73	185.4	68.0	72.6	78.5	89.3	100.2	106.1	110.7
74	188.0	70.7	75.3	81.2	92.1	102.9	108.8	113.4

Appendix A12.22: (Cont.) Percentiles for weight by age and height for U.S. adults aged eighteen to seventy-four years from the NHANES I survey (1971–1974). Data from NCHS (1979).

Height		Weight Percentiles (kg)						
in	cm	5	10	20	50	80	90	95
Females (55–64 yr)								
57	144.8	34.9	40.4	47.2	59.9	72.6	79.4	84.8
58	147.3	36.7	42.2	49.0	61.7	74.4	81.2	86.6
59	149.9	38.5	44.0	50.8	63.5	76.2	83.0	88.4
60	152.4	39.9	45.4	52.2	64.9	77.6	84.4	89.8
61	154.9	41.7	47.2	54.0	66.7	79.4	86.2	91.6
62	157.5	43.1	48.5	55.3	68.0	80.7	87.5	93.0
63	160.0	44.4	49.9	56.7	69.4	82.1	88.9	94.3
64	162.6	46.3	51.7	58.5	71.2	83.9	90.7	96.1
65	165.1	47.6	53.1	59.9	72.6	85.3	92.1	97.5
66	167.6	49.4	54.9	61.7	74.4	87.1	93.9	99.3
67	170.2	50.8	56.2	63.0	75.7	88.4	95.2	100.7
68	172.7	52.6	58.0	64.9	77.6	90.2	97.1	102.5
Males (65–74 yr)								
62	157.5	45.3	49.9	54.9	64.8	74.8	79.8	84.4
63	160.0	47.2	51.7	56.7	66.7	76.6	81.6	86.2
64	162.6	49.0	53.5	58.5	68.5	78.5	83.4	88.0
65	165.1	51.2	55.8	60.8	70.7	80.7	85.7	90.2
66	167.6	53.1	57.6	62.6	72.6	82.5	87.5	92.1
67	170.2	54.9	59.4	64.4	74.4	84.4	89.3	93.9
68	172.7	57.1	61.7	66.7	76.6	86.6	91.6	96.1
69	175.3	59.0	63.5	68.5	78.5	88.4	93.4	98.0
70	177.8	60.8	65.3	70.3	80.3	90.2	95.2	99.8
71	180.3	63.0	67.6	72.6	82.5	92.5	97.5	102.0
72	182.9	64.9	69.4	74.4	84.4	94.3	99.3	103.0
73	185.4	66.7	71.2	76.2	86.2	96.1	101.1	105.7
74	188.0	68.5	73.0	78.0	88.0	98.0	102.9	107.5
Females (65–74 yr)								
57	144.8	37.2	42.2	48.1	59.0	69.8	75.7	80.7
58	147.3	39.0	44.0	49.9	60.8	71.7	77.6	82.5
59	149.9	40.4	45.4	51.2	62.1	73.0	78.9	83.9
60	152.4	41.7	46.7	52.6	63.5	74.4	80.3	85.3
61	154.9	43.5	43.5	54.4	65.3	76.2	82.1	87.1
62	157.5	44.9	49.9	55.8	66.7	77.6	83.4	88.4
63	160.0	46.7	51.7	57.6	68.5	79.4	85.3	90.2
64	162.6	48.1	53.1	59.0	69.8	80.7	86.6	91.6
65	165.1	49.9	54.9	60.8	71.7	82.5	88.4	93.4
66	167.6	51.2	56.2	62.1	73.0	83.9	89.8	94.8
67	170.2	53.1	58.0	63.9	74.8	85.7	91.6	96.6
68	172.7	54.9	59.9	65.8	76.6	87.5	93.4	98.4

Appendix A12.22: (Cont.) Percentiles for weight by age and height for U.S. adults aged eighteen to seventy-four years from the NHANES I survey (1971–1974). Data from NCHS (1979).

Age (yr)	Frame Size from Elbow Breadth (cm)		
	Small	Medium	Large
Caucasian males			
18–24	≤6.7	>6.7, <7.5	≥7.5
25–34	≤6.7	>6.7, <7.5	≥7.5
35–44	≤6.9	>6.9, <7.6	≥7.6
45–54	≤6.9	>6.9, <7.7	≥7.7
55–64	≤6.9	>6.9, <7.7	≥7.7
65–74	≤6.9	>6.9, <7.7	≥7.7
Caucasian females			
18–24	≤5.7	>5.7, <6.4	≥6.4
25–34	≤5.8	>5.8, <6.5	≥6.5
35–44	≤5.9	>5.9, <6.6	≥6.6
45–54	≤5.9	>5.9, <6.8	≥6.8
55–64	≤6.0	>6.0, <6.9	≥6.9
65–74	≤6.0	>6.0, <6.9	≥6.9
Black males			
18–24	≤6.7	>6.7, <7.6	≥7.6
25–34	≤6.8	>6.8, <7.6	≥7.6
35–44	≤6.7	>6.7, <7.7	≥7.7
45–54	≤6.9	>6.9, <7.9	≥7.9
55–64	≤6.9	>6.9, <7.9	≥7.9
65–74	≤6.9	>6.9, <7.8	≥7.8
Black females			
18–24	≤5.8	>5.8, <6.6	≥6.6
25–34	≤5.8	>5.8, <6.7	≥6.7
35–44	≤6.0	>6.0, <7.0	≥7.0
45–54	≤6.0	>6.0, <7.1	≥7.1
55–64	≤6.1	>6.1, <7.2	≥7.2
65–74	≤6.1	>6.1, <7.0	≥7.0

Appendix A12.23: Frame size by elbow breadth of United States black and Caucasian adults. Data from the NHANES I survey (1971–1974). Adapted from Frisancho and Flegel (1983). © Am. J. Clin. Nutr. American Society for Clinical Nutrition.

Height		Weight Percentiles (kg)						
in	cm	5	10	15	50	85	90	95
			Male subjects 25–54 yr old (small frame)					
62	157	46	50	52	64	71	74	77
63	160	48	51	53	61	70	75	79
64	163	49	53	55	66	76	76	80
65	165	52	53	58	66	77	81	84
66	168	56	57	59	67	78	83	84
67	170	56	60	62	71	82	83	88
68	173	56	59	62	71	79	82	85
69	175	57	62	65	74	84	87	88
70	178	59	62	67	75	87	86	90
71	180	60	64	70	76	79	88	91
72	183	62	65	67	74	87	89	93
73	185	63	67	69	79	89	91	94
74	188	65	68	71	80	90	92	96
		Female subjects 25–54 yr old (small frame)						
58	147	37	43	43	52	58	62	66
59	150	42	43	44	53	63	69	72
60	152	42	44	45	53	63	65	70
61	155	44	46	47	54	64	66	72
62	157	44	47	48	55	63	64	70
63	160	46	48	49	55	65	68	79
64	163	49	50	51	57	67	68	74
65	165	50	52	53	60	70	72	80
66	168	46	49	54	58	65	71	74
67	170	47	50	52	59	70	72	76
68	173	48	51	53	62	71	73	77
69	175	49	52	54	63	72	74	78
70	178	50	53	55	64	73	75	79
		Male subjects 25–54 yr old (medium frame)						
62	157	51	55	58	68	81	83	87
63	160	52	56	59	71	82	85	89
64	163	54	60	61	71	83	84	90
65	165	59	62	65	74	87	90	94
66	168	58	61	65	75	85	87	93
67	170	62	66	68	77	89	93	100
68	173	60	64	66	78	89	92	97
69	175	63	66	68	78	90	93	97
70	178	64	66	70	81	90	93	97
71	180	62	68	70	81	92	96	100
72	183	68	71	74	84	97	100	104
73	185	70	72	75	85	100	101	104
74	188	68	76	77	88	100	100	104

Appendix A12.24: Percentiles for weight by frame size and height for U.S. adults aged twenty-five to fifty-four years old. Data from the NHANES I (1971–1974) and NHANES II (1976–1980) surveys. From Frisancho (1984). © Am. J. Clin. Nutr. American Society for Clinical Nutrition.

Height		Weight Percentiles (kg)						
in	cm	5	10	15	50	85	90	95
Female subjects 25–54 yr old (medium frame)								
58	147	41	46	50	63	77	75	79
59	150	47	50	52	66	76	79	85
60	152	47	50	52	60	77	79	85
61	155	47	49	51	61	73	78	86
62	157	49	50	52	61	73	77	83
63	160	49	51	53	62	77	80	88
64	163	50	52	54	62	76	82	87
65	165	52	54	55	63	75	80	89
66	168	52	54	55	63	75	78	83
67	170	54	56	57	65	79	82	88
68	173	58	59	60	67	77	85	87
69	175	49	58	60	68	79	82	87
70	178	50	54	57	70	80	83	87
Male subjects 25–54 yr old (large frame)								
62	157	57	62	66	82	99	103	108
63	160	58	63	67	83	100	104	109
64	163	59	64	68	84	101	105	110
65	165	60	65	69	79	102	106	111
66	168	60	65	75	84	103	106	112
67	170	62	70	71	84	102	111	113
68	173	63	74	76	86	101	104	114
69	175	68	71	74	89	103	105	114
70	178	68	72	74	87	106	112	114
71	180	73	78	82	91	113	116	123
72	183	73	76	78	91	109	112	121
73	185	72	77	79	93	106	107	116
74	188	69	74	82	92	105	115	120
Female subjects 25–54 yr old (large frame)								
58	147	56	63	67	86	105	110	117
59	150	56	62	67	78	105	109	116
60	152	55	62	66	87	104	109	116
61	155	54	64	66	81	105	117	115
62	157	59	61	65	81	103	107	113
63	160	58	63	67	83	105	109	119
64	163	59	62	63	79	102	104	112
65	165	59	61	63	81	103	109	114
66	168	55	58	62	75	95	100	107
67	170	58	60	65	80	100	108	114
68	173	51	66	66	76	104	105	111
69	175	50	57	68	79	105	104	111
70	178	50	56	61	76	99	104	110

Appendix A12.24: (Cont.) Percentiles for weight by frame size and height for U.S. adults aged twenty-five to fifty-four years old. Data from the NHANES I (1971–1974) and NHANES II (1976–1980) surveys. From Frisancho (1984). © Am. J. Clin. Nutr. American Society for Clinical Nutrition.

Height		Weight Percentiles (kg)						
in	cm	5	10	15	50	85	90	95
		Male subjects 55–74 yr old (small frame)						
62	157	45	49	56	61	68	73	77
63	160	47	49	51	62	71	71	79
64	163	47	50	54	63	72	74	80
65	165	48	54	59	70	80	90	90
66	168	51	55	59	68	77	80	84
67	170	55	60	61	69	79	81	88
68	173	54	54	58	70	79	81	86
69	175	56	59	63	75	81	84	88
70	178	57	61	63	76	83	86	89
71	180	59	62	65	69	85	87	91
72	183	60	64	66	76	86	89	92
73	185	62	65	68	78	88	90	94
74	188	63	67	69	77	89	92	95
		Female subjects 55–74 yr old (small frame)						
58	147	39	46	48	54	63	65	71
59	150	41	45	48	55	66	68	74
60	152	43	45	47	54	67	70	73
61	155	43	43	45	56	65	70	71
62	157	47	49	52	58	67	69	73
63	160	42	45	49	58	67	68	74
64	163	43	47	49	60	68	70	75
65	165	43	47	49	60	69	72	75
66	168	44	48	50	68	70	72	76
67	170	45	48	51	61	71	73	77
68	173	45	49	51	61	71	74	77
69	175	46	49	52	62	72	74	78
70	178	47	50	52	63	73	75	79
		Male subjects 55–74 yr old (medium frame)						
62	157	50	54	59	68	77	81	85
63	160	51	57	60	70	80	82	87
64	163	55	59	62	71	82	83	91
65	165	56	60	64	72	83	86	89
66	168	57	62	66	74	83	84	89
67	170	59	64	66	78	87	89	94
68	173	62	66	68	78	89	95	101
69	175	62	66	68	77	90	93	99
70	178	62	68	71	80	90	95	101
71	180	68	70	72	84	94	97	101
72	183	66	65	69	81	96	97	101
73	185	68	72	79	88	93	99	103
74	188	69	73	76	95	98	101	104

Appendix A12.25: Percentiles for weight by frame size and height for U.S. adults aged fifty-five to seventy-four years old. Data from the NHANES I (1971–1974) and NHANES II (1976–1980) surveys. From Frisancho (1984). © Am. J. Clin. Nutr. American Society for Clinical Nutrition.

Height		Weight Percentiles (kg)						
in	cm	5	10	15	50	85	90	95
		Female subjects 55–74 yr old (medium frame)						
58	147	40	44	49	57	72	82	85
59	150	47	49	52	62	74	78	86
60	152	47	50	52	65	76	79	86
61	155	49	51	54	64	78	81	86
62	157	49	53	54	64	78	82	88
63	160	52	54	55	65	79	83	89
64	163	51	54	57	66	78	81	87
65	165	54	56	59	67	78	84	88
66	168	54	57	57	66	79	85	88
67	170	51	59	61	72	82	85	89
68	173	52	56	59	70	83	86	90
69	175	53	57	60	72	84	87	91
70	178	54	58	61	73	85	88	92
		Male subjects 55–74 yr old (large frame)						
62	157	54	59	63	77	91	95	100
63	160	55	60	64	80	92	96	101
64	163	57	62	65	77	94	97	102
65	165	58	63	73	79	89	98	103
66	168	59	67	73	80	101	102	105
67	170	65	71	73	85	103	108	112
68	173	67	71	73	83	95	98	111
69	175	65	70	74	84	96	98	105
70	178	68	73	77	87	102	104	117
71	180	65	70	70	84	102	109	111
72	183	67	76	81	90	108	112	112
73	185	68	73	76	88	105	108	113
74	188	69	74	78	89	106	109	114
		Female subjects 55–74 yr old (large frame)						
58	147	53	59	63	92	95	99	104
59	150	54	59	63	78	95	99	105
60	152	54	65	69	78	87	88	105
61	155	64	68	69	79	94	95	106
62	157	59	61	63	82	93	101	111
63	160	61	65	67	80	100	102	118
64	163	60	65	67	77	97	102	119
65	165	60	66	69	80	98	102	111
66	168	57	60	63	82	98	105	109
67	170	58	64	68	80	105	104	109
68	173	58	64	68	79	100	104	110
69	175	59	65	69	85	101	105	110
70	178	60	65	69	85	101	105	111

Appendix A12.25: (Cont.) Percentiles for weight by frame size and height for U.S. adults aged fifty-five to seventy-four years old. Data from the NHANES I (1971–1974) and NHANES II (1976–1980) surveys. From Frisancho (1984). © Am. J. Clin. Nutr. American Society for Clinical Nutrition.

Age Group Frame Size	Median Age	Weight	Triceps Skinfold	Subscapular Skinfold	Arm Muscle Area
			Males		
25–54					
Small	39	0.074	0.016	0.080	0.030
Medium	39	0.080	0.005	0.083	0.055
Large	40	0.000	-0.024	0.049	0.026
55–74					
Small	66	-0.329	-0.036	-0.115	-0.407
Medium	67	-0.435	-0.040	-0.125	-0.521
Large	67	-0.562	-0.054	-0.185	-0.644
			Females		
25–54					
Small	37	0.165	0.166	0.142	0.087
Medium	37	0.234	0.189	0.214	0.191
Large	37	0.284	0.191	0.233	0.270
55–74					
Small	67	-0.027	-0.072	-0.013	0.036
Medium	67	-0.196	-0.210	-0.221	-0.033
Large	67	-0.466	-0.370	-0.515	-0.378

Appendix A12.26: The use of the age correction factors in the above table is illustrated in the following example: Given a fifty-seven-year-old, large-framed male who is 170 cm (67 in) tall, we wish to determine whether he is above or below the U.S. median, if he weighs 90 kg. The general equation used to determine the age-adjusted median weight (AAMW) for such an individual is: AAMW = unadjusted weight standard + (age correction) × (deviation from median age). Where: the unadjusted weight standard = 85 kg (from A12.25), the age correction factor = -0.562 (see above), the median age = 67 yr (see above), and the actual age = 57 yr. Thus:

$$AAMW = 85 + (-0.562) \times (57 - 67)$$

$$AAMW = 90.62 \text{ kg (or approximately 91 kg)}$$

Therefore, the age-adjusted weight standard indicates that this individual is actually *below* the U.S. median (90 vs 91 kg), whereas without age correction, he would appear to be about 5 kg *above* the median weight for his height and frame size. From Frisancho (1984). © Am. J. Clin. Nutr. American Society for Clinical Nutrition.

Height (cm)	'Ideal' Weights (kg) for Females			'Ideal' Weights (kg) for Males		
	Small Frame	Medium Frame	Large Frame	Small Frame	Medium Frame	Large Frame
148	46.4–50.6	49.6–55.1	53.7–59.8			
149	46.6–51.0	50.0–55.5	54.1–60.3			
150	46.7–51.3	50.3–55.9	54.4–60.9			
151	46.9–51.7	50.7–56.4	54.8–61.4			
152	47.1–52.1	51.1–57.0	55.2–61.9			
153	47.4–52.5	51.5–57.5	55.6–62.4			
154	47.8–53.0	51.9–58.0	56.2–63.0			
155	48.1–53.6	52.2–58.6	56.8–63.6			
156	48.5–54.1	52.7–59.1	57.3–64.1			
157	48.8–54.6	53.2–59.6	57.8–64.6			
158	49.3–55.2	53.8–60.2	58.4–65.3	58.3–61.0	59.6–64.2	62.8–68.3
159	49.8–55.7	54.3–60.7	58.9–66.0	58.6–61.3	59.9–64.5	63.1–68.8
160	50.3–56.2	54.9–61.2	59.4–66.7	59.0–61.7	60.3–64.9	63.5–69.4
161	50.8–56.7	55.4–61.7	59.9–67.4	59.3–62.0	60.6–65.2	63.8–69.9
162	51.4–57.3	55.9–62.3	60.5–68.1	59.7–62.4	61.0–65.6	64.2–70.5
163	51.9–57.8	56.4–62.8	61.0–68.8	60.0–62.7	61.3–66.0	64.5–71.1
164	52.5–58.4	57.0–63.4	61.5–69.5	60.4–63.1	61.7–66.5	64.9–71.8
165	53.0–58.9	57.5–63.9	62.0–70.2	60.8–63.5	62.1–67.0	65.3–72.5
166	53.6–59.5	58.1–64.5	62.6–70.9	61.1–63.8	62.4–67.6	65.6–73.2
167	54.1–60.0	58.7–65.0	63.2–71.7	61.5–64.2	62.8–68.2	66.0–74.0
168	54.6–60.5	59.2–65.5	63.7–72.4	61.8–64.6	63.2–68.7	66.4–74.7
169	55.2–61.1	59.7–66.1	64.3–73.1	62.2–65.2	63.8–69.3	67.0–75.4
170	55.7–61.6	60.2–66.6	64.8–73.8	62.5–65.7	64.3–69.8	67.5–76.1
171	56.2–62.1	60.7–67.1	65.3–74.5	62.9–66.2	64.8–70.3	68.0–76.8
172	56.8–62.6	61.3–67.6	65.8–75.2	63.2–66.7	65.4–70.8	68.5–77.5
173	57.3–63.2	61.8–68.2	66.4–75.9	63.6–67.3	65.9–71.4	69.1–78.2
174	57.8–63.7	62.3–68.7	66.9–76.4	63.9–67.8	66.4–71.9	69.6–78.9
175	58.3–64.2	62.8–69.2	67.4–76.9	64.3–68.3	66.9–72.4	70.1–79.6
176	58.9–64.8	63.4–69.8	68.0–77.5	64.7–68.9	67.5–73.0	70.7–80.3
177	59.5–65.4	64.0–70.4	68.5–78.1	65.0–69.5	68.1–73.5	71.3–81.0
178	60.0–65.9	64.5–70.9	69.0–78.6	65.4–70.0	68.6–74.0	71.8–81.8
179	60.5–66.4	65.1–71.4	69.6–79.1	65.7–70.5	69.2–74.6	72.3–82.5
180	61.0–66.9	65.6–71.9	70.1–79.6	66.1–71.0	69.7–75.1	72.8–83.3
181	61.6–67.5	66.1–72.5	70.7–80.2	66.6–71.6	70.2–75.8	73.4–84.0
182	62.1–68.0	66.6–73.0	71.2–80.7	67.1–72.1	70.7–76.5	73.9–84.7
183				67.7–72.7	71.3–77.2	74.5–85.4
184				68.2–73.4	71.8–77.9	75.2–86.1
185				68.7–74.1	72.4–78.6	75.9–86.8
186				69.2–74.8	73.0–79.3	76.6–87.6
187				69.8–75.5	73.7–80.0	77.3–88.5
188				70.3–76.2	74.4–80.7	78.0–89.4
189				70.9–76.9	74.9–81.5	78.7–90.3
190				71.4–77.6	75.4–82.2	79.4–91.2
191				72.1–78.4	76.1–83.0	80.3–92.1
192				72.8–79.1	76.8–83.9	81.2–93.0
193				73.5–79.8	77.6–84.8	82.1–93.9

Appendix A12.27: 'Ideal' weights for U.S. adults according to frame size at ages twenty-five to fifty-nine years based on lowest mortality. Weight in kilograms in indoor clothing weighing 1.4 kg (male) and 2.3 kg (female). Heights include 2.5-cm heels. Data from the 1979 Build Study, Society of Actuaries and Association of Life Insurance Medical Directors of America, 1980. From Metropolitan Height and Weight Tables (1983). Courtesy Statistical Bulletin, Metropolitan Life Insurance Company.

Age	Triceps Skinfold Percentiles (mm)						
(yr)	5	10	25	50	75	90	95
Males							
1–1.9	6	7	8	10	12	14	16
2–2.9	6	7	8	10	12	14	15
3–3.9	6	7	8	10	11	14	15
4–4.9	6	6	8	9	11	12	14
5–5.9	6	6	8	9	11	14	15
6–6.9	5	6	7	8	10	13	16
7–7.9	5	6	7	9	12	15	17
8–8.9	5	6	7	8	10	13	16
9–9.9	6	6	7	10	13	17	18
10–10.9	6	6	8	10	14	18	21
11–11.9	6	6	8	11	16	20	24
12–12.9	6	6	8	11	14	22	28
13–13.9	5	5	7	10	14	22	26
14–14.9	4	5	7	9	14	21	24
15–15.9	4	5	6	8	11	18	24
16–16.9	4	5	6	8	12	16	22
17–17.9	5	5	6	8	12	16	19
18–18.9	4	5	6	9	13	20	24
19–24.9	4	5	7	10	15	20	22
25–34.9	5	6	8	12	16	20	24
35–44.9	5	6	8	12	16	20	23
45–54.9	6	6	8	12	15	20	25
55–64.9	5	6	8	11	14	19	22
65–74.9	4	6	8	11	15	19	22
Females							
1–1.9	6	7	8	10	12	14	16
2–2.9	6	8	9	10	12	15	16
3–3.9	7	8	9	11	12	14	15
4–4.9	7	8	8	10	12	14	16
5–5.9	6	7	8	10	12	15	18
6–6.9	6	6	8	10	12	14	16
7–7.9	6	7	9	11	13	16	18
8–8.9	6	8	9	12	15	18	24
9–9.9	8	8	10	13	16	20	22
10–10.9	7	8	10	12	17	23	27
11–11.9	7	8	10	13	18	24	28
12–12.9	8	9	11	14	18	23	27
13–13.9	8	8	12	15	21	26	30
14–14.9	9	10	13	16	21	26	28
15–15.9	8	10	12	17	21	25	32
16–16.9	10	12	15	18	22	26	31
17–17.9	10	12	13	19	24	30	37
18–18.9	10	12	15	18	22	26	30
19–24.9	10	11	14	18	24	30	34
25–34.9	10	12	16	21	27	34	37
35–44.9	12	14	18	23	29	35	38
45–54.9	12	16	20	25	30	36	40
55–64.9	12	16	20	25	31	36	38
65–74.9	12	14	18	24	29	34	36

Appendix A12.28: Percentiles for triceps skinfolds (mm) by age for U.S. white persons aged one to seventy-five years. Data from the NHANES I (1971–1974) survey. Date from Frisancho (1981). © Am. J. Clin. Nutr. American Society for Clinical Nutrition.

Height		Triceps Skinfold Percentiles (mm)						
in	cm	5	10	15	50	85	90	95
		Male subjects 25–54 yr old (small frame)						
62	157				11			
63	160			6	10	17		
64	163		5	5	10	16	18	
65	165	4	5	6	11	17	19	21
66	168	5	6	6	11	18	18	20
67	170	5	6	6	11	18	20	22
68	173	5	6	6	10	15	16	20
69	175		6	6	11	17	20	
70	178			7	10	17		
71	180			7	10	16		
72	183				10			
		Female subjects 25–54 yr old (small frame)						
58	147		12	13	24	30	33	
59	150	8	11	14	21	29	36	37
60	152	8	11	12	21	28	29	33
61	155	11	12	14	21	28	31	34
62	157	10	12	14	20	28	31	34
63	160	10	11	13	20	27	30	36
64	163	10	13	13	20	28	30	34
65	165	12	13	14	22	29	31	34
66	168			12	19	30		
67	170				18			
68	173				20			
		Male subjects 25–54 yr old (medium frame)						
62	157				15			
63	160				11			
64	163		6	6	12	18	20	
65	165	5	7	8	12	20	22	25
66	168	5	6	7	11	16	18	22
67	170	5	7	7	13	21	23	28
68	173	4	5	7	11	18	20	24
69	175	5	6	7	12	18	20	24
70	178	5	6	7	12	18	20	23
71	180	4	5	7	12	19	21	25
72	183	5	7	7	12	20	22	26
73	185	6	7	8	12	20	24	27
74	188		6	9	13	21	23	

Appendix A12.29: Percentiles for triceps skinfolds (mm) by frame size and height for U.S. adults aged twenty-five to fifty-five years old. Data from the NHANES I (1971–1974) and NHANES II (1976–1980) surveys. From Frisancho (1984). © Am. J. Clin. Nutr. American Society for Clinical Nutrition.

Height		Triceps Skinfold Percentiles (mm)						
in	cm	5	10	15	50	85	90	95
		Female subjects 25–54 yr old (medium frame)						
58	147			20	25	40		
59	150	15	19	21	30	37	40	40
60	152	14	15	17	26	35	37	41
61	155	11	14	15	25	34	36	42
62	157	12	14	16	24	34	36	40
63	160	12	13	15	24	33	35	38
64	163	11	14	15	23	33	36	40
65	165	12	14	15	22	31	34	38
66	168	11	13	14	22	31	33	37
67	170	12	13	15	21	29	30	35
68	173	10	14	15	22	31	32	36
69	175		11	12	19	29	31	
70	178				19			
		Male subjects 25–54 yr old (large frame)						
65	165				14			
66	168		9		14	30		
67	170		7	7	11	23	27	
68	173		9	10	14	22	23	
69	175	6	7	8	15	25	29	31
70	178	7	7	7	14	23	25	30
71	180	6	8	10	15	25	27	31
72	183	5	6	7	12	20	22	25
73	185	5	6	7	13	19	22	31
74	188			8	12	19		
		Female subjects 25–54 yr old (large frame)						
59	150				36			
60	152				38			
61	155		25	26	36	48	50	
62	157	16	19	22	34	48	48	50
63	160	18	20	22	34	46	48	51
64	163	16	20	21	32	43	45	49
65	165	17	20	21	31	43	46	48
66	168	13	17	18	27	40	43	45
67	170	13	16	17	30	41	43	49
68	173		16	20	29	37	40	
69	175			21	30	42		
70	178				20			

Appendix A12.29: (Cont.) Percentiles for triceps skinfolds (mm) by frame size and height for U.S. adults aged twenty-five to fifty-four years old. Data from the NHANES I (1971–1974) and NHANES II (1976–1980) surveys. From Frisancho (1984). © Am. J. Clin. Nutr. American Society for Clinical Nutrition.

Height		Triceps Skinfold Percentiles (mm)						
in	cm	5	10	15	50	85	90	95
Male subjects 55–74 yr old (small frame)								
62	157			6	9	12		
63	160		5	5	10	16	17	
64	163	4	4	4	9	20	21	22
65	165	5	6	7	11	18	19	24
66	168	5	6	7	11	16	20	20
67	170	5	6	6	10	15	17	25
68	173		5	5	10	15	17	
69	175			8	10	15		
70	178				11			
71	180				9			
Female subjects 55–74 yr old (small frame)								
58	147		14	16	21	31	34	
59	150	11	13	15	21	30	31	33
60	152	10	11	13	20	29	31	35
61	155	10	12	14	22	29	29	32
62	157	11	11	12	21	29	30	32
63	160		12	13	20	29	30	
64	163		12	13	21	27	29	
65	165				18			
66	168				23			
Male subjects 55–74 yr old (medium frame)								
62	157			5	12	25		
63	160		7	7	11	20	23	
64	163	5	6	6	10	17	20	26
65	165	5	6	7	11	17	19	24
66	168	6	6	7	12	18	19	22
67	170	5	6	7	12	18	20	23
68	173	6	7	8	12	18	21	23
69	175	5	6	7	12	19	22	25
70	178	6	7	7	11	18	19	21
71	180	5	6	6	11	16	17	20
72	183		6	8	11	19	20	
73	185			8	13	16		
74	188				11			

Appendix A12.30: Percentiles for triceps skinfolds (mm) by frame size and height for U.S. adults aged fifty-five to seventy-four years old. Data from the NHANES I (1971–1974) and NHANES II (1976–1980) surveys. From Frisancho (1984). © Am. J. Clin. Nutr. American Society for Clinical Nutrition.

Height		Triceps Skinfold Percentiles (mm)						
in	cm	5	10	15	50	85	90	95
		Female subjects 55–74 yr old (medium frame)						
58	147	5	13	17	28	40	40	41
59	150	12	15	18	26	34	38	41
60	152	13	17	18	25	33	34	38
61	155	13	16	18	25	35	37	42
62	157	13	15	17	24	33	36	39
63	160	12	14	16	24	32	35	38
64	163	12	14	16	25	33	34	37
65	165	14	16	17	24	33	35	39
66	168	12	13	16	24	33	33	36
67	170		17	17	27	35	35	
68	173				25			
		Male subjects 55–74 yr old (large frame)						
63	160				15			
64	163				21			
65	165			11	14	22		
66	168		7	8	13	21	25	
67	170	6	8	9	16	21	25	27
68	173	6	7	8	13	20	21	23
69	175	6	7	8	12	18	20	23
70	178	5	6	8	14	22	25	31
71	180		6	6	13	18	22	
72	183		8	8	13	23	26	
73	185				11			
74	188				12			
		Female subjects 55–74 yr old (large frame)						
58	147				45			
59	150				36			
60	152		25	26	35	44	45	
61	155	18	22	24	33	40	44	46
62	157	19	24	24	32	40	43	50
63	160	20	24	25	33	41	43	45
64	163	18	22	23	29	42	46	50
65	165	15	17	20	30	43	44	46
66	168		18	18	27	35	40	
67	170			22	32	44		
68	173				26			

Appendix A12.30: (Cont.) Pecentiles for triceps skinfolds (mm) by frame size and height for U.S. adults aged fifty-five to seventy-four years old. Data from the NHANES I (1971–1974) and NHANES II (1976–1980) surveys. From Frisancho (1984). © Am. J. Clin. Nutr. American Society for Clinical Nutrition.

Age (yrs)	Subscapular Skinfold Percentiles (mm)								
	5	10	15	25	50	75	85	90	95
	Male children of all races								
1	4.0	4.0	4.0	5.0	6.0	7.0	8.0	8.5	10.0
2	3.0	4.0	4.0	4.5	5.0	6.5	7.0	8.0	10.0
3	3.5	4.0	4.0	4.0	5.0	6.0	6.8	7.0	9.5
4	3.0	3.5	4.0	4.0	5.0	6.0	6.0	7.0	7.0
5	3.0	3.5	4.0	4.0	5.0	6.0	7.0	7.0	8.0
6	3.0	3.0	3.5	4.0	4.5	5.0	6.0	7.0	9.0
7	3.0	3.0	3.5	4.0	4.5	6.0	7.0	9.0	11.0
8	3.0	3.0	3.5	4.0	4.5	6.0	6.0	7.5	9.0
9	3.5	3.5	4.0	4.0	5.0	8.0	11.0	14.0	14.0
10	3.5	4.0	4.0	4.0	5.5	7.0	10.0	12.0	18.0
11	4.0	4.0	4.0	4.5	6.0	8.5	13.0	15.0	19.0
12	3.5	4.0	4.5	5.0	6.0	9.0	11.0	14.0	20.5
13	3.5	4.0	4.5	5.0	6.5	9.0	13.5	17.0	26.0
14	4.0	4.5	5.0	5.0	6.5	9.0	13.0	16.0	20.0
15	4.0	5.0	5.0	5.5	7.0	10.0	13.0	15.5	23.0
16	5.0	5.5	6.0	6.5	8.0	10.5	13.5	16.5	23.5
17	5.0	5.5	6.0	7.0	8.0	10.0	13.0	16.0	23.0
	Female children of all races								
1	4.0	4.0	4.0	5.0	6.0	8.0	8.0	9.0	9.0
2	4.0	4.0	4.0	5.0	6.0	7.0	8.0	9.0	10.0
3	4.0	4.0	4.0	4.5	5.5	6.5	7.0	8.0	9.0
4	3.5	4.0	4.0	4.5	5.0	6.0	7.0	8.0	9.0
5	3.5	4.0	4.0	4.0	5.0	6.5	8.0	9.0	15.0
6	3.0	4.0	4.0	4.5	5.5	6.5	7.0	8.0	10.0
7	3.0	4.0	4.0	4.5	5.0	7.0	9.0	10.5	11.5
8	3.5	4.0	4.0	4.5	5.5	8.0	12.5	14.5	19.5
9	4.0	4.0	4.5	5.0	7.0	10.0	13.0	17.0	19.0
10	4.0	4.5	5.0	5.5	6.5	10.0	13.0	18.0	20.0
11	4.0	5.0	5.0	6.0	8.0	13.0	16.0	19.0	25.5
12	5.0	5.0	5.5	6.0	9.5	13.0	16.0	20.0	25.0
13	5.0	6.0	6.0	7.0	9.5	15.0	19.0	23.4	26.0
14	5.0	6.0	6.5	8.0	10.0	16.0	19.0	24.0	28.0
15	6.0	6.5	7.0	7.5	10.0	14.0	18.0	20.0	27.0
16	6.0	7.0	7.5	8.0	10.5	15.0	21.0	25.5	29.0
17	6.5	7.0	7.5	9.0	12.5	20.0	25.5	27.0	34.1

Appendix A12.31: Percentiles for subscapular skinfolds (mm) by single year of age for U.S. children of all races. Data from the NHANES I survey (1971–1975). From NCHS (1981).

Height		Subscapular Skinfold Percentiles (mm)						
in	cm	5	10	15	50	85	90	95
		Male subjects 25–54 years old (small frame)						
62	157				16			
63	160			8	12	20		
64	163		7	7	15	25	29	
65	165	7	8	9	14	25	28	35
66	168	7	8	8	14	26	26	32
67	170	6	7	9	15	23	25	30
68	173	7	8	9	13	24	30	40
69	175		7	7	13	24	26	
70	178			9	14	23		
71	180			8	13	22		
72	183				14			
		Female subjects 25–54 years old (small frame)						
58	147		10	12	23	34	38	
59	150	6	9	10	17	29	32	34
60	152	6	7	8	18	27	32	39
61	155	7	8	9	16	28	32	36
62	157	6	7	8	14	22	27	32
63	160	6	7	7	14	27	29	31
64	163	6	7	8	13	24	27	34
65	165	7	8	8	15	26	30	33
66	168			9	12	25		
67	170				13			
68	173				15			
		Male subjects 25–54 years old (medium frame)						
62	157				13			
63	160				18			
64	163		7	9	17	30	32	
65	165	8	9	10	16	26	29	32
66	168	7	7	9	16	25	27	33
67	170	8	9	10	18	26	30	33
68	173	7	8	9	16	25	28	31
69	175	7	8	9	16	25	27	31
70	178	7	8	9	15	24	27	30
71	180	7	8	9	14	24	27	30
72	183	7	8	9	15	26	30	32
73	185	8	9	9	15	25	29	32
74	188		7	9	14	25	30	

Table A12.32: Percentiles for subscapular skinfolds (mm) by frame size and height for U.S. adults aged twenty-five to fifty-four years old. Data from the NHANES I (1971–1974) and NHANES II (1976–1980) surveys. Data from Frisancho (1984). © Am. J. Clin. Nutr. American Society for Clinical Nutrition.

Height		Subscapular Skinfold Percentiles (mm)						
in	cm	5	10	15	50	85	90	95
Female subjects 25–54 years old (medium frame)								
58	147			15	23	38		
59	150	10	12	13	29	38	39	43
60	152	8	10	11	22	35	37	41
61	155	7	9	10	19	32	36	42
62	157	7	9	10	18	33	37	40
63	160	7	8	10	18	31	34	38
64	163	7	7	8	16	31	35	38
65	165	7	8	8	15	29	33	38
66	168	7	8	9	14	28	30	35
67	170	7	8	8	15	28	32	37
68	173	8	8	9	15	29	33	35
69	175		8	8	12	25	29	
70	178				20			
Male subjects 25–54 years old (large frame)								
65	165				21			
66	168			13	22	36		
67	170		8	11	20	36	40	
68	173		12	14	20	31	35	
69	175	9	10	11	18	31	32	38
70	178	7	10	11	17	31	35	38
71	180	9	11	11	20	35	40	46
72	183	8	9	9	19	28	30	36
73	185	7	9	9	18	27	28	30
74	188			9	18	32		
Female subjects 25–54 years old (large frame)								
59	150				35			
60	152				42			
61	155		17	17	35	48	53	
62	157	13	16	18	32	48	51	55
63	160	11	14	16	32	44	48	50
64	163	10	12	15	28	42	46	50
65	165	10	12	14	29	42	48	52
66	168	8	9	11	25	36	40	45
67	170	7	10	11	25	41	46	55
68	173		10	12	21	45	48	
69	175		11		20	43		
70	178				16			

Table A12.32: (Cont.) Percentiles for subscapular skinfolds (mm) by frame size and height for U.S. adults aged twenty-five to fifty-four years old. Data from the NHANES I (1971–1974) and NHANES II (1976–1980) surveys. Data from Frisancho (1984). © Am. J. Clin. Nutr. American Society for Clinical Nutrition.

Height		Subscapular Skinfold Percentiles (mm)						
in	cm	5	10	15	50	85	90	95
		Male subjects 55–74 years old (small frame)						
62	157			11	16	23		
63	160		6	6	12	21	22	
64	163	6	7	7	14	24	25	29
65	165	6	8	8	16	28	28	29
66	168	7	7	8	15	25	26	30
67	170	7	8	9	13	22	25	31
68	173		7	7	13	21	22	
69	175			10	16	27		
70	178				13			
71	180				10			
		Female subjects 55–74 years old (small frame)						
58	147		8	9	18	32	33	
59	150	6	7	9	19	29	30	33
60	152	5	7	8	15	27	32	36
61	155	6	7	8	17	29	31	34
62	157	7	8	9	17	25	26	30
63	160		6	7	14	25	27	
64	163		6	7	18	24	25	
65	165				13			
66	168				13			
		Male subjects 55–74 years old (medium frame)						
62	157			11	19	27		
63	160		8	10	15	26	28	
64	163	6	7	9	15	25	27	35
65	165	7	8	9	17	25	29	31
66	168	7	9	10	16	25	28	31
67	170	7	9	10	17	26	29	34
68	173	7	9	10	17	26	29	32
69	175	6	8	9	16	25	28	30
70	178	7	9	10	16	25	27	30
71	180	7	9	10	15	25	26	31
72	183		8	10	16	28	30	
73	185			10	15	26		
74	188				18			

Table A12.33: Percentiles for subscapular skinfolds (mm) by frame size and height for U.S. adults aged fifty-five to seventy-four years old. Data from the NHANES I (1971–1974) and NHANES II (1976–1980) surveys. Data from Frisancho (1984). © Am. J. Clin. Nutr. American Society for Clinical Nutrition.

658

Appendix A

Height		Subscapular Skinfold Percentiles (mm)						
in	cm	5	10	15	50	85	90	95
		Female subjects 55–74 years old (medium frame)						
58	147	3	7	10	25	37	43	48
59	150	8	9	11	23	32	36	43
60	152	8	10	12	22	34	36	40
61	155	8	10	10	20	33	36	42
62	157	7	8	10	20	33	36	38
63	160	8	8	10	18	32	37	41
64	163	7	9	10	17	30	33	38
65	165	7	8	9	17	30	35	37
66	168	6	7	8	16	30	31	34
67	170		9	10	19	35	35	
68	173				16			
		Male subjects 55–74 years old (large frame)						
63	160				20			
64	163				31			
65	165			14	19	27		
66	168		9	11	20	31	35	
67	170	8	11	12	20	35	35	38
68	173	8	10	11	18	27	30	32
69	175	7	11	11	19	27	30	33
70	178	9	11	13	20	30	33	37
71	180		8	9	15	30	30	
72	183		8	9	20	28	31	
73	185				19			
74	188				15			
		Female subjects 55–74 years old (large frame)						
58	147				44			
59	150				31			
60	152		19	21	31	42	45	
61	155	13	16	19	29	40	43	48
62	157	13	19	22	30	39	48	53
63	160	13	15	16	29	40	45	51
64	163	10	12	16	24	41	46	55
65	165	8	9	12	26	42	46	48
66	168		9	12	26	34	36	
67	170			14	25	46		
68	173				21			

Table A12.33: (Cont.) Percentiles for subscapular skinfolds (mm) by frame size and height for U.S. adults aged fifty-five to seventy-four years old. Data from the NHANES I (1971–1974) and NHANES II (1976–1980) surveys. Data from Frisancho (1984). © Am. J. Clin. Nutr. American Society for Clinical Nutrition.

Age (yr)	Mid-Upper Arm Circumference Percentiles (mm)						
	5	10	25	50	75	90	95
Males							
1–1.9	142	146	150	159	170	176	183
2–2.9	141	145	153	162	170	178	185
3–3.9	150	153	160	167	175	184	190
4–4.9	149	154	162	171	180	186	192
5–5.9	153	160	167	175	185	195	204
6–6.9	155	159	167	179	188	209	228
7–7.9	162	167	177	187	201	223	230
8–8.9	162	170	177	190	202	220	245
9–9.9	175	178	187	200	217	249	257
10–10.9	181	184	196	210	231	262	274
11–11.9	186	190	202	223	244	261	280
12–12.9	193	200	214	232	254	282	303
13–13.9	194	211	228	247	263	286	301
14–14.9	220	226	237	253	283	303	322
15–15.9	222	229	244	264	284	311	320
16–16.9	244	248	262	278	303	324	343
17–17.9	246	253	267	285	308	336	347
18–18.9	245	260	276	297	321	353	379
19–24.9	262	272	288	308	331	355	372
25–34.9	271	282	300	319	342	362	375
35–44.9	278	287	305	326	345	363	374
45–54.9	267	281	301	322	342	362	376
55–64.9	258	273	296	317	336	355	369
65–74.9	248	263	285	307	325	344	355
Females							
1–1.9	138	142	148	156	164	172	177
2–2.9	142	145	152	160	167	176	184
3–3.9	143	150	158	167	175	183	189
4–4.9	149	154	160	169	177	184	191
5–5.9	153	157	165	175	185	203	211
6–6.9	156	162	170	176	187	204	211
7–7.9	164	167	174	183	199	216	231
8–8.9	168	172	183	195	214	247	261
9–9.9	178	182	194	211	224	251	260
10–10.9	174	182	193	210	228	251	265
11–11.9	185	194	208	224	248	276	303
12–12.9	194	203	216	237	256	282	294
13–13.9	202	211	223	243	271	301	338
14–14.9	214	223	237	252	272	304	322
15–15.9	208	221	239	254	279	300	322
16–16.9	218	224	241	258	283	318	334
17–17.9	220	227	241	264	295	324	350
18–18.9	222	227	241	258	281	312	325
19–24.9	221	230	247	265	290	319	345
25–34.9	233	240	256	277	304	342	368
35–44.9	241	251	267	290	317	356	378
45–54.9	242	256	274	299	328	362	384
55–64.9	243	257	280	303	335	367	385
65–74.9	240	252	274	299	326	356	373

Table A12.34: Percentiles for mid-upper arm circumference (mm) for U.S. white persons aged one to seventy-four years old. Data from the NHANES I (1971–1974) survey. From Frisancho (1981). © Am. J. Clin. Nutr. American Society for Clinical Nutrition.

Age (yr)	Mid-Upper Arm Fat Area Percentiles (mm^2)						
	5	10	25	50	75	90	95
Males							
1–1.9	452	486	590	741	895	1036	1176
2–2.9	434	504	578	737	871	1044	1148
3–3.9	464	519	590	736	868	1071	1151
4–4.9	428	494	598	722	859	989	1085
5–5.9	446	488	582	713	914	1176	1299
6–6.9	371	446	539	678	896	1115	1519
7–7.9	423	473	574	758	1011	1393	1511
8–8.9	410	460	588	725	1003	1248	1558
9–9.9	485	527	635	859	1252	1864	2081
10–10.9	523	543	738	982	1376	1906	2609
11–11.9	536	595	754	1148	1710	2348	2574
12–12.9	554	650	874	1172	1558	2536	3580
13–13.9	475	570	812	1096	1702	2744	3322
14–14.9	453	563	786	1082	1608	2746	3508
15–15.9	521	595	690	931	1423	2434	3100
16–16.9	542	593	844	1078	1746	2280	3041
17–17.9	598	698	827	1096	1636	2407	2888
18–18.9	560	665	860	1264	1947	3302	3928
19–24.9	594	743	963	1406	2231	3098	3652
25–34.9	675	831	1174	1752	2459	3246	3786
35–44.9	703	851	1310	1792	2463	3098	3624
45–54.9	749	922	1254	1741	2359	3245	3928
55–64.9	658	839	1166	1645	2236	2976	3466
65–74.9	573	753	1122	1621	2199	2876	3327
Females							
1–1.9	401	466	578	706	847	1022	1140
2–2.9	469	526	642	747	894	1061	1173
3–3.9	473	529	656	822	967	1106	1158
4–4.9	490	541	654	766	907	1109	1236
5–5.9	470	529	647	812	991	1330	1536
6–6.9	464	508	638	827	1009	1263	1436
7–7.9	491	560	706	920	1135	1407	1644
8–8.9	527	634	769	1042	1383	1872	2482
9–9.9	642	690	933	1219	1584	2171	2524
10–10.9	616	702	842	1141	1608	2500	3005
11–11.9	707	802	1015	1301	1942	2730	3690
12–12.9	782	854	1090	1511	2056	2666	3369
13–13.9	726	838	1219	1625	2374	3272	4150
14–14.9	981	1043	1423	1818	2403	3250	3765
15–15.9	839	1126	1396	1886	2544	3093	4195
16–16.9	1126	1351	1663	2006	2598	3374	4236
17–17.9	1042	1267	1463	2104	2977	3864	5159
18–18.9	1003	1230	1616	2104	2617	3508	3733
19–24.9	1046	1198	1596	2166	2959	4050	4896
25–34.9	1173	1399	1841	2548	3512	4690	5560
35–44.9	1336	1619	2158	2898	3932	5093	5847
45–54.9	1459	1803	2447	3244	4229	5416	6140
55–64.9	1345	1879	2520	3369	4360	5276	6152
65–74.9	1363	1681	2266	3063	3943	4914	5530

Table A12.35: Percentiles for mid-upper arm fat area (mm^2) for U.S. white persons aged one to seventy-four years old. Data from the NHANES I (1971–1974) survey. From Frisancho (1981). © Am. J. Clin. Nutr. American Society for Clinical Nutrition.

Age (yr)	Mid-Upper Arm Muscle Circumference Percentiles (mm)						
	5	10	25	50	75	90	95
Males							
1–1.9	110	113	119	127	135	144	147
2–2.9	111	114	122	130	140	146	150
3–3.9	117	123	131	137	143	148	153
4–4.9	123	126	133	141	148	156	159
5–5.9	128	133	140	147	154	162	169
6–6.9	131	135	142	151	161	170	177
7–7.9	137	139	151	160	168	177	190
8–8.9	140	145	154	162	170	182	187
9–9.9	151	154	161	170	183	196	202
10–10.9	156	160	166	180	191	209	221
11–11.9	159	165	173	183	195	205	230
12–12.9	167	171	182	195	210	223	241
13–13.9	172	179	196	211	226	238	245
14–14.9	189	199	212	223	240	260	264
15–15.9	199	204	218	237	254	266	272
16–16.9	213	225	234	249	269	287	296
17–17.9	224	231	245	258	273	294	312
18–18.9	226	237	252	264	283	298	324
19–24.9	238	245	257	273	289	309	321
25–34.9	243	250	264	279	298	314	326
35–44.9	247	255	269	286	302	318	327
45–54.9	239	249	265	281	300	315	326
55–64.9	236	245	260	278	295	310	320
65–74.9	223	235	251	268	284	298	306
Females							
1–1.9	105	111	117	124	132	139	143
2–2.9	111	114	119	126	133	142	147
3–3.9	113	119	124	132	140	146	152
4–4.9	115	121	128	136	144	152	157
5–5.9	125	128	134	142	151	159	165
6–6.9	130	133	138	145	154	166	171
7–7.9	129	135	142	151	160	171	176
8–8.9	138	140	151	160	171	183	194
9–9.9	147	150	158	167	180	194	198
10–10.9	148	150	159	170	180	190	197
11–11.9	150	158	171	181	196	217	223
12–12.9	162	166	180	191	201	214	220
13–13.9	169	175	183	198	211	226	240
14–14.9	174	179	190	201	216	232	247
15–15.9	175	178	189	202	215	228	244
16–16.9	170	180	190	202	216	234	249
17–17.9	175	183	194	205	221	239	257
18–18.9	174	179	191	202	215	237	245
19–24.9	179	185	195	207	221	236	249
25–34.9	183	188	199	212	228	246	264
35–44.9	186	192	205	218	236	257	272
45–54.9	187	193	206	220	238	260	274
55–64.9	187	196	209	225	244	266	280
65–74.9	185	195	208	225	244	264	279

Table A12.36: Percentiles for mid-upper arm muscle circumference (mm) for U.S. white persons aged one to seventy-four years old. Data from the NHANES I (1971–1974) survey. From Frisancho (1981). © Am. J. Clin. Nutr. American Society for Clinical Nutrition.

| Age | Mid-Upper Arm Muscle Area Percentiles (mm^2) | | | | | | |
(yr)	5	10	25	50	75	90	95
Males							
1–1.9	956	1014	1133	1278	1447	1644	1720
2–2.9	973	1040	1190	1345	1557	1690	1787
3–3.9	1095	1201	1357	1484	1618	1750	1853
4–4.9	1207	1264	1408	1579	1747	1926	2008
5–5.9	1298	1411	1550	1720	1884	2089	2285
6–6.9	1360	1447	1605	1815	2056	2297	2493
7–7.9	1497	1548	1808	2027	2246	2494	2886
8–8.9	1550	1664	1895	2089	2296	2628	2788
9–9.9	1811	1884	2067	2288	2657	3053	3257
10–10.9	1930	2027	2182	2575	2903	3486	3882
11–11.9	2016	2156	2382	2670	3022	3359	4226
12–12.9	2216	2339	2649	3022	3496	3968	4640
13–13.9	2363	2546	3044	3553	4081	4502	4794
14–14.9	2830	3147	3586	3963	4575	5368	5530
15–15.9	3138	3317	3788	4481	5134	5631	5900
16–16.9	3625	4044	4352	4951	5753	6576	6980
17–17.9	3998	4252	4777	5286	5950	6886	7726
18–18.9	4070	4481	5066	5552	6374	7067	8355
19–24.9	4508	4777	5274	5913	6660	7606	8200
25–34.9	4694	4963	5541	6214	7067	7847	8436
35–44.9	4844	5181	5740	6490	7265	8034	8488
45–54.9	4546	4946	5589	6297	7142	7918	8458
55–64.9	4422	4783	5381	6144	6919	7670	8149
65–74.9	3973	4411	5031	5716	6432	7074	7453
Females							
1–1.9	885	973	1084	1221	1378	1535	1621
2–2.9	973	1029	1119	1269	1405	1595	1727
3–3.9	1014	1133	1227	1396	1563	1690	1846
4–4.9	1058	1171	1313	1475	1644	1832	1958
5–5.9	1238	1301	1423	1598	1825	2012	2159
6–6.9	1354	1414	1513	1683	1877	2182	2323
7–7.9	1330	1441	1602	1815	2045	2332	2469
8–8.9	1513	1566	1808	2034	2327	2657	2996
9–9.9	1723	1788	1976	2227	2571	2987	3112
10–10.9	1740	1784	2019	2296	2583	2873	3093
11–11.9	1784	1987	2316	2612	3071	3739	3953
12–12.9	2092	2182	2579	2904	3225	3655	3847
13–13.9	2269	2426	2657	3130	3529	4081	4568
14–14.9	2418	2562	2874	3220	3704	4294	4850
15–15.9	2426	2518	2847	3248	3689	4123	4756
16–16.9	2308	2567	2865	3248	3718	4353	4946
17–17.9	2442	2674	2996	3336	3883	4552	5251
18–18.9	2398	2538	2917	3243	3694	4461	4767
19–24.9	2538	2728	3026	3406	3877	4439	4940
25–34.9	2661	2826	3148	3573	4138	4806	5541
35–44.9	2750	2948	3359	3783	4428	5240	5877
45–54.9	2784	2956	3378	3858	4520	5375	5964
55–64.9	2784	3063	3477	4045	4750	5632	6247
65–74.9	2737	3018	3444	4019	4739	5566	6214

Table A12.37: Percentiles for mid-upper arm muscle area (mm^2) for U.S. white persons aged one to seventy-four years old. Data from the NHANES I (1971–1974) survey. From Frisancho (1981). © Am. J. Clin. Nutr. American Society for Clinical Nutrition.

Height (cm)	20–29	30–39	40–49	Age (yr) 50–59	60–69	70-79	80–89
Males							
146	1258	1169	1079	985	896	807	718
148	1284	1193	1102	1006	915	824	733
150	1308	1215	1123	1025	932	839	747
152	1334	1240	1145	1045	951	856	762
154	1358	1262	1166	1064	968	872	775
156	1390	1291	1193	1089	990	892	793
158	1423	1322	1222	1115	1014	913	812
160	1452	1349	1246	1137	1035	932	829
162	1481	1376	1271	1160	1055	950	845
164	1510	1403	1296	1183	1076	969	862
166	1536	1427	1318	1203	1094	986	877
168	1565	1454	1343	1226	1115	1004	893
170	1598	1485	1372	1252	1139	1026	912
172	1632	1516	1401	1278	1163	1047	932
174	1666	1548	1430	1305	1187	1069	951
176	1699	1579	1458	1331	1211	1090	970
178	1738	1615	1491	1361	1238	1115	992
180	1781	1655	1529	1395	1269	1143	1017
182	1819	1690	1561	1425	1296	1167	1038
184	1855	1724	1592	1453	1322	1190	1059
186	1894	1579	1625	1483	1349	1215	1081
188	1932	1795	1658	1513	1377	1240	1103
190	1968	1829	1689	1542	1402	1263	1123
Females							
140	858	804	754	700	651	597	548
142	877	822	771	716	666	610	560
144	898	841	790	733	682	625	573
146	917	859	806	749	696	638	586
148	940	881	827	768	713	654	600
150	964	903	848	787	732	671	615
152	984	922	865	803	747	685	628
154	1003	940	882	819	761	698	640
156	1026	961	902	838	779	714	655
158	1049	983	922	856	796	730	670
160	1073	1006	944	877	815	747	686
162	1100	1031	968	899	835	766	703
164	1125	1054	990	919	854	783	719
166	1148	1076	1010	938	871	799	733
168	1173	1099	1032	958	890	817	749
170	1199	1124	1055	980	911	835	766
172	1224	1147	1077	1000	929	853	782
174	1253	1174	1102	1023	951	872	800
176	1280	1199	1126	1045	972	891	817
178	1304	1223	1147	1065	990	908	833
180	1331	1248	1171	1087	1011	927	850

Table A16.1: Expected creatinine excretion (mg/day) in males and females of ideal weight. Data from Imbembo AL, Walser M. (1984). Nutritional assessment. In: Walser M, Imbembo AL, Margolis S, Elfert GA. (eds). Nutritional Management. The Johns Hopkins Handbook. WB Saunders Co., Philadelphia, with permission.

Antigen	Concentration	Response	Response (size at 48 hr)			
			1–5 mm Indur-ation or ≥10 mm Erythema	6–10 mm Indur-ation	11–20 mm Indur-ation	>20 mm Indur-ation
SK-SD	10 u SK - 2.5 u SD / 0.1 mL	Erythema Induration				
Mumps	2 u/0.1 mL	Erythema Induration				
Tricophytin	100 PNU/0.1 mL	Erythema Induration				
Candida	100 PNU/0.1 mL	Erythema Induration				
PPD	5 TU/0.1 mL	Erythema Induration				

Table A16.2: Forms for classifying and recording skin test response. From Bates SE, Suen JY, Tranum BL. (1979). Immunological skin testing and interpretation. A plea for uniformity. Cancer 43: 2306–2314, with permission.

Age (yr)	Hemoglobin Percentiles (g/dL)						
	5	10	25	50	75	90	95
Children							
1–2		11.3	11.6	12.2	12.6	13.0	
3–4	11.1	11.4	11.9	12.4	12.9	13.4	13.8
5–10	11.5	11.8	12.3	12.9	13.5	13.9	14.3
Males							
11–14	12.1	12.4	13.1	13.8	14.5	15.1	15.4
15–19	13.3	13.6	14.2	15.0	15.6	16.3	16.6
20–44	13.7	14.0	14.6	15.3	15.9	16.5	16.8
45–64	13.5	13.8	14.4	15.1	15.8	16.4	16.8
65–74	13.1	13.6	14.3	15.0	15.7	16.5	17.1
Females							
11–14	11.8	12.1	12.7	13.3	13.9	14.3	14.7
15–19	12.0	12.3	12.8	13.4	14.0	14.7	15.0
20–44	12.0	12.3	12.9	13.5	14.2	14.8	15.1
45–64	12.1	12.4	13.0	13.7	14.5	15.2	15.5
65–74	12.1	12.5	13.1	13.8	14.5	15.1	15.6

Table A17.1: Hemoglobin (g/dL) percentiles for persons one to seventy-four years (all races). Percentiles are for the NHANES II 'reference population'. Abstracted from more comprehensive tabulations of Pilch and Senti (1984).

Age (yr)	Mean Cell Volume Percentiles (fL)						
	5	10	25	50	75	90	95
Children							
1–2	73.3	75.3	77.2	79.6	82.2	84.6	86.7
3–4	74.3	76.0	78.4	81.0	83.7	86.6	88.5
5–10	76.4	77.8	80.3	83.0	85.6	88.6	90.7
Males							
11–14	77.6	79.0	81.1	83.9	87.3	89.8	92.8
15–19	79.7	81.7	84.3	87.2	90.1	93.1	94.5
20–44	81.3	83.2	85.8	88.8	91.8	94.8	97.2
45–64	82.8	84.0	86.9	90.2	93.9	97.5	99.2
65–74	82.6	84.6	87.4	90.7	94.2	98.1	101.0
Females							
11–14	78.6	80.1	82.7	86.0	89.1	92.6	93.8
15–19	80.6	82.5	85.4	88.5	91.6	94.8	96.6
20–44	81.9	84.1	87.2	90.4	93.8	96.6	98.9
45–64	82.5	84.1	87.1	90.3	94.1	96.9	99.3
65–74	82.6	84.1	87.0	90.3	94.0	97.8	99.8

Table A17.2: Mean cell volume (fL) percentiles for persons one to seventy-four years (all races). Percentiles are for the NHANES II 'reference population'. Abstracted from more comprehensive tabulations of Pilch and Senti (1984).

Age (yr)	Transferrin Saturation Percentiles (%)						
	5	10	25	50	75	90	95
Children							
1–2	10.1	12.0	14.2	20.3	27.6	32.9	37.6
3–4	10.4	12.6	17.2	23.0	29.6	38.7	42.2
5–10	12.4	14.6	18.7	24.1	30.3	35.7	39.4
Males							
11–14	12.8	14.9	18.9	23.9	30.7	35.2	39.1
15–19	16.7	18.7	22.8	28.6	35.1	42.5	45.6
20–44	16.6	18.4	23.3	29.1	35.9	43.7	48.5
45–64	15.2	17.6	21.8	27.8	34.2	39.7	44.4
65–74	16.3	18.3	22.8	28.5	35.3	41.9	47.1
Females							
11–14	11.7	14.8	19.9	24.8	31.5	37.8	44.1
15–19	11.4	13.4	19.7	25.5	33.6	40.9	46.5
20–44	13.6	15.7	20.2	26.0	33.4	42.3	47.4
45–64	14.4	15.8	20.4	25.7	30.6	36.7	41.3
65–74	14.4	16.9	20.8	25.9	31.2	36.9	40.7

Table A17.3: Transferrin saturation (%) percentiles for persons one to seventy-four years (all races). Percentiles are for the NHANES II 'reference population'. Abstracted from more comprehensive tabulations of Pilch and Senti (1984).

Age (yr)	Serum Ferritin Percentiles (ng/mL)						
	5	10	25	50	75	90	95
Children							
3–4		7	9	17	32	39	
5–10	5	8	12	17	25	34	40
Males							
11–14		8	13	17	28	41	
15–19	13	15	21	35	58	80	95
20–44	25	32	54	90	128	181	227
45–64	25	39	66	106	172	255	337
65–74	21	35	60	102	173	290	367
Females							
11–14		8	13	17	28	35	
15–19	3	5	10	20	35	59	69
20–44	7	9	18	30	58	98	118
45–64	5	21	33	62	113	156	193
65–74	8	28	45	73	111	158	231

Table A17.4: Serum ferritin (ng/mL) percentiles for persons three to seventy-four years (all races). Percentiles are for the NHANES II 'reference population'. Abstracted from more comprehensive tabulations of Pilch and Senti (1984).

Age (yr)	Erythrocyte Protoporphyrin Percentiles (μg/dL RBC)						
	5	10	25	50	75	90	95
Children							
1–2	40	42	47	57	66	78	86
3–4	36	39	45	53	63	75	87
5–10	36	40	45	53	62	69	76
Males							
11–14	36	37	43	50	58	67	79
15–19	33	36	40	45	50	58	64
20–44	33	36	40	45	51	58	64
45–64	34	37	41	47	54	64	75
65–74	34	37	41	49	58	67	74
Females							
11–14	35	39	45	52	59	70	74
15–19	37	38	43	49	57	66	73
20–44	37	40	45	51	60	69	76
45–64	35	39	44	51	61	72	82
65–74	38	41	46	53	62	74	83

Table A17.5: Erythrocyte protoporphyrin (μg/dL RBC) percentiles for persons one to seventy-four years (all races). Percentiles are for the NHANES II 'reference population'. Abstracted from more comprehensive tabulations of Pilch and Senti (1984).

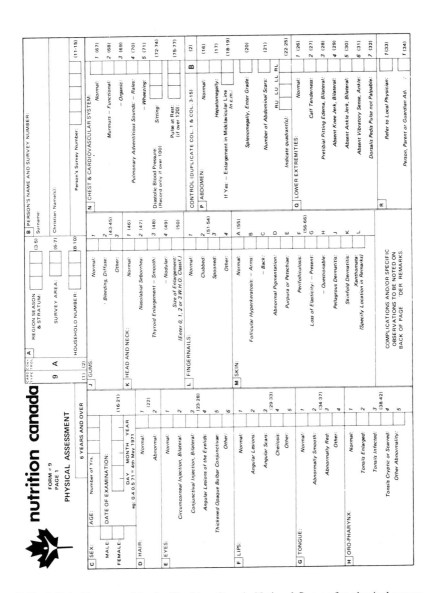

Table A25.1: Forms used in the Nutrition Canada National Survey for physical assessment. From Health and Welfare Canada (1973). Reproduced with permission of the Minister of Supply and Services Canada.

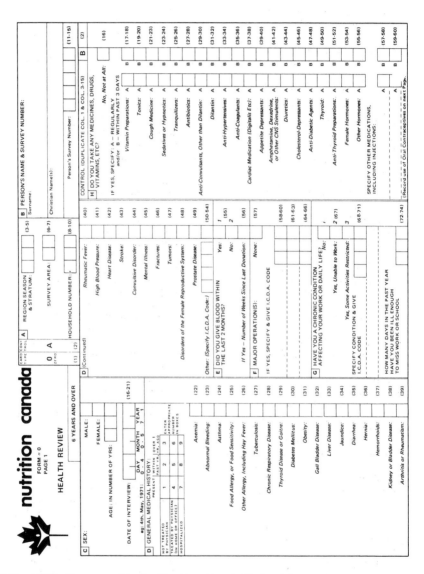

Table A25.2: Forms used in the Nutrition Canada National Survey for health review. From Health and Welfare Canada (1973). Reproduced with permission of the Minister of Supply and Services Canada.

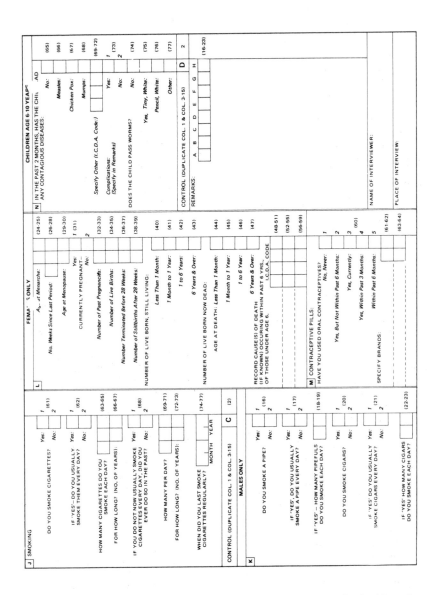

Table A25.2: Forms used in the Nutrition Canada National Survey for health review. From Health and Welfare Canada (1973). Reproduced with permission of the Minister of Supply and Services Canada.

References

Anderson SA. (1986). Guidelines for Use of Dietary Intake Data. Life Sciences Research Office, Federation of American Societies for Experimental Biology, Bethesda, Maryland.

Bates SE, Suen JY, Tranum BL. (1979). Immunological skin testing and interpretation. A plea for uniformity. Cancer 43: 2306–2314.

Department of Health and Social Security (1981). Recommended Daily Amounts of Food Energy and Nutrients for Groups of People in the United Kingdom. Second impression. Report by the Committee on Medical Aspects of Food Policy. Report on Health and Social Subjects 15. Her Majesty's Stationery Office, London.

Dibley MJ, Goldsby JB, Staehling NW, Trowbridge FL. (1987). Development of normalized curves for the international growth reference: historical and technical considerations. American Journal of Clinical Nutrition 46: 736–748.

Durnin JVGA, Womersley J. (1974). Body fat assessed from total body density and its estimation from skinfold thickness: measurements on 481 men and women aged from 16 to 72 years. British Journal of Nutrition 32: 77–97.

FAO (Food and Agriculture Organization) (1980). Food Balance Sheets 1975–77. Average and Per Capita Food Supplies 1961–65, Average 1967–77. Food and Agriculture Organization, Rome.

Food and Nutrition Board, Committee on Dietary Allowances (1980). Recommended Dietary Allowances, Ninth edition. National Academy of Sciences, Washington, D.C.

Frisancho AR. (1981). New norms of upper limb fat and muscle areas for assessment of nutritional status. American Journal of Clinical Nutrition 34: 2540–2545.

Frisancho AR. (1984). New standards of weight and body composition by frame size and height for assessment of nutritional status of adults and the elderly. American Journal of Clinical Nutrition 40: 808–819.

Frisancho AR, Flegel PN. (1983). Elbow breadth as a measure of frame size for United States males and females. American Journal of Clinical Nutrition 37: 311-314.

Gurney JM, Jelliffe DB. (1973). Arm anthropometry in nutritional assessment: nomogram for rapid calculation of muscle circumference and cross-sectional muscle and fat areas. American Journal of Clinical Nutrition 26: 912–915.

Hamill PVV, Drizd TA, Johnson CL, Reed RB, Roche AF, Moore WM. (1979). Physical growth: National Center for Health Statistics percentiles. American Journal of Clinical Nutrition 32: 607–629.

Health and Welfare Canada (1973). Nutrition Canada National Survey. Health and Welfare, Ottawa.

Health and Welfare Canada (1983). Recommended Nutrient Intakes for Canadians. Bureau of Nutritional Sciences, Health Protection Branch, Health and Welfare, Ottawa.

Imbembo AL, Walser M. (1984). Nutritional assessment. In: Walser M, Imbembo AL, Margolis S, Elfert GA (eds). Nutritional Management. The Johns Hopkins Handbook. WB Saunders Co., Philadelphia, pp. 23.

Metropolitan Height and Weight Tables (1983). Statistical Bulletin, Metropolitan Life Insurance Company, New York 64: 1–9.

NCHS (National Center for Health Statistics) (1979). Weight by height and age for adults 18–74 years: United States, 1971–1974. (Vital and health statistics: Series 11, Data from the National Health Survey; no. 208) (DHEW publication; no. (PHS) 79-1656), Hyattsville, Maryland.

NCHS (National Center for Health Statistics) (1981). Basic data on anthropometric measurements and angular measurements of the hip and knee joints for selected age groups 1–74 years of age, United States, 1971–1975. (Vital and health statistics: Series 11, Data from National Health Survey; no. 219) (DHHS publication; no. (PHS) 81-1669), Hyattsville, Maryland.

Nutrition Canada (1980). Anthropometry Report: Height, Weight, and Body Dimensions. Bureau of Nutritional Sciences, Health Protection Branch, Health and Welfare, Ottawa.

Pilch SM, Senti FR (eds). (1984). Assessment of the iron nutritional status of the US population based on data collected in the second National Health and Nutrition Examination Survey, 1976–1980. Life Sciences Research Office, Federation of the American Societies for Experimental Biology, Bethesda, Maryland.

Tanner JM. (1978). Fetus into Man. Physical Growth from Conception to Maturity. Harvard University Press, Cambridge, Massachusetts.

Appendix B

This book contains complete references to over one thousand published articles dealing with all aspects of nutritional assessment. The references are listed at the end of each chapter making it easy to scan the list of articles related to the topic of that chapter. The arrangement of the book, however, makes it difficult to find the references in the book that relate to a specific topic mentioned in several chapters — topics such as 'cancer', 'serum transferrin', or 'kwashiorkor'. These topics are listed in the index which therefore provides a starting point for locating further information. As a supplement to the index, the author is also preparing a machine-readable database containing all the references cited in the book. Readers can then search the database to locate all the references with words such as 'cancer' in the reference title. The reference list generated will provide coverage of cancer in relation to nutritional assessment.

All reference texts such as this become progressively out of date in the period following completion of the work and publication. In an effort to overcome this problem, the database described above will be supplemented by additional references that have appeared since the preparation of the book. These supplementary references will be listed separately.

A variety of database programs are in use at the present time, making it inappropriate to structure the reference database for only one program. Consequently, the information will be arranged as an ASCII file which the user can modify for use with their specific database program. Precise details of the ASCII file structure will be supplied with the database. It will be available initially in the following disk formats:

- MS-DOS IBM-PC compatible formats: 3.5 inch, 720 K bytes OR 5.25 inch, 360 K bytes

- Apple Macintosh 3.5 inch disks. 400 K bytes OR 800 K bytes

Interested readers are invited to contact the author at the address below for further details.

Rosalind S. Gibson,
University of Guelph,
Guelph, Ontario, N1G 2W1, Canada.

Index

Within the index, references to tables are shown in *italics*, and references to figures are shown in **boldface**; references to the appendix are prefaced by the letter A.